Geriatric Rehabilitation Manual

For Elsevier:

Publisher: Heidi Harrison
Associate Editor: Siobhan Campbell
Development: Veronika Krcilova
Project Manager: Anne Dickie
Design: Andy Chapman

Geriatric Rehabilitation Manual

SECOND EDITION

Edited by

Timothy L. Kauffman PT, PhD

Physical Therapist, Kauffman-Gamber Physical Therapy, Lancaster, Pennsylvania; Adjunct Assistant Professor of Rehabilitation Medicine (Physical Therapy), Columbia University, New York

John O. Barr PT, PhD

Professor, Physical Therapy Department, St. Ambrose University, Davenport, Iowa, USA

Michael Moran PT, DPT, ScD

Professor, Physical Therapy Department, College Misericordia, Dallas, Pennsylvania, USA

Foreword by

Steven L. Wolf PhD, PT, FAPTA

Emory University, Atlanta, Georgia, USA

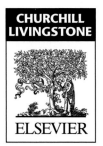

CHURCHILL LIVINGSTONE

ELSEVIER

EDINBURGH   LONDON   NEW YORK   OXFORD   PHILADELPHIA   ST LOUIS   SYDNEY   TORONTO   2007

CHURCHILL LIVINGSTONE
An imprint of Elsevier Limited

First edition 1999
Second edition 2007
  Reprinted 2008

ISBN: 978-0-443-10233-2

British Library Cataloguing in Publication Data
A catalogue record for this book is available from the British Library

Library of Congress Cataloging in Publication Data
A catalog record for this book is available from the Library of Congress

Note
Neither the Publisher nor the Authors assume any responsibility for any loss or injury
and/or damage to persons or property arising out of or related to any use of the material
contained in this book. It is the responsibility of the treating practitioner, relying on
independent expertise and knowledge of the patient, to determine the best treatment
and method of application for the patient.

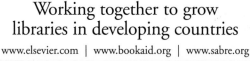

Working together to grow
libraries in developing countries

www.elsevier.com | www.bookaid.org | www.sabre.org

ELSEVIER   BOOK AID
            International   Sabre Foundation

your source for books,
journals and multimedia
in the health sciences
www.elsevierhealth.com

The
Publisher's
policy is to use
**paper manufactured
from sustainable forests**

World Aging Map on inside front cover – with permission from
Aging Successfully, Summer 2005, Vol. XV, No. 2.

Printed in China

Contents

Dedications

To my wife, Brenda, to my son, Ben, to my daughter, Emily, to my daughter-in-law, Beth, to my parents, Walter and Lillian, Bob and Lois. To the families of all the contributors. To all of our patients who teach us so much. To the students who will hopefully benefit from the combined wisdom and knowledge of all the contributors.

Timothy L. Kauffman

This work is dedicated to my dear mother, Norma S. Barr, in celebration of her 95th birthday on November 28, 2006.

John O. Barr

To my parents, John and Jane Moran: thank you for everything you taught me.

Michael Moran

Contributors

Louis R. Amundsen PT, PhD
Professor, Physical Therapy Program, EACPHS, Wayne State University, Detroit, Michigan

Cheryl Anderson PT, PhD, MBA, GSC
Director of Health Policy and Quality Management, Alexandria, Minnesota

Susan Barker PT, PhD
Associate Professor and Chair, Physical Therapy Department, College Misericordia, Dallas, Pennsylvania

John O. Barr PT, PhD
Professor, Physical Therapy Department, St. Ambrose University, Davenport, Iowa

The late E. Frederick Barrick MD
Deceased, formerly Associate Clinical Professor, Department of Orthopaedic Surgery, Georgetown University School of Medicine, Washington, DC; Director of Orthopaedic Trauma, Inova Fairfax Hospital, Falls Church, Virginia

Margaret Basiliadis DO
Owner, Family Geriatrics, PA, Fort Worth, Texas

Randy Berger Ugent MD
Dermatology Associates, Norwood, Massachusetts

Richard W. Bohannon EdD, PT, NCS, FAHA
Professor, University of Connecticut, Connecticut; Principal, Physical Therapy Consultants

Michelle Bolton MS, PT
Physical Therapist, Kauffman-Gamber Physical Therapy, Lancaster, Pennsylvania

Jennifer M. Bottomley PT, MS, PhD
Core Faculty, Harvard Division on Aging, Boston; Geriatric Rehabilitation Program Consultant, Wayland, Massachusetts

Mark A. Brimer PT, PhD
Corporate Director, Rehabilitation Services, Wuesthoff Health System, Florida

Stephen Brunton MD
Cabarrus Family Medicine Residency Program, Charlotte, North Carolina

Eli Carmeli PhD, PT
Senior Lecturer, Department of Physical Therapy, Sackler Faculty of Medicine, The Stanley Steyer School of Health Professions, Tel Aviv University, Ramat Aviv, Israel

Blaine Carmichael RN, MPAS, PA-C
Alamo City Medical Group, San Antonio, Texas

Mary M. Checovich MS
Associate Researcher, Institute on Aging, University of Wisconsin-Madison, Madison, Wisconsin

Ronni Chernoff PhD, RD, FADA
Associate Director, Geriatric Research Education and Clinical Center, Central Arkansas Veterans Healthcare System; Professor, Geriatrics, University of Arkansas for Medical Sciences, Arkansas

Charles D. Ciccone PT, PhD
Professor, Department of Physical Therapy, Ithaca College, Ithaca, New York

Meryl Cohen PT, DPT, MS, CCS
Assistant Professor, Department of Physical Therapy, Miller School of Medicine, University of Miami, Florida

Anita S.W. Craig DO
Clinical Instructor, Department of Physical Medicine and Rehabilitation, University of Michigan

Joanne Dalgleish MD
Physiotherapists, Optima Sports Medicine, Kelvin Grove Clinic, Australia

Carol M. Davis PT, EdD, MS, FAPTA
Professor, Assistant Chair, Department of Physical Therapy, Miller School of Medicine, University of Miami, Florida

Gordon Dickinson MD, FACP
Chief, Division of Infectious Diseases University of Miami Miller School of Medicine; Chief, Infectious Diseases, Miami Veterans Affairs Medical Center, Miami, Florida

Joan E. Edelstein MA, PT, FISPO
Special Lecturer, Columbia University, New York

Reenie Euhardy MS, PT, GCS
Faculty Associate, University of Wisconsin-Madison; Physical Therapist, Middleton Memorial Veteran Hospital, Madison, Wisconsin

Michael Fischer OD, FAAO
Associate Chief, Optometry Service, Northport Veterans Administration Medical Center, Northport, New York; Low Vision Clinical Consultant, Lighthouse International, New York; Adjunct Assistant Clinical Professor, State University of New York, State College of Optometry, New York

Walter R. Frontera MD, PhD
Dean, School of Medicine, University of Puerto Rico, San Juan, Puerto Rico

Wade S. Gamber PT
Physical Therapist, Kauffman-Gamber Physical Therapy, Lancaster, Pennsylvania

Emily L. Germain-Lee MD
Associate Professor, Department of Pediatrics, Division of Pediatric Endocrinology, The Johns Hopkins University School of Medicine, Baltimore, Maryland

Barbara A. Gilchrest MD
Professor and Chairman, Department of Dermatology, Boston Unviersity School of Medicine; Chief of Dermatology, Boston Medical Center, Boston, Massachusetts

Deborah Gold PhD
Duke University Medical Center, Durham, North Carolina

Stephen A. Gudas PT, PhD
Associate Professor, Department of Anatomy and Neurobiology, Physical Therapist, Cancer Rehabilitation, Virginia Commonwealth University, Medical College of Virginia, Richmond, Virginia

Brenda Hage MSN, CRNP, APRN, BC
Assistant Professor Nursing, College Misericordia, Dallas, Pennsylvania

Patricia A. Hageman PT, PhD
Director and Professor, Division of Physical Therapy Education, University of Nebraska Medical Center, Omaha, Nebraska

June E. Hanks PT, PhD
UC Foundation Associate Professor of Physical Therapy, University of Tennessee at Chattanooga, Tennessee

Marilia Harumi Higuchi dos Santos MD
Post Doctorate Fellow, School of Medicine, Sao Paulo University, Sao Paulo, Brazil

Barry Hull MD, FAAFP
The Doctor's Office, Peachtree City, Georgia

Osa Jackson Schulte PT, PhD, GCFP/AT
Director of Movement and Healing Center, Clarkson, Michigan

Robert R. Karpman MD
Vice-President of Medical Affairs, Caritas Holy Family Hospital, Methuen, Massachusetts

Benjamin W. Kauffman PTA
Physical Therapist Assistant, Facilities Manager, Kauffman-Gamber Physical Therapy, Lancaster, Pennsylvania

Beth E. Kauffman MPT, ATC
Physical Therapist, Kauffman-Gamber Physical Therapy, Lancaster, Pennsylvania

Timothy L. Kauffman PT, PhD
Physical Therapist, Kauffman-Gamber Physical Therapy, Lancaster, Pennsylvania; Adjunct Assistant Professor of Rehabilitation Medicine (Physical Therapy), Columbia University, New York

Dennis W. Klima PT, MS, GCS, NCS
Senior Lecturer, Department of Physical Therapy, University of Maryland Eastern Shore, Princess Anne, Maryland

Edmund M. Kosmahl PT, EdD
Professor, University of Scranton, Pennsylvania

Lars Larsson MD, PhD
Professor and Chair Clinical Neurophysiology, Department of Neuroscience, Uppsala University Hospital, Uppsala, Sweden

Megan Laughlin PT
Physical Therapist, Kauffman-Gamber Physical Therapy, Lancaster, Pennsylvania

Rolando T. Lazaro PT, DPT, MS, GCS
Assistant Professor, Department of Physical Therapy, Samuel Merritt College, Oakland, California

Sandra J. Levi PT, PhD
Associate Professor, Midwestern University, Illinois

David Levine PT, PhD, OCS
Cline Chair of Excellence and UC Foundation Professor of Physical Therapy, The University of Tennessee at Chattanooga, Tennessee

Rosanne W. Lewis PT, MS, GCS
Geriatric Clinical Specialist, Home Health Agency, Lodi Memorial Hospital, Lodi, California

Dario G. Liebermann PhD
Lecturer, Department of Physical Therapy, Sackler Faculty of Medicine, The Stanley Steyer School of Health Professions, Tel Aviv University, Ramat Aviv, Israel

Carleen Lindsey PT, MS, GCS
Educator, Senior Therapist, Adjunct University of Connecticut Instructor, University of Connecticut, Connecticut

Mark V. Lombardi PT, DPT, ATC
Director of Rehabilitation, Scranton Orthopaedic Specialists, Scranton, Pennsylvania

Katie Lundon PT, PhD
Assistant Professor, Department of Physical Therapy, Faculty of Medicine, University of Toronto, Ontario, Canada

Michelle M. Lusardi PT, PhD
Associate Professor, Department of Physical Therapy and Human Movement, College of Education and Health Professions, Sacred Heart University, Fairfield, Connecticut

Zoran Maric MD
Arizona Spine Center, Phoenix, Arizona

Carolyn Marshall MPH, PhD
Project Director, Teacher Enrichment Initiatives, The University of Texas Health Science Center, San Antonio, Texas

Jeff A. Martin MD
Formerly of Orthocare International, Phoenix, Arizona

David C. Martin MD
Clinical Professor of Medicine, Psychiatry, and Health Services Administration, University of Pittsburgh; Director, Geriatric Medicine Fellowship, Univeristy of Pittsburgh Medical Centre Shadyside, Pittsburgh, Pennsylvania

P. Christopher Metzger MD, FACS
Orthopaedic Surgeon, Scranton Orthopaedic Specialists, Scranton, Pennsylvania

Molly Mika MS, OTR/L
Assistant Professor, Department of Occupational Therapy, College Misericordia, Dallas, Pennsylvania

Marilyn E. Miller PhD, PT, GCS
Physical Therapy Department, California State University – Fresno, California

Stephen E. Mock PhD, FAAA
Audiologist/Clinical Director, Northeastern Hearing & Balance Centers, Scranton, Pennsylvania

Michael Moran PT, DPT, ScD
Professor, Physical Therapy Department, College Misericordia, Dallas, Pennsylvania

Richard Mowrer PTA, CSCS
Physical Therapist Assistant, Drayer Physical Therapy Institute, Harrisburg, Pennsylvania

Dominique Noë Long MD
Fellow, Department of Pediatrics, Division of Pediatric Endocrinology, The Johns Hopkins University School of Medicine, Baltimore, Maryland

Caroline O'Connell BSc (Hons) Physio, Dip Stats, MISCP
School of Physiotherapy, The University of Dublin, Trinity College, Dublin, Ireland

S. Scott Paist III MD
Clinical Associate Professor, Temple University School of Medicine, Philadelphia; Director of Geriatrics, Department of Family and Community Medicine, Lancaster General Hospital, Lancaster, Pennsylvania

Alexandra Papaioannou MD
McMaster University, Hamilton, Ontario, Canada

David Patrick PT, MS, CPO
Director, Orthotic Services, Keystone Prosthetics & Orthotics, Clarks Summit, Pennsylvania

Clive Perry MBBS, FRANZCR, FRCR
Radiologist, Lancaster Radiology Associates, Lancaster General Hospital, Department of Radiology, Lancaster, Pennsylvania

Steven Pheasant PT, PhD
Assistant Professor, Physical Therapy Department, College Misericordia, Dallas, Pennsylvania

The late Lynn Phillippi PT
Deceased, formerly Vice President, MJ Care, Racine, Wisconsin

Randolph Rasch PhD, FNP, FAANP
Vanderbilt University, Nashville, Tennessee

Pamela Reynolds PT, EdD
Associate Professor, Gannon University, Erie, Pennsylvania

James K. Richardson MD
Associate Professor, Department of Physical Medicine and Rehabilitation, University of Michigan Medical School, Ann Arbor, Michigan

Jodi Robinson MA CCC/SLP
Staff Speech Pathologist, Genesis Medical Center, Davenport, Iowa

Anita Alonte Roma PT, DPT, NCS
Physical Therapist, Kauffman-Gamber Physical Therapy, Lancaster, Pennsylvania

Maureen Romanow Pascal PT, DPT, NCS
Associate Professor, Physical Therapy Department, College Misericordia, Dallas, Pennsylvania

Bruce P. Rosenthal OD, FAAO
Chief of the Low Vision, Lighthouse International, New York; Adjunct Professor, Mount Sinai Hospital, New York; Adjunct Clinical Professor, State College of Optometry, State University of New York, New York

John Sanko PT, EdD
Associate Professor, Chair of Physical Therapy, University of Scranton, Scranton, Pennsylvania

Jane K. Schroeder PT, MA
Private Practitioner, Gifted Hands, Sarasota, Florida

Ron Scott JD, LLM, MSBA, MS, OCS
Director and Associate Professor, Physical Therapy Department, Lebanon Valley College, Annville, Pennsylvania

James Siberski MS
Coordinator, Gerontology Education, College Misericordia, Dallas, Pennsylvania

Everett L. Smith PhD
Associate Professor, Department of Population Health Sciences, University of Wisconsin-Madison, Madison, Wisconsin

Christine Stabler MD
Deputy Director, Family Medicine Residency, Lancaster General Hospital, Lancaster, Pennsylvania

William H. Staples PT, DPT, GCS
Assistant Professor, Krannert School of Physical Therapy, University of Indianapolis, Indianapolis

Emma K. Stokes BSc, MSc, PhD
Lecturer, School of Physiotherapy, The University of Dublin, Trinity College, Dublin, Ireland

Hilmar H.G. Stracke MD, PhD
University Hospital Giessen, Giessen, Germany

Lisa Tews MA, CCC/SLP
Staff Speech-language Pathologist, Genesis Medical Center, Davenport, Iowa

LaDora V. Thompson PT, PhD
Associate Professor, Program in Physical Therapy, Department of Physical Medicine and Rehabilitation, University of Minnesota, Minneapolis, Minnesota

Eeric Truumees MD
William Beaumont Hospital, Royal Oak, Michigan; Wayne State University, Detroit, Michigan

Darcy A. Umphred PT, PhD, FAPTA
Emeritus Professor, University of the Pacific, Stockton, California

Pamela G. Unger PT
Physical Therapist, Director of Clinical and Administrative Services, The Center for Advanced Wound Care, St. Joseph Medical Center, Pennsylvania

Kristin von Nieda PT, DPT, MEd
Clinical Associate Professor, Department of Physical Therapy, Temple University, Philadelphia, Pennsylvania

Chris L. Wells PT, PhD, CCS, ATC
Assistant Professor, School of Medicine, Department of Physical Therapy & Rehabilitation Science, University of Maryland, Baltimore, Maryland; Advanced Physical Therapist, Department of Rehabilitation Services, University of Maryland Medical Center, Baltimore, Maryland

Mary Ann Wharton PT, MS
Associate Professor of Physical Therapy and Curriculum Coordinator, Department of Physical Therapy, Saint Francis University, Loretto, Pennsylvania; Adjunct Associate Professor, Physical Therapist Assistant Program, Community College of Allegheny County, Boyce Campus, Monroeville, Pennsylvania

Susan L. Whitney PT, PhD, NCS, ATC
Associate Professor, Physical Therapy Department, University of Pittsburgh, Pittsburgh, Pennsylvania

Diane M. Wrisley PT, PhD, NCS
Assistant Professor, Department of Rehabilitation Science, The State University of New York, University at Buffalo, Buffalo, New York

Foreword

For age is opportunity no less
Than youth itself, though in
another dress,
And as the evening twilight
fades away,
The sky is filled with stars
invisible by the day.

Henry Wadsworth Longfellow, "Morituri Salutamus"

Grow old along with me!
The best is yet to be.
The last of life, for which the
first was made.

Robert Browning, "Rabbi Ben Ezra"

Years steal
Fire from the mind as vigour
from the limb,
And life's enchanted cup but
sparkles near the brim.

Lord Byron, "Childe Harold's Pilgrimage"

Age is a question of mind over
matter. If you don't mind, it
doesn't matter.

Satchel Page (ageless baseball pitcher)

In 1997, one out of every eight US citizens, or 34.1 million people, was over the age of 65. By the year 2030 that number could rise to one in five. In 1996, about 3.8 million people were amongst our "oldest old," the segment of our population that is the fastest growing. This number will almost double to 5.7 million in 2010. By the twenty-first century, 70 000 of our oldest members were over the age of 100. The number of centenarians is expected to double each decade in the present century. By the year 2030, adults over the age of 65 will account for 20% of our population, and this metric will stabilize as the "baby boomers" retire at about that time.

Inevitably, improvements in education, nutrition, health care, exercise options and standards of living contribute to these rising numbers. Persons of discriminating taste judge the quality of their salads not by the amount of dressing but by the freshness of the greens. Comparable palatability must be exercised when we judge the quality of our aging process. Simply to presume that knowledge about what we should eat throughout our lives to minimize cholesterol accumulation imposes the self-discipline to eat accordingly is a lesson in self-deception. The belief that we should "move, move, move" our bodies and our minds does not always combat regression toward a sedentary lifestyle. These perspectives are driven home when a multi-billion dollar pharmaceutical industry "piles on the dressing" by overtly suggesting that we persist in unhealthy behaviors and take a product to counteract the consequences. More to the point, the options to prolong life are superficial if the resultant quality of life is void of meaning. Eating without awareness of intake, engaging the mind without processing written materials, moving only our fingertips at a keyboard that emblematically denotes an inactive lifestyle in the absence of exercising our limbs, inevitably imprison our mind, body and spirit within the archives of aging rather than liberating them.

One cannot dismiss the reality that our populace is becoming older. More resources to foster a better quality of life will have to be expended because older adults can no longer be counted as a fragmented minority. Optimizing ways in which we can prevent behavioral and physiological decline or remediate processes that contribute to it are assuming progressively more significant roles among rehabilitationists.

Against this background, the *Geriatric Rehabilitation Manual* (second edition) represents the continued effort of clinicians dedicated to enhancing the lives of our older citizens so that "quality of life" becomes more than just a buzz phrase devoid of meaning. This text is written with the sensitivity that concern for the multi-dimensions of the aging process must be appreciated by those treating older adults. Furthermore, the mantra of this text seems to be that physical or behavioral decay can be delayed or prevented so that our "later years" are not synonymous with the pervasive presumption of "declining years." And among that proportion of older adults who must eventually reach the asymptote of their golden years, the inevitable end can be draped in veils of dignity crafted from hearts and minds of the most compassionate of clinicians.

Each unit contains content that blends experiential perspective with evidence. The text is intended for both clinicians and students. Although never explicitly stated, one can easily deduce, from the empathetic tone set by so many contributors and the reality gleaned from the data previously cited, that more and more practitioners will be drawn to this exponentially growing segment of our population. Given that reality, this textbook should guide clinical decisions on the one hand, while fostering creative therapies on the other. Moreover, such behaviors can be engaged while considering other important factors, such as limitations in treatment time, unique client attributes and complexities in problem solving that are so emblematic of the aging process itself.

Last, and perhaps most intriguing, the reader should be encouraged to first peruse the content of this book. After so doing, one should visualize a patient, one who possesses perhaps a comparatively less complex problem list. Then the exercise should be repeated with a more "difficult" patient. See if the result in either case is not the same. Specifically, one should find that valuable guidelines to either confirm or modify, perhaps even "create," a treatment option are not confined to any one unit or even chapter within a unit, but require absorbing information from multiple sections of this text. Therein lies the beauty of the effort ensconced within these pages ... the caring necessary to produce an optimal treatment plan is manifest in the ideas posed by so many geriatric specialists who share the reader's passion and professionalism.

Steven L. Wolf PhD, PT, FAPTA
Professor, Department of Rehabilitation Medicine
Professor of Geriatrics, Department of Medicine
Associate Professor, Department of Cell Biology
Emory University School of Medicine
Professor of Health and Elder Care
Nell Hodgson Woodruff School of Nursing
Senior Scientist, Atlanta VA Rehab R&D Center

Preface to the first edition

The passage of time . . . aging . . . brings a plethora of experiences that constitute the psychosocial, economic and medical milieu that our patients and we as healthcare practitioners face every day. To provide quality healthcare for the older person in this robust arena, given the constraints of time and healthcare payment systems, one must have easily accessible, comprehensive, and concise information. This text is written to enable the healthcare provider to review or to learn quickly the pathology of a diagnosis or condition and to present treatment ideas, especially for rehabilitation, prevention (maintenance) care and prognosis.

No two individuals experience life in identical fashion; thus, one hallmark of aging is the "uniqueness" of each person. Because aging may be viewed as an accumulation of microinsults that present as a collection of chronic diseases and one or more acute problems, the interactive relationships must be considered. This perspective is different from the isolated computerized model of labeling geriatric patients with the clean number listed in the *International Classification of Diseases*, 9th edition, *Clinical Modifications*. We as health-care providers must remain constantly vigilant to avoid this lure of simplification.

One of the issues encountered in geriatric patient care is that the symptoms and signs or responses to treatment may not be as clear as might be expected. The reward is recognizing this and determining an appropriate course of patient care in order to support each aging patient so that he or she has a sense of worth and control even in the presence of physical losses and illnesses. This textbook and, we hope, its readers will acknowledge the challenge and reward.

This book is for clinicians. Although not specifically designed to be a textbook for classroom instruction, students become practitioners; thus, it is also appropriate for the entry-level practitioner in the geriatric rehabilitation setting, including physicians, nurses, physical therapists, occupational therapists, speech pathologists, respiratory therapists and social workers.

The text is written with a dual purpose for the seasoned practitioner who will benefit from reviewing the information and recognizing that he or she is giving proper care according to today's standards. Furthermore, the seasoned practitioner will also learn because of the breadth of information presented in this text.

For the healthcare provider who is newly entering the field of geriatric care, this text will prove to be invaluable. It is clearly acknowledged that not every suggestion offered within the chapters has been put to the rigors of clinical research in order to validate efficacy; however, the suggestions are offered nonetheless because they represent potential treatment ideas, and they are the standard wisdom of the rehabilitation field at this time. Although some of the ideas have not been proven, they have not been refuted. If they had

been refuted, they would no longer represent the standard wisdom that defines the ambits of care. These treatment ideas should be employed by thinking practitioners for individual patients.

Throughout the text, the reader should recognize different writing styles that also reflect different treatment approaches. The authors were encouraged to discuss the science of geriatric rehabilitation and to infuse the art of patient care, the soft underbelly of humane medical care for persons who are undergoing involution and are closing out a life. Some of the chapters in this text have references within the material presented. Other chapters have only selected readings at the end of the chapter. The editorial board encouraged each of the writers to minimize the references so that more treatment ideas, graphs and clinical forms could be included. Readers are strongly encouraged to seek out further information from the lists of suggested readings.

The text is organized into seven separate areas. The first unit deals with some overview of geriatric care and the review of system as they relate to aging. This should be helpful for classroom instruction and review of age-related changes. Chapter 1 specifically deals with the complexity of aging, pathology and healthcare.

The second unit deals with aging pathokinesiology and is clearly directed at specific clinical conditions. It also parallels a rudimentary systems review, since the unit is subdivided into topics pertaining to musculoskeletal involvement, neuromuscular and neurological involvement, neoplasms, cardiopulmonary diseases, and finally blood vessel, circulatory and skin disorders.

The third unit deals with the aging and pathological sensorium, especially as it relates to vision, hearing and communication. The following unit (Unit IV) presents a potpourri of common specific conditions, complaints and problems and is followed by special considerations or physical therapeutic intervention techniques (Unit V). The sociopolitical, legal, and ethical considerations are addressed in Unit VI because they also impact on geriatric rehabilitation. It is important to recognize that the paradigm shifts at the end of life from the medical model to the dying model, which is more culture based. There is less concern about traditional rehabilitation constructs and greater emphasis on value of life and palliation to minimize suffering and to maintain quality for the dying patient and the family.

Unit VII, the final unit, elucidates the prominent members of the geriatric rehabilitation healthcare team. I hope that healthcare providers and others who use this manual will understand that:

1. Aging not stagnant, dull, and/or unattractive.
2. Aging is very dynamic, perhaps too fluctuating, with a wide range of responses.
3. Aging is very diverse—a hallmark is the variability of individuals.
4. Aging is very challenging.
5. Aging is very complex.
6. The study of aging is the study of life—it starts in the uterus and our intervention must be life long.
7. Aging and living are synonymous.
8. ABOVE ALL ELSE, AGING IS VENERABLE AND VALUED.

Respectfully,
Timothy L. Kauffman PT, PhD

Preface

Aging … the passage of time … brings with it an abundance of experiences within the psychosocial, economic and medical milieu that our patients and we healthcare practitioners face every day. In order to provide quality healthcare for the older person, given the constraints of time and healthcare payment systems, one must have easily accessible, concise, and yet comprehensive, information. This book will enable the busy healthcare provider to review, or to learn quickly about, a range of pathologies/conditions, examinations/diagnostic procedures and interventions that can be effectively used in the physical rehabilitation of older persons.

No two individuals experience the passage of time in identical fashion. Thus, one hallmark of aging is the uniqueness of each person. Because aging may be viewed as an accumulation of "microinsults" that present as a collection of chronic diseases affecting multiple body systems, interactive relationships must be considered in patient evaluation and treatment. These interactive, multi-system relationships are emphasized in this book.

One of the challenges encountered in geriatric patient care is that the symptoms and signs, and responses to treatment, may not be clear-cut. There is professional reward in recognizing this and in determining an appropriate course of patient care in a manner that supports each aging patient so that he or she has a sense of control and worth in the presence of physical losses and illnesses. We hope that this textbook and its readers acknowledge this challenge and reward.

This book is written for both practicing clinicians and students who are practicing to become clinicians. It is appropriate for entry-level practitioners in geriatric rehabilitation settings, including physicians, nurses, physical therapists, occupational therapists, speech pathologists, respiratory therapists and social workers. We believe that the seasoned practitioner will also benefit from the broad review of information that this book provides and by recognizing that he or she is giving proper care according to today's standards.

For the health-care provider who is newly entering the field of geriatric rehabilitation, this text will prove to be truly invaluable. In this second edition of the *Geriatric Rehabilitation Manual*, we updated evidence to support the use of specific examination and evaluation procedures, as well as interventions. However, we clearly acknowledge that not every suggestion provided in this book has been subjected to rigorous clinical research. Nonetheless, a range of suggestions are offered because they represent wisdom from the field of rehabilitation and are concepts that can be further investigated.

Throughout the text, the reader should appreciate that the different writing styles employed by our authors also reflect different evaluation and intervention approaches. The authors were encouraged to discuss the science of geriatric rehabilitation and to infuse the art of humane patient care for older persons.

This book is organized into eleven distinct, but interrelated, units. The first unit is concerned with key anatomical and physiological considerations seen with aging and having significant impact on the older individual. Also included are overviews of laboratory and imaging procedures, and pharmacologic considerations for older persons. The second and third units review important aging-related conditions and disorders of the musculoskeletal and neuromuscular/neurological systems respectively. Neoplasms commonly encountered in older persons are the focus of the fourth unit. Aging-related conditions of the cardiovascular, pulmonary, integumentary and sensory systems are presented in units five through seven. Unit eight highlights a range of specific clinical problems and conditions commonly encountered with older patients. Critically, all of these units emphasize important examination and diagnostic procedures needed for a thorough evaluation and stress interventions that can be of significant benefit to the older patient. The ninth unit presents select physical therapeutic interventions that are especially important in managing rehabilitative care. Key societal issues related to aging are discussed in the tenth unit. The concluding unit focuses on the successful rehabilitation team that includes both professional and non-professional caregiver members.

We sincerely hope that students and colleagues who utilize the *w* will appreciate that:

1. Aging is not stagnant, dull or unattractive.
2. Aging is dynamic and fluctuating, with a wide range of responses.
3. Aging is diverse—its hallmark is the variability of individuals.
4. Aging is challenging.
5. Aging is complex.
6. The study of aging is the study of life—our assessments and interventions must be lifelong.
7. Aging and living are synonymous.

ABOVE ALL ELSE, AGING IS TO BE VALUED AND VENERATED.

Respectfully, the Editors:
Timothy L. Kauffman PT, PhD
John O. Barr PT, PhD
Michael L. Moran PT, ScD

Acknowledgments

A book of this breadth cannot be conceived, nurtured and published without a host of persons making significant contributions. Foremost, a heartfelt thanks to Veronika Krcilova, Siobhan Campbell and Heidi Harrison, my publishing editors from the Kidlington office, Anne Dickie, project manager in the Edinburgh office, and Andy Chapman, designer in the London office. Also, I am grateful to Jacqui Merrell and Marion Waldman for connecting me to Kidlington. An earnest thank you is given to Karin Skeet and her associates for their diligent efforts in producing this text.

I must express immeasurable gratitude to my wife, Brenda, daughter, Emily, son, Ben, and daughter-in-law, Beth, who have contributed significantly through their support as well as administratively by collating information, assisting with editing and keeping me on track. Special recognition must go to Marieke James, whose tireless organization skills greatly facilitated this project, and to Lynn Sterkenberg, Kelly Williams, Megan Laughlin, Michelle Bolton, Tom Webb, Gretchen Manwiller, Karen King and Jamie Perrone.

Finally, this book would not have been completed without the sharing, reflecting and tireless contributing from my co-authors, John Barr and Mike Moran.

Timothy L. Kauffman PT, PhD

UNIT **1**

Anatomical and physiological considerations

UNIT CONTENTS

Chapter 1

Wholeness of the individual

Timothy L. Kauffman and Osa Jackson Schulte

INTRODUCTION

Aging is a wonderful and unique experience. The word 'wonderful' should not imply that aging includes only good things but rather that it is extraordinary and remarkable. Aging starts in the uterus at the time of conception. It represents the passage of time, not pathology. By the age of 1 year, each individual's uniqueness is evident, and, by the age of 5 years, the personality is well formed. Multiply the first 5 years of life by 15 times and expand the environmental and life experiences, and one of the hallmarks of aging becomes clear – individual uniqueness. No two people age identically. Idiosyncrasy is the norm, and it is important that the healthcare provider looks at the wholeness of the individual geriatric patient as well as the chief presenting complaint or primary diagnosis.

In the healthcare arena of America today, the wholeness of the patient is compressed into an electronic number taken from the requisite International Classification of Diseases, 9th Revision, Clinical Modification (ICD-9-CM). Unfortunately, the number does not necessarily reflect the magnitude of the patient's condition but, instead, may reflect what pays the most or what allows the most hospital or rehabilitation days. The World Health Organization has upgraded to the ICD-10-CM in order to allow for more relevant coding, but, in the United States, third-party payers, including Medicare, have not made the switch to the ICD-10.

The problem with this coding system and its failure to recognize the whole patient can be seen in the example of a cerebrovascular accident (CVA) with an ICD-9-CM code of 436 with modifiers. The outcomes from this simple group of code numbers range from good to fatal: full recovery within 1 week; full recovery within 3–6 months; partial recovery; severe limitation in physical, cognitive or communicative abilities; confined to chair, bed or institution; or death. It is not just antecedent diagnoses such as chronic obstructive pulmonary disease, diabetes mellitus or degenerative joint disease that are likely to affect the results of rehabilitation for a CVA; psychosocial factors must also be considered. For example, the grandmother of recent Russian immigrants may be labeled confused or poorly motivated when, in actuality, the language barrier is the major stumbling block in rehabilitation efforts.

Age alone is a factor to consider; however, chronological age based on date of birth is not always similar to physiological age (Nakamura et al 1998), which is based on cross-sectional measurements and comparisons with age-estimated or established norms. For example, a specific 70-year-old man may have an aerobic capacity that is similar to that of the average 60-year-old; the older man is said to have a 10-year physiological age advantage. In Chapter 15 there is a photograph of three individuals ranging in age from 60 to 93; it clearly shows differences among the three, although generalizations can be cautiously extrapolated. But far too often such an age span is grouped together as if aging changes are monolithic: they are not. It is not common to compare a 10-year-old with a 43-year-old, which also represents an age span of 33 years. When dealing with a patient who has lived for seven decades or more, the person's individuality must be acknowledged by providers, administrators and health delivery systems if optimal care is to be rendered.

VARIOUS MEDICAL MODELS OR PERSPECTIVES

The standard medical model of signs and symptoms equaling a diagnosis of disease does not fit well with the geriatric population (Fig. 1.1). Fried et al (1991) found that this medical model was able to fit actual cases in fewer than half of the geriatric patients that they studied. They developed several other models: the synergistic morbidity model, the attribution model, the causal chain model and the unmasking event model (Fried et al 1991).

The synergistic morbidity model uses a scenario in which the patient presents with a history of multiple, generally chronic diseases (represented by A, B and C in Fig. 1.2) that result in cumulative morbidity. When this hypothetical patient loses functional capacity, medical attention is sought. This may also be viewed as a cascading effect.

The attribution model uses a scenario in which a patient attributes declining capacity to the worsening of a previously diagnosed chronic health condition (see Fig. 1.2). However, physical examination and workup reveal a new, previously unrecognized condition that is causing the declining health status. This possibility is especially important to consider when evaluating or caring for a patient labeled

Medical

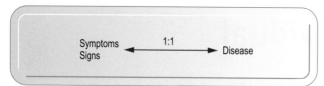

Figure 1.1   Diagnosis of illness presentation in the elderly: diagrammatic representation of the medical model.
(From Fried et al 1991, with permission of Blackwell.)

Synergistic morbidity

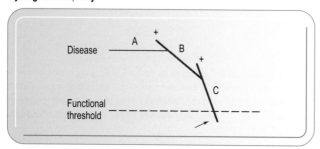

Attribution

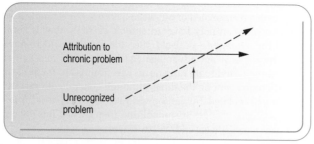

Figure 1.2   Diagrammatic representations of the synergistic morbidity model and the attribution model for diagnosis of illness presentation in a geriatric population. The description of each model is provided in the text. The arrow indicates the usual time of presentation for medical evaluation.
(From Fried et al 1991, with permission of Blackwell.)

Causal chain

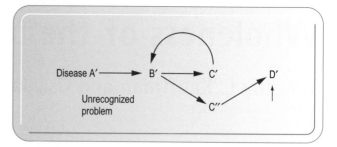

Unmasking event

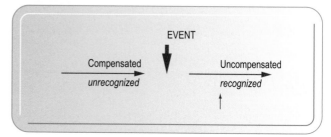

Figure 1.3   Diagrammatic representations of the causal chain model and the unmasking event model for diagnosis of illness presentation in a geriatric population. The description of each model is provided in the text. The arrow indicates the usual time of presentation for medical evaluation.
(From Fried et al 1991, with permission of Blackwell.)

with a chronic disease such as multiple sclerosis, arthritis or postpolio syndrome. Not all new complaints are attributable to the chronic condition.

The causal chain model (Fig. 1.3) uses a scenario in which one illness causes another illness and functional decline. In this case, disease A causes disease B, which precipitates a chain of additional conditions that may worsen the present medical problems and/or lead on to further medical problems. For example, a patient who has severe arthritis (Fig. 1.3, disease A') is unable to maintain good cardiovascular health, which leads to heart disease (disease B'). The cardiac condition leads to peripheral vascular disease (disease C' and C''), which may reflect back to disease B and/or lead to amputation (disease D').

The final model proposed by Fried et al (1991) is the unmasking event model (Fig. 1.3). In this situation, a patient has an unrecognized and subclinical or compensated condition. When the compensating factor is lost, the condition becomes apparent and is often viewed as an acute problem. For example, a patient who suffers from vertigo may have functional balance because the visual and proprioceptive systems compensate for the deficient vestibular system. However, when walking on soft carpet or in a darkened room, this individual may have marked balance dysfunction, which may lead to a fracture resulting from a fall.

Coming from a similar perspective, Besdine (1990) presented several important concepts that relate to the complexity of geriatric care in his introduction to the first edition of the *Merck Manual of Geriatrics*. First, he states that 'the restriction of independent functional ability is the final common outcome for many disorders in the elderly'. Like Fried et al (1991) in their attribution and unmasking event models, Besdine warns that 'deterioration of functional independence in active, previously unimpaired elders is an early subtle sign of untreated illness characterized by the absence of typical symptoms and signs of disease'. Additionally, he suggests that in geriatric medicine there is a 'poor correlation between type and severity of problem (functional disability) and the disease problem list'. Besdine warns further that finding a diseased organ or diseased tissue does not necessarily determine the degree of functional impairment that will be found. Another lesson he points out is that 'the severity of illness as measured by objective data does not necessarily determine the presence or severity of functional dependency'.

Recent research validates the need to consider the wholeness of each patient because of the complexity of treating the aging patient. Reporting on the admission of patients to a trauma center in Canada, Bergeron et al (2005) found that the proportion of patients with one or more comorbidities increased from 8.7% for patients under the age of 55 years to 92% for those over the age of 85 years. This was significant and was associated with an increase in the length of stay.

Boyd et al (2005a) studied clinical practice guidelines (CPGs) as they might apply to a hypothetical 79-year-old woman with chronic obstructive pulmonary disease, chronic heart failure, hypertension, stable angina, atrial fibrillation, hypercholesterolemia, diabetes mellitus, osteoarthritis and osteoporosis. They reported that most CPGs did not present modifications for these common geriatric comorbidities. Using the relevant CPGs, this hypothetical woman would have been prescribed 12 medications, with a high cost for the drugs and a risk of adverse drug interactions. In another study, Boyd et al (2005b) reported that hospitalization for an acute illness in moderately disabled, community-dwelling older women led to increased dependence in daily living activities that persisted for up to 18 months after hospitalization and the resolution of the acute problem. They advocate improved interventions during *and* after hospitalization.

Because of the uniqueness of each aging patient, these authors advocate an interdisciplinary team approach to effectively treat the common multiple comorbidities. The whole person must be considered and rehabilitation services should be consulted in the majority of geriatric cases.

AGING CONSIDERATIONS AND REHABILITATION

Physical exercise

Exercise, fitness and aging

From a philosophical point of view, one might consider movement to be the most fundamental feature of the animal kingdom in the biological world. Thus, life is movement. Movement is crucial not only for securing basic needs such as food, clothing and shelter but also for obtaining fulfillment of higher psychosocial needs that involve quality of life. Maintaining independence in thought and mobility is a universal desire that is, unfortunately, not achieved by all individuals.

The value of exercise and fitness is that they help to maintain the fullest vigor possible as time ages everyone. By exercising, it is hoped that one may enhance the quality of life, decrease the risk of falls and maintain or improve function in various activities. Fitness, however, is more than aerobic capacity. It is a state of mind and it involves endurance (physical work capacity determined by oxygen consumption, Vo_2), strength, flexibility, balance, and coordination and agility.

The benefits of exercise are systemic and may be viewed as being favorable for all body systems and functions provided the phenomena of overuse are abated before causing irreparable damage to the organism. The opposite is also true; the deleterious effects of immobility are profound, as Chapter 58 makes clear. Box 1.1 presents a number of the beneficial effects of exercise on the actions of various cells, tissues and systems and on the organism as a whole, as judged by comparing the findings with those of sedentary people.

The beneficial effects of the systemic response to aerobic exercise by the cardiopulmonary and cardiovascular systems as well as by the musculoskeletal system are fairly well recognized (*Merck Manual of Geriatrics* 2000, Fiatarone Singh 2004). These are presented hypothetically in Figure 1.4, which compares typical linear senescence, disease and levels of physical activity. Less well recognized is the association between fitness and mortality. A higher level of fitness is associated with a lower mortality rate (Fiatarone Singh 2004). However, many exercise enthusiasts do not extol the benefits of exercise in order to lengthen lives. Rather, the emphasis is placed on experiencing a better quality of life by maintaining robust health and physical competence.

Exercise and cancer

Over the past few decades, the death rate from heart disease has been decreasing and the incidence of cancer deaths increasing. A favorable relationship is now being shown between exercise and a

Box 1.1 Aging markers, risks and diseases modified by exercise

- Aerobic capacity[a,b,c]
- All cause of mortality[a,b]
- Breast cancer[a]
- Cognitive function[b]
- Colon cancer[a]
- Depression[a,b]
- Disability[a]
- Falls[a]
- Hyperlipidemia[a,c]
- Hypertension[a,b,c]
- Osteoporosis[a,b,c]
- Sarcopenia[a,b,c]
- Stroke[a,b]
- Total adipose tissue[a,b,c]
- Type 2 diabetes[a,c]
- Walking speed[b]

[a]From Fiatarone Singh (2004).
[b]From Bassey E 2002 Exercise for the elderly: an update. Age Ageing 31(suppl 1):3–5.
[c]From Gormley J, Hussey J 2005 Exercise Therapy: Prevention and Treatment of Disease, 1st edn. Blackwell Publishing, Oxford.

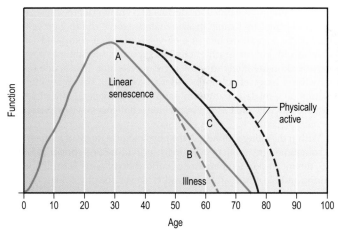

Figure 1.4 The age-related effects of exercise and illness on function. The age-related declines have been described as linear senescence and are shown in curve A. Illness such as heart disease or cancer may accentuate the decline, as shown in curve B. Physically active people benefit by delaying the declines in function, as shown in curve C. Curve D represents a higher level of fitness and the absence of misfortune.

lower risk of cancer (Kiningham 1998). The exact mechanism is not clear; however, it is possible that aerobic exercise enhances immune function, which reduces cancer risk. It appears that the favorable effect of exercise on cancer risk is found particularly in breast and colon cancers, which are the principal causes of death in women (Fiatarone Singh 2002). Conversely, the risk of skin cancer increases for those who work and play in the sun without proper protection.

The benefits of exercise for cancer rehabilitation are not to be overlooked. Exercise may control or reduce nausea during chemotherapy. It reduces muscle loss and fatigue, enhances satisfaction with life and improves psychosocial adjustment. Immune function may also be maintained or enhanced. The full relationship between exercise and cancer remains to be defined.

Exercise is extremely diverse, ranging from passive range-of-motion to strength training in order to enhance muscle hypertrophy, and includes balance and gait mobility and cardiovascular fitness. The multiple interactive physiological effects of exercise require recognition. However, the importance of looking at the whole individual goes beyond physical activity alone.

Confusion

Only a few decades ago, the simple symptom of confusion was synonymous with aging and senility. Now it is well recognized that acute confusion may be caused by drugs (diuretics, tricyclic antidepressants, antihistamines, barbiturates, sleep-inducing hypnotic drugs); sleep deprivation; infection (typically respiratory or urinary tract infections that are not always febrile); diet; dehydration; sunset syndrome; cardiac arrhythmia; environmental influences (heat, cold); and stress (psychosocial factors, depression, anxiety). Thus, when working with an acutely confused patient, one must look at a variety of potential interactive causes (*Merck Manual of Geriatrics* 2000).

Additional considerations

In addition to a lifetime of experience yielding individual variations, other gerontological considerations influence rehabilitation care. For example, integrative functions decline to a greater degree than can be communicated by simple measurements. Nerve conduction velocity may show a small decline in a 65-year-old when compared with a 25-year-old, but integrative activities such as responding to postural perturbation are likely to show a greater decline. This is one reason why the etiology of falls in the elderly is complex, involving intrinsic factors (age-related changes in neuromusculoskeletal integrity) and extrinsic factors such as environmental challenges (*Merck Manual of Geriatrics* 2000).

Within the aging individual, the physiological range of homeostasis is sometimes greater than in younger individuals. As shown in Figure 1.5, the mean skin temperature of various body parts is similar when young and old adults are compared; however, the physiological range of measurements is greater in aging individuals (Kauffman 1987).

When rehabilitating the geriatric patient, it is vital to remember that multiple chronic diseases are common and many systems may be involved. Because of the greater physiological range of homeostasis and the multiple systems and diseases that may be involved, the aging individual is more vulnerable to the stresses of rehabilitation.

A comprehensive functional assessment is crucial if treatment is to be effective. Because of the many concomitant conditions and diseases, improvement may manifest more slowly and with a greater variety of responses during the rehabilitation process. This uniqueness is not always acceptable within the scope of the present healthcare delivery system and the classic medical model, as shown by Fried et al (1991) in Figure 1.1.

THEORETICAL PERSPECTIVES

Since antiquity, humans have developed models and theories about the causes of aging. It is not the intent of this text to explore all of these causes; however, it may be helpful to perceive them at work in the fields of gerontology, which is the study of aging, and geriatrics, which is the medical treatment of aging persons. The intention of this book is to combine gerontology and geriatrics. For more extensive reviews of different theories of aging, the reader is referred to Matteson & McConnell (1988), Moody (1994) and Bonder & Wagner (2001).

Hippocrates, sometime around 400 BC, and Aristotle, in approximately 350 BC, were in agreement when they wrote about health, medicine and old age. They reasoned that the human body consists of many structures which deal with the four conditions of heat, coldness, moistness and dryness. The following statement is attributed to Hippocrates in his work *On Ancient Medicine*: 'Whoever pays no attention to these things or paying attention does not comprehend them, how can he understand the diseases which befall a man?' Humankind was seen '... in relation to the articles of food and drink, and to his other occupations'. Aristotle, in his short physical treatise *On Youth and Old Age, On Life and Death, On Breathing*, wrote: 'Hence, of necessity, life must be coincident with the maintenance of heat, and what we call death is its destruction'. These perspectives remain viable today because we know that the loss of moistness (dehydration) and loss of heat (hypothermia) are serious conditions for all human beings.

Montaigne, the French philosopher of the 16th century, may be seen as arguing for the present day progressive decline model or wear and tear theory. In his *Book One*, Essay 1.19 he notes '... how nature deprives us of light and sense of our own bodily decay. What remains to an old man of the vigour of his youth and better day?' He saw withered bodies with decrepit motion. In his Essay 1.57, Montaigne noted that few people live to the age of 40 years and, 'To die of old age is a death rare, extraordinary, and singular, and, therefore, so much less natural than the others ... and the more remote, the less to be hoped for'. He believed it to be '... an idle conceit to expect to die as a decay of strength which is the effect of extremist age ...'. But rather, death was the result of everyday occurrences such as injuries, accidents, pleurisy or the plague and, hence, he calls these natural deaths.

More contemporary theories can be divided into social theories and biological theories. One social theory that created a tremendous amount of research is called the disengagement theory. Basically, this theory holds that the relationship between an aging person and society is changed because of the inevitable events within our life cycle and eventually ends with death, which is universal. This can easily be seen as life's central roles change, such as employment for men and motherhood for women. Disengagement for males and females is different and may be the result of individual ego changes or changes imposed by society such as mandatory retirement. This theory has mostly been rejected by research; however, it provided a foundation for the study of the social process of aging, including changing roles (Achenbaum & Bengtson 1994).

The activity theory is another social perspective that has been criticized but which has nonetheless provided a stimulus for research into a valid theory of aging. In essence, this theory states that, as people age, life satisfaction will be greater in those with activities. Those who maintain activities or add new activities, especially social activities, seem to have better morale and satisfaction (Bonder & Wagner 2001). A 10-year longitudinal study conducted in Stockholm, Sweden, found that those who had frequent mental, social or productive activities were less likely to develop dementia. Conversely, those who were isolated and, in essence, disengaged socially were more likely to develop dementia (Wang et al 2002). It is important to note that, as presented earlier, there are many benefits to physical exercise; however, a rehabilitation specialist should not forget the importance of social activity as well.

There are several biological theories of aging which have generated considerable interest. The first and probably most widely accepted by general society is the progressive decline model. This indicates that

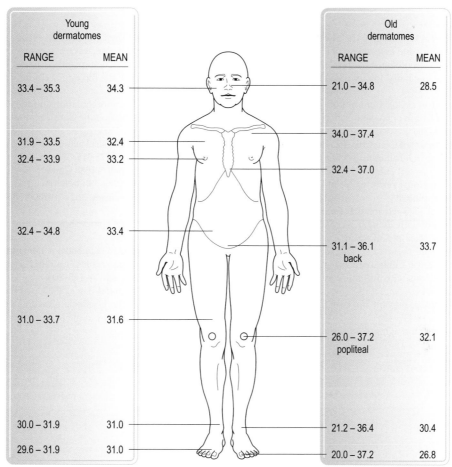

Young dermatomes				Old dermatomes	
RANGE	MEAN			RANGE	MEAN
33.4 – 35.3	34.3			21.0 – 34.8	28.5
				34.0 – 37.4	
31.9 – 33.5	32.4				
32.4 – 33.9	33.2			32.4 – 37.0	
32.4 – 34.8	33.4			31.1 – 36.1 back	33.7
31.0 – 33.7	31.6			26.0 – 37.2 popliteal	32.1
30.0 – 31.9	31.0			21.2 – 36.4	30.4
29.6 – 31.9	31.0			20.0 – 37.2	26.8

Figure 1.5   A sample of skin temperatures of young and old adults. Measurements of skin temperature were made by various investigators with different instruments under resting conditions without extreme ambient temperatures or humidity. When possible, range and mean temperatures (°C) are reported.
(From Kauffman 1987, with permission.)

the longer we live, the more wear and tear there is; everything progressively declines. From a gerontological perspective, it is well recognized that there are indeed changes with the passage of time. The research model of 40–50 years ago fits this perspective well, as most aging research was based on cross-sectional data in an attempt to define the age-related diminutions in nearly all measurements.

Another theory is the biological time clock, which postulates that aging is directed by biological time and specifically cell replication. Research has demonstrated that, in some cells, there are a finite number of replications after which apoptosis or programmed cell death occurs. This theory is used to support the concept that the human lifespan (the maximum number of years an individual can live) has not changed. In other words, we have a biological clock which says that the maximum number of years that a human being can live is somewhere between 120 and 130 years.

The free radical theory posits that, during the normal biological process of oxidative phosphorylation, free radicals are generated. This oxidative damage increases with age and can cause changes in cell function and tissues. Oxygen radicals contribute to the pathophysiological changes associated with aging and thus may be a factor in determining the lifespan of a species (Beckman & Ames 1998).

The cross-linkage theory suggests that aging takes place because of chemical reactions that create irreparable damage to DNA and cause subsequent cell death. This concept is easily used to explain the clinical complaint of increased stiffness that is common among elderly people.

The immune theory of aging indicates that a breakdown in the immune system leads to a greater risk of disease and cancer. As the body ages, it becomes less able to recognize itself, so the immune system produces antibodies which are detrimental to the host organism.

The error catastrophe theory of aging, sometimes referred to as the Orgel hypothesis, postulates that there are errors in cellular RNA transcription leading to faulty structures, especially proteins (Gafni 2002). This was considered to be a plausible explanation as to why earlier research demonstrated poor potential for muscle hypertrophy with increasing age. However, research by Fiatarone Singh (2004) and others (see Chapter 16) has indicated that the potential for muscle hypertrophy is sustained with increasing age and is achievable through proper exercise stimulus.

CONCLUSION

Aging is life's journey, leading to changes, uniqueness and, usually, multiple diagnoses. It ends in death. It is incumbent upon healthcare providers to recognize these complexities and thus, when rendering care, the whole patient must be considered, including societal and cultural implications. Each patient is more than a number or code.

References

Achenbaum W, Bengtson V 1994 Re-engaging the disengagement theory of aging: on the history and assessment of theory development gerontology. Gerontologist 34:756–763

Beckman K, Ames B 1998 The free radial theory of aging matures. Physiol Rev 78:547–581

Bergeron E, Lavoie A, Moore L et al 2005 Comorbidity and age are both independent predictors of length of hospitalization in trauma patients. Can J Surg 48:361–366

Besdine R 1990 The Merck Manual of Geriatrics, 1st edn (Introduction). Merck Sharp & Dohme Research Laboratories, Rahway, NJ, pp 2–4

Bonder B, Wagner M 2001 Functional Performance in Older Adults, 2nd edn. FA Davis, Philadelphia, PA

Boyd C, Xue Q, Guralnik J et al 2005a Hospitalization and development of dependence in activities of daily living in a cohort of disabled older women: The Women's Health and Aging Study I. J Gerontol Biol Sci 60A:888–893

Boyd C, Darer J, Boult C et al 2005b Clinical practice guidelines and quality of care for older patients with multiple comorbid diseases. J Am Med Assoc 294:716–724

Fiatarone Singh M 2002 Exercise to prevent and treat functional disability. Clin Geriatr Med 18:431–462

Fiatarone Singh M 2004 Exercise and aging. Clin Geriatr Med 20:201–221

Fried LP, Storer D, King D, Lodder F 1991 Diagnosis of illness presentation in the elderly. J Am Geriatr Soc 39:117–123

Gafni A 2002 Protein Structure and Turnover. In: Masoro E, Austad S (eds) Handbook of the Biology of Aging, 5th edn. Academic Press, San Diego, CA

Kauffman T 1987 Thermoregulation and the use of heat and cold. In: Jackson O (ed) Therapeutic Considerations for the Elderly. Churchill Livingstone, New York, p 72

Kiningham RB 1998 Physical activity and the primary prevention of cancer. Primary Care 25:515–536

Matteson M, McConnell E 1988 Gerontological Nursing Concepts and Practice. WB Saunders, Philadelphia, PA

Merck Manual of Geriatrics, 3rd edn 2000. Merck, Whitehouse Station, NJ

Moody HR 1994 Aging Concepts and Controversies. Pine Forge Press, Thousand Oaks, CA

Nakamura E, Moritani T, Kanetaka A 1998 Further evaluation of physical fitness age versus physiological age in women. Eur J Appl Physiol Occup Physiol 78:195–200

Wang H, Karp A, Winblad B et al 2002 Late-life engagement in social and leisure activities is associated with a decreased risk of dementia: a longitudinal study from the Kungsholmen project. Am J Epidemiol 155(12):1081–1087

Chapter **2**

Skeletal muscle function in older people

Marilia Harumi Higuchi dos Santos, Walter R. Frontera and Lars Larsson

Table 2.1 The effects of aging at different levels of the human motor unit

Motor unit	↓ Number and ↑ size
Contractile properties	↑ Contraction and 50% relaxation times
Anterior horn	↓ Number of cells
Peripheral nerves	↓ Motor nerve conduction velocity
Neuromuscular junction	↓ More complex and irregular
Muscle	
Strength	↓ Upper and lower extremities
Contractility	Slow contraction
Mass	↓ Segmental and whole body
Fiber number	↓ Types I and II
Fiber area	↓ Type II fiber area
Fiber type	No change; increased coexpression of myosin isoforms
Local muscular endurance	↓ Endurance; earlier onset of fatigue

INTRODUCTION

Impairment of neuromuscular performance evidenced by muscle weakness, slowing of movement, loss of muscle power and early muscle fatigue is a prominent feature of old age in humans. This impairment is often accompanied by inactivity or chronic diseases that will further impair neuromuscular performance. As a result, many elderly men and women have functional limitations on walking, lifting and maintaining postural balance and on recovering from impending falls, leading to disability.

The mechanisms underlying these limitations are complex, but alterations in the components of the motor units play an important role. By the age of 80, 40–50% of muscle strength, muscle mass, alpha motoneurons and muscle cells are lost. The independence associated with mobility is critical in achieving a longer lifespan and, especially, a high quality of life. The increasing number and overall percentage of elderly people, and the social and economic consequences of this increase, underline the importance of understanding geriatric neuromotor performance. In this chapter, we will briefly discuss the age-associated changes in the motor unit, skeletal muscle functional properties and skeletal muscle structural characteristics (Table 2.1).

MOTOR UNIT

In the elderly, there is a decrease in the number of functional motor units associated with a concomitant enlargement of the cross-sectional area of the remaining units. This motor unit remodeling is achieved by selective denervation of muscle fibers, especially type IIb fibers, followed by reinnervation by axonal sprouting from juxtaposed innervated units. This process leads not only to a net loss of fibers and functional motor units but also to an increase in motor unit size (fibers dispersed throughout a larger territory) and amplitude and duration of the motor unit potential. Besides this partial switch of motor unit innervation, there are other neurological changes that could contribute to the development of sarcopenia (defined as the loss of muscle mass associated with aging) such as: (i) a decrease in the number of nerve terminals; (ii) fragmentation of the neuromuscular junction; (iii) a decrease in neurotransmitter release; and (iv) a decreased number of acetylcholine receptors.

MUSCLE STRENGTH

Muscle weakness is an important determinant of physical function in older people. In general, the decline in strength starts during the third decade of life and accelerates during the sixth and seventh decades. The overall rate of decline is approximately 8% per decade

(Schiller et al 2000). Thus, during the course of daily living, older people may be working at relatively close to their maximal capacity, and additional impairments in muscle function associated with acute or chronic diseases, hospitalization resulting from trauma or surgery, and inactivity may accelerate the decline in strength. This concept of 'close to maximal capacity' is important during rehabilitation when the aim is not only to regain muscle strength but also to enhance functional reserve. Thus, when treating an elderly woman recovering from a humeral fracture who needs to lift a 1-kg (2 lb) box of sugar onto a cupboard shelf, her functional reserve can be enhanced by performing the activity 10 times with a 1-kg (2 lb) weight or several times with a 1.5-kg (3 lb) weight.

Some features that are prominent among the aged include decreases in both muscle mass and muscle strength and also changes in the muscle composition with increasing infiltration of fat and connective tissue. These age-related alterations can be modified with behavioral and pharmacological interventions including exercise training, nutritional interventions and, in some cases, hormonal supplementation. Strength training in frail older people is accompanied by improvements in physical function.

PHYSIOLOGY OF MUSCLE WEAKNESS

Physiologically, muscle weakness may be due to a decrease in the ability to activate the existing muscle mass, a reduction in the quantity of muscle tissue and therefore in the number of force-generating crossbridges interacting between thin and thick filaments, a decrease in the force developed by each crossbridge, or a combination of all three factors. It seems that the ability to maximally activate the remaining motor unit pool is well preserved in the aged. Muscle atrophy and loss of myofibrillar protein, on the other hand, are caused by a reduction in the number of motor neurons in the spinal cord and an incomplete reinnervation of denervated muscle cells, which results in a decrease in the number and size of muscle fibers.

Changes in neural mechanisms include undefined changes in the central nervous system, a delay in the conduction velocity of motor nerve fibers, a delayed transmission in the neuromuscular junction, or all three. Alterations in the proportions of motor units and myofibers of different types, particularly a decrease in the number or the relative cross-sectional area of type II fast fibers, are also noticeable. Finally, losses in the ability of the sarcoplasmic reticulum to handle calcium within the fibers, changes in the myosin molecule, an increased passive resistance of the connective tissue structures, or a combination of factors may contribute to altered contractile behavior.

SPEED OF CONTRACTION AND MUSCLE POWER

An important characteristic of neuromuscular performance is the time-course of muscle actions. This characteristic can be studied in vivo with measurements of the speed of contraction of individual muscles or muscle groups and in vitro by measuring the maximal shortening velocity of single muscle fibers (Larsson & Moss 1993). This property is important because the velocity of movement (and thus power generation) can have greater relevance than absolute muscle strength on the ability to perform a number of the activities of daily living, independence and functional capacity (Foldvari et al 2000).

In the elderly, the in vivo muscle twitch (evoked by electrical stimulation) is characterized by prolonged contraction and 50% relaxation times. Thus, fused tetanic forces occur at lower stimulation frequencies, an adaptation that increases muscle efficiency. However, this adaptation also lengthens the time for muscle relaxation, thus impairing the ability to perform rapid powerful alternating movements. Human studies have shown that the time to produce the same absolute and relative forces during voluntary contractions is lengthened in the elderly and, therefore, the ability to generate explosive force (power) and to accelerate a limb is reduced (Foldvari et al 2000, Frontera et al 2000). These alterations have a negative effect on the protective reactions used before or during a fall. Several studies have shown that, in the elderly, differences in skeletal muscle power could explain more of the variability in function and disability, particularly during lower intensity tasks such as walking compared with higher intensity activities such as climbing stairs or rising from a chair.

MUSCLE ENDURANCE

Muscle fatigability is another important component of performance. Fatigue is typically measured as a loss of force during repeated or continuous activation. The effect of age on local muscular endurance is controversial and probably reflects different experimental approaches. The results of some investigations suggest that older men and women fatigue more than younger subjects, which is consistent with studies in animal models. Other investigators, however, have demonstrated similar fatigability in young and old subjects, whereas still others have observed that older adults fatigue less than younger. Even less clear than the effect of old age on the magnitude of fatigue is its effect on the potential mechanisms that contribute to fatigue. Human aging is accompanied by a number of changes in the neuromuscular system (Stackhouse et al 2001) that might affect fatigue, including motor unit remodeling, reduced maximal motor unit discharge rates and a general shift toward a greater type I fiber composition. The extent of these age-related alterations appears to vary by muscle group and level of habitual physical activity.

Alterations in muscle with advanced adult age that may contribute to a decrease in muscle endurance include reduced blood supply and capillary density, impairment of glucose transport and therefore substrate availability, lower mitochondrial density, decreased activity of oxidative enzymes and decreased rate of phosphocreatine repletion.

MUSCLE MASS

Lower muscle mass has been correlated with poor physical function. A large recent study, including more than 4400 older participants, demonstrated that the likelihood of physical disability (measured as ability to perform activities of daily living) was increased when the skeletal muscle index (SMI, determined by estimating whole body muscle mass and dividing by height in meters squared) values were lower than $5.75 \, kg/m^2$ in women and $8.50 \, kg/m^2$ in men (Melton et al 2000). According to the authors, these cut-off points could be used to determine the degree of sarcopenia.

The factors contributing to the loss of muscle mass with age seem to be a reduction in the numbers of both type I and type II muscle fibers and a decline in cross-sectional area, predominantly of type II fibers; the cross-sectional area of type I fibers seems to be well maintained. As mentioned above, the relative area (percentage of type II fibers $\times$ mean fiber area of type II fibers) occupied by type II fibers is significantly reduced with age. This may contribute to the changes in contractile behavior mentioned above.

PROTEIN METABOLISM AND INFLAMMATION

It is commonly held that age-related changes in the processes that regulate muscle protein mass contribute to sarcopenia as protein is the primary structural and functional macromolecule in muscle. Muscle protein content is determined by the balance between protein synthesis and breakdown and some studies in humans have shown that postabsorptive muscle protein synthesis declines with age. Although not all studies concur, it seems that mixed muscle and myofibrillar protein synthesis rates decline with advanced adult age (Welle et al 1993, Toth et al 2005) and increase in response to exercise training (Hasten et al 2000).

Age-related changes in the physiological systems that regulate skeletal muscle protein metabolism could also contribute to sarcopenia. Specific skeletal muscle proteins and groups of proteins, with important structural and functional roles, have different rates of metabolism. From both quantitative and functional perspectives, myosin heavy chain (MyHC) is the most important protein in skeletal muscle and its synthesis is reduced with age. In addition to the overall mass of MyHC protein, the type of MyHC isoforms expressed has relevance for both the metabolism and functionality of aging muscle. Because the isoforms are synthesized at different rates, a change in MyHC isoform distribution with age could contribute to altered MyHC protein synthesis rates. Additionally, a shift in MyHC isoform distribution can alter muscle performance given the different functional properties of each isoform. At present, however, conflicting reports exist regarding the effect of age on skeletal muscle MyHC isoform distribution (Hasten et al 2000, Marx et al 2002).

Aging is associated with increased cytokine levels/production and reduced circulating insulin-like growth factor (IGF)-1 concentrations. Studies in cultured myocytes and animal models have demonstrated the catabolic effects of cytokines and the anabolic effects of IGF-1 on skeletal muscle. Because aging is associated with increased levels of inflammatory markers, it is thought that immune activation may contribute to the development of sarcopenia. There is a growing body of evidence suggesting that chronic inflammation is one of the most important biological mechanisms underlying the decline in physical function that is often observed over the aging process. The plasma concentration of interleukin 6 (IL-6), a cytokine that plays a central role in inflammation, tends to increase with age and high serum levels of IL-6 predict disability in the elderly (Taafe et al 2000). Also, some preliminary data suggest that IL-6 is associated with accelerated sarcopenia (Taafe et al 2000). Further, several studies suggest that IGF-1 is an important modulator of muscle mass and function across the entire lifespan and recent findings show that low plasma IGF-1 levels are associated with poor knee extensor muscle strength, slow walking speed and self-reported difficulties with mobility tasks, thus suggesting a role for IGF-1 in the causal pathway leading to disability in the elderly. There are some data which show that IL-6 inhibits the secretion of IGF-1 and its biological activity and it has been shown that higher plasma IL-6 levels and lower plasma IGF-1 levels were associated with lower muscle strength and power (Hasten et al 2000). Thus, the balance between the catabolic effect of cytokines and the anabolic effect of IGF-1 may play an important role in the development of sarcopenia (Barbieri et al 2003).

MUSCLE FAT

Fat infiltration of skeletal muscle is common among the elderly and has been associated with a greater incidence of mobility limitations. In a recent study, muscle attenuation (indicative of fat infiltration) remained an independent determinant of incident mobility limitations. People in the lowest quartile of muscle attenuation (with the greatest amount of fat infiltration into the muscle) were 50–80% more likely to develop mobility limitations during follow-up, which was independent of muscle area, muscle strength or total body fat mass.

References

Barbieri M, Ferrucci L, Ragno E et al 2003 Chronic inflammation and the effect of IGF-1 on muscle strength and power in older persons. Am J Physiol 284:E481–487

Foldvari M, Clark M, Laviolette LC et al 2000 Association of muscle power with functional status in community-dwelling elderly women. J Gerontol Biol Med Sci 55A:M192–199

Frontera WR, Hughes VA, Fielding RA et al 2000 Aging of skeletal muscle: a 12-yr longitudinal study. J Appl Physiol 88:1321–1326

Hasten DL, Pak-Loduca J, Obert KA et al 2000 Resistance exercise acutely increases MyHC and mixed muscle protein synthesis rates in 78–84 and 23–32 yr olds. Am J Physiol 278:E620–626

Larsson L, Moss RL 1993 Maximum velocity of shortening in relation to myosin isoform composition in single fibres from human skeletal muscles. J Physiol 472:595–614

Marx JO, Kraemer WJ, Nindl BC et al 2002 Effects of aging on human skeletal muscle myosin heavy-chain mRNA content and protein isoform expression. J Gerontol 57:B232–238

Melton JL III, Khosla S, Crowson C et al 2000 Epidemiology of sarcopenia. J Am Geriatr Soc 48:6215–6230.

Schiller B, Casas Y, Tarcy B et al 2000 Age-related declines in knee extensor strength and physical performance in healthy Hispanic and Causian women. J Gerontol Series A Bio Med 55:B563–569

Stackhouse SK, Stevens JE, Lee SC et al 2001 Maximum voluntary activation in nonfatigued and fatigued muscle of young and elderly individuals. Phys Ther 81:1102–1109

Taaffe DR, Harris TB, Ferrucci L et al 2000 Cross-sectional and prospective relationships of interleukin-6 and C-reactive protein with physical performance in elderly person: MacArthur studies of successful aging. J Gerontol Biol Med Sci 55:M706–708

Toth MJ, Matthews DE, Tracy RP et al 2005 Age-related differences in skeletal muscle protein synthesis: relation to markers of immune activation. Am J Physiol 288:E883–891

Welle S, Thornton C, Jozefowicz R et al 1993 Myofibrillar protein synthesis in young and old men. Am J Physiol 264:E693–698

Chapter 3

Effects of aging on bone

Emily L. Germain-Lee, Mary M. Checovich, Everett L. Smith and Katie Lundon

INTRODUCTION

Bone is a tissue that gives form to the body, supporting its weight, protecting organs and facilitating movement by providing attachments for muscles so that they can act as levers. Although the general anatomy of the skeleton is genetically determined, skeletal strength and shape can be influenced by a variety of factors, including mechanical loading, pharmacological agents and nutritional intake. The skeleton consists of specialized connective tissue made up of cells including osteoblasts, osteocytes, bone-lining cells and osteoclasts that produce, maintain and organize the cellular matrix (Marks & Popoff 1988).

BONE STRUCTURE

Macroscopic anatomy

Bones vary in their shape but can be broadly divided into two general categories: flat bones (skull bones, scapula, mandible, etc) and long bones (tibia, femur, humerus, etc).

Long bones are designed for bearing weight and consist of a thick and dense outer layer (cortex) of compact bone, of which 90% by volume is calcified. The long bone is composed of the central diaphysis, or midshaft, the metaphysis and the epiphysis, which is capped with articular cartilage.

Although there is only one mechanism of bone formation, it may occur within cartilage (endochondral), within an organic matrix membrane (intramembranous) or by means of deposition of new bone onto existing bone (appositional). The bones of the vertebral column, the base of the skull and the appendicular skeleton (other than the clavicle) are formed by endochondral ossification. Most of the bones of the face, the vault of the skull and the pelvis are formed by intramembranous ossification. The formation of periosteal bone and bone modeling and remodeling depend on the process of appositional bone formation. All three types of bone formation occur throughout life and can contribute to the repair of the skeleton after injury or disease or to the treatment of skeletal deformity.

The degree of bone mass attained is governed by hormonal, nutritional and mechanical factors. At all ages, women have a lower bone mass than men and, with increasing age, this gap widens. For cortical bone, a slow loss of bone mass (0.3–0.5% per year) begins at about age 40 in both sexes (Mazess 1982). Additionally, women generally experience an accelerated period of bone loss around the menopause. Bone loss rates of 5–6% per year for up to 10 years are not unusual. This accelerated loss is associated with the withdrawal of estrogen (Avioli & Krane 1990, Dempster 2003, Downey & Siegel 2006). The role of estrogen deficiency appears to involve an increase in bone resorption as well as a diminution of bone formation. Thus, in females and males, estrogen has both a catabolic and an anabolic effect on bone throughout life, even into the eighth and ninth decades. In older men, osteoporosis is more closely related to low estrogen than to low androgen levels (Raisz 2005).

Microscopic anatomy

Gross inspection shows that there are two forms of bone tissue: cortical (compact) bone and trabecular (cancellous) bone. Cortical and trabecular bone have the same matrix composition and structure but the mass of the cortical bone matrix per unit of volume is much greater.

Cortical bone constitutes about 80% of the mature skeleton. Dense cortical tissue forms the diaphysis (midshaft) of long bones and there is little or no trabecular bone in this region. The thick cortical walls of the diaphysis become thinner and increase in diameter as they form the metaphysis, where plates of trabecular bone orient themselves to provide support for a thin shell of subchondral bone that underlies the articular cartilage.

Trabecular bone is a network of mineralized bone that forms the greater part of each vertebral body and the epiphyses of long bones and is present at other sites such as the iliac crest. It constitutes 20% of the total skeletal mass. In humans, cancellous bone consists of 5–30% of hard bone tissue and the rest is soft tissue including marrow and blood vessels (Banse 2002). Trabecular bone provides a large surface area and is the most metabolically active part of the skeleton, with a high rate of turnover and a blood supply that is much greater than that of cortical bone. It acts as a reservoir for calcium; it is negatively affected by immobility, systemic acidosis (Arnett 2003) and some pharmaceutical agents (e.g. glucocorticoids, corticosteroids, anticonvulsant therapy), and positively affected by other pharmaceutical agents [e.g. estrogen replacement therapy (ERT), calcitonin, bisphosphonates].

Cortical bone fulfills mainly the mechanical and protective function, and trabecular bone fulfills the metabolic function of the skeleton. In long bones, the thick dense cortical bone of the diaphysis provides maximum resistance to torsion and bending. In the metaphyses and epiphyses, the thinner cortices allow greater deformation to occur under the same load.

Cortical or trabecular bone may consist of woven (primary) or lamellar (secondary) bone. Woven bone forms the embryonic skeleton and is replaced by mature bone. Fracture callus formation follows the same sequence. Woven bone is rarely present after the age of 4 years in humans. However, it can appear at any age in response to an osseous or soft-tissue injury. Woven bone is more flexible and more easily deformed than lamellar bone. For this reason, replacement of woven bone with mature lamellar bone is essential to restore the normal mechanical properties of bone tissue. Lamellar bone consists of highly orientated, densely packed collagen fibrils. These fibrils lend strength to bone.

To carry out the diverse functions of bone formation, bone resorption, mineral homeostasis and bone repair, bone cells assume specialized forms characterized by morphology, function and characteristic location. They originate from two cell lines: a mesenchymal stem-cell line and a hematopoietic stem-cell line. The mesenchymal stem-cell line consists of undifferentiated cells or preosteoblasts, osteoblasts, bone-lining cells and osteocytes. The hematopoietic stem-cell line consists of circulating, or marrow, monocytes, preosteoclasts and osteoclasts.

Undifferentiated mesenchymal cells that have the potential to become osteoblasts reside in bone canals, endosteum, periosteum and marrow. These cells, under the right conditions, will undergo proliferation and differentiate into preosteoblasts and then mature osteoblasts. Osteoblasts never appear or function individually but are always found in clusters along the bone surface. Active osteoblasts may follow one of three courses. They may remain on the surface of the bone, decrease their synthetic activity and assume the flatter form of bone-lining cells; they may surround themselves with matrix and become osteocytes; or they may disappear from the site of bone formation.

Osteoclasts are large multinucleated cells found on the surface of bone. They are the cells responsible for bone resorption. Specific hormones and growth factors influence their development. Osteoclasts are very efficient in destroying bone matrix. They begin by binding themselves to the surface of the bone, creating a sealed space between the cell and the bone matrix. Endosomes containing membrane-bound proton pumps transport protons into the sealed space, decreasing the pH from about 7.0 to about 4.0. The acidic environment solubilizes the bone mineral. Excess organic matrix is degraded by acid proteases secreted by the cells (Urist 1980).

BONE REMODELING

Throughout life, physiological remodeling (removal and replacement) of bone occurs without affecting the shape or density of the bone. Remodeling occurs on the surface of the bone as well as within the bone. It includes osteoclast activation, resorption of bone, osteoblast activation and formation of new bone at the site of resorption. Internal, or osteonal, remodeling begins when osteoclasts create a tunnel through bone. These cutting cones create large resorption cavities. Within the cutting cones, groups of osteoblasts follow the advancing osteoclasts. Layers of osteoblasts arrange themselves along the surface of the resorption cavity behind the osteoclast and

deposit successive lamellae of new bone matrix. These layers mineralize and fill in the canal. It appears that physiological remodeling serves to replace bone matrix in which defects may have developed because of normal use. It may also have a role in mineral homeostasis.

In normal adult bone, remodeling is usually a tightly controlled physiological process in which bone resorption equals bone formation, achieved through teams of osteoblasts and osteoclasts forming basic multicellular units (BMUs) or bone remodeling units (BRUs) (Dempster 2003). This homoeostasis may change under pathological conditions in which bone resorption and formation are stimulated. Primary osteoporosis is an uncoupling of the balance between resorption and formation. Imbalances of bone remodeling lead to persistent deficits of bone mass, which translate into fracture susceptibility.

CALCIUM AND MECHANICAL HOMEOSTASIS

Bone cells respond to changes in hormonal levels to maintain calcium homeostasis and to changes in mechanical loading to maintain mechanical competence (Smith & Gilligan 1996). Serum calcium is maintained through regulation of calcium absorption from the gastrointestinal tract, reabsorption by the kidney and resorption from bone. Lowered blood calcium levels increase parathyroid hormone levels, which draws calcium from the skeletal reservoir. Increased mechanical loading stimulates greater bone mass. Osteocytes appear to detect strain and transmit messages to the preosteoblasts and preosteoclasts to increase the bone-forming activities relative to the bone-resorbing activities. These signals, generated by hormones and growth factors, are integrated by the cells and their response leads to overall maintenance of skeletal integrity and calcium homeostasis.

Abnormal bone

Osteomalacia is a metabolic bone disorder that affects the adult skeleton by means of abnormal mineralization and results in skeletal deformity. It is a state of high bone turnover and is characterized primarily by excessive amounts of inadequately mineralized osteoid (unmineralized bone tissue). Specifically, this increase in osteoid is associated with prolonged mineralization time. In cancellous bone, this osteoid presents in the form of large seams that coat the trabeculae and contribute to overall preserved bone volume. In cortical bone, intracortical bone resorption, or tunneling, as well as increased amounts of osteoid lining the haversian canals may be observed.

Biochemical features

Mineralization of newly formed bone requires the deposition of adequate concentrations of calcium and phosphate. In general, the combination of moderate hypocalcemia and clear hypophosphatemia are hallmarks of adult osteomalacia. When there is vitamin D3 deficiency because of dietary considerations or malabsorption, the serum calcium level is low, the serum phosphate level is very low (because of decreased intestinal phosphate absorption and increased renal phosphate clearance caused by secondary hyperparathyroidism induced by the low serum calcium levels) and urinary calcium excretion is also very low. There may also be elevated alkaline phosphatase and osteocalcin (also known as bone Gla protein or BGP) levels (Hutchinson & Bell 1992).

FUTURE DIRECTIONS

Recent advances in our understanding of the molecular signals that regulate bone and muscle growth have identified new strategies for enhancing bone mass either directly or indirectly. One example of a direct strategy is to promote bone formation by increasing the activities of signaling molecules named bone morphogenetic proteins (BMPs). The discovery of BMPs arose from the now classic studies by Urist and colleagues (Urist 1965, Reddi & Huggins 1972, Urist et al 1973) demonstrating that extracts prepared from demineralized bone could induce ectopic de novo bone formation when implanted either subcutaneously or intramuscularly in rodents. Subsequent biochemical and gene cloning studies identified the active molecules in these extracts to be a group of related secretory proteins collectively referred to as BMPs (Wozney et al 1988). Each of these BMPs has been demonstrated to be capable of inducing new bone formation, and several have been shown to have beneficial effects in enhancing fracture repair in human patients (Moghadam et al 2001, Kain & Einhorn 2005). The remarkable ability of these proteins to promote bone growth has also led to the suggestion that these proteins may be useful for increasing bone mass in patients with osteoporosis, although clinical efficacy in human trials has yet to be demonstrated.

An alternative to strategies aimed at directly promoting bone growth is to indirectly enhance bone mass by increasing the mechanical load on bone. An example of such a strategy is to increase muscle mass by targeting pathways that normally suppress muscle growth. Recent work has identified a molecule named myostatin as a potent inhibitor of skeletal muscle growth (McPherron et al 1997). Myostatin is normally made by skeletal muscle cells, circulates in the blood and acts to maintain muscle satellite cells in a quiescent state

(for review see Lee 2004). When the activity of myostatin is blocked, these satellite cells are activated, proliferate and fuse to existing myofibers causing the fibers to hypertrophy. Although the mechanisms by which myostatin activity is regulated in vivo are still being elucidated, activity can be blocked artificially by a variety of both naturally occurring and engineered myostatin-binding proteins. One engineered binding protein is a neutralizing monoclonal antibody directed against myostatin, and this monoclonal antibody is currently being tested in clinical trials in patients with muscular dystrophy. A successful outcome of these trials in terms of promoting muscle growth would open the possibility of exploiting such agents for other clinical applications, including increasing bone mass.

CONCLUSION

The rapid increase in the understanding of the mechanisms that control bone cell function has led to many advances in musculoskeletal research. The ability to manipulate formation and resorption of bone as needed will substantially improve the treatment of musculoskeletal disorders. Interventions that exploit this knowledge of bone cell function offer the potential to treat numerous diseases.

Acknowledgment

Thanks to Dr S.J. Lee for his review of this manuscript.

References

Arnett T 2003 Regulation of bone cell function by acid–base balance. Proc Nutr Soc 62:511–520

Avioli LV, Krane SM 1990 Metabolic Bone Disease and Clinically Related Disorders. WB Saunders, Philadelphia, PA

Banse X 2002 When density fails to predict bone strength. Part II: structural organization of the trabeculae. Acta Orthop Scand 73 (suppl303):11–22

Dempster DW 2003 The pathophysiology of bone loss. Clin Geriatr Med 19:259–270

Downey PA, Siegel MI 2006 Bone biology and the clinical implications for osteoporosis. Phys Ther 86:77–91

Hutchinson R, Bell N 1992 Osteomalcia in rickets. Semin Nephrol 12:127–145

Kain MS, Einhorn TA 2005 Recombinant human bone morphogenetic proteins in the treatment of fractures. Foot Ankle Clin 10(4):639–650

Lee SJ 2004 Regulation of muscle mass by myostatin. Annu Rev Cell Dev Biol 20:61–86

Marks SC Jr, Popoff SN 1988 Bone cell biology: the regulation of development, structure, and function in the skeleton. Am J Anat 183:1–44

Mazess RB 1982 On ageing bone loss. Clin Orthop 165:239–252

McPherron AC, Lawler A, Lee SJ 1997 Regulation of skeletal muscle mass in mice by a new TGF-beta superfamily member. Nature 387(6628):83–90

Moghadam HG, Urist MR, Sandor GK et al 2001 Successful mandibular reconstruction using a BMP bioimplant. J Craniofac Surg 12(2):119–127

Raisz LG 2005 Pathogenesis of osteoporosis: concepts, conflicts, and prospects. J Clin Invest 115:3318–3325

Reddi AH, Huggins C 1972 Biochemical sequences in the transformation of normal fibroblasts in adolescent rats. Proc Natl Acad Sci USA 69(6):1601–1605

Smith EL, Gilligan C 1996 Dose-response relationship between physical loading and mechanical competence of bone. Bone 18:455–508

Urist MR 1965 Bone: formation by autoinduction. Science 150(3698):893–899

Urist MR 1980 Fundamental and Clinical Bone Physiology. JB Lippincott, Philadelphia, PA

Urist MR, Iwata H, Ceccotti PL et al 1973 Bone morphogenesis in implants of insoluble bone gelatin. Proc Natl Acad Sci USA 70(12):3511–3515

Wozney MR, Rosen V, Celeste AJ et al 1988 Novel regulators of bone formation: molecular clones and activities. Science 242(4885):1528–1534

Chapter **4**

Effects of age on joints and ligaments

Louis R. Amundsen

INTRODUCTION

With the passage of time, many micro- and macrochanges take place in the axial and appendicular skeletal joint structures and periarticular connective tissue. The changes may be due to aging, trauma, pathological processes or, most likely, a combination of factors. These factors may alter joint movement, posture and function. It is important for the clinician to be cognizant of the typical changes that occur in joints and ligaments and to modify treatment procedures accordingly.

JOINTS AND LIGAMENTS

Joints (articulations or arthroses) are the connections between bones of the skeleton. Some joints are designed to hold bones together without allowing movement and others are designed for efficient movement. Joints are classified as synovial (diarthroses) or nonsynovial (synarthroses). The synovial joints allow maximal movement and minimal stability. Nonsynovial joints, classified as fibrous or cartilaginous, allow limited or no movement and maximum stability. Fibrous suture joints, which join the bones of the skull, generally become more stable with age and are often classified as truly immovable joints. As a person ages, these fibrous joints become calcified or coated with bone matrix. Fibrous gomphosis joints, which hold the teeth in their sockets in the mandible or maxilla, often become less stable with age because of changes in the bony sockets or in the fibrous connective tissue. Fibrous syndesmosis joints, which hold the radius and ulna or the tibia and fibula together with interosseous ligaments, allow considerable movement. Stiffening of the ligaments limits the extent and speed of movement of these joints in the elderly. Cartilaginous joints include the synchondrosis joints (hyaline cartilage growth centers of adolescents) and the symphysis joints of the pubic symphysis, the manubriosternal joint and the intervertebral joints between bodies of vertebrae. Changes in the cartilaginous

intervertebral disks, such as loss of hydration, increased rigidity and degeneration of collagen, contribute significantly to the loss of range of motion or mobility of the spine with age (Carola et al 1992, Digiovanna 1994, Levangie & Norkin 2005).

Synovial joints

Diarthroses, or synovial joints, are designed to allow smooth efficient movement by means of hyaline cartilage at the ends of the articulating bones, lubrication by synovial fluid and the flexible articular capsule enclosure. The inner linings or synovial membranes of the capsule are the source of synovial fluid. The outer layer of the capsule is a fibrous membrane that is attached to the articulating bones and encloses the joint and offers limitation to the separation of the articulating bones. Fibrous thickenings of the capsule form ligaments, which are pliable but are designed to limit movement of the joint by preventing excessive separation of the articulating bones. Most joints of the upper and lower extremities are synovial joints, as are those between the ribs and vertebrae, between the ribs and costal cartilages and the sternum, and between the articular processes of adjacent vertebrae as well as the atlantooccipital joint, the medial and lateral atlantoaxial joints, and the temporomandibular joint. In general, the movement of synovial joints is limited by the tension of ligaments, which do not stretch, muscle tension and body structures, such as the thorax, the limbs and the pelvis, etc. (Carola et al 1992, Digiovanna 1994, Levangie & Norkin 2005).

Cartilage

In synovial joints, articular cartilage or hyaline cartilage covers the ends of articulating bones. The outer surface consists of collagen fibers arranged parallel to the surface; it looks like a moist, polished pearl. This smooth surface minimizes resistance to sliding and gliding. The outer surface is attached to a transitional layer of collagen fibers and eventually to the bone by calcified cartilage. The middle layer is relatively thick and will absorb shock. The cartilage itself has no nerve or blood supply. Pain and position, or proprioception, receptors are located in the capsule and in the ligaments of the joint. When compressed, the articular cartilage exudes fluid through pores in the outer layer and, when the compression ceases, synovial fluid is drawn back into the cartilage. This intermittent pressure is essential for nourishing the articular cartilage. Prolonged periods of compression or lack of compression cause deterioration of the articular cartilage. Social expectations of reduced physical activity, diminished sensation of pressure and pain, illness, hospitalization, decreased muscle strength and coordination, falls and hip fractures, for example, result in elderly individuals being less likely to move at optimal intervals and more likely to have deteriorated articular cartilage. Articular cartilage has a limited ability to repair itself and this capacity is further diminished in the elderly (Digiovanna 1994, Bautch et al 1997, Hamerman 1998, Brandt 2003, Ahmed et al 2005, Levangie & Norkin 2005). Normal aging also causes a reduction in the amount and quality of synovial fluid, which contributes to the deterioration of articular cartilage (Boxes 4.1 and 4.2) (Digiovanna 1994, Bautch et al 1997, Hamerman 1998, Brandt 2003, Ahmed et al 2005, Levangie & Norkin 2005).

Box 4.1   Age-related changes in synovial joints and ligaments

↓ Flexibility of the joint capsule
↑ Stiffness of ligaments
↓ Quality and quantity of synovial fluid
↓ Quality of information from joint receptors
↓ Relative number of elastic fibers

Box 4.2   Age-related changes in articular cartilage

↓ Water content
↓ Chondroitin sulfate quality and content of glycosaminoglycans
↓ Quality and content of proteoglycans
↑ Articular surface roughness
↑ Resistance to gliding
↓ Thickness
↓ Synovial fluid perfusion

Joint capsules and ligaments

The joint capsules and ligaments become stiffer with age because of the increase in the formation of crosslinks in collagen fibers and the loss of elastic fibers. The stiffening of the capsules and ligaments has direct and indirect effects on the extent and quality of movement. This stiffening directly hampers joint motion which, in turn, causes a deterioration in the quality of afferent information from the joint receptors. The end result is slower and more uncertain or uncoordinated movements. This combination makes the elderly less likely to move spontaneously through the complete range of motion (Amiel et al 1991, Digiovanna 1994, Barros et al 2002, Hewitt et al 2002, Iida et al 2002, Levangie & Norkin 2005).

CONCLUSION

With aging, the loss of range of motion diminishes the ability to perform the basic activities of daily living and higher level occupational and recreational activities. Loss of range of motion is likely to occur in the following joint movements: cervical flexion, extension and lateral bending; thoracic and lumbar flexion, extension and lateral bending; shoulder flexion, abduction and rotation; elbow flexion

and extension; forearm pronation and supination; all movements of the hand and wrist; hip flexion, extension, abduction, adduction and rotation; knee flexion and extension; ankle dorsiflexion and plantar flexion; and all movements of the foot. Table 4.1 includes examples of the range of motion that can be expected from elderly subjects. Although adult women usually have a greater range of motion than men, it is not consistent for all joints or within all age groups. For this reason, no attempt was made to separate values by gender. The range of motion required for normal movement has been reported for many activities (Johnston & Smidt 1970, Laubenthal et al 1972, Colby & May 1999, Norkin & White 2003, Magermans et al 2005). Elderly individuals are especially likely to have difficulty walking rapidly, climbing ladders, squatting and recovering from a loss of balance. Lack of range of motion for all low back movements; hip extension, flexion and rotation; knee flexion; and ankle dorsiflexion contribute to these problems. In the upper extremities, limited range of motion is likely to make it difficult or impossible to reach high shelves and eventually to perform routine activities of daily living such as dressing, eating and personal hygiene. Exercise and physical activities should be used to prevent, delay or minimize these problems (Dunlop et al 1998, Escalante et al 1999a, 1999b, Beissner et al 2000, Escalante et al 2001, Bennett et al 2002, Booth et al 2002).

Table 4.1   Range of motion for selected joints

Motion (in degrees, mean ± SD)	Age	
	<40	75+
Shoulder abduction	184 ± 7[a]	118 ± 20[b]
Hip flexion	122 ± 12[c]	105 ± 10[d]
Hip extension	22 ± 8[c]	17 ± 8[e]
Knee flexion	134 ± 9[c]	100 ± 20[d]
Ankle dorsiflexion	25 ± 6[f]	8 ± 8[d]
Ankle plantar flexion	56 ± 6[a]	35 ± 15[d]
Cervical flexion	50 ± 9[g]	38 ± 9[g]
Cervical extension	82 ± 15[g]	50 ± 15[g]
Lumbar flexion	47 ± 7[h]	25 ± 10[h]
Lumbar extension	18 ± 10[h]	10 ± 6[h]

Created using data from the following sources:
[a] Boone DC, Azen SP, 1979 Normal range of motion of joints in male subjects. J Bone Joint Surg 61: 756
[b] Bassey EJ, Morgan K, Dallosso HM et al 1989 Flexibility of the shoulder joint measured as range of abduction in a large representative sample of men and women over 65 years of age. Eur J Appl Physiol 58: 353
[c] Roach KE, Miles TP 1991 Normal hip and knee active range of motion: The relationship to age. Phys Ther 71: 656
[d] James B, Parker AW 1989 Active and passive mobility of lower limb joints in elderly men and women. Am J Phys Med 68: 162
[e] Same as reference (c), but the age range is 60–74 years
[f] Greene WB, Heckman JD 1994 The Clinical Measurement of Joint Motion. American Academy of Orthopedic Surgeons, Rosemount, IL
[g] Youdas JW, Garrett TR, Suman VI et al 1992 Normal range of motion of the cervical spine: An initial goniometric study. Phys Ther 72: 770
[h] Amundsen LR 1993 The effect of aging and exercise on joint mobility. Orthopedic Physical Therapy Clinics of North America 2: 241

References

Ahmed MS, Matsumura B, Cristian A et al 2005 Age-related changes in muscles and joints. Phys Med Rehabil Clin North Am 16(1):19–39

Amiel D, Kuiper SD, Wallace CD et al 1991 Age-related properties of medial collateral ligament and anterior cruciate ligament: a morphologic and collagen maturation study in the rabbit. J Gerontol 46(4)B159–B165

Barros EM, Rodrigues CJ, Rodrigues NR et al 2002 Aging of the elastic and collagen fibers in the human cervical interspinous ligaments. Spine J 2(1):57–62

Bautch JC, Malone DG, Vailas AC et al 1997 Effects of exercise on knee joints with osteoarthritis: a pilot study of biologic markers. Arthritis Care Res 10(1):48–55

Beissner KL, Collins JE, Holmes H et al 2000 Muscle force and range of motion as predictors of function in older adults. Phys Ther 80(6):556–563

Bennett SE, Schenk RJ, Simmons ED et al 2002 Active range of motion utilized in the cervical spine to perform daily functional tasks. J Spinal Disord Tech 15(4):307–311

Booth FW, Chakravarthy MV, Manu V et al 2002 Exercise and gene expression: physiological regulation of the human genome through physical activity. J Physiol 543(part 2):399–411

Brandt KD 2003 Response of joint structures to inactivity and to reloading after immobilization. Arthritis Rheum 49(2):267–271

Carola R, Harley JR, Noback CR 1992 Human Anatomy and Physiology, 2nd edn. McGraw-Hill, New York

Colby LA, May BJ 1999 Therapeutic exercise in the home setting: a functional perspective. In: May BJ (ed) Home Health and Rehabilitation: Concepts of Care, 2nd edn. FA Davis, Philadelphia, PA

Digiovanna AG 1994 Human Aging: Biological Perspectives. McGraw-Hill, New York

Dunlop DD, Hughes SL, Edelman P et al 1998 Impact of joint impairment on disability-specific domains at four years. J Clin Epidemiol 51(12):1253–1261

Escalante A, Lichtenstein MJ, Dhanda R et al 1999a Determinants of hip and knee flexion range: results from the San Antonio Longitudinal Study of Aging. Arthritis Care Res 12(1):8–18

Escalante A, Lichtenstein MJ, Hazuda HP et al 1999b Determinants of shoulder and elbow flexion range: results from the San Antonio Longitudinal Study of Aging. Arthritis Care Res 12(4):277–286

Escalante A, Lichtenstein MJ, Hazuda HP et al 2001 Walking velocity in aged persons: its association with lower extremity joint range of motion. Arthritis Rheum 45(3):287–294

Hamerman D 1998 Biology of the aging joint. Clin Geriatr Med 14(3):417–433

Hewitt JD, Glisson RR, Guilak F et al 2002 The mechanical properties of the human hip capsule ligaments. J Arthroplasty 17(1):82–89

Iida T, Abumi K, Kotani Y et al 2002 Effects of aging and spinal degeneration on mechanical properties of lumbar supraspinous and interspinous ligaments. Spine J 2(2):95–100

Johnston RC, Smidt GL 1970 Hip motion measurements for selected activities of daily living. Clin Orthop Related Res 72:205–215

Laubenthal KN, Smidt GL, Kettelkamp DB 1972 A quantitative analysis of knee motion during activities of daily living. Phys Ther 52(1):34–43

Levangie PK, Norkin CC 2005 Joint Structure and Function: A Comprehensive Analysis. FA Davis, Philadelphia, PA

Magermans DJ, Chadwick EK, Veeger HE et al 2005 Requirements for upper extremity motions during activities of daily living. Clin Biomech 20(6):591–599

Norkin CC, White DJ 2003 Measurement of Joint Motion: A Guide to Goniometry, 3rd edn. FA Davis, Philadelphia, PA

Chapter 5

Aging and the central nervous system

Darcy A. Umphred and Rolando T. Lazaro

INTRODUCTION

Changes that occur in the central nervous system (CNS) with age can be discussed at a cellular level, a system level such as the size of a nuclear mass, a functional level such as the ability to stand up, or a social level in terms of the ability to interact and communicate. Identification of specific changes can be found throughout the research literature, including studies that show statistically significant differences when older people are compared with young adults. At the same time, these differences do not necessarily reflect functionally significant differences when the activities of daily living of healthy older adults are analyzed. Thus, discussing changes that occur with increasing age is a difficult task especially when differentiating healthy adults from those with chronic pathologies or significant acute diseases. Recent work investigating the changes in the CNS that occur as the individual ages suggests that neuroplasticity is a strong and significant driver in the variability of functional performance in these individuals (Gorman 2006, Umphred & El-Din 2006).

As humans age, their activity level changes and their choices of activities vary tremendously, as does their nutritional intake and general health. All these factors relate directly to the function of the CNS and to its ultimate control over the entire body. Genetic predisposition as well as environmental factors account for how the CNS acts and reacts in an aging individual. With aging, humans become more diverse rather than more homogeneous so it becomes difficult to compare one adult with another. There has been time in each life for many experiences – the accumulation of minor and major traumas, exposure to toxins, overuse and disuse of major body systems – all of which affect the functioning of the CNS. Therefore, difficulties arise when asking, 'What is expected with normal aging?'. Yet, when one looks specifically at the CNS, certain changes are observed with aging. These changes by themselves do not create disease, subsystem problems, functional limitations or limitations in life activities, but their cumulative effects may dramatically influence an aging adult's ability to compensate and relearn once a specific pathology or disease has created functional loss and a decrease in quality of life.

NERVOUS SYSTEM CHANGES WITH AGING

Recent studies have established that, in the brain, there is an age-related decrease in weight and gyral thickness with an increase in ventricular size. However, in the healthy aging human, there is no conclusive research showing that this is related to a decline in function (Guccione 2000). Evidence exists that changes in neurotransmitters occur with aging but again, this is not related to dysfunction in the healthy aging human (Guccione 2000). Loss of conduction velocity in sensory and motor nerves within the central and peripheral nervous systems as well as loss of myelin sheaths and the large myelinated fibers with advancing age have been reported (Bottomley & Lewis 2003). Although these losses might appear to explain a propensity for falling as a result of slower entry of sensory information into the system or delayed motor response time, a connection between a deficiency in one part of the system and the overall function of an individual has not been clearly proven. Further, it is not understood why some individuals can function well into very old age without severe functional loss whereas others cannot.

Sensory changes

Documented changes also occur in both the visual and auditory systems with aging. Visual acuity declines with age gradually until the sixth decade, then decreases rapidly in many individuals between the ages of 60 and 80. Traditional testing of acuity is valid for reading but not for functional tasks such as observing a step in a darkened room (Guccione 2000). For an individual to respond appropriately, it requires receiving an input, processing that input both perceptually and cognitively at an intellectual level or automatically at a motor level and, finally, selecting the motor response that best matches the environmental requirements. Thus, the client whose visual acuity is corrected with glasses for reading may be impaired when evaluated for motor function. An individual who wears bi- or trifocals and glances down for visually augmented feedback may see a distorted image, so inaccurate information is sent to the CNS. Thus, the motor response may be appropriate for the input being received but inappropriate for the actual environment. The nervous system functions on consensus and thus, if available, will always use other sensory systems and prior learning to determine whether to respond to visual information. Similarly, an individual with visual impairment may respond adequately to environmental demands and show no signs of motor limitation.

Hearing loss is also common among the elderly: the causes of such dysfunction are either peripheral or central deficits generally associated with disease. It is important for the therapist working with the geriatric patient to be aware of the client's hearing abilities before giving auditory cues. Whether the individual's auditory difficulty is caused by a peripheral conduction problem or an auditory processing problem plays a critical role in the selection of interventions and the methods of patient–clinician interaction. Although hearing loss itself does not lead to motor impairment, often, when the auditory portion of the eighth cranial nerve is involved, the vestibular portion is also affected. This potentially results in vertigo and balance impairments and increases an individual's risk of falling. Similarly, loss of auditory acuity means that an individual may have difficulty hearing or carrying on a normal conversation within a noisy environment. This variable may be a primary explanation for why an individual is isolated and chooses not to be part of group activities.

The processing of information in the cognitive and emotional areas of the CNS cannot be ignored when considering CNS changes with age, with or without pathology. Healthcare providers must remember that when the processing or the learning of cognitive materials becomes a problem, this avenue for assistance in motor learning may be lost. Without cognitive assistance, procedural learning of motor programs will become the only avenue to regain functional control over movement. The principles of motor learning then become paramount in optimizing the therapeutic environment for patient improvement (Gorman 2006).

Changes in the limbic system

The healthcare provider must also consider the emotional system in all patients, especially when looking at CNS function. Emotions are controlled and modified by the limbic system. This system has extensive connections to the hypothalamus, so emotion is often expressed through regulation of the autonomic nervous system as well as in the tone of the striated muscle system (Umphred et al 2006).

Hormone levels increase with stress and that the amount of hormones elicited increases with age (McEwen 2002). By virtue of advanced age, a patient may be very close to multiple-system failure. Such an individual would be considered frail. The hypothalamus regulates the areas of the brainstem that control the heart, lungs, internal organs and immune system (Umphred et al 2006).

Many behavioral syndromes have been attributed to this area of the brain. The most pertinent to the elderly was described by Hans Selye in 1956 and is called the general adaptive syndrome (GAS) (Umphred et al 2006). Today, it is considered a response to stress and it can be observed in any frail individual, such as a premature infant, an individual with severe CNS damage or an elderly individual with fragile bodily systems. The GAS response is paradoxical to the anticipated response. Under stress, an individual generally has a sympathetic response, with an increase in heart rate and blood pressure and a fight–flight reaction. In the GAS, the same environmental conditions initially cause a sympathetic response but, over time, and sometimes quickly, the individual switches to a parasympathetic reaction. Blood pressure drops, heart rate decreases, blood pools in the periphery and the level of consciousness can drop (Umphred et al 2006). The GAS is a survival response to stress because, without such a response, the increase in heart rate and blood pressure would cause heart failure or vascular rupture. Once an individual responds in such a paradoxical manner, treatment based on the signs and symptoms may be aimed at

increasing the sympathetic response, which, in this particular case, may cause an even greater paradoxical reaction.

A client may have recently developed a disease that adds stress to the already frail system. If the corresponding treatment is interpreted by the individual as creating more stress, it may result in a GAS, which has the potential of evolving into a life-threatening situation. The patient's response may be to withdraw, and the healthcare provider's reaction generally would be to increase the level of input in order to motivate or wake up the patient. In the GAS, the patient withdraws further and could potentially die from heart failure resulting from diminished heart rate and blood pressure. For that reason, the healthcare provider should evaluate the patient's emotional response to the environment and try to keep a homeostatic autonomic balance. This requires being sensitive to all the systems of the body: respiration, blood pressure and level of alertness as well as specific motor responses to interventions. All of these systems are ultimately under the control of the limbic system (Umphred et al 2006).

Changes in the motor system

The motor system, with the guidance of prior learning and experience as well as analysis by the CNS of current needs, modulates the state of the motor pools in the brainstem and spinal cord in order to drive peripheral nerves and orchestrate synergistic interactions of muscle groups to create functional behavior and mastery of the environment. Ultimate control of the end product called functional behavior is the result of the consensus of a variety of areas within the motor system. Understanding how this motor system regulates and controls movement is the key to identifying motor impairments and understanding why an individual exhibits functional limitations.

The areas typically considered to be part of the motor system are the premotor and motor areas of the frontal lobes, the basal ganglia, the cerebellum, the brainstem, the spinal cord and all the interneurons that link these systems together. The thalamus plays a key role as a relayer and modulator whereas the limbic or emotional system has the ability, directly and indirectly, to alter the state of motor responses (Kandel et al 2000). Obviously, the sensory areas also guide and alter existing motor programs. Where the motor system begins and ends is not clear because there are so many interdependent systems that loop between one area and another; therefore, a linear analysis is not appropriate. There is not one single area that controls motor output, yet certain areas, or nuclear masses, are responsible for specific aspects of motor function. When any one of these areas is diseased or injured, specific clinical symptoms manifest. Similarly, some motor components such as base tone in striated muscles are regulated by many areas, so a deficit does not automatically reflect the involvement of a specific area. The CNS is made up of many connected neuronal loops, so a deficit in one loop might present a clinical problem that would make it appear as if a nuclear mass or system were damaged. Advanced age is not a reason for CNS problems: disease and injury are. Thus, CNS motor changes that occur with aging do not necessarily indicate functional motor deficits (Bottomley & Lewis 2003).

Research does show that the motor system changes with age (Guccione 2000). For example, head-turning plays a greater role in electromyographic activity in synergistic upper- and lower-extremity muscle groups in an aging human brain than in a young individual. This suggests that the CNS no longer has the refined regulating ability over preprogrammed synergistic patterning that might be called a stereotypic or abnormal movement pattern. A child gains control over all preprogrammed movement patterns and refines that regulation; an older adult possible begins to lose some of the refinement. Whether this is because of disuse or aging is not clear. Again, it must be emphasized that these changes, although statistically significant, do not represent measurable functional changes. The significance of these changes may be more meaningful following injury or disease. If the aging CNS loses some of its plasticity or ability to adapt, then it may take more time to learn new programs or alter existing ones. This might explain why aging adults seem to exhibit synergistic patterns very quickly following injury, whereas younger adults may take more time to develop the same abnormal patterns.

If new learning is impossible, then the need to create an environment that optimizes old learning should be clearly identified and used in the therapeutic setting to achieve optimal functioning. However, it is important to consider current literature on learning and plasticity of the CNS, which states that new learning is possible, before deciding that adaptation of the environment is the best solution. The challenge with the elderly is that change can create confusion, stress and limit new learning, whereas novelty, motivation and repetitive practice will enhance the brain's ability to learn and respond appropriately to functional demands (Gorman 2006).

As a team, the patient, therapist and caregiver first need to identify outcomes relevant to the patient and the patient's functional desires. Second, practice of those functional activities is critical but variance within that environment is crucial in order to allow for correction of error within the movement itself. Maintenance of novelty to motivate attention and learning of the task is also important. For example, if the patient is reaching for something within a cabinet while standing at a sink, the exact standing position in relation to the sink will result in challenges to stability and, simultaneously, the level of reaching while standing will shift the center of gravity. Both of these factors can be used to create challenges to the task, vary the activity and specific muscle and joint range interactions and introduce novelty. Reaching for large, small or weighted objects, placing them from one shelf level to another or asking the patient to do additional activities such as washing their face, brushing their teeth, picking up soap and washing their hands are all variations on the original motor activities but allow the environment to change and the novelty to remain.

A complete explanation of the specifics of the motor control system (Shumway-Cook & Woollacott 2000, Schmidt & Lee 2005) is not within the scope of this chapter, but a brief overview of the system might help the reader to understand and appreciate the complexity of the system. The frontal lobe of the brain not only helps process the motivation to move (prefrontal) but also modulates or regulates information that travels between primary motor centers such as the basal ganglia and cerebellum (Kandel et al 2000). In addition, it plays a primary role in regulating fine motor function through the corticospinal and corticobulbar systems. Normal movement results from the coordinated work of multiple areas that influence the final common pathways of motor neurons.

The frontal lobe plays a primary but not a dictatorial role in the modulation of fine motor as well as gross motor behavior. After summating and modulating messages from other areas of the CNS, the frontal lobe sends messages concurrently to the basal ganglia and cerebellum (Kandel et al 2000). In turn, these centers formulate new motor plans or draw upon existing plans to correctly modulate the motor system. If either center or the loops connecting them is damaged or diseased, then motor function may neither be smooth, coordinated and effortless nor will it match the environmental context of the activity. The cerebellum, unlike the basal ganglia, is simultaneously aware of the peripheral kinematics through the input from proprioceptors in the limbs and trunk, and based on the position of the head in space as judged by the vestibular system. Similarly, the cerebellum is aware of existing states of the motor pool through a variety of ascending tracts that send that information directly to the anterior lobes of the cerebellum. For this reason, the cerebellum is considered a synergistic programmer and plays a key role in feed-forward movement or regulation of a movement activity over time.

The role of the cerebellum in high center regulation of motor programming certainly interfaces with the limbic system as well as the frontal lobe and basal ganglia (Melnick 2006a, 2006b, Umphred et al 2006). Deficits within the frontal lobe, limbic system or the basal ganglia can affect cerebellar function and have been shown to trigger what looks like cerebellar neuronal damage (Melnick 2006b). The cerebellum is not only responsible for helping to write new programs, it also makes sure that the programs being used at any one moment match the environmental context. The cerebellum will run that desired program until it is told to do something else. If there is a mismatch between the desired movement sequence and the environmental input stimuli, the cerebellum will try to readjust the synergistic patterns and run the program that matches the environmental demands. For example, if an individual is walking on a level cement surface and suddenly the surface changes because of a crack or a hole, the cerebellum will adjust balance strategies in order to regain homeostasis of the center of gravity, which allows the person to keep walking. If the crack or hole in the cement creates such a large pertubation that the cerebellum cannot correct the patterns being run, it will be up to consensus of the CNS to determine what new program should be initiated.

The basal ganglia are responsible for changing the plan of movement and initiating new programs, whereas the cerebellum, in preparation for the changes to take place, regulates the state of the motor generators (base tone) and controls the force, speed and direction of movement. For example, if an individual is rising to a standing position and goes beyond vertical and starts to fall, the basal ganglia change the motor setting from rising to vertical to falling. Both the basal ganglia and the cerebellum play roles in modulating posture but the specific roles are different. The basal ganglia and aspects of the cerebellum play key roles in the development of new motor programs and the refinement of existing ones. They relay specific motor programming to the frontal lobes by way of the thalamus, and they relay programming down through the brainstem to the motor generators of the cranial and spinal neurons. Therefore, changes in any of these structures or in the pathways between them that occur with aging could have critical effects on normal movement. The changes do not necessarily create identifiable alterations in motor performance but, along with other pathology, they could become cumulative, with the end result being loss of function. For example, a reported loss with age of Purkinje cells in the cerebellum has not been related to loss of function. However, this change along with cerebellar degeneration or a cerebellar stroke would be cumulative and the result might be a greater deficit than would occur in a younger individual without Purkinje cell loss who develops a similar medical pathology (Melnick 2006b).

In summary, research has shown changes in the anatomy and physiology of the brain with aging but has not shown that these changes affect function directly in the healthy elderly human. Pathology and disease are the causes of functional limitations. Thus, structural or anatomical changes due to aging do not necessarily correlate with functional loss. Similarly, lack of structural or anatomical changes does not necessarily reflect normal functional ability. The aging process may affect the potential of the nervous system to adapt with plasticity but age is only one factor that influences that potential. Aging should never be considered the primary cause of functional limitations or restriction of normal life activities (McEwen 2002, Bottomley & Lewis 2003).

MODELS OF REHABILITATION FOR THE ELDERLY

Utilizing a model to understand the relationship between the medical diagnosis, consequent abnormalities in body structure and function

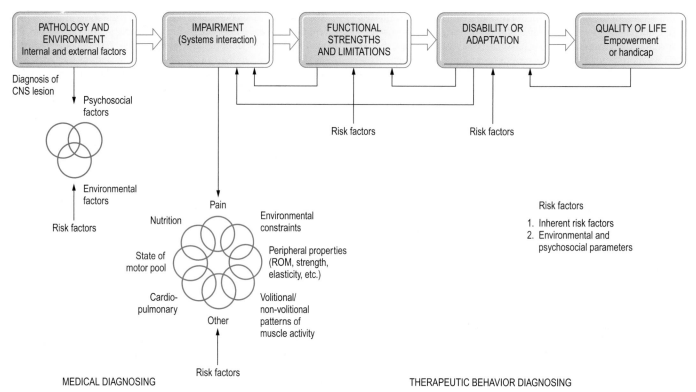

Figure 5.1   Behavioral model for evaluation and intervention of human movement performance. ROM, range of motion.

and their impact on an individual's physical and societal functioning facilitates the development of efficient and effective interventions. As physical therapy practice becomes more complicated, previously advocated rehabilitation models appear to be inadequate for capturing the best picture of this practice. The World Health Organization's (WHO) International Classification of Impairments, Disabilities and Handicaps (ICIDH) model (1980) and Nagi's model of Impairments/ Functional Limitations/Disability (1965) have been accepted and widely used for at least two decades. The Top/Down model was introduced during the last decade by James Gordon and the International Classification of Body Function and Structures, Activity and Participation (ICF) was introduced by the WHO in 2002. Each model has a place and a categorization system that can help the clinician organize and differentiate various system and subsystem problems that lead to limitations in function and quality of life (Gordon et al 2006).

Integration of the Nagi and ICIDH models

Therapists are expected to identify the specific components that have led to functional problems, predict how long it will take to correct or develop compensation for the problem and establish an intervention protocol that will allow the patient to become functional in the shortest time possible. This responsibility of differential diagnosis is closely interrelated with the concept of impairment/disability/handicap as described in the WHO model of 1980. The Nagi model follows the same conceptual process but uses impairments/ functional limitations/disability as the three-step sequence following disease or pathology. Figure 5.1 illustrates these models and shows that they do not proceed in a linear fashion.

Therapists first evaluate functional skills, both attainable and with limitations, by looking at daily living activities. What allows an individual to demonstrate normal functional skills are the interactions of many body systems and their abilities to function adequately to allow for a normal motor response to a specific task. A breakdown in

any part of one of these systems or subsystems can lead to functional limitations. These system or subsystem problems are considered to be impairments within an area and need to be addressed in order to regain function. Not all impairments lead to disabilities and often it is the sum of the impairments that create the greatest problems. Therapists need to evaluate how impairments are affecting movement and whether the central and/or peripheral systems have the potential to be corrected. This conclusion will guide the therapist in the direction of creating a learning environment that will give normal function back to the individual or teach the patient to compensate for the problem, which always leads to a change in motor control.

Top/Down model

The Top/Down model (Fig. 5.2) reverses the direction of clinical problem solving. It does not start with disease but rather with the larger roles a patient plays in life, and it continues with the specificity of physiological problems and potential for recovery. Once the roles are identified and it is confirmed that the patient still wants to participate in them, the therapist analyzes the functional skills necessary to maintain or resume those roles. These skills need bodily system resources, including physical, cognitive and emotional resources, to work together.

In this model, the last area of focus is termed recovery. This identifies the active and interactive physiological mechanisms necessary to support recovery and prevent future degrading of quality of life. This model focuses on the individual first before looking at pathology as a potential cause or explanation for the limitations in roles that a person wishes to maintain. The individual and those specific life roles identified as being important to that individual become the parameters that direct and set the specifications for the evaluation, movement science prognosis/diagnosis and the intervention strategies selected (Gordon et al 2006).

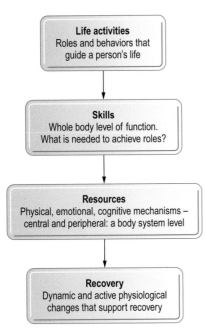

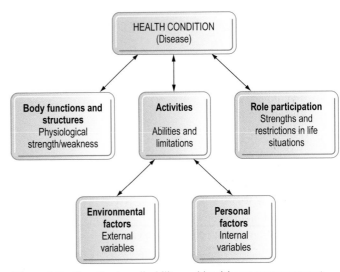

Figure 5.3   Functioning, disability and health: an empowerment model. Available: http://www.who.int/classification/icf.

Figure 5.2   Top/Down model: identification of parameters starting from life activities and ending with recovery intervention.

International Classification of Function (ICF) model

The ICF model is the second WHO model and was introduced to the international community in 2002. This model is considered to be an empowerment model and is based on the strengths of the individual. It replaces the previous disablement model (ICIDH), which identified the healthy individual from one who was disabled. This new model replaces the terminology of impairment, disability and handicapped with more positive words that define bodily functions and structures, activities and participation. It is hoped that the ICF model will replace the previous model throughout the world and will introduce a universal language for functioning, disability and health.

In this model, the identification of functional bodily systems and problems replaces the concept of impairment (Fig. 5.3). Activity is defined as those tasks, functional behaviors and activities of daily life that can be executed by the individual as well as those activities that are limited. Participation in life identifies the social or family engagements that the individual would choose to engage in, and the restrictions that limit the individual from engaging in those activities. Often therapists begin their examination at either an activity or life participation entry point. The patient presents with changes in normal activities and the desire to return to a better quality of life motivates the individual to participate in the rehabilitation process. Thus, the arrows within the figure can go in either direction. As the therapist examines the functional activities category, environmental and personal variables that may affect activity and function must be considered within the framework of the whole person (Gordon et al 2006). The goal is always to guide the patient to or toward the desired participation activities which will allow the quality of life that the person expects (Gorman 2006, Lazaro et al 2006, Umphred & El-Din 2006).

Summary of models

In the elderly, there exists the potential for problems in many systems and subsystems, such as joint changes resulting in a smaller range of motion, muscular weakness, lack of endurance resulting from disease or disuse, cardiac insufficiency, pulmonary dysfunction and central and peripheral nervous system impairments. Children and young adults can also have these problems, but the elderly have had many additional decades to traumatize their bodies, to compensate for earlier diseases and pathologies and to be exposed to environmental hazards that younger people have not. It is the interaction of all these systems and experiences within their respective lives that ultimately leads to functional limitations. Many impairments that occur within the motor system of aging adults originate within the CNS, whether or not the patient's acute problems are centrally driven.

THEORIES OF MOTOR LEARNING, MOTOR CONTROL AND NEUROPLASTICITY

Physical and occupational therapists are movement specialists who receive referrals regarding patients with movement problems that affect quality of life, including both activities of daily living and activities of life participation such as golf, hiking, swimming, playing card games, gardening, dancing, fishing, birdwatching or any other identified skill that is valued by the patient. Because of the complexity of the human organism, there are many systems and subsystems that interact to drive the observed motor behavior. There are three distinct categories that must be differentiated when analyzing motor behavior as an expression of CNS response to environmental demands or task-specific goals. These concepts are motor control, motor learning and neuroplasticity (Shumway-Cook & Woollacott 2000, Gorman 2006).

Motor control as a system includes components that are differentiated into biomechanical, musculoskeletal (power, strength and muscle elasticity) and central (state of the motor pool, availability of synergistic programming, postural integrity, balance, force, speed, trajectory and automatic versus anticipatory programming). All of these components interact and must be evaluated within the context of the environment in which the activity is occurring. That context will determine whether the CNS can adapt or must be accommodated by changes within the external environment. Movement should never be analyzed by considering only one variable such as the biomechanical, musculoskeletal or central basis. If only one part is considered to the exclusion of a large portion of the whole, the person

Box 5.1   Motor control components and system interactions: classification of system and subsystem impairments

Systems traditionally considered central

1. State of the motor pool
   Hypotonicity
   Hypertonicity
   Rigidity
   Tremor

2. Synergies (volitional or reflexive)
   Pattern of motor program
   Flexibility over programming

3. Postural integration
   Agonist/antagonist co-activation
   Automatic prolonged holding against gravity in all
      spatial positions

4. Balance
   Limits of stability
   Sensory integration of somatosensory, visual, vestibular
      inputs
   Interaction of ankle, hip, stepping strategies
   Interaction with postural function
   Interaction with task/environmental context

5. Speed of movement
   Ability to alter rate of movement throughout entire task
   Movement responses to speed demands

6. Timing
   Ability to start, stop and change a motor plan
   Interaction with environmental context
   Timing of muscle sequencing relationship to task

7. Reciprocal movements
   Ability to change direction
   Rotatory components present/absent
   Turnaround time/delay
   Smoothness of agonist/antagonist

8. Trajectory or pattern of movement
   Trajectory, velocity, acceleration curve
   Smoothness throughout range

9. Accuracy
   Placement of entire body or a component part at a
      specific point in space
   Changes with demand for speed, difficulty of task,
      direction, distance

10. Task content
    New versus old learning

11. Emotional influences
    Value placed on activity
    Differentiation of procedural and declarative learning
    Fear factor
    Motivation

12. Sensory organization
    Intact, deficient, compensation, conflict

13. Perception/cognition
    Interaction of sensory organization with perceptual
       processing
    Ability to use cognition to assist in motor learning
    Short, intermediate, long-term cognitive abilities

14. Hormonal and nutritional levels of consciousness
    Daily biorhythms and levels of alertness throughout day
    Drug and nutritional interactions on central and
       peripheral function

Systems traditionally considered peripheral or environmental

1. Range of motion
   Specific joint limitation
   Causation within joint structure

2. Muscle strength or power
   Muscle endurance
   Muscle power

3. Cardiac function
   Output
   Pacing
   Endurance
   Interaction with respiratory system

4. Respiratory function
   Input/output
   Exchange
   Interaction with cardiac system

5. Circulatory function
   Ability to supply muscles with foodstuffs, oxygen,
      minerals, etc
   Ability to eliminate waste

6. Other organ and system interactions
   Skin integrity and pliability
   Kidney, liver, intestinal function

7. Environmental context
   The specific task or functional activity
   Familiarity with existing task or environment (hospital
      versus home)

8. Endurance
   Differentiation of disuse from system failure or
      inefficiency

9. Psychosocial factors
   Family demands
   Ethnicity, cultural beliefs and stressors
   Past experiences and role identification
   Religious beliefs and their interaction with healthcare
      delivery
   Individual's belief in and acceptance of a healthcare
      system and its expectations

is forgotten. The end result of forgetting the patient will impact on both prognosis and treatment (Umphred et al 2006).

Movement is always a combination of interactions of all of the variables that determine the motor patterns observed. These patterns assist a therapist in determining whether the movement expressions are caused by degeneration due to age, disuse over time or disease. Box 5.1 illustrates the variables under motor control that are considered to originate within the nervous system and those that do not. Thus, motor control is the study of how an individual controls movement already acquired.

To understand the distinctions between a system or subsystem function and physiological mechanism problem (impairment) and a functional activity or limitation (disability), it is necessary to analyze how the various systems function together in the healthy elderly individual. For the most part, the human body has been provided with large physiological reserves within each system. Thus, a deficit in a portion of one system may have little or no effect on the whole organism because the reserves in other areas can substitute for small deficiencies.

It has been postulated that, with aging, many areas of physiological reserve may be close to a critical level of maximal adaptation. In this scenario, the whole organism functions normally, using all its capability to adapt and learn until the occurrence of an acute problem in one area. Similar to a domino or cascading effect, one small problem forces the entire motor system beyond its capability to adapt or learn and the end result is loss of function in specific activities affected by the given pathology or disease. Established motor control mechanisms become insufficient to run smoothly and adequately for motor expression of the entire system. In some instances, there can be improvement within systems or subsystems as a result of impairment training, functional training and environmental manipulations. Healing or establishment of homeostasis can also result from medication, surgery and the body's response to disease, as well as therapeutic interventions that enhance system and subsystem function. This is especially true if some reserve is still available and the patient is motivated to learn and regain function.

If the clinician correctly relates specific impairments to certain functional movement problems and creates an optimal environment for relearning, then even with depleted reserves, function often can be improved (Rossini & Dai 2004). In other instances, the therapist cannot change the impairment but can find an alternative way for the patient to use intact systems to perform the desired function. For example, an aging individual who chooses to become more sedentary over time may no longer need to keep his or her vestibular system at a high level of sensitivity. The lack of movement may lead to some joint limitation in the ankles and hips, which may decrease the limits of stability of balance and increase a fear of falling. As the individual ages, his or her visual system may also become compromised. None of these minor impairments necessarily leads to balance dysfunction or to falls. If, however, this same person then suffers a vascular insult with acute residual motor impairments, the additional preexisting impairments become compounded and interact with the new problem.

Motor learning is the study of how an individual acquires, modifies and retains motor memory patterns so that programs can be used, reused and modified during functional activities. The critical elements of motor learning deal with the stages of learning, the practice context that optimizes the learning, the practice schedule used and the reinforcement strategies employed to optimize that learning (Shumway-Cook & Woollacott 2000, Schmidt & Lee 2005).

Neuroplasticity can be defined as the brain's ability to adapt and use cellular adaptations to learn or relearn functions previously lost because of cellular death caused by trauma or disease at any age. These changes occur in response to a variety of both external and internal demands placed upon the CNS. In reality, neuroplasticity occurs throughout life and does not stop once an individual reaches old age. The CNS internally adapts to occurrences in life whether they result from normal changes or from chronic disease, trauma, metabolic imbalances, dietary or external demands.

Until the more recent scientific discoveries regarding neuroplasticity, the medical and research environments believed that, once a neuron was damaged or died, the only mechanism able to replace the function of that specific cell was adaptation of other neurons, and that adaptation ultimately leads to a decrease in the function of the CNS. As observant clinicians, therapists have recognized that patients learn after trauma and that, just because someone is elderly and suffers a stroke, the potential for learning cannot be determined through a medical protocol. Neuroplasticity has shown that change and cellular growth can occur, especially when the external and internal environment nurtures that change and the activity has some novelty (Ito et al 2005, Gorman 2006). Motivation of the individual, environmental tasks that allow the motor functions of the CNS to succeed and optimizing the potential change by focusing and integrating aspects of motor learning create the best environment to encourage neuroplasticity (Umphred et al 2006). As clinicians, educators and researchers, the authors have always believed that, 'If a motor behavior looked right to us or other people, was easy and enjoyable for the patient; then somehow the intervention was creating change in the direction of normality and functional recovery no matter the theory'. Neuroplasticity has given the basic science efficacy to that statement.

SYSTEM INTERACTIONS AND REHABILITATION

It is the total interaction of all systems that the therapist must consider when establishing goals with a patient. Some systems that have changed over a long period of time will probably not readapt quickly, such as joint contractures. If range of motion is regained but power is not available, then function is not regained, and the therapist has just shifted to a new impairment.

Some systems that have changed may no longer have the ability to adapt. Vision is a good example of this phenomenon. Still others, for example the CNS, may have undergone both chronic and acute injury such as disuse prior to a stroke. The therapist will have to determine through an assessment process which systems are trying to compensate for the systems with deficits, thus not showing the dysfunction themselves, and which systems are permanently damaged and no longer have the ability to compensate and learn.

Loss of primary sensory input from peripheral damage and diminution of that sensory information on the primary somatosensory parietal receiving lobes is more devastating to the nervous system than loss of associative areas, which can be replaced by other areas (Kandel et al 2000). The difficulty therapists have with assessment is determining whether the primary system is nonfunctional or whether the amount of incoming sensory information is not at a level at which awareness is recognized. This same phenomenon exists within the motor system. If a system is overpowered by the tone of another system, the initial behavior will be masked. For example, if an individual suffers a stroke and has residual hypotonia within the involved upper extremity, the natural inclination of a therapist is to try to increase proximal tone for better stabilization. But, if the tone is increased without functional control of fluid and relaxed movement patterns, the tone is often asymmetrical and hypertonic. This increase of proximal tone through the ventral, medial and lateral descending tracts often overpowers the descending corticospinal tract and, thus, hand function is minimal if present.

If the visual system is deficient and compensation is not available, increasing awareness of the vestibular and somatosensory systems

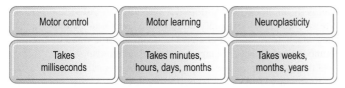

Figure 5.4   Time variables for motor control, motor learning and neuroplasticity.

will allow for retention of motor programs for balance. If this specific training is not a focus, then balance impairments and a potential for future falls exist. Disuse, fear of falling or falling itself can lead to a functional limitation and a decrease in participation in most social activities (Umphred & El-Din 2006). Although disuse and muscle weakness, affective fear and reinforced fear following a fall are not permanently damaged physiological mechanisms, they can certainly lead to chronic motor problems.

The acute physiological reason for a fall, such as a stroke, heart attack or acute hypotension, needs to be addressed by a medical team. The prognosis of impairments resulting from disuse or fear can be integrated into intervention for the acute CNS damage (Chen et al 2005). All three (visual, vestibular and somatosensory) impairments individually and collectively alter balance and the end result is a high risk of falls and future impairments from a fall. The physiological category of impairment is balance; the specific impairments fall under musculoskeletal and central mechanisms of motor and limbic systems. If sensory deprivation in any one or more of the sensory systems responsible for balance is also affected, that system is also considered a deficit in a physiological mechanism. Central impairments may include state of the motor pool, synergistic patterning, postural control, perceptual distortion of position in space, anxiety or other systems that work for consensus when controlling movement. Each mechanism can be evaluated as it is identified and quantitatively measured. The number and magnitude of impairments will determine prognosis and clearly direct the therapist toward intervention strategies that will guide the patient toward desired functional outcomes.

The therapist can determine whether motor control, motor learning or neuroplasticity is the primary mode used by the patient's CNS. Figure 5.4 indicates the time variable for each of these potential areas of CNS response. Spontaneous control following intervention suggests that the therapist has created an environment within which the patient can control responses. Thus, future interventions need to broaden the variability of that environment to facilitate variability in control and learning. If the patient progresses slowly following each treatment session, the therapist may be assisting in correcting physiological impairments and/or encouraging motor learning. Given this as a prognosis, more time will be needed and determination of the stage of motor learning is important in order to optimize the learning. If the progress of the patient is very slow but continuous and over a long period of time and the patient still exhibits flexibility in learning and control, neuroplasticity has probably occurred.

When the therapist introduces an activity and motor learning becomes necessary, the specific stage of learning must be identified: acquisition, refinement or retention. Stage one, acquisition, requires extra reinforcement, which can be internally driven through normal inherent sensory feedback systems or externally driven through augmented feedback from someone else. As the individual increases their skill in the activity, less feedback is necessary and internal self-correction should become more observable. Similarly, the type of practice schedule selected by the therapist can range from mass practice (daily and structured) to distributed (scheduled by the therapist or patient with larger gaps between treatment) or random (part of an activity of daily living) practice. Acquisition of a skill requires mass practice whereas retention depends more on random practice (Shumway-Cook & Woollacott 2000, Schmidt & Lee 2005, Gorman 2006).

When the therapist introduces the activity, another concept must be considered. The task itself will determine whether it will be practiced as a cohesive activity, taught in separate parts and then put together as a whole, or taught as a progressive sequence of parts. This is the practice context. Simple and discrete tasks like standing from a chair are more easily taught as whole activities, whereas a complex skill is generally learned best as an activity that is broken into parts and then reassembled as a whole. Intermediate skills and serial tasks are often best learned progressively.

Much of the research from a decade ago regarding aging, changes within the nervous system and motor control identified that, as humans age, they lose cognitive function, memory and motor skills. These results, which were statistically significant from a research perspective, did not necessarily prove significant when functional behaviors such as sit to stand, eating using utensils and standing balance were analyzed. It has become evident that, as an individual ages, changes occur within the CNS. Whether they progress to functional loss or to neuroplasticity has more to do with the novelty of the task (Ito et al 2005), the motivation of the learner (Umphred et al 2006), the environmental variables and the state (i.e. healthy or not) of the components of the body.

Current research suggests that changes in function are almost always related to disease or pathology. However, disuse is another variable that drives decline. Thus, elderly people who have the good fortune of maintaining their health, who stay physically and mentally active, who participate in life activities and engage in new, novel learning should not show functionally significant changes in motor behavior. The brain will engage in neuroplasticity under normal healthy environments when cellular change is occurring. It will also engage in reorganizing, restructuring and reconnecting neuronal activity between and within nuclei whenever possible. Variables that help to nurture that plasticity and learning are motivation, attention to the task, maintenance of metabolic health, ability to successfully use multiple sensory input systems as part of maintaining and relearning motor function, and challenging the CNS both physically and mentally on a consistent level. Thus, declines in motor skills, executive functioning and memory may be better correlated with a long pattern of disuse over decades rather than chronological age. Elderly individuals show declines in many abilities but the causes of those declines are multifactorial and should not be labeled as 'aging' (Rossini & Dai 2004).

CLINICAL EXAMPLES

In many instances, improvement of impairments, such as those involved in range of motion, muscle power or balance, can be achieved through therapeutic activities. If the therapist correctly relates the subsystem or physiological mechanisms that are affected to specific functional activities valued by the patient, both the subsystem mechanisms as well as the functional activity skill will improve, giving the patient a better quality of life. In other instances, the therapist cannot change the impairment problem but can find an alternative that allows the patient to compensate and use intact systems to perform the desired function, again giving the individual more control and greater opportunities to participate in life.

In the first scenario, the patient has a high probability of going beyond skill acquisition through refinement and may even retain and carry the skill learned into other functional activities. In the second scenario, compensation is being taught and thus the skill learned is activity-specific and may have little carryover to other functional behaviors. Given the plasticity of the CNS, there is usually untapped potential within the client and empowering that person with hope will play a key role in unlocking the limbic aspect of neuroplasticity. As soon as hope is taken away, the CNS loses its drive to change and thus the likelihood of any neuroplasticity developing is low.

An example of the first instance is Mr Smith, who recently had a cerebrovascular accident (CVA) with residual motor problems in both his right upper and lower extremities. The therapist worked with him, putting him into postures and situations or activities involving sitting, which demanded that his trunk and hip muscles respond with balance and weight shifting. These responses activated existing neurological mechanisms to regain power, strength, balance and range that might have been lost because of hospitalization or disuse at home. The therapist also used a partial body weight support system to allow the patient to practice walking and meet the need for normal power in walking, posture and co-activation during walking. Initially, the therapist placed the patient's right foot on each step but within two weeks the patient was able to bring the right foot through during the swing phase of gait and walk short distances using a quad cane. The CNS was learning to regain and control all the mechanisms necessary for normal ambulation without compensatory gait patterns. Motor learning was occurring because, although it had taken weeks, it was progressively improving over time. The patient, through whole–part learning, was able to stand–pivot–transfer from bed to chair to toilet to shower to chair independently before leaving rehabilitation. Although the patient had motor control over the upper extremities, his power was poor. Initially, the therapist supported the shoulder during reaching and hand-to-mouth activities in order to prevent the development of an abnormal shoulder pattern. The patient practiced effortless reaching with his shoulder supported over a ball, again to reduce the need for power while encouraging functional arm movement with controlled hand dexterity.

Once it was determined that Mr Smith had hand and arm function, the therapist, with consent from the patient, encouraged him to only use his right limb. This might be considered constraint-induced therapy but the patient was volitionally making the decision, which encouraged emotional buy-in and increased the possibility of neuroplasticity. Although he was discharged from the rehabilitation program, he came back in for a follow-up visit 6 months later. At that time, his right upper extremity function was still not normal but he could use his hand to write his name and the entire extremity to assist in any upper extremity functional activity of his choice. This follow-up improvement probably resulted from neuroplasticity within the CNS. Along with the trauma from the CVA, Mr Smith drove that change.

As a clinician, whether the change was due to learning, spontaneous return or neuroplasticity is irrelevant. Both the therapist and the patient's goals are functional recovery and, as long as that was the outcome, the exact neuromechanism seems unimportant. It is up to researchers to help determine how the CNS adapts and changes so that future therapeutic programs can be more effective and efficacious. In this example, it is important for the therapist to identify by early testing what previously learned motor programs are intact within the neuromusculoskeletal loop systems. Initially, that determination may be made by eliciting responses or guiding movement and feeling the programs as they come in to assist in a functional movement. If alternative loops or synaptic sensitivities exist, recovery potential is high and the prognosis is good, as long as the treatments are consistent with appropriate environmental contexts, practice scheduling, practice context and the goals and expectations of the patient.

The second scenario involves Mrs Jones, an elderly client with a recent amputation following prolonged diabetic instability and eventual gangrene. The therapist was never going to change the physiological mechanism that was the cause of limb amputation or

the medical condition of diabetes. The amputation had, by itself, altered the state of the CNS. The sensory system had changed, as had the posture, balance and motor programming needed to ambulate with a prosthetic device. The inherent sensory feedback necessary to create new programs had to be evaluated. The sensory physiological mechanisms may have been progressively deteriorating because of the diabetes. However, if new learning could occur and new programs written, this elderly individual might be able to run the programs, even with progressive sensory deterioration. Thus, the therapist had to work with the patient in using a prosthesis to regain normal gait programming. Strengthening the residual limb muscles would not necessarily translate into a smooth and normal gait using a prosthesis.

To match the context of the environment with the task, the programming necessary and the patient-specific impairment, the therapist wanted to work on standing and walking. Additional considerations such as skin integrity, pain and range of motion had to be interfaced with the practice environment. The therapist was potentially optimizing the environment for early and maximal function. Knowing that the gait training would be considered a new learning situation allowed the therapist to guard for error while the patient walked.

The old programs for walking that were learned by the client as a small child and practiced for decades would function with the remaining muscle groups but not as a total program that encompassed the prosthesis. In this situation, the therapist wanted the patient to concentrate on the task at first to bring in somatosensory awareness and sensory–motor planning. Once the patient demonstrated that the program was present, the therapist needed to distract the patient's attention on the walking motor activity and allow the motor system to practice running the program. In order for the client to be truly successful in this new variation of ambulation, she had to practice it as a feed-forward automatic task. At first, the practice had to be performed on a mass-practice level before, finally, it was performed as an activity of daily living, in which walking was part of life and practiced on a random schedule. As Mrs Jones began to regain her participation in life, with walking as an expected outcome, she started to challenge herself in many environments, which further increased her ability to adapt and change. Varying the lighting or surface, or distracting with conversation, are examples of challenges a therapist might use and eventually recommend to a caregiver.

Gait is a preprogrammed pattern that develops variability in relationship to different contexts, so practicing the gait pattern as a whole would be the context of choice. In this example, the therapist has created an environment that has changed the CNS, even though the original physiological mechanism that was damaged was not centrally induced.

CONCLUSION

The CNS is a complex conglomerate of nuclear masses that communicates with all bodily systems and expresses thoughts, feeling and desires to the world through motor behavior. This function, or the goals it represents, does not change with advancing age, nor does a specific age imply that the CNS is no longer functioning adequately or normally or that it has a diminished ability to adapt and learn. Yet, through life's experiences, age itself does potentially affect all bodily functions, including that of the nervous system. Life's physical traumas, habits and environmental stressors can all become additive and cause slow progressive deterioration of one or all of the body's anatomical systems over time. One system, the CNS, has the capability to adapt and change depending upon internal and external environmental demands. This plasticity is dependent upon other systems for oxygen, nutritional demands, or delivery of both substances and removal of waste. It is also dependent upon homeostasis of a large number of neurochemicals, intracranial pressure and healthy communication between and within the internal and external environments. Change and novelty can create neuroplasticity. On the other hand, change and novelty, when beyond the systems' capabilities to adapt, can cause functional motor problems. The nervous system adapts more easily when change occurs slowly. Unfortunately, many geriatric patients suffer a variety of CNS trauma or pathologies that dramatically affect functional movement. Whether these problems cause specific impairments, functional limitations or decrease the person's participation in life are often client-specific and directly correlate more with the disease than the specific age. Therapists should evaluate the interactions of the various physiological mechanisms or impairments and relate them to functional behavior in order to identify the intervention protocols that will lead to optimal performance in the shortest time frame. Application and generation of knowledge regarding motor control, motor learning and neuroplasticity play key roles in the effectiveness of a clinician and ultimately the quality of life of the individuals who are recipients of clinical services.

References

Bottomley JM, Lewis CL 2003 Geriatric Physical Therapy: A Clinical Approach, 2nd edn. Prentice Hall, Englewood Cliffs, NJ

Chen KM, Chen WT, Wang JJ et al 2005 Frail elders' views of Tai Chi. J Nurs Res 13(1):11–20

Gordon J, Hodges P, Jette AM 2006 Models for neurological rehabilitation. III STEP: Symposium on Translating Evidence into Practice. July 15–21, 2005, Salt Lake City, Utah. APTA, Alexandria, VA

Gorman SL 2006 Contemporary issues and theories of motor control/motor learning and neuroplasticity: assessment of movement and posture. In: Umphred DA (ed.) Neurological Rehabilitation, 5th edn. Elsevier, St Louis, MO

Guccione AA (ed) 2000 Geriatric Physical Therapy, 2nd edn. Elsevier, Philadelphia, PA

Ito M, Fukuda M, Suto T et al 2005 Increased and decreased cortical reactivation in novelty seeking and persistence: a multichannel near-infrared spectroscopy in health subjects. Neuropsychobiology 52(1):45–54

Kandel ER, Schwartz JH, Jessell TM 2000 Principles of Neural Science, 4th edn. Elsevier, New York

Lazaro RT, Roller ML, Umphred DA 2006 Differential diagnosis phase 2: examination and evaluation of functional movement activities and system/subsystem impairments. In: Umphred DA (ed.) Neurological Rehabilitation, 5th edn. Elsevier, St. Louis, MO

McEwen BS 2002 Sex, stress and the hippocampus: allostasis, allostatic load and the aging process. Neurobiol Aging 23(5):921–939

Melnick ME 2006a Metabolic, hereditary, and genetic disorders in adults with basal ganglia movement disorders. In: Umphred DA (ed.) Neurological Rehabilitation, 5th edn. Elsevier, St Louis, MO

Melnick ME 2006b Clients with cerebellar dysfunction. Movement dysfunction associated with cerebellar problems. In: Umphred DA (ed.) Neurological Rehabilitation, 5th edn. Elsevier, St. Louis, MO

Rossini PM, Dai FG 2004 Integration technology for evaluation of brain function and neural plasticity. Phys Med Rehabil Clin North Am 15(1):263–306

Schmidt RA, Lee TD 2005 Motor Control and Learning: A Behavioral Emphasis, 4th edn. Human Kinetics Books, Champaign, IL

Shumway-Cook A, Woollacott MH 2000 Motor Control: Theory and Practical Application. Williams & Wilkins, Philadelphia, PA

Umphred DA, Hall M, West TM 2006 Limbic system: influence over motor control, and learning. In: Umphred DA (ed.) Neurological Rehabilitation, 5th edn. Elsevier, St. Louis, MO

Umphred DA, El-Din D 2007 Theoretical foundations (2006) for clinical practice. In: Umphred DA (ed.) Neurological Rehabilitation, 5th edn. Elsevier, St. Louis, MO

Chapter **6**

Cardiac considerations in the older patient

Meryl Cohen

INTRODUCTION

The determination of health and wellness among young individuals is relative, varying from person to person. Similarly, the effects of an aging cardiovascular system vary among the elderly. There is controversy in the literature regarding the application of a single model to the influence of aging on heart function. Structural changes that occur with aging are more consistent and more easily identifiable than physiological changes. The latter findings are difficult to distinguish for several reasons, including the interrelatedness of dynamic variables contributing to myocardial performance, the pathophysiology and symptomatology of heart disease, and the concept of hypokinesis in American society, of which the older person is considered to be partly entitled (Lakatta 1993, Susic 1997). In addition, comparisons between studies are limited because of measurement inconsistencies and varying definitions of 'elderly' and 'heart disease'. Many of the pioneering studies of the 1950s and 1960s continue to be reproduced, using new definitions of 'old' and paying more deliberate attention to the presence of heart disease in study populations.

Nevertheless, there is a general consensus regarding the effects of aging on several factors that influence cardiac performance. These factors have been studied in older individuals who are healthy and in those with heart disease, both at rest and during various levels of exertion. This chapter presents these findings as a model of declining cardiac performance with increasing age. Comparisons are made to the baseline 'young' model in an attempt to define a 'healthy older' model. The unique influences of exercise and disease on this model are then discussed, with emphasis on the clinical implications of these physiological changes.

CARDIOVASCULAR STRUCTURE

Age-related changes in cardiovascular tissue can be found in cardiac contractile fibers, conducting tissue and valvular structure (Lakatta & Levy 2003a). Although the actual number of myocytes decreases, the myocyte volume per nucleus increases in both ventricles. Commonly, the coronary microvasculature is unable to accommodate this increase in tissue volume, which raises the likelihood of myocardial ischemia. In addition, there is an increase in nondistensible fibrous tissue and an accumulation of senile amyloid deposits (see Box 6.1). In the elderly, the loss of pacemaker cells (sinoatrial node tissue) and the increase in fibrous tissue in conducting pathways combine to increase the risk of cardiac arrhythmias.

Box 6.1 Age-related changes in cardiovascular tissue

Cardiac

- ↓ Number of myocytes (myofibrils and pacemaker cells)
- ↑ Size of myocytes (myocellular hypertrophy)
- ↑ Lipid deposition in myocytes
- ↑ Lipofuscin deposition in myocytes
- ↓ Mitochondrial oxidative phosphorylation
- ↑ Amyloid deposition in the heart
- ↓ Rate of protein synthesis in internodal tracts
- ↑ Fibrosis and calcification of valves (especially the mitral annulus and aortic valve)

Vascular

- ↑ Endothelial cell heterogeneity (size, shape, axial orientation)
- ↑ Nondistensible collagen, fibrous tissues and calcium in media
- ↑ Thickness of smooth muscle cells in media
- ↓ Release of nitric oxide by coronary endothelium

↑, Increased; ↓, decreased.

Table 6.1 Age-related cardiovascular responses to exercise

Response	Effects of aging	After exercise training
Resting		
Oxygen consumption	↔	↔
Heart rate	↔	↔
Stroke volume	↔	↔
Arteriovenous oxygen difference	↑	?
Submaximal exercise		
Oxygen consumption	↔	
Heart rate	↔	↓
Stroke volume	↔	?
Arteriovenous oxygen difference	↑	?
Maximal exercise		
Oxygen consumption	↓	↑
Heart rate	↓	↔
Stroke volume	↓ or ↑	↑
Arteriovenous oxygen difference	↓ or ↔	↑ or ↔
Cardiac output	↔ (?) or ↑	↔

Reprinted from Protas E 1993 Physiological change and adaptation to exercise in the older adult. In: Guccione A (ed) Foundation of Geriatric Physical Therapy, 2nd edn. Mosby, St Louis, MO, with permission from Elsevier. ↑, Increased; ↓, decreased; ↔, no change; ?, insufficient data on elderly subjects.

resting heart rate, but they do typically decrease the maximal heart rate after exercise (Fleg et al 1994).

CO is maintained in the older individual if the SV is able to increase and compensate for any blunted HR response. This is the case if the individual remains physically fit, but usually the resting and submaximal CO tend to decrease with age because of a decrease in SV. This reduction in SV may occur as a result of alterations in a number of variables (see Box 6.2).

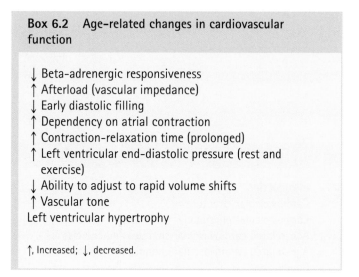

Box 6.2 Age-related changes in cardiovascular function

↓ Beta-adrenergic responsiveness
↑ Afterload (vascular impedance)
↓ Early diastolic filling
↑ Dependency on atrial contraction
↑ Contraction–relaxation time (prolonged)
↑ Left ventricular end-diastolic pressure (rest and exercise)
↓ Ability to adjust to rapid volume shifts
↑ Vascular tone
Left ventricular hypertrophy

↑, Increased; ↓, decreased.

Simultaneous age-related changes occur in coronary arteries and systemic vasculature. These changes tend to increase the stiffness of the vessel walls (see Table 6.1, Fig. 6.1) (Priebe 2000). Typically, proximal segments of the arteries change first, and the left coronary artery changes before the right. Together, the locations of the changes and the increased vessel rigidity cause an increase in peripheral vascular resistance. The heart attempts to adapt to this increased afterload (see discussion below) with myocellular hypertrophy, which probably accounts for the increase in myocyte volume previously mentioned. Alterations found in endothelial cells lining the arterial lumen cause a decrease in laminar blood flow, possibly establishing sites for lipid deposition, and further increase cardiac afterload. In addition, decreased nitric oxide release from the coronary endothelium further reduces vasodilator capacity in the older individual (Susic 1997, Lakatta & Levy 2003b).

CARDIOVASCULAR PHYSIOLOGY

The purpose of the heart is to pump blood rich with oxygen to body tissues. The ability of the heart to do this work efficiently is closely affected by three other systems: the lungs, the vasculature and the blood. Age- or disease-related changes occurring in these systems will directly affect cardiac function (see related Chapters 7, 9 and 13).

Cardiac output (CO), or the volume of blood pumped to body tissues each minute, depends on the frequency of cardiac contractions (heart rate, HR) and the volume of blood ejected with each contraction (stroke volume, SV). HR can be influenced by many external factors; however, intrinsically, the HR depends on pacemaker tissue function and autonomic nervous system stimulation. In addition to the loss of pacemaker cells in older people, there is also a decreased sensitivity to beta-adrenergic stimulation (see Box 6.2). These two age-associated changes in heart rate control may or may not affect the

SV is influenced by ventricular filling (preload), ventricular contractility and peripheral vascular resistance (afterload). Ventricular filling occurs early during diastole and is rapid and mostly passive, with the last part of filling attributed to atrial contractions. However, with aging, a prolonged contraction–relaxation time and decreased myocardial compliance (because of the increase in nondistensible fibrous tissue) cause a greater dependency on slower, active atrial contraction for the majority of diastolic filling (see Fig. 6.2).

Myocardial contractility is directly affected by sympathetic nervous system stimulation, specifically, beta-adrenergic receptors. Older individuals are less responsive to catecholamine stimulation, which results in a blunted inotropic response. In addition, if diastolic filling volumes are inadequate, contractile tension can be diminished, as a consequence of the Frank–Starling law of the heart, which states that the *energy of contraction is proportional to the initial length of the cardiac muscle fiber.*

The final component of SV determination is cardiac afterload (opposition to left ventricular ejection). As discussed above, afterload increases with aging because of increased vascular rigidity. Vascular stiffness is a result not only of loss of elastic elements but also of decreased responsiveness to catecholamine stimulation, which enables prolonged vasoconstriction.

It is important to note that, in the aging heart's attempt to maintain CO, the consequent left ventricular hypertrophy can account for the onset of myocardial ischemia independently of coronary atherosclerosis (see Fig. 6.3). On a purely physiological basis, several factors may contribute to the older heart's increased predisposition to developing ischemia:

● a disproportionate increase in myocyte size relative to the available circulation, resulting in a demand by tissues for more oxygen than the blood can supply;

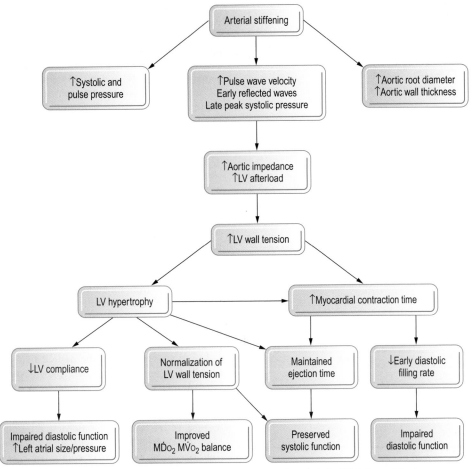

Figure 6.1 Cardiac adjustments to arterial stiffening during aging. L, left; LV, left ventricular. MḊo₂, myocardial oxygen supply; MV̇o₂, myocardial oxygen demand.
(Reproduced with permission from Priebe HJ 2000. © The Board of Management and Trustees of the British Journal of Anaesthesia. Reproduced by permission of Oxford University Press/British Journal of Anaesthesia.)

- an inability of aging coronary vessels to dilate because of increasing stiffness and prolonged sympathetic-mediated vasoconstriction, resulting in an inadequate blood supply for cardiac demand;

- the prolonged time for ventricular relaxation, which utilizes more energy and oxygen than a rapid relaxation period, thus creating a supply–demand imbalance;

- myocardial ischemia caused by any of these physiological processes of aging, which further decreases myocardial compliance and worsens ischemia, ventricular filling and, finally, systolic function, *potentially resulting in heart failure.*

AGE-RELATED CARDIOVASCULAR CHANGES AND EXERCISE

The decline in cardiac performance that occurs with aging reduces cardiac reserves. The healthy older individual is less able to accommodate to the added stress of exertion and fatigues more easily than the healthy younger individual with comparable workloads. Maximal oxygen consumption [$V_{O_2(max)}$], a measure of total body oxygen intake at exhaustion and an index of overall cardiovascular and pulmonary fitness, tends to decrease with aging (Dehn & Bruce 1972,

Schulman et al 1996). Oxygen consumption (V_{O_2}) can be expressed by the following formula (the Fick equation):

$$V_{O_2} = CO \times (a - v)_{O_2}; \text{ or}$$

Oxygen consumption = cardiac output × arteriovenous oxygen difference

The decline in $V_{O_2(max)}$ may be partially attributed to a decrease in CO. The age-related decrease in skeletal muscle mass and consequent decrease in oxygen extraction may also contribute to the decrease in $V_{O_2(max)}$ (see Table 6.1).

Elderly individuals who exercise regularly and maintain an active lifestyle show less of a decrease in $V_{O_2(max)}$ and may be able to reverse a number of age-associated changes in cardiovascular function (see Table 6.1). In general, daily light to moderate aerobic-type activities may be adequate to achieve cardiovascular benefit. It is of interest to note that many of the benefits of exercise training enjoyed by older people are similar to those found in the younger population. For example, compared with sedentary elderly individuals, older individuals who are exercise-conditioned tend to have a lower resting HR and blood pressure, improved diastolic function, lower peripheral vascular resistance and improved peripheral oxygen utilization. In addition, 'trained' elderly individuals demonstrate lower

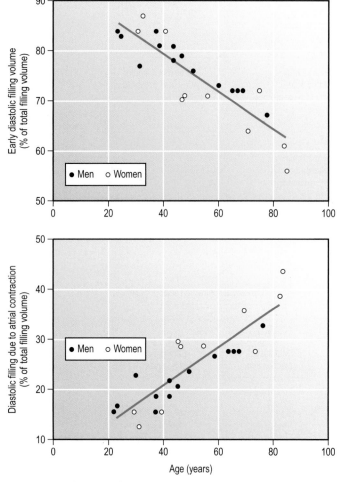

Figure 6.2 Age-associated decrease in early diastolic filling rate is compensated for by an increase in filling due to atrial contraction. (Reprinted from Swinne CJ et al 1992, with permission from Excerpta Medica.)

rates of myocardial infarction, heart failure and overall morbidity and mortality because of disease. Strength training also contributes to improved endurance and efficiency in daily activities (Nied & Franklin 2002). As long as it is medically safe, both high resistance/low repetition and low resistance/high repetition training can contribute to improved cardiovascular health.

AGE-RELATED CARDIOVASCULAR CHANGES AND DISEASE

Advancing age is associated with increased morbidity. More than 50% of all individuals over 60 years of age have heart disease. The combination of age-related changes in the cardiovascular system and the impact of heart disease on cardiac performance makes physiological responses during rest and exercise difficult to anticipate. Isolation of the effects of aging on the heart is inconclusive in the presence of heart disease. For example, myocardial scarring caused by the chronic ischemia of coronary artery disease decreases ventricular

compliance and slows ventricular filling, eventually promoting diastolic dysfunction. As discussed previously, the senescent heart also exhibits increased myocardial wall stiffness, which slows ventricular filling and can similarly lead to diastolic dysfunction. Diastolic dysfunction is the primary cause of heart failure in elderly patients (Gardin et al 1998). More than 50% of patients older than 80 years who have heart failure have 'normal' systolic function. Table 6.2 lists additional examples of the clinical consequences of age-related cardiovascular changes, some of which cannot be distinguished from preexisting disease. Clinical measures that may assist the practitioner in recognizing these changes are also listed in Table 6.2.

In addition, older individuals with comorbidities of the lung or circulation can show significantly reduced exercise capacities. Failure of the lungs to diffuse oxygen into the blood effectively or failure of the blood to transport oxygen and exchange it in the tissue creates a greater demand for cardiac efficiency. The older individual may not have the reserve capacity to increase either the HR or the SV to meet this demand. This may stimulate compensatory mechanisms in cardiac performance, such as ventricular hypertrophy, or prevent the individual from tolerating physical activity.

It is worth noting that the older individual typically takes medication for the management of heart disease or other illnesses. Many of these agents directly alter the physiological performance of the heart at rest, during exercise or both. Often, the prescribed dosage of a drug does not achieve the desired therapeutic outcome and may contribute to polypharmacy, which increases the risk of drug toxicity. For example, digoxin, a drug commonly prescribed for the management of congestive heart failure and atrial arrhythmias, can be toxic in an older individual. Digoxin tends to accumulate in the blood because of the reduced glomerular filtration rate through the kidneys, a common finding with aging. When quinidine, an antiarrhythmic drug, is taken in combination with digoxin, the serum digoxin level may double, further increasing the risk of digoxin toxicity, a potentially fatal condition. Hence, knowledge of the indications and pharmacokinetics of commonly prescribed drugs is essential for caregivers working with a geriatric population (see Chapter 12).

Dehydration is a common finding in older individuals. The direct cardiovascular effects of dehydration, including reduced ventricular filling volume, can impair cardiac performance and result in hypotension. The combination of dehydration and the delay in autonomic responses to position change that is commonly seen in the older individual often results in orthostatic hypotension, a significant risk factor for falls that may go unrecognized until a fall occurs.

CONCLUSION

Cardiac performance is a dynamic interplay of compensatory mechanisms, some of which may not be available in the older individual. The senescent cardiovascular system, stressed by the presence of disease of the heart or other organs and commonly supported by pharmacological agents, appears to be vulnerable to decompensation. Although the aging process cannot be stopped, healthcare providers are challenged not only to help the healthy older individual to safely slow or reverse the progressive decline but also to consider these changes when implementing a demanding rehabilitation program. The value of an exercise program for older individuals should not be underestimated. Minimal improvements in cardiovascular and pulmonary fitness can enable an older person to continue to live independently.

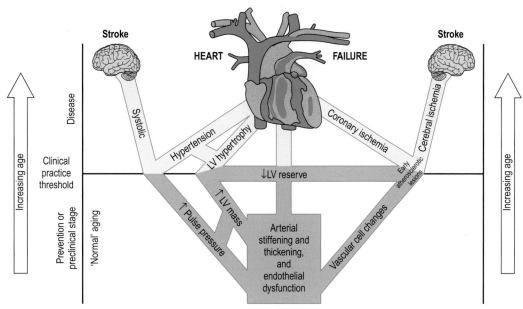

Figure 6.3 Changes in the vasculature and heart associated with aging. Changes below the bisecting line tend to occur with 'normal' aging and without clinical symptoms. Above a certain aging threshold, these changes tend to produce clinical symptoms. LV, left ventricular. (From Lakatta & Levy 2003b, with permission from Lippincott Williams & Wilkins.)

Table 6.2 Clinical consequences of age-related cardiovascular changes and clinical measurements

Age-related change[a]	Clinical consequences	Clinical measure/symptom[b]
↑ Beta-adrenergic responsiveness	Blunted heart rate response to exercise	HR, BP, RR, RPE
	Orthostatic hypotension	HR, BP, lightheadedness, change in color
	Longer to reach steady state	HR, RR
	Longer to recover from exercise	HR, RR
↑ Vascular tone; ↑ vascular stiffness	Systolic hypertension	BP
	Signs of ventricular hypertrophy	Laterally placed PMI
(↑ afterload)	Symptoms of myocardial ischemia	RPP, ECG, chest pain, change in color
	Arrhythmias (e.g. sss[c])	HR, BP, ECG, rhythm
↓ Pacemaker and conducting tissue cells	Conduction blocks	HR, BP, ECG, rhythm
↓ Ventricular compliance	Diastolic dysfunction, heart failure	S4, BP (may be normal)
↓ Early diastolic filling	Left atrial hypertrophy, atrial arrhythmias	HR, ECG, rhythm
Prolonged relaxation time	Symptoms of ischemia	RPP, ECG, chest pain, change in color

[a] ↑, Increase; ↓, decrease.
[b] HR, heart rate; BP, blood pressure; RR, respiratory rate; RPE, rating of perceived exertion; PMI, point of maximal impulse; RPP, rate–pressure product; S4, fourth heart sound.
[c] sss, sick sinus syndrome.

References

Abrams WB, Berkow R 1990 The Merck Manual of Geriatrics. Merck, Rahway, NJ.

Dehn MM, Bruce RA 1972 Longitudinal variations in maximal oxygen intake with age and activity. J Appl Physiol 33(6):805–807

Fleg JL, Schulman S, O'Connor F et al 1994 Effects of acute beta-adrenergic receptor blockade on age-associated changes in cardiovascular performance during dynamic exercise. Circulation 90:2333–2341

Gardin JM, Arnold AM, Bild ED 1998 Left ventricular diastolic filling in the elderly: Cardiovascular Health Study. Am J Cardiol 82:345–351

Lakatta EG 1993 Cardiovascular regulatory mechanisms in advanced age. Physiol Rev 73(32):413–467

Lakatta EG, Levy D 2003a Arterial and cardiac aging: major shareholders in cardiovascular disease enterprises. Part II: the aging heart in health: links to heart disease. Circulation 107:346–354

Lakatta EG, Levy D 2003b Arterial and cardiac aging: major shareholders in cardiovascular disease enterprises. Part I: aging arteries: a 'set up' for vascular disease. Circulation 107:139–146

Nied RI, Franklin B 2002 Promoting and prescribing exercise for the elderly. Am Fam Physician 65:419–427

Priebe HJ 2000 The aged cardiovascular risk patient. Br J Anaesth 85:763–778

Schulman SP, Fleg JL, Goldberg AP et al 1996 Continuum of cardiovascular performance across a broad range of fitness levels in healthy older men. Circulation 94:359–367

Susic D 1997 Hypertension, aging and atherosclerosis: the endothelial interface. Med Clin North Am 81(5):1231–1240

Swinne CJ, Shapiro EP, Lima SD et al 1992 Age-associated changes in left ventricular diastolic performance during isometric exercise in normal subjects. Am J Cardiol 69:823–826

Chapter **7**

Pulmonary considerations in the older patient

Meryl Cohen

CHAPTER CONTENTS

INTRODUCTION

Age-related changes in the pulmonary system of a healthy individual are slow and progressive. Often, the decline in pulmonary function is not noticed until the person reaches 60, 70 or even 80 years of age. Unlike the cardiovascular system, the pulmonary system has large reserves available to compensate for the structural and physiological consequences of aging. However, in the presence of pulmonary disease, these ventilatory reserves are often inadequate and can impose severe limitations on the performance of physical activities (see Chapter 47 for a discussion of pathological lung conditions). In addition, exposure to environmental toxins over a lifetime can contribute to a more rapid decline in pulmonary function in the older person.

The age-related changes that occur in lung tissue and in the 'musculoskeletal pump' are discussed in this chapter. A clear distinction between the effects of aging, subclinical disease and prolonged exposure to air pollutants on the pulmonary system is difficult to establish as all three cause similar structural and physiological abnormalities (Chan & Welsh 1998). General observations regarding the senescent lung and the effects of exercise and pulmonary disease on age-related changes in pulmonary function are also discussed. The clinical effects of aging on the pulmonary system and the implications for caregivers of older individuals are identified.

PULMONARY STRUCTURE

Age-associated changes can be found in the anatomical structures of the pulmonary system. Both the gas-exchanging organ (the lung tissue) and the musculoskeletal pump (the thoracic cage and its muscular attachments) show decline in the older individual when they are compared with the organs of a healthy younger person (see Box 7.1).

Box 7.1 Age-related changes in pulmonary system structure

Airways

- ↑ Rigidity of trachea and bronchi
- ↓ Elasticity of bronchiolar walls
- ↓ Cilia

Replacement of smooth muscle fibers in bronchioles with noncontractile tissue

Lungs

- ↑ Mucus layer (thickening) and ↑ mucus glands
- ↑ Thinning of alveolar walls (↓ alveolar collagen)
- ↓ Functional respiratory surface resulting from destruction of alveolar septa (loss of fibrous supporting network)
- ↑ Alveolar diameter with a ↓ in alveolar surface area
- ↓ Alveolar–capillary interface (because of ↑ alveolar size and ↓ capillary bed)
- ↑ Lung compliance
- ↓ Lung parenchymal weight

Vascular walls stiffen as media and intima thicken
Probable ↓ surfactant-producing cells

Respiratory muscles

- ↓ Contractile protein
- ↑ Noncontractile protein
- ↑ Connective tissue
- ↓ Capillary numbers relative to muscle fibers
- ↑ Contraction and relaxation times

Alteration in diaphragm position and efficiency

Skeleton

- ↓ Loss of bone mineralization
- ↓ Disk spaces
- ↓ Costal movements resulting from reduced sternal and costovertebral motion (↑ stiffness at joints)
- ↑ Anterior–posterior thoracic diameter
- ↑ Kyphosis resulting from a decrease in thoracic length

↑, Increased; ↓, decreased.

The lung

Changes in the alveolar membrane, including loss of the alveolar–capillary interface and increase in alveolar size due to the destruction of walls of individual alveoli, are the major forms of damage found in the aging lung (Brandstetter & Kasemi 1983). The general disintegration of the supporting fibrous network of the lung and the septa of the alveoli is considered a consequence of aging, but these changes can also result from repeated inflammatory injuries caused by lifelong exposure to environmental oxidants and cigarette smoke. Importantly, Pelkonen et al (2001) have demonstrated that when older individuals stop smoking, the rate of alveolar membrane destruction is slower when compared with that of older individuals who continue to smoke.

The musculoskeletal pump

Many of the age-related changes in the thoracic cage result from the loss of mineral and bone matrix and the increased cross-linking of collagen fibers (see Chapter 24), which, along with osteoporotic vertebral changes, contribute to the characteristic thoracic kyphosis and barrel chest of the older individual. The decreased mobility of the bony thorax and the less efficient resting position of the muscles of respiration alter lung performance and further contribute to the decline in pulmonary function with age (Polkey et al 1997, Janssens et al 1999). In fact, one thoracic vertebral compression fracture can lead to a loss of forced vital capacity (FVC) of up to 9% (Leech et al 1990).

PULMONARY PHYSIOLOGY

The primary functions of the pulmonary system are to exchange gas between the blood and atmospheric air and to protect the body from airborne invaders. Resting lung function results from a balance of elastic tissue forces pulling inward and musculoskeletal pump forces pulling outward. This dynamic and mostly involuntary interplay between lung tissue and chest wall musculoskeletal components depends on the compliance of both. Age-related changes in lung tissue compliance result from structural changes in the alveoli. The decrease in efficiency of pulmonary function is not generally perceived in healthy elderly people because the compromise of other systems with less reserve usually accounts for the alterations in their activity patterns.

The decline in alveolar structure and the pulmonary capillary bed contributes to the changes seen in ventilation (movement of gas to and from the alveoli) and gas distribution. Effective diffusion of oxygen and carbon dioxide into and out of the bloodstream depends on the integrity of the alveolar membrane and on adequate vascularity. Because alveolar membranes and capillary interfaces are compromised in the older individual, the ventilation–perfusion mismatching that is normally found in young individuals worsens with advancing age (Chan & Welsh 1998, Janssens et al 1999). As a result, there are larger ventilated areas relative to perfused parts of the lung (physiological dead space), which leads to a noticeable reduction in diffusing capacity (see Box 7.2).

The loss of elastic recoil in alveolar and conducting tissue and the disintegration of the fibrous supporting network also contribute to an increase in ventilation–perfusion imbalance. Smaller airways are unable to stay patent at low lung volumes (with expiration), leading to early airway closure. The resulting collapse of distal airways creates an imbalance in ventilation–perfusion. In addition, the excessive decrease in ventilation as compared with circulation causes a lowering of arterial oxygen pressure (P_aO_2) (see Box 7.3 and Fig. 7.1).

Box 7.2   Age-related changes in pulmonary function

↑ Ventilation–perfusion mismatch (less homogeneous)
↓ Diffusing capacity
↑ Physiological dead space
↓ Lung emptying
↑ Respiratory muscle oxygen consumption (rest)
↑ Minute ventilation (rest)
↓ Inspiratory muscle strength

↑, Increased; ↓, decreased.

Box 7.3   Age-related changes in pulmonary function measures

↑ Residual volume (RV)
↓ Functional residual capacity (FRC)
↓ Or ↔ total lung capacity (TLC)
↑ Closing volume
↓ Maximal voluntary ventilation (MVV); ↓ 30% between 30 and 70 years of age
↓ Vital capacity (VC); ↓ 25% between 30 and 70 years of age
↓ Forced expiratory volume (FEV$_1$)
↓ Arterial pressure of oxygen (P_aO_2); 75 mmHg is normal for individual aged 70
↓ Oxygen saturation
↓ Diffusing capacity of carbon monoxide (DLCO)

↑, Increased; ↓, decreased; ↔, no change.

An increase in closing volume caused by small airway collapse and poor lung emptying because of increased alveolar compliance and decreased elastic recoil helps to account for the increase in functional residual capacity (FRC). This is the volume at which the lung comes to rest at the end of quiet expiration. Residual volume (RV), the volume that remains in the lung after maximal expiration, also increases. The increases in lung volume tend to flatten the diaphragm, the major muscle responsible for inspiration, as it is unable to return to its original resting position. The altered mechanics of the diaphragm cause an increase in the anterior–posterior diameter of the rib cage. Changes in the position of the diaphragm and the dimensions of the thorax increase the work of breathing, and the muscle primarily responsible for inspiration is at a mechanical disadvantage when it comes to performing the increased work (Fig. 7.2).

The progressive decrease in chest wall compliance and the consequent stiffness also increase the energy expended when breathing. More oxygen is consumed by the respiratory muscles and the minute ventilation increases to meet this demand. In addition, there are age-related decreases in the strength and endurance of ventilatory muscles that are similar to those seen in skeletal muscle (see Chapter 2). Inspiratory and abdominal muscle weakness can also compromise cough efficacy. This becomes more significant with

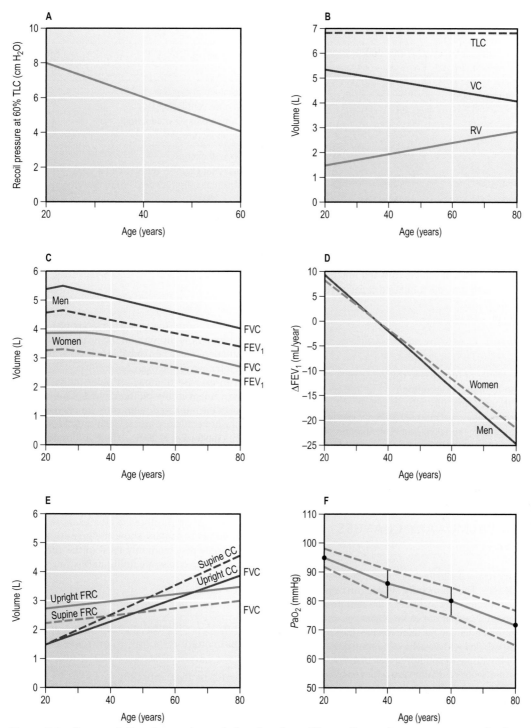

Figure 7.1   Representative changes in respiratory function with age. Curves show mean or generalized changes, and there may be considerable variation among individuals. Note the varying age scales on the horizontal axes. (A) Changes in lung elastic recoil with age; (B) changes in static lung volume with age; (C) changes in FVC (solid lines) and FEV_1 (dashed lines) with age in men and women; (D) changes in the rate of loss of FEV_1 with age in men (solid line) and women (dashed line); (E) changes in CC (defined as RV plus CV) and in FRC with age: solid lines, upright posture; dashed lines, supine posture; (F) changes in Pao_2 (at sea level) with increasing age: dashed lines represent ± 2 SD from the mean for the subjects studied. CC, closing capacity; CV, closing volume; FEV_1, forced expiratory volume; FRC, functional residual capacity; FVC, forced vital capacity; Pao_2, arterial oxygen pressure; RV, residual volume; TLC, total lung capacity; VC, vital capacity.

(From Pierson DJ 1992 Effects of aging on the respiratory system. In: Pierson DJ, Kacmarek RM (eds) Foundations of Respiratory Care. Churchill Livingstone, New York, with permission from the publishers.)

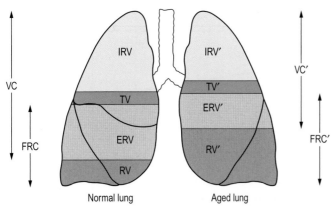

Figure 7.2 Schematic representation of lung volume changes associated with aging. Note that with senescence, there is a decrease in the inspiratory reserve volume (IRV), the expiratory reserve volume (ERV) and the vital capacity (VC). There is a corresponding increase in residual volume (RV) and functional residual capacity (FRC) such that the total lung capacity remains about the same. TV, tidal volume.

(From Chan & Welsh 1998, with permission.)

Table 7.1 Age-related pulmonary changes with exercise

	Effects of aging	After endurance exercise training
Submaximal exercise		
Minute ventilation ($\dot{V}_E$)	↑	↓
Carbon dioxide production	↑	↓
Blood lactate	↑	↓
Maximal exercise		
Maximal exercise ventilation [$\dot{V}_{E(max)}$]	↓	↑
Maximal voluntary ventilation (MVV)	↓	↑
$\dot{V}_{E(max)}$/MVV	↓	↑

From Protas E 1993 Physiological change and adaptation to exercise in the older adult. In: Guccione A (ed) Geriatric Physical Therapy. Mosby, St Louis, MO, p 42, with permission from Elsevier.
↑, Increased; ↓, decreased.

aging as the mucous layer of lung tissue thickens and a more forceful cough is required to mobilize secretions.

The decrease in thoracic mobility also results in decreased vital capacity (the maximum amount of air that can be exhaled following a maximum inhalation) and maximal voluntary ventilation (the volume of air breathed when an individual breathes as fast and as deeply as possible for a given time). This decline in pulmonary function can have a negative impact on an older individual's ability to exercise.

AGE-RELATED PULMONARY CHANGES AND EXERCISE

In general, pulmonary responses to low and moderate exercise are the same in people of all ages. The pulmonary system can respond to the increased demands of exercise by increasing the minute ventilation (the amount of air moved into or out of the lungs per unit of time). Minute ventilation is dependent on the tidal volume (the volume of air normally inhaled and exhaled with each breath during quiet breathing) and the frequency of breathing (respiratory rate). In the older individual, initial increases in minute ventilation are achieved by increases in tidal volume. These increases result from greater abdominal excursion in the older individual as the decreased compliance of the musculoskeletal pump limits significant thoracic movement. Dyspnea is perceived when the increase in tidal volume reaches 55–60% of vital capacity (Altose et al 1985, Janssens et al 1999). As already discussed, vital capacity decreases with advancing age. Hence, the ability to increase minute ventilation may be reduced at higher exercise intensities.

In addition, the older individual tends to perform work less efficiently, generating more blood lactate. The resultant acidosis is compensated for by an increased ventilatory effort to expire more carbon dioxide. Often, this results in early fatigue and a higher rating of perceived exertion (RPE) for a given workload compared with a younger or more fit older individual.

At low exercise workloads, an older individual continues to demonstrate ventilation–perfusion mismatching and decreased diffusing capacity. However, during vigorous exercise, pulmonary artery pressure increases. This tends to increase the alveolar capillary blood flow throughout the lungs. With improved perfusion, the ventilation–perfusion imbalance lessens and lung function and exercise tolerance improves (Zadai 1992).

With exercise training, an older individual is able to show some improvement in the pulmonary response to exercise (see Table 7.1). Most of the improved pulmonary function results from the greater efficiency of ventilatory and skeletal muscle performance (Pelkonen et al 2003, Watsford et al 2005). This is indicated by the decreased production of lactate and carbon dioxide when undertaking a given workload. The individual is able to work at a lower percentage of maximal voluntary ventilation and has an increased ventilatory response for a given oxygen uptake ($\dot{V}_E/\dot{V}O_2$) and less perceived dyspnea. Improved pulmonary function may also be attributed to the increase in thoracic mobility typically seen after exercise training. Individuals who are initially sedentary show the greatest improvement in function. Measurements commonly used in the clinic to monitor pulmonary response to exercise are found in Box 7.4.

Box 7.4 Clinical measurements used to monitor pulmonary responses to exercise

- Respiratory rate (RR)
- Oxygen saturation (Sao_2)
- Rating of perceived exertion (RPE)
- Heart rate (HR)
- Oxygen consumption ($\dot{V}o_2$)
- Anaerobic threshold (AT)
- Arterial blood gases (ABG)
- Oxygen tension (Pao_2)
- Carbon dioxide tension ($Paco_2$)
- pH
- Peak expiratory flow rate (PEFR)
- Breath sounds
- Cough
- Color (lips, fingernails)

Exercise can also help to mobilize secretions because it increases minute ventilation. Secretion retention can predispose an older individual to disease, hence exercise may further prevent decline of pulmonary function.

AGE-RELATED PULMONARY CHANGES AND DISEASE

The weakening of pulmonary structure and the decline in performance that occur with advancing age tend to have minimal impact on the functional ability of the healthy older individual. In the presence of chronic lung disease, pulmonary performance may be the limitation to exercise. Although the physiological changes in chronic obstructive pulmonary disease (COPD) are similar to those observed with aging, any lung disease that alters alveolar cell function or thoracic cage mobility can negatively impact on lung function.

The cumulative effects of COPD on the pulmonary changes normally seen with aging include a range of physiological outcomes. During rest, an individual may or may not show an increase in minute ventilation. At low workloads, an early increase in minute ventilation is observed as the lungs attempt to improve the ventilation–perfusion imbalance. Clinically, the older individual with COPD may be chronically short of breath but accepts it as a normal part of aging. As the intensity of work increases or as the disease progresses, the growing work of breathing causes an increase in the relative percentage of oxygen delivered to the respiratory muscles. Often, in the presence of thoracic cage rigidity and a significant loss of diffusing capacity, the extra energy required for pulmonary muscle function is obtained from inefficient anaerobic processes. This is seen clinically as a significant increase in dyspnea and heart rate and a decrease in arterial oxygen tension, which creates an even greater minute ventilation. In an attempt to meet this increased demand for oxygen, the heart tries to increase its performance. In some patients with compromised heart reserve, a decline in heart function can occur and, when combined with increased performance efforts, can lead to heart failure and further compromise of the oxygen delivery system.

Age-related changes in the lungs may increase an older person's risk of developing pulmonary disease. The thickening of the mucous layer, the loss of cilia and ciliary function within airways, decreased cough effectiveness due to muscle weakness and early airway closure combined with increased closing volume may contribute to the increased risk of pneumonia that is seen in the older population (Puchelle et al 1979). In addition, the age-associated decline in the physiological performance of the immune system may further predispose senescent lungs to infection.

CONCLUSION

Age-related changes occur in lung tissue and in the musculoskeletal pump. Pathological conditions potentiate the effects of these changes.

Although the objective benefits of exercise training are difficult to measure, older individuals with pulmonary disease are able to recognize an improved physical work capacity and sense of well-being. Respiratory and peripheral muscle conditioning and increased thoracic cage mobility improve the mechanical efficiency of the musculoskeletal pump and of oxygen extraction by the tissues. This may interrupt the declining cycle of dyspnea, inactivity and worsening dyspnea, and enable an individual to remain independent and active. In addition, the improved strength and endurance of respiratory and abdominal muscles can facilitate cough effectiveness and assist in the management of retained secretions, thus decreasing the risk of pulmonary infection.

References

Altose MD, Leitner J, Cherniak NS 1985 Effects of age and respiratory efforts on the perception of resistive ventilatory loads. J Gerontol 40:147–153

Brandstetter RD, Kasemi H 1983 Aging and the respiratory system. Med Clin North Am 67(2):419–431.

Chan ED, Welsh CH 1998 Geriatric respiratory medicine. Chest 114:1704–1733

Janssens JP, Pache JC, Nicod LP 1999 Physiological changes in respiratory function associated with ageing. Eur Respir J 13:197–205

Leech JA, Dulberg C, Kellie S et al 1990 Relationship of lung function to severity of osteoporosis in women. Am Rev Respir Dis 141(1):68–71.

Pelkonen M, Notkola IL, Tukianinen H et al 2001 Smoking cessation, decline in pulmonary function and total mortality: a 30 year follow-up study among Finnish cohorts of the Seven Countries Study. Thorax 56:703–707

Pelkonen M, Notkla IL, Lakka T et al 2003 Delaying decline in pulmonary function with physical activity: a 25-year follow-up. Am J Respir Crit Care Med 168:494–499

Polkey MI, Harris ML, Hughes PD et al 1997 The contractile properties of the elderly human diaphragm. Am J Respir Crit Care Med 155(5):1560–1564

Puchelle E, Zahm JM, Bertrand A 1979 Influence of age on bronchial mucociliary transport. Scand J Respir Dis 60:307–313

Watsford M, Murphy AJ, Pine MJ et al 2005 The effect of habitual exercise on respiratory-muscle function in older adults. J Aging Phys Activity 13:34–44

Zadai CC (ed) 1992 Pulmonary Management in Physical Therapy. Churchill-Livingstone, New York

Chapter **8**

Effects of aging on the digestive system

Ronni Chernoff

The gastrointestinal (GI) tract serves two major functions in the body; the first is the digestion, absorption and excretion of nutrients and their by-products, and the second is as an organ that filters and defends against pathogens. The ingestion, digestion and absorption of nutrients are essential processes that are part of the maintenance of nutritional status. The function of the GI tract is, therefore, intricately involved in nutrition and a factor in an individual's nutritional status. Because of the physiological changes that occur with advancing age, older people may have difficulties in meeting their nutritional requirements and fighting microorganisms.

The physiological changes associated with advancing age include the loss of lean body mass and body protein compartments, a decrease in total body water, reduction in bone density and a proportional gain in total body fat. These changes affect both nutritional requirements as well as the GI tract and other organs and tissues. In an older individual, adequate nutrition is an important factor for the maintenance of health and recovery from disease. It is important to note that many studies that describe changes in the GI tract with aging are conducted on subjects who have chronic conditions that may affect GI physiology or function (Moskovitz et al 2006).

NUTRITIONAL REQUIREMENTS IN AGING

Energy

The maintenance of health status and the provision of adequate nutrition in elderly people requires an understanding of the impact of age on nutritional requirements. The most well-documented change that occurs over time is the decrease in energy metabolism. This reduction in energy requirements is related to a decrease in total protein mass rather than a reduction in the metabolic activity of aging tissue.

Basal energy requirements reflect the energy needed for all of the metabolic processes that are involved in maintaining cell function; the reduction of active metabolic mass will result in lowered energy needs.

Protein

Protein requirements in elderly individuals might be expected to decrease to accommodate a lower total lean body mass. However, studies appear to indicate that protein requirements may be slightly higher in older subjects. One explanation is that a lower calorie intake contributes to reduced retention of dietary nitrogen, therefore requiring more dietary protein to achieve nitrogen balance (Campbell et al 2006).

Protein needs are also affected by immobility, which contributes to negative nitrogen balance. Elderly people who are bed-bound, wheelchair-bound or otherwise immobilized will require higher levels of dietary protein to achieve nitrogen equilibrium. Surgery, sepsis, long-bone fractures and unusual losses, such as those that occur with burns or GI disease, increase the need for dietary protein.

Some clinicians have been wary of providing high levels of protein for fear of precipitating renal disease in elderly individuals. Research has shown that there is no evidence that dietary protein induces deterioration of renal function in individuals who have no evidence of renal disease. For elderly patients who have a measurable decline in renal function, therapeutic regimens should be followed.

Fat

The major contribution of fat in the diet is energy, essential fatty acids and fat-soluble vitamins. Because only small amounts of fat are needed to provide essential fatty acids, and fat-soluble vitamins are available from other dietary sources, the primary contribution from dietary fat is the provision of calories. For older people, restricting dietary fat, thereby reducing caloric intake, is a reasonable strategy to maintain caloric balance without restricting intake of other nutrients; however, in some individuals, too rigid restrictions on dietary fat may contribute to energy deficits.

Altering the type and amount of dietary fat in the diet of older adults is somewhat controversial. As a controllable variable in the reduction of the risk of heart disease, there are major differences in opinion regarding the need for dietary fat alteration in adults over 65.

Carbohydrates

Carbohydrate intake in the diets of elderly people should be approximately 55–60% of the total caloric intake, with an emphasis on complex carbohydrates. The ability to metabolize carbohydrates appears to decline with advancing age.

It is important to encourage complex carbohydrate intake in elderly people because it provides fiber, a constituent of the diet that enhances bowel motility, which tends to decrease over time. Fresh fruits and vegetables are difficult to chew if oral health status is not optimal or dentures do not fit properly, and these foods are expensive when they are out of season. Cereal fibers should be encouraged as an alternative; however, it is difficult to obtain adequate fiber from cereal foods alone.

Vitamins

Vitamin requirements for adults over 65 are mostly speculative at present, although there is much ongoing research. Vitamin deficiencies may exist subclinically in the elderly, particularly for some of the water-soluble vitamins. In times of stress, after illness or injury, a depleted reserve capacity may not be able to compensate for rapid depletion of tissue stores and the individual may become overtly deficient. Subclinical deficiencies may exist in people who have adequate but not excess dietary intake, because the absorption and utilization of these vitamins may be compromised by the use of multiple medications or single nutrient supplements or by the declining efficiency of the small bowel to absorb micronutrients.

The water-soluble vitamins that are often the focus of attention are vitamin C and vitamin B_{12}. Although there appears to be no age-related alteration in vitamin C (ascorbic acid) absorption, this vitamin is often linked with wound-healing problems or a tendency to bruise easily. Vitamin C is an essential factor needed to make collagen, the protein matrix that holds cells together, and is therefore required when new tissue is being made. The recommended daily allowance (RDA) for vitamin C is 60 mg/day, a level that is far exceeded in most American diets. With large doses of supplemental vitamin C, tissue saturation is reached rapidly and the excess vitamin is excreted in urine. Very large doses (greater than 1 g/day) may contribute to some serious side effects such as the formation of kidney stones or chronic diarrhea in sensitive individuals. There is little evidence that massive doses of vitamin C aid in wound healing, ward off the common cold or cure cancer.

Vitamin B_{12} is a vitamin for which many older adults may be at risk for deficiency. The major dietary source of vitamin B_{12} is red meat and organ meats, which many elderly people have eliminated from their diets because of the fat and cholesterol content. In addition to dietary inadequacy, some older adults have a condition called atrophic gastritis, in which gastric acid production is decreased. Gastric acid is necessary for the release of vitamin B_{12} from a series of protein carriers; it is then linked to an intrinsic factor that forms a complex with the vitamin, allowing it to be absorbed. Production of intrinsic factor is also decreased with atrophic gastritis. Symptoms of vitamin B_{12} deficiency are generally non-specific but include irritability, lethargy and mild dementia.

It is less likely that elderly people will be deficient in fat-soluble vitamins (A, D, E, K) because of the ability to store these vitamins in liver tissue. The greatest risk is for deficiency of vitamin D, particularly for homebound or institutionalized elderly. Limited exposure to sunlight, the use of sunscreens and an inadequate intake of dairy products contribute to this risk. It is also known that the amount of vitamin D precursor in skin, which is stimulated by sunlight, particularly ultraviolet rays, decreases with age. Dietary vitamin D goes through several conversions in the liver and kidney, resulting in production of the active form of the vitamin; the kidney becomes less efficient at the final step of conversion with advanced age. Because vitamin D is an important nutrient in bone mineralization and immune function, it is wise to encourage the inclusion of foods rich in vitamin D in the diets of elderly individuals who may be at risk of deficiency.

For vitamin A, the risk of vitamin toxicity is greater than the risk of deficiency. This is especially true of older people who are taking over-the-counter vitamin supplements, many of which have very high levels of vitamin A. Beta-carotene, a vitamin A precursor, has received a great deal of attention in recent years because of its apparent protective effect against various types of neoplasm. The long-term effects of high doses of beta-carotene have not been adequately explored.

Minerals

The requirements for most minerals do not change with age. An exception is iron, for which there is a decreased requirement because of a tendency to increase tissue iron stores with advancing age and a cessation of menstrual blood loss in women. Calcium requirements have attracted much attention in recent years. Investigators have suggested that the recommendations for dietary calcium intake increase from 800 mg/day to 1200 or 1500 mg/day to reduce the risk of osteoporosis. However, the controversy surrounding calcium requirements in older people has not yet been settled, with many investigators believing that the recommendations should not be changed.

For most other major minerals, such as sodium and potassium, requirements are not changed by the aging process but are affected by the presence of acute or chronic diseases and their treatment.

Water

Water is an important nutrient for older people. Inadequate fluid intake may lead to rapid dehydration and precipitate associated problems: hypotension, elevated body temperature, constipation, nausea, vomiting, mucosal dryness, decreased urine output and mental confusion. It is particularly noteworthy that these problems are rarely attributed to fluid imbalances, which can be easily corrected.

Fluid intake should be adequate to compensate for normal losses (through kidneys, bowel, lungs and skin) and for unusual losses associated with increased body temperature, vomiting, diarrhea or hemorrhage. A reasonable estimate of fluid needs is approximately 1 mL of fluid/kcal ingested or 30 mL/kg actual body weight. The minimum intake for all older adults regardless of their size or caloric intake should be approximately 1500 mL/day. Fluid needs can be met with water, juices, beverages such as tea or coffee, gelatin desserts and other foods that are liquid at room temperature. Tube-feeding formulas contain approximately 750 mL water/L of solution; it is wise to compensate for the solid displacement by adding 25% of the volume of the tube feeding as additional free water.

Meeting all of these changes is often challenging. Encouraging older adults to consume an adequate diet may be linked to a functional and healthy GI tract. Age does have an impact on GI structure and function and it is worth assessing GI function in older adults.

AGE AND THE GI TRACT

The aging oral cavity

The changes associated with the aging process affect the structures of the mouth. Bone loss is a common problem and, in the oral cavity, where the alveolar bone is more prone to brittleness and fragility, there is an increased likelihood of tissue damage occurring because of oral trauma, periodontal disease and loss of teeth. Nutritional deficiencies are also manifested in periodontal and perioral tissue, which can impair chewing and normal ingestion of food.

As lean body mass decreases, gum tissue may be lost because of disease and atrophy. This process, along with bone resorption, leads to an increased risk of root caries, periodontal disease and loss of structure to support dentures. These changes, along with others in oral musculature and the mucous membranes, contribute to difficulty in chewing food adequately. Many individuals alter their dietary intake to compensate for their diminished efficiency in chewing, thereby putting themselves at risk for malnutrition. Malnutrition is associated with negative outcomes and adds an additional burden to the challenge of rehabilitation.

Other changes that may occur in the mouth and affect nutritional status include decreased taste and smell sensitivity, loss of taste and smell, and decreased salivary flow, which may be associated with disease conditions or the effects of medications. In chronically ill patients, the possibility that this condition may be present should be investigated. It is important to assess the ability of an individual to consume adequate nutrients to restore or maintain nutritional status through a period of rehabilitation.

The esophagus

The esophagus is the conduit that serves to transport food from the mouth to the stomach. Although it may not seem to be a very important part of the GI tract, esophageal dysfunction may have a profound impact on nutritional status and, therefore, on the recovery from an illness or other physiological problem.

The most common dysfunction of the esophagus is swallowing disorders (Tracy et al 1989). Swallowing problems may be characterized by pain, choking, spitting or vomiting. These symptoms are usually associated with an obstruction, cerebrovascular accident, neurological disease or degenerative muscular disease. Gastroesophageal reflux may be a secondary problem resulting from weakness in the lower esophageal sphincter, failure of peristalsis, or an injury or illness in the stomach (Dunn-Walters et al 2004).

Diagnosis and correction of esophageal problems are key to safe ingestion of food and liquids. Depending on the etiology and severity of the dysfunction, dietary modification may be the appropriate treatment. More severe problems require medical, pharmacological or surgical interventions. In either case, consideration of nutritional status is important to ensure adequate nutrient intake.

The stomach

The stomach serves several functions in the digestive process: its mechanical action breaks up food; it digests food through chemical and enzymatic actions; and it serves as a reservoir to hold partially digested food until it can be released into the small intestine. There is no evidence that age has a significant effect on gastric function; however, age-related conditions and diseases may result in altered gastric function.

The gastric conditions most commonly seen in elderly individuals are atrophic gastritis, peptic ulcer disease and gastroesophageal reflux disease (Saltzman & Russell 1998). Atrophic gastritis may contribute to a perception of food intolerance but, more importantly, it may be a major factor in vitamin B_{12} deficiency because gastric acid is required for the digestion process that allows this vitamin to be absorbed. Folic acid may also be malabsorbed with this condition.

Peptic ulcer disease is increasing among the elderly although the incidence in the general population appears to be declining (Newton 2004). Medications, such as H_2 (histamine) antagonists and antacids, may have multiple side effects, which could lead to other problems, including constipation, obstruction, osteomalacia, diarrhea, dehydration and electrolyte disturbances.

Gastroesophageal reflux disease is usually associated with the incompetence of the lower esophageal sphincter. There is no evidence that this is an age-related condition but some older individuals do experience this condition.

The pancreas

There is no strong evidence that age affects the pancreas in any significant way; however, glucose intolerance seems to increase and insulin secretion tends to decrease with advanced age and there appears to be a reduction in secretory output (Elahi et al 2002). This reduction is not considered clinically significant until pancreatic output is less than 10% of normal or these changes become symptomatic.

Diseases of the pancreas do commonly occur in older people. Acute pancreatitis occurs in older patients and may have severe consequences, resulting in sepsis and shock. An uncomplicated course may have a brief period of pain, nausea and vomiting, and tends to occur in individuals who have biliary tract disease. A more severe occurrence may result in abscesses, other septic symptoms or shock, and may require surgery and stress metabolic management.

Chronic primary inflammatory pancreatitis is a disease of older people. Symptoms include steatorrhea, diabetes, pancreatic calcification and weight loss. This is often a pain-free condition with an unpredictable response to therapy.

The aging liver

The liver tends to get smaller in mass with advancing age, which can lead to changes in structure and function. This may be important because many of the functions of the liver (synthesis, excretion and metabolism) are crucial for the maintenance of health. These functions are more affected by systemic disease and liver disease, both of which are common in elderly people.

The changes which occur that are important consider-ations in elderly people include alterations in drug metabolism and a decrease in the rate of protein synthesis. Both of these factors contribute to a diminished ability to respond appropriately to drug therapy or to the physiological burden associated with disease.

The small bowel

The GI tract, beginning at the mouth and ending at the anus, is a large muscle that propels food and its digested products through the body. Food is ingested and almost immediately acted upon by digestive enzymes, chemicals and mechanical actions. Many of the critical digestion and absorption functions occur in the small bowel. Age and disease can have an impact on the normal function of the small bowel.

The most common disorder of carbohydrate metabolism is disaccharidase deficiency of lactase. Lactase deficiency occurs with age and with common GI diseases such as viral gastroenteritis, Crohn's disease, bacterial infections and ulcerative colitis. Symptoms are associated with the ingestion of milk and milk products, and occur when the ingestion of lactose exceeds the production of lactase in the small bowel.

Another disorder with vague symptoms is celiac disease; this involves sensitivity to gluten, a protein commonly found in wheat products. It frequently results from an injury to the small bowel from exposure to gluten, which contributes to malabsorption and steatorrhea. The treatment is to eliminate gluten from the diet. Replacement of malabsorbed nutrients (iron, folic acid, calcium, vitamin D) should be part of the therapy.

Another source of malabsorption in older individuals is bacterial overgrowth. This may be associated with the decrease in gastric acid production by the stomach and the age-related decrease in bowel motility. Generalized malabsorption may result from this condition; vitamin B_{12} is a nutrient that is at risk of being malabsorbed.

Other conditions that may damage the small bowel and impair its ability to digest and absorb essential nutrients include radiation enteritis and inflammatory bowel diseases. Radiation enteritis is often a consequence of treatment for cancer of the cervix, uterus, prostate, bladder or colon. Because of their rapidly dividing characteristics, the cells in the small intestine are vulnerable to damage from radiation. Symptoms of diarrhea, nausea, cramping and distension often occur years after the period of therapy and may go unreported. Malabsorption and dehydration are potential nutritional consequences.

Inflammatory bowel disease may occur, with its symptoms attributed to other conditions because it is more commonly seen in younger people. Careful diagnosis is important for early treatment and adequate nutritional intervention.

Along with the digestive and absorptive bowel functions is a mucosal immune system that exists independently of the peripheral immune system and functions separately from the nutritional functions of the bowel mucosa. Age-related deterioration of immune function has been well recognized in older adults; the incidence of infection, autoimmune diseases and cancer is higher among older adults. Although immunosenescence in both host and cell-mediated systems is well described, mucosal immunity is less well understood (Fujihashi & McGhee 2004).

The large intestine

The primary function of the large intestine is the absorption of water, electrolytes, bile salts and short-chain fatty acids. The major conditions related to the large intestine that are experienced by older people are colon cancer, diverticulosis and constipation. If diagnosed early enough, colon cancer is treatable with surgery and radiation therapy. Diverticular disease may be asymptomatic in elderly patients until an infection occurs and the individual becomes symptomatic. Dietary treatment is the same for older patients as it is for younger patients.

Constipation is a common complaint among older adults. It may occur as a result of many conditions: neurological disease, drug effects, systemic disease, inadequate fluid intake, lack of dietary bulk and physical inactivity. However, the primary issue may be aging smooth muscle; there has been very little exploration of this physiological process and extensive research is needed (O'Mahoney et al 2002, Bitar & Patil 2004). Treatment should be based on the etiology of the condition and include adequate hydration, dietary fiber and physical activity.

Dietary management of malnutrition

As with other nutritional problems, the patient who is in rehabilitation should be encouraged to eat as much as possible. Underlying disease conditions should be treated first with nutritional adequacy encouraged as appropriate. Smaller, frequent meals may be accepted more readily by elderly patients with smaller appetites and early satiety. Oral liquid supplements can be added to solid food if fluid overload is not a contraindication. The goal of refeeding should be to provide 35 kcal/kg of the patient's actual weight and at least 1 g of protein/kg. Our experience has demonstrated that only 10% of elderly people who have protein energy malnutrition can consume adequate calories orally to correct their nutritional deficiencies; most subjects therefore require more aggressive nutritional intervention, such as enteral or parenteral feeding.

CONCLUSION

The impact of aging on GI tract function happens slowly over time but will often contribute to nutritional challenges that may affect the ingestion, digestion and absorption of nutrients. In older individuals, the ability to maintain nutritional status will also be affected by chronic conditions and episodes of acute illness that require adequate nutritional reserve. For most of the changes encountered, nutritional solutions can be devised; the greatest challenge is to recognize that there is a problem and to start interventions as soon as possible.

References

Bitar KN, Patil SB 2004 Aging and smooth gastrointestinal smooth muscle. Mech Ageing Dev 125:907–910

Campbell WW, Carnell NS, Thalacker AE 2006 Protein metabolism and requirements. In: Chernoff R (ed) Geriatric Nutrition: The Health Professional's Handbook. Jones & Bartlett, Boston, MA

Dunn-Walters DK, Howard WA, Bible JM 2004 The ageing gut. Mech Ageing Dev 125:851–852

Elahi D, Muller DC, Egan JM et al 2002 Glucose tolerance, glucose utilization and insulin secretion in ageing. Novartis Found Symp 242:222–242

Fujihashi K, McGhee JR 2004 Mucosal immunity and tolerance in the elderly. Mech Ageing Dev 125:851–852

Moskovitz DN, Saltzman J, Kim Y-I 2006 The aging gut. In: Chernoff R (ed) Geriatric Nutrition: The Health Professional's Handbook. Jones & Bartlett, Boston, MA

Newton JL 2004 Changes in upper gastrointestinal physiology with age. Mech Ageing Dev 125:867–870

O'Mahoney D, O'Leary P, Quigley EM 2002 Aging and intestinal motility: a review of factors that affect intestinal motility. Drugs Aging 19(7):515–527

Saltzman JR, Russell RM 1998 The aging gut. Nutrition issues. Gastro Clin North Am 27(2):309–324

Tracy F, Logemann JA, Kahrilas PJ et al 1989 Preliminary observations on the effects of age on oropharyngeal deglutition. Dysphagia 4:90–94

Chapter 9

Effects of aging on vascular function

Kristin von Nieda

INTRODUCTION

The study of aging has grown significantly in recent years. Several factors, such as an increase in the aging population, the increase in life expectancy and the increase in health expenditure, contribute to this growth. Studies concerned with aging have also evolved in scope. Earlier studies focused on identifying a single cause or explanation for aging. More recently, aging has been viewed as a complex process in which many factors and processes interrelate. Thus, a single cause or process is no longer sufficient to address the intricacies of the aging process (Weinert & Timiras 2003).

Age-associated changes occur in the musculoskeletal, neuromuscular, cardiovascular, pulmonary and integumentary systems. This chapter addresses a subset of the cardiovascular and pulmonary systems and focuses on the effects of aging on the vascular system. Just as these systems function interdependently, it is impossible to isolate and limit aging effects to the vascular system without an awareness of concomitant age-associated changes in other systems.

REVIEW OF THE STRUCTURE AND FUNCTIONS OF THE VASCULAR SYSTEM

The oxygen transport system is the biological system responsible for (i) bringing oxygen into the body from the ambient environment; (ii) circulating oxygen throughout the body; (iii) supplying oxygen at the tissue level; and (iv) ultimately removing the waste products created as a result of utilizing oxygen. The vascular system is the means by which oxygen and nutrients are delivered to the working tissues, and by which the metabolic by-products are removed from the tissues. The vascular network supplies a steady stream of oxygen-rich blood that allows working tissues and muscles to function at optimal levels. The ability to shunt blood preferentially and to deliver oxygen to the areas of greatest metabolic demand makes the vascular system an essential component of the oxygen transport system.

The vascular system is made up of three basic types of blood vessel: the arteries, capillaries and veins. The thickness of each layer of the vessels varies throughout the vascular system depending on the location and function of the specific vessel. Figure 9.1 summarizes the relative differences among the arterial, capillary and venous vessels.

The arterial system functions to accommodate the large volume of blood received as cardiac output and to propel it forward using the property of elastic recoil. The presence of smooth muscle in the arterial system allows it to control and direct the flow of blood throughout the vascular system via autonomic and endothelial controls and in response to local metabolic demand.

The normal structure of the arteries includes three layers. The adventitia is the outermost layer and attaches the vessel to the surrounding tissue. It consists of longitudinally oriented connective tissue with varying amounts of elastic and collagenous fibers. The middle layer or the media is usually the thickest and is a highly elastic, circumferentially oriented fibromuscular layer. Its function is to provide vascular support and to regulate blood flow and blood pressure by facilitating changes in diameter. The intima, the innermost layer, is composed of a single, continuous layer of endothelial cells that separates blood from the vessel wall. The endothelium serves as a barrier between the circulating blood and the underlying interstitium and cells, allowing selective transport of macromolecules in the blood to meet metabolic demands in surrounding tissues. The endothelium responds to regulatory substances released by physical and chemical stimuli and has many important functions, including regulation of vascular tone and growth, thrombosis and thrombolysis, and interaction with platelets and leukocytes.

The capillaries are the smallest and most numerous of the blood vessels, forming the connection between the arteries and the veins. The capillaries are thin and fragile in comparison to arteries and veins, and there is little resistance to the diffusion of oxygen and other metabolic products. The capillary wall is one endothelial cell thick, which allows for the exchange of nutrients and waste products at the tissue level.

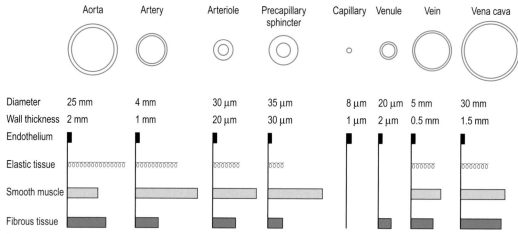

Figure 9.1   Internal diameter, wall thickness and relative amounts of the principal components of the walls of the various blood vessels that compose the circulatory system. Cross-sections of the vessels are not drawn to scale because of the huge range in size from aorta and vena cava to capillary.
(From Berne RM, Levy MN 1981 Cardiovascular Physiology, 4th edn. CV Mosby, St Louis, MO, p 2, with permission.)

The veins have the same three layers as the arteries; however, the walls are thinner and less rigid because there is less smooth muscle and connective tissue. The veins are capacitance vessels, which serve as collecting tubules for blood as it exits the capillary beds. At any given time, the majority of the blood volume is located in the venous circulation. The maintenance of a large reservoir of venous blood allows for adequate venous return as well as a necessary reserve during periods of increased oxygen demand.

Venous return is the principal determinant of cardiac preload, and sufficient venous return is necessary to ensure sufficient cardiac output. This function is accomplished by a combination of venous smooth muscle contraction, external muscle compression and a series of unidirectional internal venous valves.

AGE–ASSOCIATED VASCULAR CHANGES

Advancing age, with its associated vascular changes described below, is recognized as being a major risk factor for cardiac disease. Aging in the presence of cardiovascular disease accelerates structural and physiological changes, and the presence of other risk factors further influences the rate at which the changes occur. Hence, physiological aging and chronological aging cannot be considered equivalent.

In addition to the alteration of the underlying cardiovascular structures and functions, the increase in life expectancy also lengthens the exposure time to certain risk factors. In this sense, age-associated cardiovascular changes in structure and function are 'partners' with cardiovascular disease mechanisms. More specifically, it is the interaction between age, disease and several additional factors, such as lipid levels, diabetes, sedentary lifestyle and genetics, that determines the threshold, severity and prognosis of the disease in older people (Lakatta & Levy 2003). The presence of risk factors such as abdominal obesity, which is associated with metabolic risk factors, such as insulin resistance, metabolic syndrome and impaired glucose tolerance, compounds the effects of aging on the vascular system (Scuteri et al 2005).

Age-related cardiovascular changes occur in healthy, unhealthy and seemingly healthy older people. Lakatta & Levy (2003) differentiated between 'successful' and 'unsuccessful' aging. 'Successful' aging refers to healthy individuals, for whom the age-associated changes pose little or no threat to the development of disease. 'Unsuccessful' aging encompasses individuals who do not have or have not yet experienced clinical cardiovascular disease, but whose age-related cardiovascular changes put them at risk for future disease.

STRUCTURAL CHANGES ASSOCIATED WITH AGING

Structural changes associated with aging occur throughout the vascular system. Significant changes occur within the walls of the large elastic arteries, in which the intimal medial thickness increases two- to threefold between the ages of 20 and 90 years (Nagai et al 1998). The adventitia is most affected by a decrease in the number of elastic fibers and an increase in collagen, resulting in a loss of distensibility and a reduction in elastic recoil, essential for accommodating blood volume and propelling the blood into the vascular system. Both within the intima and the media, there is increased calcification, a loss of elastin content because of increased thinning and fragmentation of the elastin, and an increase in collagen. Lipid deposits in the intima further contribute to vascular wall thickening. These structural changes appear to be similar to the atherosclerotic changes seen in disease states, but occur even in the absence of occult disease and within populations with a low incidence of atherosclerosis (Moore et al 2003).

Aging is linked to significant changes in the microcirculation, resulting in age-associated endothelial dysfunction. The endothelial cells become irregularly shaped and are no longer longitudinally oriented along the vessels. Endothelial permeability is increased (Ferrari et al 2003), disrupting the selective transport system and resulting in concentrations of macromolecular materials and proinflammatory substances that further contribute to plaque formation. Within the media, vascular smooth muscle cells proliferate, migrate and infiltrate into the subendothelial space (Lakatta & Levy 2003). The irregular alignment and the increase in intimal medial thickness affect the dynamics of and resistance to blood flow, thereby affecting the transport of oxygen and other nutrients.

The age-associated increase in vascular wall thickness is accompanied by dilatation of the large arteries, loss of compliance and an increase in arterial stiffness, which may not be uniform throughout the vascular system (D'Alessio 2004). In peripheral vessels, there is less of an increase in the diameter of the vessels and more of an increase in wall thickening. In large arteries there is an age-dependent loss of capacitive compliance, whereas the reduction in small artery compliance is oscillatory or reflective (McVeigh et al 1999). Both types of compliance changes contribute to modifications in the generation, propulsion and reflection of pulse waves in the aging vascular system.

Pulse wave velocity (PWV), a noninvasive measure of vascular stiffness, increases with age in populations with little or no atherosclerosis, indicating that the increase in stiffness can develop independent of atherosclerotic changes (Lakatta & Levy 2003). The increase in PWV is associated with changes in vascular structure, most notably the increased collagen, decreased elastin, increased elastin fragments and calcification in the media. Lakatta & Levy (2003) also reported that arterial stiffness may be influenced by endothelial regulation of vascular smooth muscle tone. The age-associated changes in endothelial function further contribute to vascular stiffness both in the large and peripheral arteries, thereby hindering the normal contractile capability of vascular smooth muscle.

Age-associated changes also affect the venous vessels. There is an overall increase in stiffness and a decrease in venous compliance (Hernadez & Frank 2004). The venous valves begin to lose their integrity and the efficiency of unidirectional flow is lessened. It becomes more difficult to maintain venous return, and there exists the potential for venous stasis and retrograde flow. In a study of cross-sectional area (CSA) of the femoral and long saphenous veins, CSA was found to be associated with body mass index, gender and the presence of varicose veins but not necessarily with age (Kroeger et al 2003).

Varicose veins are more commonly found in the lower extremities and are characterized by tortuous dilatation and changes in the smooth muscle composition and extracellular matrix in the vessel walls, resulting in venous stasis and venous back flow (Jacob 2003). Peripheral edema formation is common. The incidence of varicose veins increases with age and is also affected by body mass index, prior or family history, and the presence of the disease during pregnancy. The estimated incidence of varicose veins in women increases from 41% to 73% between the fifth and seventh decades. For the same timespan, the incidence for men increases from 24% to 73% (Statistics about Varicose Veins 2006). Although recognized as the most common vascular disease, the presence of varicose veins is not clearly linked to disease development. Results from the Normative Aging Study population, taken over more than 35 years of follow-up, showed that men with varicose veins were less likely to develop symptomatic congestive heart failure than men without varicose veins (Scott et al 2004).

PHYSIOLOGICAL CHANGES ASSOCIATED WITH AGING

The age-associated structural alterations in blood vessels are further influenced by physiological changes that have a significant impact on the cardiovascular system. It is difficult to elucidate the intricacies of all of the interrelationships, and this section addresses only some of the interactions between the systems.

Systolic blood pressure (SBP) is known to increase with age. Blood pressure analysis of 2036 subjects over a period of 30 years in the Framingham Heart Study indicated age-related increases in systolic blood pressure (SBP), pulse pressure (PP) and mean arterial pressure (MAP), with an early rise (until 50 years of age) and a late fall (after 60 year of age) in diastolic blood pressure (DBP) (Franklin et al 1997). The increase in MAP is attributed to the progressive increase in vascular resistance associated with aging, but vascular resistance after the age of 50 is thought to be underestimated. The change in PP is a function of left ventricular ejection, large artery stiffness, early pulse wave reflection and heart rate. The rise in SBP is a result of both the increase in vascular resistance and increased stiffness in the large arteries. Under normal conditions and when arterial tone

and PWV are normal (before the influence of age-associated changes on the vascular system), the reflected pulse wave reaches the heart after the aortic valve closes, thereby enhancing DBP. With the age-associated increases in arterial stiffness and PWV, the reflected pulse wave reaches the heart before the aortic valve closes, resulting in an increase in SBP and the loss of the diastolic pressure enhancement. The late fall in DBP is associated with large artery stiffness. Franklin et al (1997) concluded that large artery stiffness rather than vascular resistance becomes the predominant factor for blood pressure changes as aging progresses. As the arterial walls become stiffer, they also become less distensible, and the lumen diameter of large central arteries increases to help accommodate blood volume as it is ejected from the left ventricle.

The loss of the elastic recoil together with the increased stiffness precipitates a decrease in the ability of the vessel to compress and propel the blood forward through the vascular system. A higher PP must then be generated to move a given volume of blood through a vessel. Because the heart is the pump that generates the initial propelling force, a decrease in the compliance of the arterial system results in an increase in the workload being placed on the heart.

At the level of the arterioles, capillaries and endothelium, alterations in structure result in alterations in function. Endothelial dysfunction has an enormous impact on the vascular system because the actions of endothelial cells are complex and involve several systems. With aging, the integrity of the endothelium is damaged and there is decreased activity of endothelium-derived relaxing factors (EDRF), including nitric oxide (NO), bradykinin and hyperpolarizing factor. Release of EDRF normally results in vasodilation and serves to counter the actions of endothelium-derived constricting factors (EDCF) (e.g. endothelin, angiotensin II), both on vascular tone and on the stimulation of growth factors derived from endothelial cells. With the decrease in EDRF activity, the vessels remain more narrowed, thus contributing to the increase in resistance to flow and the increase in PP and SBP. NO has an inhibitory effect on growth factors affecting vascular smooth muscle cells. The age-related alteration in NO activity results in an increase in the growth and proliferation of these cells, which accumulate and add to vascular wall thickening and platelet formation (Taddei et al 2001).

Another important function of the endothelium that changes with aging is the mediation of proinflammatory and antiinflammatory responses through a complex series of reactions to changes in EDRF and EDCF activity, growth factors, adhesion molecules, monocytes, cytokines, lipids and enzymes. Proinflammatory substances are no longer adequately inhibited, resulting in local inflammation, plaque formation, thrombosis and plaque rupture. With endothelial dysfunction there is an increase in plasma C-reactive protein, which is both a mediator and a marker of inflammation.

A variable pattern in the distribution of blood flow at rest is noted. Much of this decrease may be attributed to the diminished ability of the smaller arteries and arterioles to vasodilate. The net change toward vasoconstriction in these vessels also increases the turbulence of the blood flow. The endothelium responds to mechanical forces, such as the shear force of turbulent blood flow, promoting inflammation and its related sequelae. The shear forces from normal laminar flow act in a protective manner against atherogenesis. Turbulent flow is significantly more resistive than laminar flow, and the work required by the cardiovascular system to overcome the increased resistance intensifies.

Age-associated hormonal changes play a role in the development of vascular changes. In men, circulating testosterone levels decrease with age. Low testosterone is associated with arterial stiffness and is recognized as a cardiovascular risk factor (Hougaku et al 2006). Endothelial dysfunction occurs earlier in men than in women. Estrogen appears to have a protective effect on the endothelium, and there is a sharp decline in endothelial function after the onset of the menopause (Taddei et al 1996).

Given the structural and functional changes in aging blood vessels, it is not surprising to recognize aging as a major risk factor for cardiovascular disease.

AUTONOMIC SYSTEM CHANGES WITH AGING

Autonomic control declines with age, primarily reflecting an enhancement of sympathetic nervous system activity and a suppression of parasympathetic nervous system activity (Harris & Matthews 2004). Because of changes in the interplay between the autonomic nervous system and the cardiovascular system, it becomes more difficult to maintain hemodynamic stability. There is a decrease in β-adrenoreceptor responsiveness in the vasculature. The vascular responses of α_1-adrenoreceptors are either unaltered or may be increased with age (Priebe 2000). The loss of responsiveness to β-adrenergic stimuli with or without an increase in α_1-adrenoreceptor stimulation results in the predominance of α_1-adrenergic-mediated responses. Without sufficient vasodilatory input from β-adrenoreceptors, the autonomically mediated vasoconstriction compounds the vasoconstriction resulting from the previously described mechanisms.

A significant decrease in the reactivity of cardiopulmonary reflexes, especially the reflex mediated by the baroreceptors, occurs with advancing age. Baroreceptor activity is directed by the stretch demanded of vascular walls in the aorta and the carotid arteries by the blood flowing through the vessels. A decrease in the required stretch, and thus in baroreceptor activity, normally results in signals ordering restoration of cardiac output to increase blood pressure. This reflex activity is essential to prevent the orthostatic hypotensive response that can occur when moving from the reclining to the upright position. The pressor effect on SBP and PP, which normally occurs when moving into an upright position, changes with aging. The reduction in autonomic control may result in orthostatic hypotension if the elevated PPs do not adequately compensate (Cleophas & Van Marum 2003). A decrease in overall baroreceptor activity coupled with the decreased compliance of the vessel wall hinders the short-term regulation that normally occurs in the cardiac and vascular systems as a result of body position changes.

Deconditioning is another physiological state that results in an exaggerated orthostatic response. Many elderly individuals are sedentary and therefore deconditioned. This state results in less efficient oxygen transport and poorly functioning skeletal muscles. A deconditioned person needs more energy to perform tasks and is less able to adapt quickly and efficiently to alterations in the body's homeostasis. Thus, the exaggeration of the orthostatic response during body position changes can be great. Any health professional working with an elderly patient must be aware of this potential for an increased orthostatic response and know how to monitor and treat it.

TYPICAL ALTERATIONS IN THE VASCULAR RESPONSE TO EXERCISE WITH AGING

The ability to adapt and respond to the changing needs of the body during exercise is an essential function of the vascular system. One of the primary differences in the response to exercise in the elderly is the more rapid onset of fatigue, resulting from the demands placed on the cardiovascular system. The structural and functional changes in the vascular system impede the ability of the vasculature to supply the tissues with the increased oxygen needed during exercise. Maximal aerobic power refers to the body's ability to transport and use oxygen [$\dot{V}O_{2(max)}$]. Oxygen consumption increases linearly with the intensity and magnitude of exercise. With aging, $\dot{V}O_{2(max)}$ decreases as a function of body weight and age-related changes in the oxygen transport system, including the reduced ability to use oxygen and to shunt blood flow to active muscles. This deficit often causes an older individual to reach fatigue more quickly when exercising (see Chapter 6).

In a study comparing the responses of young and old adults to peak exercise, Stratton et al (1994) reported differences in several measured variables. There was a lower heart rate response and a smaller increase in ejection fraction. Systolic, diastolic and mean blood pressures were higher in the old than in the young. During submaximal exercises, there were no differences in ejection fraction between young and old.

Under normal circumstances, exercise or any other period of increased activity is sympathetically mediated and results in an increased release of the adrenergic mediators. This in turn raises the activity level in most body systems and triggers an increase in cardiac output and oxygen transport during exercise. The age-associated changes in β-adrenergic receptors in the vascular system lessen the ability of the vessels to facilitate the increased need for oxygen delivery during exercise (Stratton et al 1994).

At a more local level, the peripheral vessels are less responsive to alterations in metabolic activity. Normally, increased metabolic activity in skeletal muscle results in vasodilation to meet the oxygen demand of the tissue. The stimulation of skeletal muscle vascular adrenergic receptors during exercise also results in vasodilation. Older individuals have less ability to vasodilate in response to increased metabolic activity. These same individuals also have decreased activity mediated through the adrenergic receptors. The inability to increase blood supply quickly coupled with a decrease in structural ability to vasodilate prevents blood from being shunted quickly from areas of low metabolic activity to areas of more active muscle metabolism. Loss of this mechanism decreases an older individual's ability to do skeletal muscle work (Evans 1999).

When exercising, older individuals have been shown to have a higher percentage of their cardiac output shunted to the skin and viscera and a lower percentage directed toward working muscle. Thermoregulation is decreased in the elderly as a function of the loss of muscle mass associated with age and inactivity (Marks 2002). Normal thermoregulation relies on the processes of conduction, convection and evaporation. Sweating decreases with aging (Marks 2002). Evaporation, which is sympathetically mediated, is the predominant mechanism for heat loss during exercise. Older individuals attempt to compensate for this loss by shunting more cardiac output to the skin to regulate heat loss via conduction and convection, which are not efficient mechanisms for adequate heat loss at rest or during exercise. This shunting also prevents the delivery of an adequate blood volume to skeletal muscle.

With aging, muscle capillary density decreases and further limits the blood supply available to working muscle. An important measure of the oxygen transport function is the arteriovenous oxygen difference, which is a measure of the utilization of oxygen by working muscle. Changes in skeletal muscle tissue structure, mitochondria and metabolic enzymes result in a decreased arteriovenous oxygen difference, which indicates that less oxygen is being extracted from the capillary bed for use during exercise.

TYPICAL ALTERATIONS IN THE VASCULAR RESPONSE TO EXERCISE TRAINING WITH AGING

Stratton et al (1994) showed that exercise training had significant effects on all vascular variables except end-systolic volume index.

They also showed that the increases in maximal oxygen consumption and workload and the percentage increases were not significantly different between old and young. They concluded that, despite differences in the response to a single episode of exercise, similar changes in cardiovascular functions in old and young men occurred as a result of endurance exercise training.

Marks (2002) reported a decrease in $\dot{V}O_{2(max)}$ associated with aging, specifically a loss of 9–15% between the ages of 45 and 55, with accelerations in losses between the ages of 65 and 75 and further accelerations from 75 to 85. This decline in aerobic power can be improved by 10–25% in older individuals who participate regularly in aerobic exercise. The loss of $\dot{V}O_{2(max)}$ in women is greater than in men. Marks (2002) reported on studies indicating that an increase in walking of two miles per day may be as effective as traditional exercises for lowering blood pressure in women.

In a cross-sectional study of healthy men, DeSouza et al (2000) concluded that regular aerobic exercise can prevent age-associated loss of endothelium-dependent vasodilation (EDV). Aerobic exercise can also restore EDV in previously sedentary middle-aged and older healthy men. The aerobic exercise intervention consisted primarily of walking.

Carotid artery compliance decreases by 40–50% in healthy sedentary men and women between the ages of 25 and 75 years. Regular aerobic exercise attenuates this loss and compliance restores it to some degree (Seals 2003).

CONCLUSION

Age-associated changes occur in all of the various components of the oxygen transport system, including the vasculature. In rehabilitation, it is important to note that strength and fitness training programs in the elderly have been shown to decrease the amount of decline in function of many bodily systems, including the vascular system. Although training will not entirely eliminate the inevitable decline that occurs with advancing age, the severity of the decline will be lessened.

References

Cleophas TJ, Van Marum R 2003 Age-related decline in autonomic control of blood pressure: implications for the pharmacological management of hypertension in the elderly. Drugs Aging 20:313–319

D'Alessio P 2004 Aging and the endothelium. Exp Gerontol 39:165–171

DeSouza CA, Shapiro LF, Clevenger CM et al 2000 Regular aerobic exercise prevents and restores age-related declines in endothelium-dependent vasodilation in healthy men. Circulation 102:1351–1357

Evans WJ 1999 Exercise training guidelines for the elderly. Med Sci Sports Exerc 31:12–17

Ferrari AU, Radaelli A, Centola M 2003 Invited review: aging and the cardiovascular system. J Appl Physiol 95:2591–2597

Franklin SS, Gustin W 4th, Wong ND et al 1997 Hemodynamic patterns of age-related changes in blood pressure. The Framingham Heart Study. Circulation 96:308–315

Harris KF, Matthews KA 2004 Interactions between autonomic nervous system activity and endothelial function: a model for the development of cardiovascular disease. Psychosom Med 66:153–164

Hernadez JP, Frank WD 2004 Age and fitness differences in limb venous compliance do not affect tolerance to maximal lower body negative pressure in men and women. J Appl Physiol 97:925–929

Hougaku H, Fleg JR, Najjar SS et al 2006 Relationship between androgenic hormones and arterial stiffness, based on longitudinal hormone measurements. Am J Physiol Endocrinol Metab 290:E234–E242

Jacob MP 2003 Extracellular matrix remodeling and matrix metalloproteinases in the vascular wall during aging and pathological conditions. Biomed Pharmacother 57:195–202

Kroeger K, Rudofsky G, Roesner J et al 2003 Peripheral veins: influence of gender, body mass index, age and varicose veins in cross-sectional area. Vascular Med 8:249–255

Lakatta EG, Levy D 2003 Arterial and cardiac aging: major shareholders in cardiovascular disease enterprises. Part I: aging arteries: a 'set-up' for vascular disease. Circulation 107:139–146

Marks BL 2002 Physiologic responses to exercises in older women. Top Geriatr Rehabil 18:9–20

McVeigh GE, Bratelli CW, Morgan DJ et al 1999 Age-related abnormalities in arterial compliance identified by pressure pulse contour analysis: aging and arterial compliance. Hypertension 33:1392–1398

Moore A, Mangoni AA, Lyons D, Jackson SH 2003 The cardiovascular system. Br J Clin Pharmacol 56:254–260

Nagai Y, Metter EJ, Earley CJ et al 1998 Increased carotid artery intimal-medial thickness in asymptomatic older subjects with exercise-induced myocardial ischemia. Circulation 98:1504–1509

Priebe HJ 2000 The aged cardiovascular risk patient. Br J Anaesth 85:763–768

Scott TE, Mendez MV, LaMorte WW et al 2004 Are varicose veins a marker for susceptibility to coronary artery disease in men? Results form the Normative Aging Study. Ann Vascular Surg 18:459–464

Scuteri A, Najjar SS, Morrell CH et al 2005 The metabolic syndrome in older individuals: prevalence and prediction of cardiovascular events: the Cardiovascular Health Study. Diabetes Care 28:882–887

Seals DR 2003 Habitual exercise and the age-associated decline in large artery compliance. Exerc Sport Sci Rev 31:68–72

Statistics about Varicose Veins. Available: http://www.cureresearch.com/v/varicose_veins/stats_printer.htm. Accessed 18 February 2006

Stratton JR, Levy WC, Cerquireira MD et al 1994 Cardiovascular responses to exercise. Effects of aging and exercise training in healthy men. Circulation 89:1648–1655

Taddei S, Virdis A, Ghiadoni L et al 1996 Menopause is associated with endothelial dysfunction in women. Hypertension 28:576–582

Taddei S, Virdis A, Ghiadoni L et al 2001 Age-related reduction of NO availability and oxidative stress in humans. Hypertension 38:274–279

Weinert BT, Timiras PS 2003 Physiology of aging. Invited review: theories of aging. J Appl Physiol 95:1706–1716

Chapter **10**

Thermoregulation: considerations for aging people

John Sanko

INTRODUCTION

Internal body temperature is a relatively stable physiological function and one of the most frequently measured vital signs. Core temperature normally does not vary by more than ±0.55°C (±1°F) unless a febrile illness develops. Healthy unclothed people who were experimentally exposed to ambient temperatures as low as 12.6°C (55°F) and as high as 59.4°C (140°F) were able to maintain near constant core temperatures in spite of these extreme environmental conditions (Guyton & Hall 2000, Gonzalez et al 2001).

Humans are classified as homeotherms: they must maintain their internal temperature within a very narrow range (Gonzalez et al 2001). The critical temperature range, which is around 37°C (98.6°F), must be maintained so that the life-sustaining biochemical processes and other bodily functions can proceed at the appropriate rate, frequency and duration. Internal temperatures above 45–50°C (113–122°F) destroy the protein structure of various enzymes, which results in biochemical breakdown, tissue destruction, severe illness and death (Fig. 10.1). If the internal core temperature drops below 34.1°C (94°F), the ability of the hypothalamus to regulate body temperature is also severely impaired (Gonzalez et al 2001). Body temperatures below 33.9°C (93°F) slow metabolism to dangerously low levels and disrupt nerve conduction, which, in turn, results in decreased brain activity. If the body temperature continues to fall unchecked, loss of motor control, sensation and consciousness will be followed by ventricular fibrillation and death (see Fig. 10.1).

In essence, all warm-blooded animals, including human beings, live out their entire lives within a few degrees of death (Rhodes & Tanner 2003). Core temperatures falling outside of the normal range

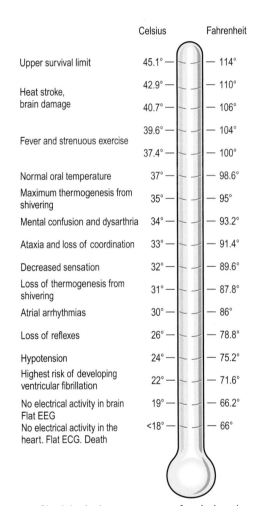

	Celsius	Fahrenheit
Upper survival limit	45.1°	114°
Heat stroke, brain damage	42.9°	110°
	40.7°	106°
Fever and strenuous exercise	39.6°	104°
	37.4°	100°
Normal oral temperature	37°	98.6°
Maximum thermogenesis from shivering	35°	95°
Mental confusion and dysarthria	34°	93.2°
Ataxia and loss of coordination	33°	91.4°
Decreased sensation	32°	89.6°
Loss of thermogenesis from shivering	31°	87.8°
Atrial arrhythmias	30°	86°
Loss of reflexes	26°	78.8°
Hypotension	24°	75.2°
Highest risk of developing ventricular fibrillation	22°	71.6°
No electrical activity in brain Flat EEG	19°	66.2°
No electrical activity in the heart. Flat ECG. Death	<18°	66°

Figure 10.1 Physiological consequences of variations in core temperature. Core temperature has a direct effect on physiological function. Extreme core temperature will seriously challenge homeostasis, which can have fatal consequences. EEG, electroencephalogram; ECG, electrocardiogram.
(Data from Guyton & Hall 2000 and Rhodes & Tanner 2003).

are indicative of some pathology or the failure of the thermoregulatory system to maintain thermal balance. The complexity of the physiological mechanisms involved in thermoregulation is shown in Figure 10.2.

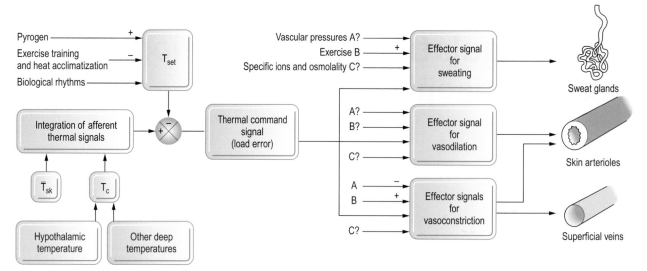

Figure 10.2   Physiological mechanisms for maintaining thermoregulatory homeostasis. Breakdown or impairment in any of the thermoregulatory mechanisms can lead to serious problems in maintaining homeostasis. T_c, core temperature; T_{set}, body's set temperature and the factors that affect it; T_{sk}, skin temperature.
(From Pandolf KB, Sawka MN, Gonzalez RR (eds) 1988 Human Performance Physiology and Environmental Medicine at Terrestrial Extremes. Benchmark, Indianapolis, p 106, with permission from the McGraw-Hill Companies.)

HYPERTHERMIA

Hyperthermia is the condition in which the internal core temperature exceeds the normal range. Hyperthermia can be caused by infections, brain lesions, environmental conditions or heavy exercise. When caused by an infection, the responsible microorganisms release toxins called pyrogens into the bloodstream; on reaching the temperature control centers of the brain, they raise the thermal setpoint. This state, known as fever, is actually beneficial and is part of the immune system's response. Higher core temperatures adversely affect the invading microorganisms' ability to replicate. This generally limits the extent of the infection and leads to its suppression.

In the older adult, the fever response is often diminished or absent, which may explain the increased morbidity and mortality rates associated with infections in the elderly (McCance & Huether 2001). When the ambient temperature rises above 30°C (86°F), progressive vasodilation of the cutaneous vasculature commences and is followed by sweating and evaporation (Gonzalez et al 2001). Factors such as high humidity and physical activity magnify the effects of ambient temperature, taxing the thermoregulatory mechanisms. This is an especially important factor in home healthcare when treating debilitated patients. Unlike fever, nonfebrile rises in body temperature are not beneficial and threaten homeostasis. If normal thermal regulation is impaired in any way, these increases can reach dangerous levels. At core temperatures above 40.7°C (106°F), heat stroke and irreversible brain damage become imminent (see Fig. 10.1).

HYPOTHALAMUS AND THERMAL REGULATION

The hypothalamus normally acts as the body's thermostat, initiating heat-dissipating, heat-conserving or heat-generating mechanisms in relation to internal core and body surface temperatures (Gonzalez et al 2001). The temperature-reduction mechanisms include vasodilation, sweating, inhibition of shivering and decreased chemical thermogenesis. When body temperature begins to rise, sympathetic outflow from the hypothalamus to the cutaneous vasculature is inhibited, allowing for vasodilation and increased heat transfer from the skin to the external environment. This mechanism is capable of increasing heat dissipation through the skin by as much as 800%. Sweating and evaporative loss further enhance the skin's ability to dissipate heat. When the body is subjected to cold, the hypothalamus conserves or generates body heat by measuring sympathetic tone, which results in vasoconstriction of the cutaneous circulation, piloerection, shivering and increased metabolism through the secretion of thyroxine (Guyton & Hall 2000, Gonzalez et al 2001, Rhodes & Tanner 2003). The efficiency of these mechanisms may be altered by skin atrophy, diminished vascular tree and reduced muscle mass and is discussed in greater detail below.

MOBILITY AND PSYCHOSOCIAL FACTORS

In spite of the exquisite physiological mechanisms that are available for dealing with temperature change, behavioral modifications may be the greatest defense against environmental challenges to thermoregulatory homeostasis. When our surroundings become too warm or too cold, we try to avoid such conditions by moving to a more comfortable location. In addition, we may add or remove clothing as conditions warrant. Because 30–40% of the body's heat can be lost through the head, the simple act of wearing a hat can have a profound influence on the thermoregulatory process (McArdle et al 2001). The very young and the elderly are at the greatest risk when exposed to extremes of environmental conditions. This may be partly because of their inability to recognize the magnitude of the situation and take appropriate action.

Older adults often find themselves dependent upon others for their well-being, commonly as a result of deficits in physical or cognitive function. The incidence of chronic disease increases dramatically with age. More than 50% of those over 65 years of age report some limitation in mobility due to arthritis and another 16% have other orthopedic problems that limit their ability to carry out the normal activities of daily living (ADLs) (Guccione 2000). In older individuals, musculoskeletal and neurological conditions often reduce their functional level to a point where they become partially, if not fully, dependent upon others to carry out the ADLs. Thermoregulatory stress may be one of many reasons why elderly people who are dependent on others for help with ADLs have a four times greater chance of dying within a two-year period than those who are totally independent. Approximately 15% of the population aged over 65 are in some way cognitively impaired. The incidence of cognitive impairment rises rapidly with age. Some deterioration in mental function is seen in nearly 50% of those individuals who are 85 years of age or older (Guccione 2000). These physical and mental impairments, combined with a reduction in the functional capacity of various organ systems, make the older adult particularly vulnerable to thermoregulatory stress.

Thermal injury

Heat stroke, heat exhaustion and hypothermia are most prevalent among the elderly and are inversely related to socioeconomic status. When elderly individuals on fixed incomes turn the heat down in the winter because they cannot pay high heating bills, they are certainly predisposing themselves to hypothermia. Conversely, elderly people who are unable to afford air conditioning are 50 times more likely to die of heat stroke than those who have access to air conditioning (Wongsurawat 1994). Although it has been stated that numerous predisposing physiological factors contribute to failure of the thermoregulatory system to maintain thermal balance, many temperature-related threats to health could undoubtedly be prevented if elderly individuals stayed indoors, adjusted the heating or air conditioning and dressed more appropriately (Gonzalez et al 2001, Powers & Howley 2003). In cases in which economic status or physical or mental condition makes these actions impossible, those involved should be referred to the appropriate agencies for the protection of their welfare.

PHYSIOLOGICAL FACTORS

Skin receptors and circulatory response

Even when healthy and mentally alert, the elderly are less able to sense changes in skin temperature and this makes them more susceptible to thermoregulatory problems (Kauffman 1987, Gonzalez et al 2001). Skin temperature, unlike core temperature, is extremely variable. Thermoreceptors for both heat and cold are found in the skin, the spinal cord and the hypothalamus itself (Powers & Howley 2003). Receptors in the skin provide the hypothalamus with important feedback regarding the need to dissipate, conserve or generate heat. Numerous bare nerve endings just below the skin are sensitive to heat and cold. They are classified as warm or cold receptors, depending on their rate of discharge when exposed to variations in temperature; there are approximately 10 times more cold receptors than hot receptors (Rhodes & Tanner 2003). It is not known whether the effectiveness of these thermoreceptors declines with age; however, because their function depends on an adequate oxygen supply, it seems reasonable to assume that any age-associated impairments in cutaneous circulation will reduce their effectiveness (Collins et al 1977).

It is known that the dermis becomes thinner and less vascularized with age (Claremont et al 1976). The changes in skin thickness and circulation along with reduced autonomic nervous system function alter the effectiveness of the vasomotor response. The vasomotor mechanism can alter cutaneous blood flow from near zero when exposed to extreme cold to increases of 500–1000% when exposed to vigorous warming. The evaporative loss of sweat from the skin surface helps to dissipate heat in the cutaneous circulation. A study that compared men of 45–57 years with men of 18–23 years during moderate intensity exercise found that the older men took twice as long to start sweating. Subsequent studies of older women showed even greater impairments in the sweating mechanism. The number of sweat glands does not appear to change significantly with aging (Finch & Schneider 1985). Therefore, it is reasonable to assume that the age-related decline in autonomic nervous system function reduces the performance of sweat glands and alters the body's ability to dissipate excess heat. In addition, the hypothalamus appears to become less sensitive to temperature variations (Guyton & Hall 2000).

It is unclear how much of the thermoregulatory impairment seen in the elderly is age-related and how much is the result of chronic disease processes and a sedentary lifestyle. Several investigators have found little or no difference in thermoregulation during exercise in physically fit younger and older subjects (Drinkwater & Horvath 1979). The ability of the cardiovascular system to dissipate body heat is enhanced by aerobic fitness. Resistive exercise has been found to be particularly beneficial in maintaining or retarding muscle loss in the elderly and should be considered when not contraindicated. Muscle is a significant tissue not only for heat generation, but also for the mobility needed for thermoregulation.

Other physiological factors

The ingestion of food and alcohol and medications to control blood pressure, cardiac function, depression and pain all exert an influence on thermal balance and regulation. A sufficient, well-balanced diet is essential to provide the calories needed to generate heat and maintain adequate levels of metabolically active muscle. Muscle, which is the major organ of metabolism and heat generation, can decrease by 10–12% in the older adult. One-third of the US population over 65 has some form of nutritional deficit, often eating inappropriate quantities of foods that are low in nutritional values. Because 80% of the calories consumed go toward the maintenance of body temperature, this deficit can further contribute to the thermoregulatory inadequacies experienced by some older individuals. The shivering mechanism, which can increase metabolism and heat generation by 300–500%, is also adversely affected by the loss of muscle tissue (Gonzalez et al 2001, Rhodes & Tanner 2003).

POSSIBLE EFFECTS OF MEDICATION

Although there is still a great deal to be learned about the effects of aging on thermoregulatory function, it appears that physical conditioning and adequate nutrition help to preserve this function in healthy older adults. However, not all older individuals are healthy or physically fit. Many have chronic conditions that interfere with their ability to respond to even mild variations in temperature. In addition, various medications can interfere with the normal physiological responses necessary to maintain thermal homeostasis. Dehydration may occur in individuals taking diuretics for the management of congestive heart failure or hypertension. A loss as small as 1% of an individual's total body fluid can lead to consequential increases in core temperature, decreased sweating, reduced cardiac output and a reduction in skin blood flow. In one study, a diuretic-induced 3% loss of body fluid resulted in a significant reduction in plasma volume and a 15–20 beat per minute increase in heart rate (Claremont et al 1976).

Beta-antagonists are another category of medication commonly prescribed for elderly individuals with heart disease and hypertension. In a Swedish study, 54% of patients taking beta blockers complained of cold hands and feet, and 35% of patients on diuretics complained of this problem (Claremont et al 1976). Additionally, individuals using beta blockers were found to rate their perception of exertion for a given workload significantly higher than would be predicted for that workload.

Although the use of illicit drugs is lowest among the elderly, the misuse of prescription drugs is a major problem in this group. In one survey of elderly people living independently in the community, 83% reported using two or more prescription drugs, with an average of 3.8 medications per person (Hooyman & Kiyak 2004). Many elderly individuals have been found to misuse prescription and nonprescription over-the-counter drugs. Surveyed individuals reported taking two to three times the recommended dosages of aspirin, laxatives and sleeping pills. Misuse of laxatives could further increase the rate and severity of dehydration, and sedatives impair the autonomic nervous system's ability to react to environmental conditions.

Alcohol also inhibits the body's ability to regulate temperature by interfering with the vasomotor system and altering cutaneous blood flow, which impairs the body's ability to dissipate or conserve heat. The dehydrating effects of alcohol can also contribute to an inadequate thermoregulatory response by reducing plasma volume and decreasing the sweat response. Combined with prescription and nonprescription medications, alcohol can create serious problems for any individual.

POSTSURGICAL CONSIDERATIONS

A number of geriatric patients receiving physical therapy in acute- and extended-care facilities are postsurgical patients. The tremendous advancements and successes in joint replacement surgery have made these procedures relatively commonplace. Plasma lost during surgery may result in some degree of dehydration, but anesthetics present the greater challenge to thermoregulation in these patients. Most anesthetics and sedatives impair the body's ability to maintain core temperature by blocking the normal heat-generating activity. There are some benefits of mild hypothermia for the surgical patient but there are also increased risks for the elderly. A 2°C (3.6°F) drop in core temperature has been shown to substantially increase blood loss during hip arthroplastic surgery. The incidence of ischemic myocardial events increases for a 24-h period following intraoperative hypothermia. Higher rates of wound infection, delayed healing and immunosuppression are also seen following anesthesia-induced hypothermia. The elderly appear to be at the greatest risk for developing one or more of these complications because of their predisposition to hypothermia even when exposed to only moderately cold conditions (Mayer & Sessler 2004).

CLINICAL CONSIDERATIONS

In spite of the fact that numerous age-correlated alterations in thermoregulation have been identified, the ability to regulate internal core temperature appears to remain within acceptable limits in the healthy, fit older adult. Furthermore, few of the changes seen in autonomic, circulatory and thermal function are solely the result of biological aging. Reduced physical work capacity, body composition changes, chronic illness, the use and misuse of various medications, and alterations in cognitive function become more prevalent with advancing age and influence the function of various body systems involved with thermoregulation. Studies on thermoregulation and aging have generally shown that aging reduces sweat gland output, skin blood flow, cardiac output, peripheral vasoconstriction and muscle mass. Gender may also play an important role; although both males and females lose muscle mass as they age, females tend to have a greater increase in percent body fat, which may account for their

ability to better maintain core temperature when exposed to cooler ambient temperatures (Kenney & Munce 2003).

Whenever treating any individual with exercise or thermal modalities, age should be a consideration. Ideally, the ambient temperature in exercise areas should be 19.8–22°C (68–72°F) with a relative humidity of 60% or less. When exercise is to be performed outdoors, appropriate clothing is necessary. Planning outdoor activities during moderate weather is also important. It would not be prudent to exercise in mid-afternoon on a hot summer's day or late in the evening on a cold winter's day. Because older adults may build up heat more quickly and take longer to dissipate it than their younger counterparts, frequent rest periods in well-ventilated areas should be incorporated into any exercise regimen.

CONCLUSION

The safe and effective use of exercise, heat, cold or hydrotherapy requires a thorough assessment of the individual's condition, medical history and ability to withstand thermal or cryogenic stress. A

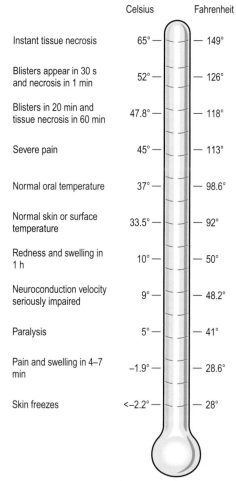

	Celsius	Fahrenheit
Instant tissue necrosis	65°	149°
Blisters appear in 30 s and necrosis in 1 min	52°	126°
Blisters in 20 min and tissue necrosis in 60 min	47.8°	118°
Severe pain	45°	113°
Normal oral temperature	37°	98.6°
Normal skin or surface temperature	33.5°	92°
Redness and swelling in 1 h	10°	50°
Neuroconduction velocity seriously impaired	9°	48.2°
Paralysis	5°	41°
Pain and swelling in 4–7 min	–1.9°	28.6°
Skin freezes	<–2.2°	28°

Figure 10.3   Effect on body tissues of direct exposure to heat and cold. Surface temperature may be very different from core temperature. Extremes in local tissue temperature will lead to cell death and tissue necrosis, regardless of core temperature. Local thermoregulatory impairments can lead to systemic consequences if not corrected.

(From Guyton & Hall 2000 and Rhodes & Tanner 2003.)

past medical history of hypersensitivity to heat or cold, Raynaud's disease, urticaria, wheals, diabetes or heart disease requires further consideration before intervention. Pain and temperature sensation should also be assessed.

The normal effects of direct heating and cooling of the tissue may be altered in some elderly individuals (Fig. 10.3). Vital signs should be monitored along with skin temperature, sensation, color, sweat rate and rate of perceived exertion (RPE). Additional care should be taken with individuals on medication and those who have impaired cognitive and mental function.

Should a thermoregulatory crisis occur, standard emergency and medical procedures should be followed (Tables 10.1 and 10.2). A few simple precautions can help to prevent many of these crises (Boxes 10.1 and 10.2). Additional research in the area of thermoregulation and aging is needed to resolve the many contradictory findings. Until these questions have been answered, the clinician must carefully consider the use of modalities and exercises with people of various ages, based on experience, common sense and the current body of knowledge.

Table 10.1   Heat-related emergencies

Condition	Signs and symptoms	Treatment
Heat edema	Swollen feet and ankles	Elevate the lower extremities and wear support stockings. If symptoms are a consequence of a cardiovascular condition, drug therapy may be required
Heat cramps	Severe muscle spasm, particularly in the lower extremities	Allow patient to rest in a cool place, cool with moist towels and drink electrolyte replacement fluids
Heat syncope	Pooling of blood in veins resulting in decreased cardiac output; symptoms ranging from lightheadedness to loss of consciousness; typically cool and wet skin	Allow patient to lie down, rest and drink electrolyte fluids. This condition is caused by physical exertion in a warm environment by an individual not acclimatized to that environment
Heat exhaustion	Loss of volume in the circulatory system as a result of excessive sweating; cool and clammy skin; nausea, headache, confusion, weakness and low blood pressure	Rest and fluid replacement; fluids with electrolytes may be necessary. Unconsciousness occurs rarely
Heat stroke	High skin and core body temperature; loss of consciousness; possible convulsions; dry skin, indicating loss of the sweating mechanism for cooling	This is the most severe heat-related condition. Cool the body as rapidly as possible. Seek immediate medical care

From Judd RL, Dinep MM 1986 Environmental emergencies. In: Judd RL, Warner CG, Shaffer MA (eds) Geriatric Emergencies. Aspen Publishers, Rockville, MD, p 255.

Table 10.2   Cold-related emergencies

Condition	Signs and symptoms	Treatment
Chilblains	Skin lesions that occur after prolonged exposure of the skin to temperatures below 15.4°C (60°F)	Protect the injured area and prevent re-exposure
Trench foot	Swollen body part (usually foot); waxy, mottled appearance of skin; complaints of numbness; caused by prolonged exposure to cool water	Remove wet shoes and socks. Gently rewarm. Cover any blisters with sterile dressings
Frostnip	Reddened skin that becomes blanched; numbness or tingling; ears, nose, lips, fingers and toes most commonly affected	Gently warm the involved area. If the condition does not resolve itself, treat the individual for frostbite
Frostbite	Waxy appearance of skin; may turn mottled	Gently warm but do not rub or squeeze the injured part. Transport patient immediately for advanced medical treatment
Hypothermia	Shivering in early stages; drowsiness and lethargy; slow breathing and bradycardia; possible loss of consciousness	Gently rewarm the individual in mild cases. Immediately transport for advanced medical care in moderate to severe cases
Cold allergy	Urticaria, erythema, itching and edema; systemic reactions, including hypotension, tachycardia, syncope and gastrointestinal dysfunction	Gently warm and acclimatize the individual

From Judd RL, Dinep MM 1986 Environmental emergencies. In: Judd RL, Warner CG, Shaffer MA (eds) Geriatric Emergencies. Aspen Publishers, Rockville, MD, p 255.

Box 10.1   How to avoid hyperthermia

- Wear loose-fitting, light clothing during periods of high heat and humidity
- Take cool baths or showers during periods of high heat and humidity
- Drink adequate amounts of fluids, even when not thirsty
- Use air conditioning or fans to cool and circulate the air
- Avoid excessive exercise during peak temperatures of the day, especially when humidity is high and fans and air conditioning are not available. This is particularly important in the home healthcare setting
- When performing physical activity or exercise outdoors, use caution. Avoid working in direct sunlight on hot days. Take frequent breaks in cool or shady areas

---

Box 10.2   How to avoid hypothermia

- Wear several layers of loose-fitting clothing and a hat
- Stay dry
- Maintain an adequate balanced diet
- Drink adequate amounts of fluids, but limit alcohol consumption
- Turn up the heating when the weather is cool
- Frequently check on elderly individuals in the community who live alone
- When performing physical activities or exercise outdoors, use caution. A great deal of heat loss can occur even when the temperatures are only moderately cool. Always consider windchill

---

References

Claremont AD, Costill DL, Fink W et al 1976 Heat tolerance following diuretic-induced dehydration. Med Sci Sports Exerc 8:239

Collins K, Dore C, Exton-Smith A et al 1977 Accidental hypothermia and impaired temperature homeostasis in the elderly. Br Med J 1:353

Drinkwater BL, Horvath SM 1979 Heat tolerance and aging. Med Sci Sports Exerc 1:49

Finch CE, Schneider EL (eds) 1985 Handbook of the Biology of Aging, 2nd edn. Van Nostrand Reinhold, New York

Gonzalez EG, Myers SJ, Edelstein JE et al (eds) 2001 Downey and Darling's The Physiological Basis of Rehabilitation Medicine, 3rd edn. Elsevier, St Louis, MO

Guccione AA (ed) 2000 Geriatric Physical Therapy, 2nd edn. Elsevier, St Louis, MO

Guyton AC, Hall JE 2000 Textbook of Medical Physiology, 10th edn. Elsevier, St Louis, MO

Hooyman NR, Kiyak HA 2004 Social Gerontology: A Multidisciplinary Perspective, 7th edn. Allyn & Bacon, Boston, MA

Kauffman T 1987 Thermoregulation and use of heat and cold. In: Jackson OL (ed) Clinics in Physical Therapy XIV. Churchill Livingstone, New York, p 69

Kenney WL, Munce TA 2003 Invited review: aging and human temperature regulation. J Appl Physiol 95:2598

Mayer SA, Sessler DI (eds) 2004 Therapeutic Hypothermia. Marcel Dekker, New York

McArdle WD, Katch FI, Katch VL 2001 Exercise Physiology: Energy, Nutrition, and Human Performance, 5th edn. Lippincott Williams & Wilkins, Baltimore, MD

McCance KL, Huether SE 2001 Pathophysiology: The Biologic Basis for Disease in Adults and Children, 4th edn. Elsevier, St Louis, MO

Powers SK, Howley ET 2003 Exercise Physiology: Theory and Application to Fitness and Performance, 5th edn. McGraw-Hill, New York

Rhodes RA, Tanner GA (eds) 2003 Medical Physiology, 2nd edn. Lippincott, Williams & Wilkins, Baltimore, MD

Wongsurawat N 1994 Temperature regulation in the aged. In: Felsenthal G, Garrison SJ, Steinberg FU (eds) Rehabilitation of the Aging and Elderly Patient. Williams & Wilkins, Baltimore, MD

Chapter 11

The aging immune system

Gordon Dickinson

INTRODUCTION

Humans possess an elaborate array of host defenses against the many potential pathogens in their environment. Among these protective mechanisms are important mechanical and physiological guards such as skin and mucosal barriers, valvular structures like the epiglottis and the urethral valves, cleansing fluids (tears and respiratory tract mucus) and involuntary activities such as coughing. These defenses are, however, frequently breached and it is the immune response that is the final and most potent form of protection. 'Immune response' generally refers to internal cellular and humoral defense mechanisms, especially those that are acquired.

INNATE AND ACQUIRED IMMUNITY

Immunity can be categorized as innate or acquired. The components of innate immunity are generally present from birth and do not require exposure to a pathogen for their development. Innate immunity includes the macrophage/phagocyte cell lines, which act as nonspecific scavengers within the body, engulfing and killing invaders that have breeched the skin or mucosal barriers. To assist the macrophages, there are substances in the serum called complement and acute-phase reactants that facilitate the attachment and ingestion of pathogens. The macrophages, as well as the complement and acute-phase reactants, are poised to function as an immediate response system against virtually all bacteria; however, even in the presence of complement and acute-phase reactants, phagocytic cells often have difficulty promptly and efficiently ingesting pathogens. Some bacteria, for example *Streptococcus pneumoniae* and *Haemophilus influenzae*, form a polysaccharide capsule that shields them from these defenses. Moreover, many pathogens are either too large for ingestion by macrophages

(e.g. parasites) or thrive in an intracellular location (e.g. viruses, mycobacteria and an assortment of other pathogens). To bolster these defenses, an acquired immune system has evolved, which is extremely potent and pathogen-specific, but which must be primed by a first-time exposure to the pathogen. Once in place, acquired immunity is permanent. The term 'immunity' generally refers to the activity of the acquired immune system.

T and B lymphocytes

The principal components of the acquired immune system are the T and B lymphocytes. All lymphocytes originate from progenitors in the bone marrow. Some evolve into B lymphocytes, so-called because in birds these cells originate in the bursa of Fabricius. The B lymphocytes become antibody factories when activated by helper/inducer T lymphocytes. T lymphocytes circulate through the thymus gland and develop the ability to recognize foreign matter (an antigen), retain memory of the antigen and influence B lymphocytes to produce antibodies against this antigen. These highly specific antibodies attach themselves to the invader, either killing it directly or facilitating the process of phagocytosis, and ultimately cause the destruction and clearance of the invader from the body. Because the lymphocytes retain a memory of the invader, the next exposure to this invader prompts a specific and immediate response. This ability of the immune system to develop and maintain a highly effective and specific response is the basis of vaccination.

When activated, natural killer cells, another subset of lymphocytes, have the ability to select and destroy abnormal host cells (i.e. malignant cells) and destroy intracellular pathogens such as viruses by destroying the cells harboring them. Other T lymphocytes, the T-suppressor lymphocytes, have the ability to down-regulate and turn off the immune response once an invader is repelled. The macrophages and lymphocytes interact with one another by secreting soluble products known as cytokines. There are many unique cytokines, and presumably others remain to be discovered.

IMMUNE FUNCTION CHANGES AND RISKS OF INFECTION

The aging process is associated with changes in immune function, particularly in those functions directed or carried out by the lymphocyte system (Schwab & Callegari 1992, Adler & Nagel 1994, Miller 1999, Allman & Miller 2005, Gomez et al 2005, Goronzy & Weyand 2005, Hodes 2005, Sebastian et al 2005). Although some research has suggested that the aging process itself may be the result of the immune system turning against the body, at present such a theory remains speculative. Most observations of age-associated altered immune function concern failure of or deficiency in function. The increased incidence of malignancies results partly from a loss of the immune system's surveillance and eradication of abnormal cells as they arise. Aging is also associated with increased activity or loss of control of some aspects of the immune system. For example, the incidence of monoclonal gammopathies (multiple myeloma) rises in the older population and the frequency of both antiidiotypic (antibodies directed against other antibodies) and autoimmune antibodies increases as a person ages. Long before our understanding of the intricacies of the cellular immune system and the specialized properties of its various components began, it was known that the thymus gland progressively atrophies until it becomes virtually a vestigial organ in later life (Adler & Nagel 1994, Miller 1999). Investigation of immune function suggests that the most dramatic changes occur within the cellular arm of the immune system (Akbar & Fletcher 2005, Allman & Miller 2005, Gomez et al 2005, Goronzy & Weyand 2005, Hodes 2005, Sadighi Akh & Miller 2005). B lymphocytes, the cells involved in the production of antibodies ('humoral immunity'), function relatively well, even in the very old. Specific changes in immune function that have been described as being associated with aging are listed in Box 11.1.

Box 11.1   Changes in immune function associated with aging

- Atrophy of the thymus with decreased production of thymic hormones
- Decreased in vitro responsiveness to interleukin-2
- Decreased cell proliferation in response to mitogenic stimulation
- Decreased cell-mediated cytotoxicity
- Enhanced cellular sensitivity to prostaglandin E_2
- Increased synthesis of antiidiotypic antibodies
- Increase in autoimmune antibodies
- Increased incidence of serum monoclonal immuno-proteins
- Decreased representation of peripheral blood B lymphocytes in men
- Diminished delayed hypersensitivity
- Enhanced ability to synthesize interferon-γ, interleukin-6, tumor necrosis factor-α

Clinically, the aging individual is at an increased risk both for infection and for a negative outcome of infection. The origin of some of this risk may be in diminished immune function. For example, the incidence and mortality rate of pneumococcal pneumonia, low throughout adolescence and most of the adult years, rises dramatically in people over the age of 65. The consequences of influenza are also enhanced in the elderly, with a dramatically increased risk of death. Primary varicella (chickenpox) is a dreaded infection in older people because of the potential for severe pneumonitis and encephalitis, which often have fatal outcomes in this population. The elderly are also at risk for reactivation of latent infections. For example, varicella zoster and reactivation tuberculosis are seen with increased frequency in older people. Conversely, there is some evidence that the senescence of the immune system correlates more closely with the quantity of comorbid diseases rather than with chronological age (Castle et al 2005).

RISKS OF INFECTION RELATED TO OTHER PATHOLOGIES

Not all of the increased risks of infection are attributable to changes in immune function. Indeed, many diseases afflicting the elderly result in increased vulnerability to infection that is unrelated to changes in the immune system. For example, the pulmonary edema of congestive heart failure is frequently a contributing factor to the development of pneumonia, presumably because the edema enhances bacterial growth and compromises clearance mechanisms. Peripheral vascular disease causes ischemic breakdown of skin and soft tissue, allowing direct invasion of microbes while impairing the blood flow necessary to carry host defenses to the site of invasion. Another example is a cerebrovascular accident, which leaves the patient with an impaired cough mechanism and malfunctioning epiglottic closure, with an attendant risk for aspiration. What is usually transient colonization with aspirated oral bacterial flora may progress, if not cleared, to cause bronchitis or pneumonia. Malignancies, which occur more frequently in the elderly, increase the risk of infection by a number of mechanisms. They can interfere with the cleansing effects of body fluids by interrupting normal flow – as seen with endobronchial carcinoma or laryngeal carcinoma, for example – thereby setting the stage for entrapment of bacteria normally swept away by mucus flow. Malignancies also frequently erode normal cutaneous or mucosal barriers, providing a direct invasion route into soft tissues and body cavities. The inanition that frequently accompanies metastatic malignancy is, moreover, associated with impaired cellular immunity.

All of these diseases may contribute indirectly to the risk of infection simply because the patient is hospitalized in a facility where the opportunity of acquiring a virulent multidrug-resistant pathogen is much increased.

IMPLICATIONS OF IMMUNE DYSFUNCTION

As noted above, the major clinical significance of immune dysfunction in the elderly is an increased risk of infection and, all too frequently, severe morbidity when an infection occurs. A number of infections are recognized to occur more frequently in the elderly (Box 11.2). The implications for health professionals are obvious. Because infections may rapidly overwhelm the immune defenses and initiate an irrevocable course, clinicians must monitor patients closely. Early warning signals may be subtle: a sensation of being unwell, a change in mentation (lethargy, confusion), a decrease in appetite or a diminution of physical activity. Such clinical signs and

---

Box 11.2   Infections that occur with increased frequency among the elderly

- Pneumonia
- Tuberculosis
- Bacteremia
- Infectious diarrhea
- Septic arthritis
- Urinary tract infection
- Skin and soft-tissue infections
- Infective endocarditis
- Meningitis

symptoms of infection may be muted in the older patient; crucial clues may be easily overlooked or attributed to other conditions. Fever, the hallmark of infection, may be subdued or even replaced by a drop in temperature in the older patient and chills may be absent. Caregivers should pay attention to subtle clinical hints and investigate by questioning and examining the patient followed by the use of laboratory and radiographic studies as appropriate. Because the elderly patient frequently has other diseases that may cause these signs and symptoms, a timely and accurate diagnosis is often difficult to establish.

Therapeutic intervention

Because bacteriological analysis to detect the causative pathogen takes hours or days, empiric treatment is frequently necessary to avoid undue morbidity and mortality associated with serious infections. The decision to initiate empiric anti-microbial treatment is often problematic when the presence of an infection has not yet been proven and the causative organism is not known. To diagnose and choose treatment, the clinician must weigh all available evidence, searching carefully for clues at typical sites of infection: respiratory tract, urinary tract, pressure sores on the skin, catheter insertion sites, and the biliary and gastrointestinal tracts. If a decision is taken to initiate empiric treatment, knowledge of a patient's prior infections and recent experiences with nosocomial pathogens within the facility will help the physician choose appropriate antibiotics. This process of determining the probable causative organism and starting empiric treatment is particularly difficult in the extended-care facility and the homecare setting and when the patient is being transferred between different treatment facilities. Effective and timely communication among the healthcare team members is a necessity if patients in such circumstances are to receive optimal care. As in all areas of healthcare, prevention is greatly preferred to treatment. Of primary importance is attention to the seemingly mundane details of daily care to avoid situations that are known to place a patient at risk for infection. Malnutrition exacerbates the frailty of the elderly, so monitoring the patient's nutritional needs and intervening to ensure that they are met are important. Such nutritional intervention may require no more than assistance with meals. Although nutritional supplements are commercially available, balanced meals prepared to accommodate the patient's taste and any impairment of mastication are usually sufficient. Measures to avoid skin breakdown should also be followed meticulously: for example, frequent turning of the immobile patient, cleaning of skin soiled by incontinence and attending to bowel and urinary habits to minimize incontinence. Discontinuation of unnecessary medical devices such as intravenous catheters and urinary catheters also eliminates two of the greatest iatrogenic sources of serious infection.

Basic to the prevention of nosocomial infections is strict attention to good infection control practices that are universally recommended but seldom scrupulously followed. In many centers, the problem of nosocomial spread of pathogens has been exacerbated by the emergence of multidrug-resistant pathogens, a phenomenon likely to continue in the future. Outbreaks of infection within hospitals and nursing homes caused by methicillin-resistant *Staphylococcus aureus* and multidrug-resistant Enterobacteriaceae, streptococci and even *Mycobacterium tuberculosis* have been documented. However, most, if not all, outbreaks are avoidable.

Exercise and the immune system

It is clear that appropriate physical exercise is of benefit to the elderly, and there are data to suggest that exercise is beneficial to immune function (Drela et al 2004, Kohut et al 2005). What is not clear is whether this is a direct benefit of exercise or an indirect benefit through psychosocial factors (Kohut et al 2005). The exercise stimulus is clearly an important factor to consider. Natural killer cell activity has been shown to increase with 10 weeks of resistance training using three sets of 10 repetitions. The graded weight training, involving 10 different exercises, was performed on machines and used an intensity of one repetition maximum (1 RM) (McFarlin et al 2005). Regardless, it is easy to suggest that regular exercise, consistent with the cardiovascular and musculoskeletal constraints of the individual, is beneficial for the aging immune system as well as the global health of the elderly.

Vaccines

No discussion of preventive medicine for the elderly is complete without mention of vaccination against two important pathogens: influenza and *S. pneumoniae*. Influenza vaccines are updated yearly to include antigens from the most recent endemic strains and are typically given in the autumn to elicit antibodies in the recipient in time for the winter influenza epidemic. The pneumococcal vaccine, containing type-specific antigens from 23 of the most prevalent *S. pneumoniae* capsular types, is recommended for all individuals over the age of 65.

The pneumococcal vaccine is not without its critics, however. In elderly recipients, particularly among subgroups with liver, renal and other chronic diseases, response is suboptimal. Moreover, the component antigens can vary considerably in their immunogenicity, with some eliciting very low antibody responses or none at all and others producing predictably good antibody titers. The emergence of penicillin-resistant *S. pneumoniae* in the past decade has, however, enhanced the potential benefit of vaccination against this pathogen. Because the antibody levels produced tend to decrease with time, revaccination every 5–10 years is recommended.

CONCLUSION

Changes in the immune systems of elderly people add to the complexity and challenge of providing appropriate healthcare to the elderly. Comorbidities further complicate this problem. Because an elevation in body temperature is not always seen, clinicians and care providers must be aware of the subtle manifestations of infection such as a sense of being unwell, lethargy, confusion and diminished appetite or physical activity. The choice of medical intervention is not always obvious, but good nutrition and infection control are necessary. Vaccinations are helpful, although their use is not without controversy.

References

Adler WH, Nagel JE 1994 Clinical immunology and aging. In: Hazzard WRY, Bierman EL, Blass JP et al (eds) Principles of Geriatric Medicine and Gerontology, 3rd edn. McGraw-Hill, New York

Akbar AN, Fletcher JM 2005 Memory T cell homeostasis and senescence during aging. Curr Opin Immunol 17:480–485

Allman D, Miller JP 2005 B-cell development and receptor diversity during aging. Curr Opin Immunol 17:463–467

Castle SC, Uyemura K, Rafi A et al 2005 Comorbidity is a better predictor of impaired immunity than chronological age in older adults. J Am Geriatr Soc 53:1565–1569

Drela N, Kozdron E, Szczypiorski P 2004 Moderate exercise may attenuate some aspects of immunosenescence. BMC Geriatr 4:8

Gomez CR, Boehmer ED, Kovacs EJ 2005 The aging innate immune system. Curr Opin Immunol 17:457–462

Goronzy JJ, Weyand CM 2005 T-cell development and receptor diversity during aging. Curr Opin Immunol 17:468–475

Hodes RJ 2005 Aging and the immune system. Curr Opin Immunol 17:455–456

Kohut ML, Lee W, Martin A et al 2005 The exercise-induced enhancement of influenza immunity is mediated in part by improvements in psychosocial factors in older adults. Brain Behav Immun 19:357–366

McFarlin BK, Flynn M, Phillips M et al 2005 Chronic resistance training improves natural killer cell activity in older women. J Gerontol A Biol Sci Med Sci 60:1315–1318

Miller RA 1999 Aging and immune function. In: Paul WE (ed) Fundamental Immunology. Lippincott-Raven, Philadelphia, PA, p 947–966

Sadighi Akh AA, Miller RA 2005 Signal transduction in the aging immune system. Curr Opin Immunol 17:486–491

Schwab EP, Callegari PE 1992 How aging impacts the immune system. Intern Med 13:34–41

Sebastian C, Espia M, Serra M et al 2005 Macrophaging: a cellular and molecular review. Immunobiology 210:121–126

Chapter **12**

Pharmacology considerations for the aging individual

Charles D. Ciccone

INTRODUCTION

Elderly people receiving physical rehabilitation services are commonly taking medications to help resolve acute and chronic ailments. These medications are intended to improve the patient's health but they frequently cause side effects that can have a negative impact on the patient's response to physical rehabilitation. Older adults are more susceptible to adverse effects of drugs because of many factors, including excessive drug use, declining function in various physiological systems and altered drug metabolism and excretion.

In particular, age-related physiological changes in liver and kidney function can profoundly affect drug metabolism and excretion (Mangoni & Jackson 2004). Most medications are metabolized and inactivated to some extent in the liver, and age-related decreases in liver size, hepatic blood flow and enzymatic capacity can impair the body's ability to metabolize these medications. Likewise, the kidneys are the primary site of drug excretion, and progressive decreases in renal mass, renal blood flow, filtration capacity and nephron function can reduce the body's ability to remove various drugs and their metabolites from the bloodstream. Because of these age-related physiological changes, the body is not able to eliminate drugs in a timely and predictable manner, thus leading to drug accumulation and an increased risk of adverse drug reactions.

Deficiencies in other physiological systems may also increase the likelihood of adverse drug reactions in older adults (Turnheim & Alexopoulos 2004). For example, an older adult with impaired balance reactions will be more likely to fall when taking hypnotic agents and other drugs that impair balance. An older patient who has cognitive deficits might become more confused when taking opioids and other medications that affect cognition. Hence, problems related to a decline in any physiological system will almost certainly be magnified by drugs that adversely affect that system.

Nonetheless, older adults often rely on medications to help improve their health and quality of life. It follows that therapists should be aware of the primary medications being taken by their elderly clients and how those medications can affect patients' participation in rehabilitation.

Some of the primary medications used to treat conditions commonly seen in older adults are addressed here. This discussion is not meant to be all-inclusive but should help clinicians to recognize and understand how medications taken by the elderly can affect their response to rehabilitation.

TREATMENT OF PAIN AND INFLAMMATION

Opioid analgesics

Opioid (narcotic) medications such as morphine and meperidine (Table 12.1) are powerful analgesics that bind to neuronal receptors in the spinal cord and brain. These medications reduce synaptic activity in pain-transmitting pathways, thereby decreasing pain perception. Common side effects of opioids include sedation, respiratory depression, constipation and postural hypotension. Therapists should also be aware that older adults are more susceptible to opioid-induced psychotropic reactions such as confusion, anxiety, hallucinations and euphoria/dysphoria (Wilder-Smith 2005). Opioids can also increase the risk of falls in older adults, by either increasing sedation or causing dizziness from orthostatic hypotension. These reactions are especially common in elderly patients recovering from surgery, perhaps because of opioid side effects being magnified by the residual effects of the general anesthetic and because of the disorientation and wooziness that often occur after surgery.

Non-opioid analgesics

Nonsteroidal antiinflammatory drugs (NSAIDs) are the primary group of non-opioid analgesics. NSAIDs include aspirin, ibuprofen and similar agents (see Table 12.1) and these drugs are often effective in treating mild to moderate pain. These medications actually produce four clinically important effects: decreased pain, decreased inflammation, decreased fever and decreased blood coagulation. There is also considerable evidence that NSAIDs may decrease the risk of certain cancers, including colorectal cancer. All of these effects are mediated through inhibition of the biosynthesis of lipid compounds called prostaglandins. Certain prostaglandins mediate painful sensations by increasing the nociceptive effects of bradykinin.

Table 12.1 Analgesic and antiinflammatory medications

Category	Common examples	
	Generic name	Trade name
Opioid analgesics	Hydromorphone	Dilaudid
	Meperidine (pethidine)	Demerol
	Morphine	Many trade names
	Oxycodone	OxyContin, others
	Propoxyphene	Darvon
Nonopioid analgesics NSAIDs	Aspirin	Many trade names
	Ibuprofen	Advil, Motrin, others
	Ketoprofen	Orudis
	Ketorolac	Toradol
	Naproxen	Aleve, others
	Piroxicam	Feldene
COX-2 inhibitors	Celecoxib	Celebrex
Acetaminophen	–	Tylenol, others
Glucocorticoids	Cortisone	Cortone, others
	Dexamethasone	Decadron
	Hydrocortisone	Many trade names
	Methylprednisone	Medrol
	Prednisone	Deltasone, others

COX-2, cyclooxygenase type 2; NSAIDS, nonsteroidal antiinflammatory drugs.

NSAID-mediated inhibition of prostaglandin synthesis therefore helps reduce painful sensations in a variety of clinical conditions. The primary problem associated with NSAIDs is gastrointestinal distress, including gastric irritation and ulceration. These medications may also cause damage to the liver and kidneys, especially in older adults who have preexisting hepatic or renal dysfunction.

In addition to traditional NSAIDs, newer drugs known as COX-2 inhibitors have been developed (Savage 2005). These drugs are so named because they inhibit the cyclooxygenase (COX)-2 enzyme that synthesizes prostaglandins during pathological conditions. The COX-2 enzyme synthesizes prostaglandins that cause pain, inflammation and other harmful effects, whereas the COX-1 enzyme synthesizes prostaglandins that are beneficial and often help protect various tissues and organs. Whereas traditional NSAIDs (e.g. aspirin, ibuprofen) inhibit both isoforms of the COX enzyme, the COX-2 drugs are designed to inhibit only the production of harmful prostaglandins (reducing pain and inflammation) while sparing the production of beneficial prostaglandins in the stomach, kidneys, and other organs and tissues. Indeed, the incidence of gastric problems is lower with COX-2 drugs, and some older adults have used these drugs successfully for extended periods to treat osteoarthritis and similar problems with minimal side effects. The COX-2 drugs, however, may also produce serious cardiovascular problems including heart attack and stroke in susceptible patients. Hence, these drugs should be avoided in those at risk for cardiovascular disease (Savage 2005). Currently, celecoxib (Celebrex) is the only COX-2 drug that remains on the market, and future studies will be needed to determine if this drug and newer COX-2 inhibitors can be used safely in older adults who have an acceptable risk profile.

Acetaminophen (paracetamol), the active ingredient in Tylenol and other products, is another type of non-opioid analgesic. This agent is different from the NSAIDs in that it does not produce any appreciable antiinflammatory or anticoagulant effects. Likewise, acetaminophen does not produce gastrointestinal irritation, but this medication can cause severe hepatotoxicity in those with liver disease or after an overdose.

Antiinflammatory medications

Treatment of inflammation consists primarily of the NSAIDs and antiinflammatory steroids. As indicated earlier, NSAIDs inhibit the synthesis of prostaglandins and this inhibition reduces the proinflammatory effects of certain prostaglandins. NSAIDs tend to be effective in treating a variety of conditions that exhibit mild to moderate inflammation. More severe inflammatory conditions often require the use of antiinflammatory steroids known as glucocorticoids. Medications such as prednisolone and cortisone (see Table 12.1) inhibit a number of the cellular and chemical aspects of the inflammatory response, often producing a dramatic decrease in the symptoms of inflammation. However, glucocorticoids cause many severe side effects including breakdown of collagenous tissues, hypertension, glucose intolerance, gastric ulcer, glaucoma and adrenocortical suppression. Tissue breakdown (catabolism) can cause severe muscle wasting and osteoporosis, especially in older people who may already be somewhat debilitated.

PSYCHOTROPIC MEDICATIONS

Antianxiety drugs

Treatment of anxiety has traditionally consisted of benzodiazepines, including diazepam and similar agents (Table 12.2) (Flint 2005). These drugs work by increasing the inhibitory effects of γ-aminobutyric acid (GABA), an endogenous neurotransmitter, in areas of the brain that control mood and behavior. The primary side effect of benzodiazepine agents is sedation. These drugs may also cause tolerance and physical dependence when used continually for prolonged periods (more than 6 weeks). Benzodiazepines also have extremely long metabolic half-lives in older adults, which means that it takes a very long time to metabolize and eliminate these drugs. As a result, benzodiazepines can accumulate in older patients and reach toxic levels, shown by symptoms of confusion, slurred speech, dyspnea, incoordination and pronounced weakness.

A newer type of non-benzodiazepine antianxiety medication has been developed, which is known as buspirone (Buspar) (Flint 2005). This agent, chemically classified as an azapirone, increases serotonin activity in the brain, thus decreasing symptoms of anxiety. Buspirone has been used increasingly in older adults because this agent does not appear to produce sedation or cause tolerance and physical dependence. However, it may take longer to exert its antianxiety effects, and may not be as effective in treating severe anxiety compared with the benzodiazepines.

Finally, certain antidepressants such as paroxetine (Paxil) and venlafaxine (Effexor) may reduce anxiety even in people who are not depressed (Flint 2005). These drugs affect the function of amine neurotransmitters that are important for mood and behavior (see below), and they may provide an effective alternative for older adults who do not respond adequately to more traditional antianxiety agents.

Antidepressants

Several different types and categories of antidepressant medication exist (see Table 12.2) (Alexopoulos 2005). These drugs all share the common goal of trying to increase activity at synapses in the brain that use amine neurotransmitters, including catecholamines

Table 12.2 Psychotropic medications

Category	Common examples	
	Generic name	Trade name
Antianxiety drugs		
Benzodiazepines	Alprazolam	Xanax
	Chlordiazepoxide	Librium, others
	Diazepam	Valium
	Lorazepam	Ativan
Azapirones	Buspirone	Buspar
Antidepressants		
Tricyclics	Amitriptyline	Elavil, others
	Doxepin	Sinequan, others
	Imipramine	Tofranil, others
	Nortriptyline	Pamelor, others
MAO inhibitors	Isocarboxazid	Marplan
	Tranylcypromine	Parnate
Second-generation drugs	Buproprion	Wellbutrin
	Citalopram	Celexa
	Fluoxetine[a]	Prozac
	Maprotiline	Ludiomil
	Paroxetine[a]	Paxil
	Sertraline[a]	Zoloft
Antipsychotics	Chlorpromazine	Thorazine
	Clozapine[b]	Clozaril
	Haloperidol	Haldol
	Prochlorperazine	Compazine, others
	Risperdone[b]	Risperdal
	Thioridazine	Mellaril

[a]Selective serotonin-reuptake inhibitors.
[b]Atypical antipsychotics.
MAO, monoamine oxidase.

(norepinephrine), 5-hydroxytryptamine (serotonin) and dopamine. Although the details remain unclear, depression is thought to be caused by a defect in the release of, or sensitivity to, these amine neurotransmitters in specific areas of the brain that control mood (i.e. the limbic system). Most antidepressants are nonselective and cause increased activity at synapses that use norepinephrine, serotonin and dopamine. However, certain antidepressants are more selective for serotonin pathways than other amine synapses. These drugs, also known as selective serotonin-reuptake inhibitors (SSRIs), include fluoxetine (Prozac), sertraline (Zoloft) and paroxetine (Paxil). There is still considerable debate whether SSRIs are more effective than their nonselective counterparts, but these drugs may produce a more acceptable side effect profile in older adults (see below).

The primary side effects of traditional (nonselective) antidepressants are sedation, postural hypotension and the results of decreased acetylcholine function (anticholinergic effects), such as dry mouth, urinary retention, constipation, tachycardia and confusion. These side effects are often much more pronounced in older people because of age-related declines in various physiological systems combined with the fact that some of these drugs have much longer metabolic half-lives in older adults. For example, the elimination half-life of amitriptyline (a traditional nonselective antidepressant) is normally around 16h in young individuals, whereas it may be twice as long (31h) in healthy older adults. More selective agents such as the SSRIs

tend to have fewer sedative, hypotensive and anticholinergic effects, and these drugs may therefore be used preferentially in older adults. Another primary concern about antidepressants is that there is typically a 1- to 2-week time lag between initiation of drug treatment and improvement of depression, and some patients may need up to 6 weeks before receiving the full benefit from these drugs. Depression may actually worsen in some patients during this period, and therapists should be especially careful to note any increase in depressive symptoms while waiting for these drugs to take effect.

Antipsychotics

Psychosis seems to be caused by increased activity in certain dopamine pathways of the brain (Masand 2004). As a result, antipsychotic medications block postsynaptic receptors in these pathways to help normalize dopaminergic influence. Common antipsychotics are listed in Table 12.2. These agents typically cause side effects such as sedation, postural hypotension, anticholinergic effects and movement disorders including tardive dyskinesia, pseudoparkinsonism, severe restlessness (akathisia) and various other dystonias and dyskinesias. Tardive dyskinesia is characterized by oral–facial movements such as extending the tongue, grinding the jaw, puffing the cheeks, and various other fragmented movements of the neck, trunk and extremities. This problem is often regarded as being the most serious side effect of antipsychotic medications because symptoms of tardive dyskinesia may take several months to disappear or may remain indefinitely after the antipsychotic drug is discontinued. Some of the newer antipsychotics are regarded as 'atypical' because they are as effective as traditional agents but pose a lower risk of tardive dyskinesia and other side effects and are better tolerated; hence, these atypical antipsychotics may be used preferentially in older adults (Masand 2004). Nonetheless, therapists should be cognizant of any aberrant movement patterns in patients taking antipsychotic medications, especially symptoms of tardive dyskinesia.

NEUROLOGICAL DISORDERS

Parkinson's disease

The motor symptoms of Parkinson's disease (bradykinesia, rigidity, resting tremor) are related to the loss of dopami-nergic neurons in the basal ganglia (Nutt & Wooten 2005). The primary method of drug treatment is levodopa (L-dopa), which is the metabolic precursor to dopamine. Although dopamine will not cross the blood–brain barrier, levodopa will enter brain tissues where it is subsequently converted to dopamine, thus helping to restore the influence of dopamine in the basal ganglia. Levodopa is often administered with carbidopa, a drug that prevents premature conversion of levodopa to dopamine in the peripheral circulation. Combining levodopa with carbidopa in preparations such as Sinemet allows levodopa to reach the brain before undergoing conversion to dopamine.

Levodopa is associated with several side effects including gastrointestinal irritation, hypotension and psychotic-like symptoms. Other movement problems, including dyskinesias and dystonias, may also occur, especially at higher dosages. However, the most devastating problems are typically related to a decrease in long-term effectiveness; patients who respond well to levodopa initially, commonly experience progressively diminishing benefits after 4–5 years of continual use. This phenomenon is probably related to a progressive increase in the severity of Parkinson's disease; that is, drug therapy cannot adequately resolve the motor symptoms because of the advanced degeneration of dopaminergic neurons in the basal ganglia. Helping patients and their families to deal with the physical as well

Table 12.3 Neurological medications

Category	Examples	Rationale for use
Treatment of Parkinson's disease		
Dopamine precursors	Levodopa (Sinemet)[a]	Are converted to dopamine in the brain; help resolve dopamine deficiency
Anticholinergic drugs	Benztropine (Cogentin), biperiden (Akineton)	Normalize acetylcholine imbalance caused by dopamine loss
COMT inhibitors	Entacapone (Comtan), tolcapone (Tasmar)	Prevent levodopa breakdown in bloodstream
Dopamine agonists	Bromocriptine (Parlodel), pergolide (Permax)	Directly stimulate dopamine receptors in brain
MAO$_B$ inhibitors	Selegiline (Eldepryl)	Decrease dopamine breakdown in brain
Antiseizure medications		
Barbiturates	Phenobarbital (Solfoton), mephobarbital (Mebaral)	Increase inhibitory effects of GABA in brain
Benzodiazapines	Clonazepam (Klonopin), clorazepate (Tranxene)	Increase inhibitory effects of GABA in brain
Carboxylic acids	Valproic acid (Depakene)	May increase GABA concentrations in brain
Hydantoins	Phenytoin (Dilantin), ethotoin (Peganone)	Decrease sodium entry into hyperexcitable neurons
Iminostilbenes	Carbamazepine (Tegretol)	Similar to hydantoins
Succinimides	Ethosuximide (Zarontin), methsuximide (Celontin)	May decrease calcium entry into hyperexcitable neurons
Second generation antiseizure drugs	Lamotrigine (Lamictal), gabapentin (Neurontin), tiagabine (Gabitril)	Various effects; generally either increase effects of inhibitory neurotransmitters (e.g. GABA) or decrease the effects of excitatory neurotransmitters (e.g. glutamate, aspartate)
Treatment of Alzheimer's dementia		
Cholinergic stimulants	Donepezil (Aricept), galantamine (Reminyl), rivastigmine (Exelon), tacrine (Cognex)	Increase acetylcholine influence in the brain

COMT, catechol-O-methyltransferase; GABA, γ-aminobutyric acid; MAO$_B$, monoamine oxidase type B.
[a]Sinemet is the trade name for levodopa combined with carbidopa.

as psychological impact of decreased levodopa effectiveness is one of the more difficult tasks that therapists face.

Several other types of medications are used as supplemental drug therapy in Parkinson's disease (Table 12.3). These agents are typically used to supplement levodopa therapy or they serve as the primary agent when levodopa is poorly tolerated or no longer effective. A common strategy is to combine several agents in low to moderate doses to obtain optimal benefits while avoiding the excessive side effects that would occur with large amounts of any single drug.

Seizures

Some of the medications commonly used to control seizure activity are listed in Table 12.3. These agents act on the brain to selectively reduce excitability in neurons that initiate seizures (Bergey 2004); however, it is often difficult to reduce excitation in these neurons without producing some degree of general inhibition throughout the brain. This is especially true in the older patient who has had a previous cerebral injury such as a cerebrovascular accident or closed head injury. As a result, older patients taking antiseizure medications are especially prone to side effects such as sedation, fatigue, weakness, incoordination, ataxia and visual disturbances (e.g. blurred vision and diplopia) (Bergey 2004). Therapists should pay particular attention to patients taking antiseizure medication because they are in a position to help determine whether dosages are too high (as indicated by excessive side effects) or too low (as evidenced by an increase in seizure activity).

Alzheimer's disease

Donepezil (Aricept), tacrine (Cognex) and several other medications (see Table 12.3) were developed fairly recently to help improve cognition and intellectual function in patients with Alzheimer's disease (Potyk 2005). These drugs are cholinergic stimulants; they decrease acetylcholine breakdown at synapses in the brain, thereby helping to maintain acetylcholine influence in areas of the brain that are undergoing the neuronal degeneration associated with Alzheimer's disease. These drugs do not cure Alzheimer's disease, but preliminary evidence indicates that they may help patients retain more intellectual and functional ability during the early stages of the disease. The primary side effects associated with these drugs include loss of appetite and gastrointestinal distress (diarrhea, nausea and vomiting).

CARDIOVASCULAR DRUGS

Antihypertensive medications

Several drug categories (Table 12.4) are used to treat high blood pressure in older adults and reduce the chance of hypertensive-related incidents such as stroke, myocardial infarction and kidney disease (Dickerson & Gibson 2005). Angiotensin-converting enzyme (ACE) inhibitors prevent the formation of angiotensin II, which is a powerful vasoconstrictor and stimulant of vascular smooth muscle growth. Agents such as alpha blockers, beta blockers and other sympatholytic drugs decrease sympathetic nervous system stimulation of the heart and vasculature, thereby decreasing myocardial contraction force and peripheral vascular resistance. Calcium-channel blockers reduce myocardial contractility and vascular smooth muscle contraction by limiting calcium entry into these tissues. Diuretics increase sodium and water excretion, thereby decreasing blood pressure by reducing fluid volume in the vascular system. Certain direct-acting vasodilators (see Table 12.4) reduce vascular resistance by inhibiting vascular smooth muscle contraction.

Table 12.4 Cardiovascular medications

Category	Examples	Rationale for use
Antihypertensive drugs		
ACE inhibitors	Captopril (Capoten), enalapril (Vasotec)	Decreases angiotensin II synthesis; promotes vasodilation and increases vascular compliance
Alpha blockers	Doxazosin (Cardura), prazosin (Minipress)	Promotes vasodilation by decreasing sympathetic stimulation of vasculature
Beta blockers	Metoprolol (Lopressor), nadolol (Corgard), propranolol (Inderal)	Decreases myocardial contractility by decreasing sympathetic stimulation of the heart
Calcium-channel blockers	Diltiazem (Cardizem), nifedipine (Procardia, others), verapamil (Calan, others)	Promotes vasodilation and decreased myocardial contractility by limiting calcium entry into vasculature and heart
Diuretics	Chlorothiazide (Diuril), furosemide (Lasix), spironolactone (Aldactone)	Decreases intravascular fluid volume; reduce workload on heart
Vasodilators	Hydralazine (Apresoline), minoxidil (Loniten)	Promotes vasodilation by inhibiting contraction of vascular smooth muscle
Treatment of congestive heart failure		
Digitalis glycosides	Digoxin (Lanoxin)	Increases myocardial contractility by increasing calcium entry into heart muscle
Others	Diuretics, ACE inhibitors, beta blockers, vasodilators	See above
Treatment of hyperlipidemia		
Statins	Atorvastatin (Lipitor), fluvastatin (Lescol), lovastatin (Mevachor), pravastatin (Pravachol), simvastatin (Zocor),	Decreases total cholesterol, LDL-cholesterol, and triglyceride levels
Fibric acids	Clofibrate (Abitrate, Atromid), gemfibrozil (Lopid)	Primarily decreases triglyceride levels; may also decrease LDL breakdown
Others	Cholestyramine (Questran), niacin (Nicotinex, others), probuchol (Lorelco)	Decreases total cholesterol

LDL, low-density lipoprotein.

Elderly people with hypertension are treated routinely with diuretic agents because these drugs are fairly safe and well tolerated. ACE inhibitors have also been used increasingly in older patients because these agents reduce blood pressure and prevent adverse structural changes in the heart and vasculature. In contrast, sympatholytics and vasodilators tend to produce a variety of unfavorable side effects in older patients so these drugs are typically used only in severe cases. Calcium-channel blockers can also be used to treat hypertension in older adults, but the short-acting forms of these drugs should be avoided because they may decrease blood pressure too rapidly and increase the risk of myocardial infarction in certain patients. Hence, sustained- or continuous-release versions of the calcium-channel blockers should be used preferentially in older patients with hypertension.

Antihypertensive drugs produce various side effects, depending on the specific agent; however, it is important that therapists are aware that hypotension and postural hypotension are always possible whenever blood pressure is reduced pharmacologically. Blood pressure may fall by more than 10–20 mmHg, especially when an older patient sits or stands up suddenly. Likewise, physical therapy interventions that cause extensive peripheral vasodilation (e.g. warm water in the Hubbard tank or therapeutic pool) must be used very cautiously because these interventions add to the hypotensive drug effects and produce dangerously low blood pressure in older adults. Finally, some antihypertensive agents, for example beta blockers, blunt the cardiac response to exercise and this effect may limit physical work capacity during activities that require high cardiac output, such as climbing stairs and exercise training.

Treatment of congestive heart failure

Congestive heart failure (CHF) occurs commonly in older adults and is characterized by a progressive decline in myocardial pumping ability (Rich 2005). The primary medications used to treat CHF are the digitalis glycosides such as digoxin (see Table 12.4). These agents increase calcium entry into myocardial tissues, thereby increasing contractile force. Digitalis drugs often produce temporary hemodynamic improvements that decrease the symptoms of CHF, but these agents do not alter the progression of the disease or decrease the rather high morbidity and mortality rates associated with heart failure. These agents have a small safety margin and can accumulate rapidly in the bloodstream causing toxicity in older patients. Digitalis toxicity is associated with symptoms such as gastrointestinal distress, confusion, blurred vision and cardiac arrhythmias. Therapists should be alert for these symptoms because digitalis-induced arrhythmias can be quite severe or fatal.

Because of the problems related to digitalis, other medications have been used alone or with digitalis drugs to help treat patients with CHF. Diuretics and vasodilators have been used to decrease the workload on the failing heart by reducing fluid volume or decreasing vascular resistance respectively. More recently, ACE inhibitors have been recognized as being very beneficial in patients with CHF. These agents decrease angiotensin II-mediated vasoconstriction and vascular hypertrophy so that cardiac workload is reduced. Unlike digitalis drugs, ACE inhibitors appear to improve the prognosis of patients with heart failure and decrease the morbidity and mortality associated with CHF. ACE inhibitors are tolerated fairly well by older adults and have relatively minor side effects such as a mild allergic reaction (skin rash) or a dry persistent cough. As a result, ACE inhibitors continue to gain acceptance as a primary treatment of CHF in the elderly.

Treatment of hyperlipidemia

Several drugs have been introduced to the market to help improve plasma lipid profile and reduce the adverse effects of atherosclerosis on the cardiovascular system (Eimer & Stone 2004). The primary category of lipid-lowering drugs is the statins (see Table 12.4). Statin drugs inhibit an enzyme known as 3-hydroxy-3-methylglutaryl coenzyme A (HMG-CoA) that is responsible for synthesizing cholesterol in the body. This reduces endogenous cholesterol biosynthesis and also facilitates a number of other beneficial effects on plasma lipids (reduced low-density lipoproteins, reduced triglycerides). A second category of antihyperlipidemia agents is the fibric acids. Although the exact mechanism of their action is not known, fibric acids can reduce triglyceride levels and increase low-density lipoprotein breakdown. An eclectic group of other agents (e.g. niacin, probuchol) are also available, and these agents work in various ways to treat hyperlipidemia.

Drugs used to treat hyperlipidemia produce various side effects including gastrointestinal disturbances (nausea, cramping, diarrhea).

In rare cases, statins can also produce muscular pain, weakness and inflammation. This so-called 'statin-induced myopathy' can be quite severe in some people and even lead to breakdown of skeletal muscle tissues (rhabdomyolysis). Therefore, if muscle pain occurs spontaneously in older adults or any individual taking lipid-lowering drugs, clinicians should refer the patient back to the physician immediately to determine the source of the pain. If statin-induced myopathy is the suspected cause, the drug is usually discontinued and the patient is allowed several weeks to recover from the muscle damage before resuming exercise or other vigorous activities.

CONCLUSION

Medications often produce favorable as well as adverse responses in elderly patients receiving rehabilitation. Therapists must be aware of the types of medication commonly taken by older adults and of the possible side effects associated with these medications. Geriatric patients are more susceptible to adverse drug effects and clinicians often play an important role in helping to identify problematic drug responses in the elderly. Likewise, therapists must be able to plan and modify rehabilitation strategies to capitalize on beneficial drug effects while minimizing or avoiding adverse effects.

References

Alexopoulos GS 2005 Depression in the elderly. Lancet 365:1961–1970

Bergey GK 2004 Initial treatment of epilepsy: special issues in treating the elderly. Neurology 63(suppl4):S40–48

Dickerson LM, Gibson MV 2005 Management of hypertension in older persons. Am Fam Physician 71:469–476

Eimer MJ, Stone NJ 2004 Evidence-based treatment of lipids in the elderly. Curr Atheroscler Rep 6:388–397

Flint AJ 2004 Generalised anxiety disorder in elderly patients: epidemiology, diagnosis and treatment options. Drugs Aging 22:101–114

Mangoni AA, Jackson SH 2004 Age-related changes in pharmacokinetics and pharmacodynamics: basic principles and practical applications. Br J Clin Pharmacol 57:6–14

Masand P 2004 Clinical effectiveness of atypical antipsychotics in elderly patients with psychosis. Eur Neuropsychopharmacol 14(suppl4):S461–469

Nutt JG, Wooten GF 2005 Clinical practice. Diagnosis and initial management of Parkinson's disease. N Engl J Med 353:1021–1027

Potyk D 2005 Treatments for Alzheimer disease. South Med J 98:628–635

Rich MW 2005 Office management of heart failure in the elderly. Am J Med 118:342–348

Savage R 2005 Cyclo-oxygenase-2 inhibitors: when should they be used in the elderly? Drugs Aging 22:185–200

Turnheim K Alexopoulos GS 2004 Drug therapy in the elderly. Exp Gerontol 39:1731–1738

Wilder-Smith OH 2005 Opioid use in the elderly. Eur J Pain 9:137–140

Chapter **13**

Laboratory assessment considerations for the aging individual

Christine Stabler

INTRODUCTION

Of all people who have ever lived to 65, over half are alive today. This striking statement has significant implications for the ongoing care of the elderly. Until now, little research has been conducted to evaluate the specific differences seen in the laboratory assessment of the older individual.

The Human Genome Project has finally been completed and the genetic basis of many biological functions has been identified; however, there is still much to learn about the biology of aging. It is known that cells and tissues have finite lifespans, and that growth and replication slows with age. However, it seems that many metabolic and biological functions remain constant over the lifetime of humans. Extrapolating these data from tissue to human is somewhat risky but it is accurate to do so in that aging itself is not marked by predictable biochemical changes. As people age they become more dissimilar, belying any stereotype of aging. Abrupt declines in system functions or marked changes in laboratory values should be attributed to the effects of disease, not normal aging. Finally, in the absence of disease or modifiable risk factors, the concept of healthy old age is absolutely valid. This chapter will review the laboratory differences between the well young adult and the well older individual and identify the known variations that occur in the absence of disease.

AGE-RELATED CONSIDERATIONS

Certain basic tenets apply when evaluating the elderly patient. In the process of aging, there is a decline in metabolic reserves in most organ systems, particularly in the cardiovascular, central nervous, gastrointestinal, hematopoietic and endocrine systems. Disease states will affect these vulnerable systems and become evident through laboratory value changes more rapidly than in younger adults. The fragile renal and hepatic systems of older adults are more susceptible to the effects of pharmacological agents and less tolerant of their side effects.

Normal laboratory values are derived from analyses of what are considered to be disease-free healthy populations (Huber et al 2006). Normal ranges are based on plus or minus two standard deviations from the mean value. The populations analyzed are heterogeneous for age and assume that aging individuals are the same as young adults. In many cases this may be true, but adequate reference ranges for laboratory testing in the elderly are generally lacking (Brigden & Heathcote 2000). Specific differences may be caused by the loss of certain biological reserves in those over 75, ironically the fastest growing segment of the elderly population. There are some predictable changes in laboratory values that occur with age which can be attributed to the normal aging process and not to disease states. Although there is significant variation from one individual to the next, these changes begin in the fourth decade of life and continue in a linear fashion into old age. With these exceptions, it is important to understand that most laboratory values in the elderly are similar to those of the healthy young.

In blood chemistry, the level of serum alkaline phosphatase, an enzyme found in bone and liver, increases with age. In men, it increases by up to 20% between the ages of 40 and 80. In women, slightly greater (0–37%) increases are seen. Serum albumin, traditionally a marker of nutrition, decreases slightly with age, despite adequate nutrition. Levels of serum prealbumin, a marker of current nutrition, should be equivalent to those of healthy young individuals (16–35 mg/dL) (Beck & Rosenthal 2002). In healthy individuals, serum magnesium decreases by about 15% between the ages of 30 and 80. Uric acid, a metabolic product of purine metabolism, increases slightly in normal aging individuals without disease. Other chemistries, such as serum electrolytes, serum bilirubin, liver enzymes and total proteins, remain unchanged with age (Feld & Schwabbauer 2000).

Lipid values also change with aging. In both women and men, total cholesterol levels increase by 30–40 mg/dL from 30 to 80 years of age. High-density lipoprotein (HDL), which is thought to be protective against atherosclerosis, increases by approximately 30% in men, but falls by up to 30% in women after menopause. This is attributed to the fact that, during the reproductive years, women have significantly higher levels of HDL than men because of the positive effect of estrogen on lipid production in the liver. Triglycerides, or blood fats, increase by 30–50% in both men and women from age 30 to 80. Serum levels of low-density lipoprotein (LDL), cholesterol molecules associated with accelerated atherosclerosis, are unchanged by age (McKnight 2002).

Fasting blood glucose levels increase by 2 mg/dL for each decade over the age of 30. Glucose metabolism, as measured by postprandial glucose levels, increases by up to 10 mg/dL for each decade over the age of 30. The risk of developing diabetes mellitus in individuals with insulin resistance caused by either genetic predilection or obesity increases with age.

Thyroid function is measured by serum triiodothyronine (T_3) and thyroxine (T_4) levels as well as levels of the pituitary hormone thyroid-stimulating hormone (TSH). Both TSH and T_3 levels may decrease slightly with age; a marked or progressive development of abnormal values indicates a disease state in the elderly. Serum T_4 levels remain unchanged in healthy elderly individuals.

Levels of serum creatinine do not change with age but less creatinine is produced and serum creatinine clearance, a measurement of renal function, declines by approximately 10 mL/min/1.73 m^2 for each decade over the age of 40. This phenomenon is explained by an age-related reduction in muscle mass in older individuals and by a decrease in protein by-products like creatinine being delivered to the kidney. Creatinine clearance can be calculated using a simple formula including the patient's serum creatinine value, gender, weight and age. Therefore, a normal serum creatinine level does not necessarily indicate normal renal function. Like creatinine, many drugs require renal clearance during metabolism; the age-related decline in renal function therefore necessitates adjustments in the dosing of these drugs. If too large a dose of medication is delivered to an even minimally impaired kidney, incomplete clearance occurs leaving potentially toxic metabolites in the kidney tissue (parenchyma). This can build up and further damage the kidney in a process called interstitial nephritis. This can be reversed with immediate withdrawal of the drug but, occasionally, permanent impairment can occur. The most common drugs responsible for this phenomenon are nonsteroidal antiinflammatory agents and antibiotics (Mantha 2005).

Hematological assessment of the elderly is achieved by white blood cell, hemoglobin, hematocrit, platelet and red blood cell counts. White blood cell counts may decrease slightly in the healthy older individual, whereas it is thought that hemoglobin, hematocrit and platelet counts should remain constant with aging. However, anemia is quite common in the elderly. It can be associated with many chronic diseases of aging such as arthritis, diabetes, renal impairment and bone marrow suppression by drugs and environmental chemicals. The World Health Organization has established norms of 13 g/dL or more for men and 12 g/dL for women for hemoglobin levels. In the elderly, some experts accept slightly lower values as normal (11.5 g/dL in men and 11 g/dL in women); if they remain constant, these values should not trigger extensive investigations.

Serum vitamin B12 levels may decrease with age (Park & Johnson 2006). Normal values in young adults are >190 pg/mL; levels of >150 pg/mL are acceptable in older adults in the absence of macrocytic changes to the red blood cells. Levels of vitamins C, E, D and B6 also show a slight age-related decrease.

The erythrocyte sedimentation rate (ESR) increases with age by approximately 22 mm/h from a norm of 20–25 mm/h to acceptable rates of up to 40 mm/h (in men) and 45 mm/h (in women) in the elderly. Levels greater than these are indicative of inflammatory or neoplastic conditions, which commonly occur in the geriatric population. Isolated increases in ESR are associated with increases in all causes of mortality. By definition, those with elevated ESRs have a higher death rate than age-matched individuals, regardless of the cause of death. Increases in ESR mandate workup for disease states. Normal values for serum C-reactive protein (CRP), another measurement of overall inflammation, remain unchanged, regardless of age.

The assessment of nutritional status has been studied extensively. In normal healthy ambulatory elderly individuals, serum protein and albumin levels are relatively unchanged with age. Nutritional status is assessed by the measurement of serum prealbumin and albumin levels, and indirectly by the numbers of white blood cells known as lymphocytes. Nutritional deficiencies, however, are common in the elderly and are caused by a multitude of factors including poor intake, a reduction in the acuity of taste, loss of appetite, depression, malabsorption from intestinal surgery or disease, and interactions with

Table 13.1 Selected normal laboratory values

	Normal values
Serum electrolytes	
Carbon dioxide	23–31 mEq/L
Chloride	98–107 mEq/L
Potassium	3.5–5.1 mEq/L
Sodium	136–145 mEq/L
Metabolic indicators	
Calcium	8.6–10.0 mg/dL
Cholesterol	240 mg/dL
Creatinine	0.8–1.5 mg/dL
Free thyroxine (T_4)	0.8–2.3 mg/dL
Glucose, fasting	80–110 mg/dL
Glucose, 2 h postprandial	80–110 mg/dL
Protein	
Total	6.0–8.0 g/dL
Albumin	3.5–5.5 g/dL
Globulin	2.0–3.5 g/dL

medications. It is important to consider nutritional status when caring for the elderly to maximize the potential for rehabilitation.

INDICATIONS FOR LABORATORY ASSESSMENT

When is laboratory assessment necessary? Routine laboratory testing should be determined by a patient's presentation, history and current use of medication. For example, a patient who must use diuretics requires a regular assessment of serum electrolytes, especially serum potassium. Simple alterations in diet, such as increased sodium levels, may cause potassium wasting in the elderly kidney and precipitate hypokalemia, a cause of muscle weakness. A patient on anticholesterol medication such as the 3-hydroxy-3-methylglutaryl coenzyme A (HMG-CoA) reductase inhibitors requires regular assessment of liver functions, whereas a patient receiving ticlopidine (Ticlid), a platelet inhibitor used in patients with transient ischemic attacks and stroke, requires a regular blood count.

Laboratory assessment is especially important in the evaluation of a patient who presents with new physical findings. The workup for dementia and delirium is particularly vital. Neurosyphilis, vitamin B_{12} and folic acid deficiencies, and acute infection can be detected by laboratory assessment and are precipitants of acute delirium and dementia. Radiological findings and other physical diagnostic tests such as lumbar puncture can quickly identify reversible causes for a patient's neurological changes.

Lethargy and altered levels of consciousness may also be presenting symptoms in a patient with abnormal laboratory values. Hypoglycemia, hyponatremia, acidosis, hypoxia and hypocalcemia are direct causes of central nervous system depression and can be identified through commonly used laboratory tests. Neuromuscular irritability, tetany and muscle spasms may present in severe cases of hypocalcemia.

A patient who presents with peripheral, sensory or motor deficits may be suffering from a disease that is identifiable by analysis of blood chemistries. Peripheral neuropathies are caused by diabetes mellitus (hyperglycemia), heavy metal ingestion and medication toxicities, and biochemical assessment can identify these problems.

Box 13.1   Effect of aging on laboratory values

Increased	Unchanged	Decreased
Serum copper	Hemoglobin	Creatinine clearance
Serum ferritin	RBC count	Serum calcium
Serum immunoreactive parathormone	WBC count	Serum iron
Parathormone	Serum vitamin A	Serum phosphorus
Serum cholesterol	Leukocyte zinc	Serum thiamine
Serum uric acid	Serum pantothenate	Serum zinc
Serum fibrinogen	Serum riboflavin	Serum 1,25-dihydroxycholecalciferol
Serum norepinephrine	Serum carotene	Serum vitamin B_6
Serum triglycerides	Erythrocyte sedimentation rate	Serum vitamin B_{12}
Serum glucose	Serum IgM, IgG, IgA	Plasma vitamin C
Prostate-specific antigen (PSA)	Blood urea nitrogen	Serum selenium
	Serum creatinine[a]	Plasma gammatocopherol (vitamin E)
	Serum alkaline phosphatase	Triiodothyronine (T_3)
		Serum testosterone
		Dihydroepiandrosterone

From Beers MH, Berkow R (eds) 2000 The Merck Manual of Geriatics p 1384. Copyright 2000 by Merck & Co, Inc., Whitehouse Station, NJ, with permission.
[a]Serum creatinine may be normal even though creatinine clearance is decreased with aging as a result of an age-related decrease in creatinine production.

Deteriorating renal function as indicated by an elevation in the levels of serum creatinine and blood urea nitrogen may place the patient at a greater risk of medication toxicity. Frequent assessment of drug serum levels and adjustment of doses is the hallmark of safe continued usage in the face of renal insufficiency. Abnormalities in thyroid hormone levels may present differently in the elderly than in younger adults. Cardiac arrhythmias and weight loss may be the presenting symptoms of hyperthyroidism in the elderly, whereas hypothyroidism may present more insidiously, with the typical symptoms of myxedema occurring less frequently. Alterations in mental status, lethargy, weight gain and thought disorders may be caused by hypothyroidism in the elderly.

Table 13.1 indicates the normal values of routinely used laboratory assessments and Box 13.1 shows the possible age-related effects on these values. Significant deviations from these values may indicate the presence of disease or deterioration of organ systems.

CONCLUSION

In summary, the clinical use of laboratory testing for the assessment of geriatric patients is a useful tool when combined with physical assessment. Laboratory values, although traditionally derived from middle-aged populations, can be applied to elderly populations, with rare exceptions. Abnormal laboratory values should not be attributed to age alone but be investigated for the presence of disease states. Reductions in physiological reserves account for the earlier presence of abnormal values in asymptomatic disease states in the elderly.

References

Beck FK, Rosenthal TC 2002 Prealbumin: a marker for nutritional evaluation. Am Fam Physician 65(8):1575–1578

Brigden M, Heathcote J 2000 Problems in interpreting laboratory tests. What do unexpected results mean? Postgrad Med 107(7):145–162

Feld R, Schwabbauer M 2000 Clinical Chemistry in the Physician's Office. Peer Review; June 2000, University of Iowa College of Medicine, Iowa City, IA

Huber K, Mostafaie N, Strangl G et al 2006 Clinical chemistry reference values for 75-year-old apparently healthy persons. Clin Chem Lab Med 44:1355–1360

Mantha S 2005 The usefulness of preoperative laboratory screening. J Clin Anaesthesiol 17(1):51–57

McKnight E 2002 American Association for Clinical Chemistry, 54th Annual Meeting. July 2002, Orlando, FL

Park S, Johnson M 2006 What is an adequate dose of vitamin B_{12} in older people with poor vitamin B_{12} status? Nutr Rev 64:373–378

Chapter 14

Imaging

Clive Perry

INTRODUCTION

This chapter will review the current position of medical imaging, the general principles of imaging and the way it can be used to solve clinical questions.

With the discovery of X-rays by Wilhelm Conrad Roentgen in 1895, the age of medical imaging was born. With the advent of the technological age, new discoveries have added other modalities, providing unique information regarding anatomy, pathology and the function of living organs. The relatively low cost and power of modern computers has allowed very large image data sets to be generated quickly. New software allows multiple display formats including three-dimensional, multiplanar, real-time, fused and functional images. This has enabled imaging to remain a relevant and essential part of modern clinical decision-making, resulting in increased efficiencies and better outcomes. The digital nature of modern images allows the efficient storage and dissemination of information to the referring physician and radiologist via local networks and the internet.

BASIC PRINCIPLES

All medical imaging has the same basic requirements. The first is an energy source which interacts benignly with biological tissue and is capable of representing the structure and/or function of this tissue. The second is an ability to capture and store the energy or data that result from this interaction and display them as an image. As an example, let us look at the photograph. The energy source, light, is reflected from the subject and captured on photographic film or digitally to produce an image, the photograph (Fig. 14.1).

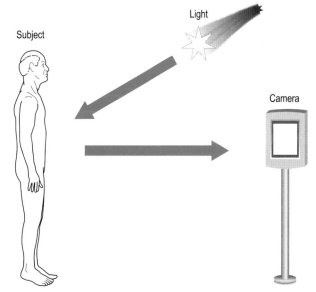

Figure 14.1 **Basic principles of imaging.** Light is reflected from the subject and the energy (light) enters the camera where it is captured by the photographic film to produce an image – the photograph.

IMAGING MODALITIES

X-rays

X-rays, like light, are part of the electromagnetic spectrum but have a higher energy and shorter wavelength, which allows them to pass into and through the human body (Fig. 14.2). Different tissue types absorb different amounts of the X-ray beam; bone, a very dense tissue, absorbs most of the beam whereas lungs, consisting mainly of air, do not. As a result, varying amounts of X-rays exit the body, reflecting the different tissue types that the X-ray beam has passed through. As Roentgen discovered, the X-rays will stimulate a fluorescent screen to produce light, which can be captured on specialized photographic film to produce an image of the body part. This is referred to as a radiograph or X-ray. Obtaining a good radiograph has many similarities to obtaining a good photograph. For example, if the subject moves, the photographic image will be blurred; if not enough light is available, the image will be dark. Similarly, if the radiograph is not exposed correctly, the image will be limited. This is particularly

Chest stand

Patient

X-ray tube

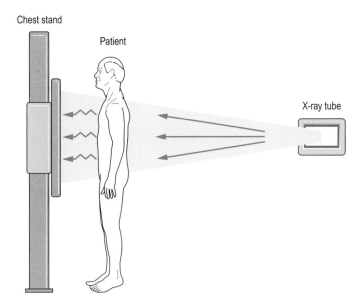

Figure 14.2 X-rays are produced by the X-ray tube. X-rays have a higher energy than light and pass through the patient; they are captured by the X-ray film contained within the chest stand. The X-rays are absorbed to a different degree by different tissues as explained in the text. The end result is a chest radiograph as seen in Fig. 14.3A. Note the X-rays enter the patient posteriorly and exit anteriorly. This orientation produces the best image and is a posterior to anterior radiograph, better known as PA, chest x-ray (CXR).

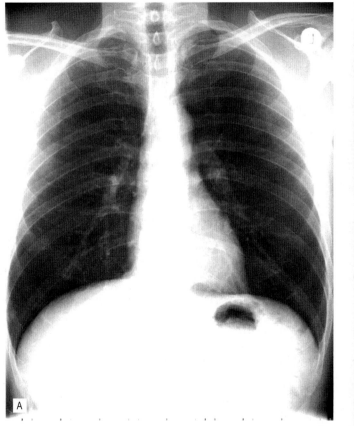

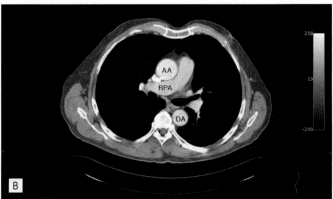

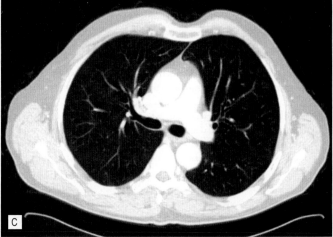

Figure 14.3 **Normal chest images.** (A) Chest radiograph. The radiograph provides a quick and inexpensive overall view of the chest. The air-containing lungs are black because of little attenuation of the X-ray beam. The central pulmonary arteries and heart are well defined by the surrounding lung. However, the chest wall soft tissue structures are poorly seen because of similar attenuation of the beam, i.e. lack of contrast. The denser bones, e.g. clavicles and ribs, are white. The heart overlies and obscures the thoracic spine in this view. (B and C) Axial CT chest. In (B) the viewing settings are optimized (i.e. window and level) to show the soft tissues to best affect. AA, ascending thoracic aorta; DA, descending thoracic aorta; RPA, right pulmonary artery. (C) Same patient and same level. However, by changing the viewing settings the lungs are now seen in exquisite detail. Note the improved anatomical depiction and improved tissue contrast in the CT images. CT solves the problem of overlapping structures obscuring the anatomy. The mediastinal and chest wall structures are now well seen.

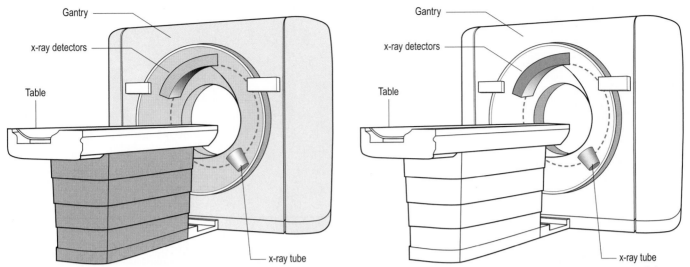

Figure 14.4 **CT scanner.** (A) The table on which the patient lies and the gantry through which the patient passes during a CT scan. (B) The position of the X-ray tube and detectors within the gantry. The X-ray tube and detectors rotate around the patient. The X-rays pass through the patient and are collected by the detectors which lie opposite. An electrical signal is produced by the detectors, which is fed into a computer to construct a cross-sectional image.

a problem with large patients. These issues are the same for all imaging studies.

Radiographs are relatively inexpensive, quick to perform and widely available. As a result, they continue to make up the bulk of imaging studies. Similar to the camera, radiographic images have moved away from film and are now mainly of digital format.

Image quality depends on the ability to discriminate between two adjacent objects, also called spatial resolution; with X-rays, this is very good. However, the ability to see a structure also depends on the difference in the attenuation of the X-ray beam between different tissues, i.e. tissue contrast. For example, bone, which attenuates most of the beam, is well outlined against adjacent soft tissue such as muscle, which does not attenuate the beam as much. Similarly, the lung parenchyma and cardiac silhouette is differentiated well from the surrounding air (Fig. 14.3A). However, differentiating soft tissue is a problem because of a similar attenuation of the beam; this means that the tissues all have a similar gray appearance, i.e. little or no contrast (Fig. 14.3A). This can be overcome to some extent by using contrast agents. Oral contrast with a barium solution, e.g. a barium enema, is used for evaluating the gastrointestinal tract. Intravenous and intra-arterial iodinated contrast agents for evaluating blood vessels and organs are used in arteriography and intravenous urograms.

Fluoroscopy uses continuous X-rays (in reduced doses) to allow real-time images. A device known as an image intensifier allows you to view the images on a TV screen. Although the radiation dose used to produce a particular image is much reduced compared with a standard radiograph, care must be taken not to prolong the procedure and cause unwanted exposure of the patient to high doses. Types of procedures using this technique include barium studies, arteriograms and internal fixation of fractures in the operating room.

Standard X-ray images produce a two-dimensional display of a three-dimensional structure; this means that there is an overlap of structures resulting in part of the anatomy being hidden. For example, on a frontal chest radiograph, the overlying heart obscures the spine (compare the chest radiograph in Fig. 14.3A with the chest CT in Fig. 14.3B and C). This can be alleviated somewhat by obtaining additional views such as a lateral view. However, the problem of overlapping structures has been overcome following the introduction of computerized axial tomography (CAT or CT scan) in the 1970s, made possible with the advent of the computer and the ability to capture and store data digitally.

Computed tomography

A CT scan also utilizes X-rays to produce images but, instead of being stationary, the X-ray tube rotates around the patient (Fig. 14.4). Specialized detectors collect the emerging X-rays and produce an electrical signal that is fed into a computer; this information is then used to construct a cross-sectional image (Fig. 14.3B). The initial CT technique took several hours to acquire the data and several days for the computer to reconstruct the images. Modern scanners are very fast and can image the entire abdomen and pelvis in seconds. Multislice CT scanners are now replacing single-slice technology and, as the name indicates, multiple slices can be produced per rotation of the X-ray tube. This has the advantage of covering more territory and shortening scan times. This technology can produce very thin axial slices allowing the production of isotropic data sets, i.e. it has the ability to acquire a volume of data that can be viewed in any plane without distorting the image. Until this innovation, CT scans were generally limited to an axial display; now, images can routinely be displayed in any plane giving multiplanar (MPR) and three-dimensional reconstruction capabilities. This allows more information to be gleaned from the study and improves diagnostic accuracy (Figs 14.5 and 14.6), particularly with complicated pathology such as complex fractures (see Fig. 14.7).

CT scanning is used to image all parts of the body. The speed of the examination makes this a particularly attractive investigation for older patients who may find it difficult to lie still for long periods of time. It also makes it the preferred method for examining very sick and injured patients when time is of the essence (Figs 14.5 and 14.6). The relatively large size of the gantry (the part of the machine that the patient passes through) has almost eliminated the problem of claustrophobia (Fig. 14.4). As with standard X-rays, CT scanning shows superb lung and bone detail (Figs 14.3C and 14.7). Fluids such as ascites and cystic structures are well defined, as are calcifications and acute and subacute hemorrhage (see Fig. 14.12A–C). Fat, particularly in the abdomen, is a natural contrast agent and is useful in defining adjacent organs and inflammation (Fig. 14.6); however, CT still requires additional contrast agents to improve visualization. Oral contrast, usually in the form of dilute barium, aids visualization of the bowel (Fig. 14.6), and intravenous contrast is used to optimize the evaluation of veins and arteries and the vascularity of organs. The addition of intravenous contrast material also allows further uses of CT, for example pulmonary embolism is now routinely evaluated by this method (see Fig. 14.5).

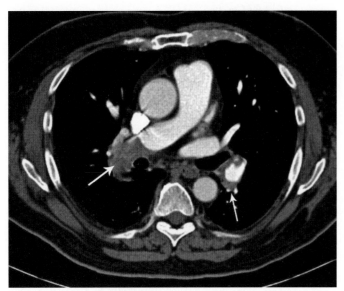

Figure 14.5 **Acute chest pain.** CT is now being used increasingly for evaluating acute chest pain. Here is an example of an acute pulmonary embolus. This 72-year-old male presented with bilateral leg pain and swelling, chest pain and shortness of breath. The lower limb ultrasound (not shown) demonstrated bilateral deep vein thrombosis. The CT (above) was obtained following intravenous contrast. Note that the contrast in the right pulmonary artery shows an abrupt cut-off, and low attenuating gray material (representing the embolus) is seen in the proximal right lower lobe pulmonary artery (right arrow). Compare with normal chest CT in Fig. 14.3. This represents a large pulmonary embolus. A smaller embolus is seen on the left side (left arrow). CT plays a major role in evaluating chest disease. The scan takes a few seconds, making it an ideal modality for emergency situations such as this.

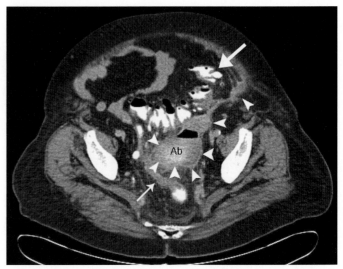

Figure 14.6 **Abdominal pain.** This can be difficult to evaluate on clinical grounds alone in the elderly as illustrated in this case of diverticulitis and diverticular abscess. This is a CT scan of the pelvis of a 70-year-old woman with minimal abdominal pain. Acute intra-abdominal processes can be a diagnostic dilemma in the elderly as symptoms and signs may be minimal or absent as in this case; CT is very helpful in this situation. The CT demonstrates diverticular disease involving the barium-filled sigmoid colon (large arrow). The arrow heads show the track of the perforation leading to the abscess in the pelvis (Ab). The rectum is seen to the right and posterior to the abscess (small arrow). The abscess was drained surgically along with resection of the sigmoid colon. Note how the intra-abdominal and subcutaneous fat acts as a natural contrast, allowing separation and good delineation of adjacent soft tissues; this is one of the few advantages of being overweight.

The speed of the new multislice scanners even allows the beating heart and coronary arteries to be evaluated. The ability of CT to demonstrate arteries is now as good as the more invasive procedure of diagnostic arteriography and, in complex anatomical situations, may be better. As a result, many arterial lesions, such as aneurysm, dissection and stenosis, are diagnosed and evaluated with CT (Fig. 14.8), and the more invasive diagnostic arteriogram is now mainly used for therapy (e.g. treatment of a narrowed artery and aortic aneurysm with specially designed stents, which can be placed percutaneously via adjacent non-diseased vessels).

Ultrasound

Ultrasound has been used since the 1950s to produce medical images using sound waves. The frequency of the wave used to produce the images is in the range of 1–20 MHz. It is called ultrasound because this frequency is above the human audible range of 2–20 kHz. The probe or transducer used during the examination is responsible for both producing the sound and collecting the sound waves reflected from the patients' organs and tissues. The received sound is converted to an electrical signal and, from this, an image is developed by a computer and displayed in real time on a TV monitor. In addition, by using the Doppler effect, the returning sound waves can be used to evaluate blood flow. It is excellent for imaging soft tissues and has a long list of uses, including imaging of the major abdominal and pelvic organs. Superficial structures are particularly well seen, for example, the thyroid, superficial tendons, muscles, veins and arteries (see Fig. 14.14C and Fig. 14.15E and F).

The combination of real-time, multiplanar and vascular imaging makes ultrasound an excellent tool for imaging the heart. The lack of ionizing radiation and substantiated adverse effects have made it a popular imaging technique in all age groups. The relatively inexpensive equipment costs and portability have added to this. It is an excellent tool for guiding percutaneous needle biopsies, especially superficially located lesions such as breast masses. There are some negative aspects of ultrasound. Unlike all other imaging methods, it relies heavily on the expertise of the sonographer/sonologist to produce diagnostic images. Sound is reflected by bone and air, limiting evaluation of the chest; abdominal organs, which may be hidden by overlying gas-filled loops of bowel; and the brain, which is surrounded by the protective cranium.

Magnetic resonance imaging

The phenomenon of magnetic resonance was discovered in the 1930s and initially used to determine the composition of chemical compounds. In the 1970s, it was realized that the same techniques could be used in medical imaging and, by the 1980s, magnetic resonance imaging (MRI) units were in clinical use. Magnetic resonance uses radio waves and a strong magnetic field to produce the image; as with ultrasound, it does not use ionizing radiation. The technique relies on the fact that some atomic nuclei have magnetic properties that act like microscopic magnets when placed in a strong magnetic field. The human body has an abundance of these in the form of the hydrogen ion that makes up water. These align with the direction of

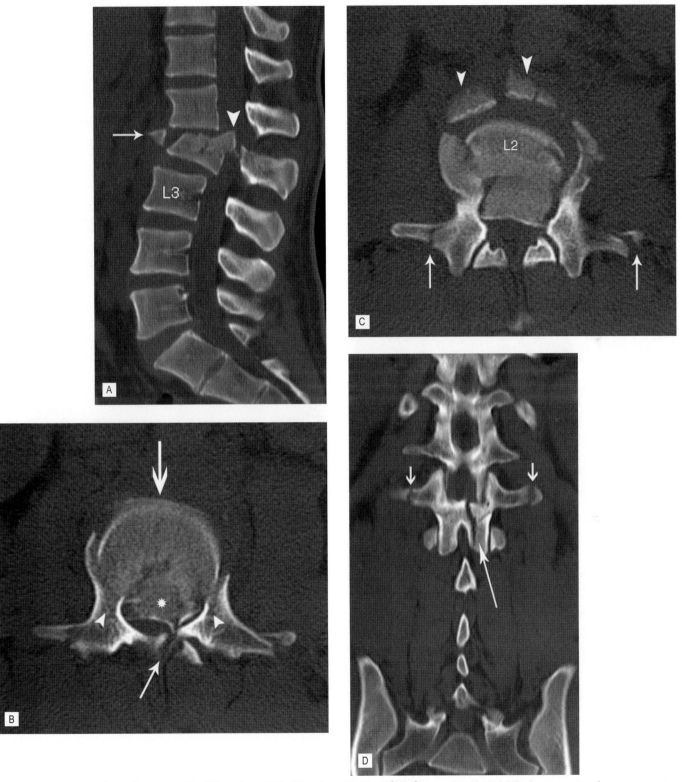

Figure 14.7   **Severe burst fracture with dislocation at L2.** CT with multiplanar (MPR) reconstruction vividly demonstrates the components of this complex fracture, which resulted following a motor vehicle accident. (A) The sagittal MPR shows posterior displacement of the body of L2. There is a large, central, superior retro-pulsed fragment. An anterior and superior fragment has been avulsed. (B) The axial image at the level of the retro-pulsed fragment (*) demonstrates severe narrowing of the spinal canal. The vertebral body has been driven between the pedicles with fractures at the junction of the vertebral body and pedicles. (C) Just caudal to (B) shows the avulsed anterior fragments (arrow head) and fractures through both transverse processes (arrows). (D) There is widening of the interpedicle distance and a sagittal fracture through the lamina best seen on this coronal MPR. The fracture is unstable with disruption of all three columns. The patient had a significant neurological deficit and was treated with spinal decompression and instrument fixation.

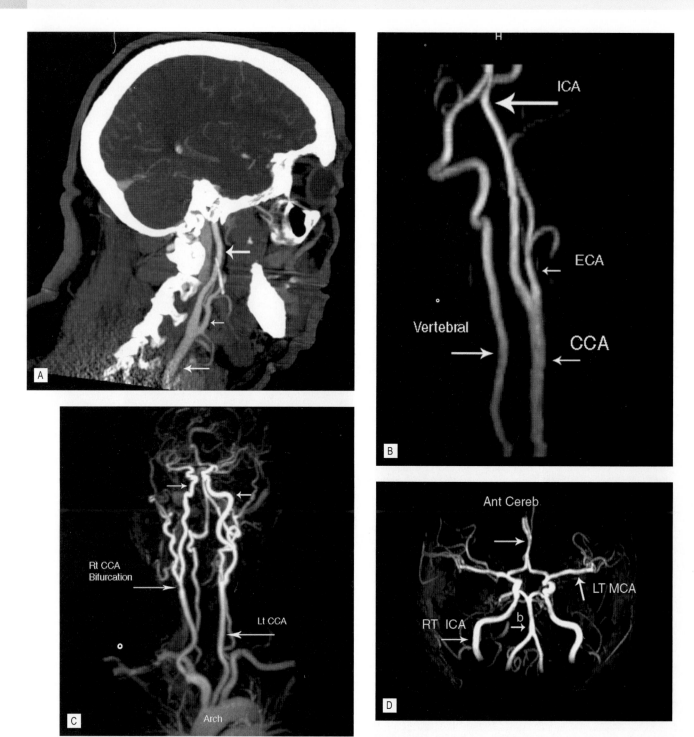

Figure 14.8 **Non-invasive vascular imaging.** Examples of noninvasive imaging of the carotid arteries and intracranial arteries using CT (CTA) and MR (MRA). (A) CTA following intravenous contrast shows a sagital MPR image of the common carotid artery (CCA; lower arrow) and the cervical portion of the internal carotid artery (ICA; upper arrow) and external carotid artery (ECA; middle arrow). (B) 2D time of flight MR image of the cervical carotid artery and its branches. This sequence does not use intravenous contrast. (C) 3D MRA following intravenous gadolinium allows a larger area to be evaluated. Here the aortic arch (Arch) and the three great vessels and both carotid arteries are seen. The cervical and intracranial (upper arrows) portions of both ICAs are seen. Note the narrowing at the right CCA bifurcation. (D) 3D time of flight MRA showing the intracranial vessels and central circle of Willis. Ant cereb, anterior cerebral arteries; b, basilar artery; LT MCA, left middle cerebral artery; RT ICA, right internal carotid artery. Atherosclerosis is a common problem in the elderly and can cause severe narrowing of the carotid artery particularly at the CCA bifurcation. This is a common cause of stroke and is a treatable condition. In the past this was diagnosed with angiography, an invasive procedure. The cervical portions of the carotid arteries are usually evaluated with ultrasound first. However both CT and MR allow evaluation of the whole carotid system including the aortic arch and intracranial vessels. Noninvasive imaging of other vessels in the body is now routine, and the individual circumstances will determine which of the three modalities is used.

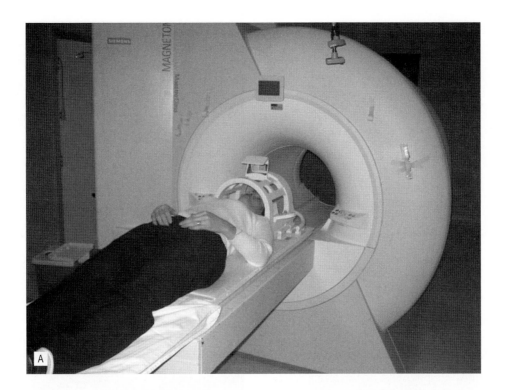

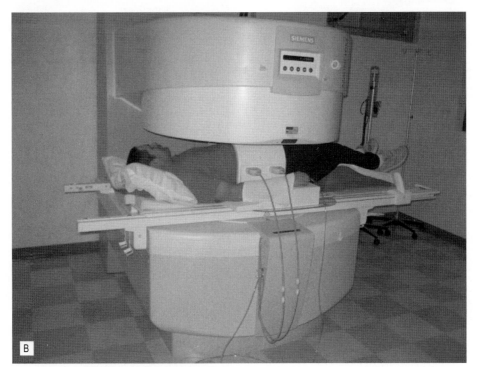

Figure 14.9 **Examples of MRI machines.** (A) This patient is getting ready for a head scan in this closed, high field strength MRI scanner. The cage around the head contains the radiofrequency (RF) coils. Note that the bore of the magnet is fairly long and not that wide. This can be a problem for large patients and patients who suffer from claustrophobia. Elderly patients may become disorientated in this enclosure. (B) Example of an open MR scanner. These scanners may not be capable of all the imaging sequences and can take longer to acquire the images but image quality is good and they are usually well tolerated by patients who suffer from claustrophobia. The large belt around the patients abdomen is an RF coil.

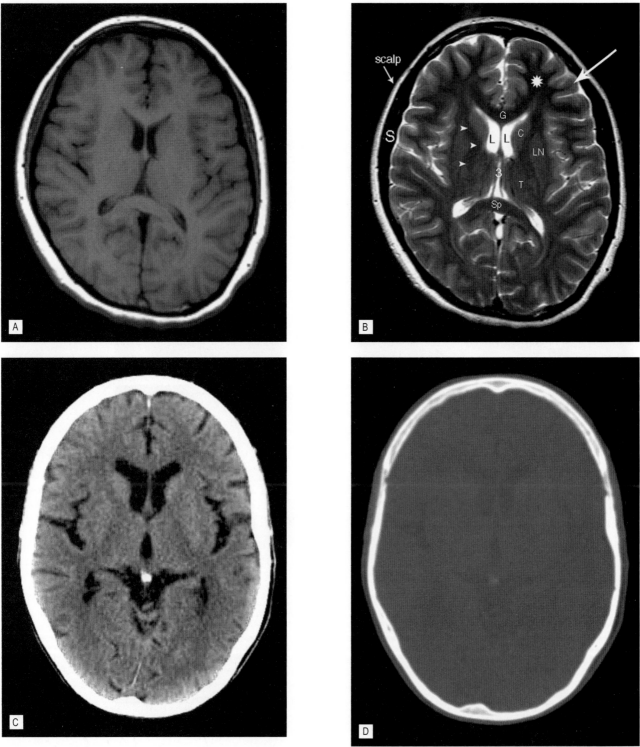

Figure 14.10   Normal MRI and CT brain. (A) T1-weighted spin echo (SE) image (T1WI) and (B) T2-weighted turbo spin echo (TSE) image (T2WI). (C) CT optimized for viewing soft tissues. (D) Same CT optimized for viewing bone. All obtained without intravenous contrast and taken through the level of the lateral (L) and third (3) ventricle. The T1 and T2 images are the basic sequences used in MRI, but there are several other sequences that are used which display certain pathologies to greater effect. CT, however, has only one sequence but by altering the level of attenuated tissues displayed the bony skull is seen to better effect. This is demonstrated in (D), which shows the same CT scan with the view settings (level and window) optimized to demonstrate bone. Note the improved tissue contrast with MR allowing improved definition of the gray matter in the cerebral cortex (arrow) versus the white matter in the adjacent left frontal lobe(*). CSF in the third, lateral ventricles and sulci on the T2WI is bright and dark on the T1WI and CT. Note the skull is bright on CT, indicating increased attenuation of the X-ray beam. Calcium in the pineal gland is also bright (image C). The bright area surrounding the brain on the two MRI images, however, is subcutaneous fat in the scalp. Cortical bone does not produce a signal and the signal void (black area) between the scalp and the brain is the skull (S). G, genu and Sp, spenium of the corpus callosum; C, head of the caudate nucleus; L, lentiform nucleus; T, thalamus; arrow heads, internal capsule.

the bore of the magnet when the patient lies in the MRI machine (Fig. 14.9). If these nuclei are stimulated by a radio wave at a specific frequency, known as the resonant frequency, they gain energy and move into a transverse plane, perpendicular to the main magnetic field. This results in a radio wave being emitted by the rotated nuclei, which allows their position to be recognized. The radio waves are emitted and received by a device called a radio frequency (RF) coil, analogous to the ultrasound transducer that transmits and receives the sound waves. The coils are placed close to the patient. The head coil, used to image the brain, looks like a cylindrical cage that surrounds the patient's head (Fig. 14.9A). As with ultrasound, the received signal, in this case radio waves, creates an electrical signal, which is fed into a computer to produce an image (Fig. 14.10A and B).

The high tissue contrast (i.e. the difference in signal between tissue types) afforded by magnetic resonance is responsible for the excellent depiction of soft tissue anatomy. There are two main types of pulse sequences used in MRI, which produce images of the same area but with a different contrast; these are known as T1- and T2-weighted images. This is achieved by varying the time when the RF pulse is emitted and when the returning RF wave is received. Fluid gives a low signal on T1 images and a bright signal on T2 images, whereas fat gives a high signal on T1 and T2 images [when using the faster T2 turbo spin echo (TSE) sequence]. Unique to MRI is the ability to selectively remove or null particular tissues from the image. For example, fat, which is bright and may obscure pathology, can be removed by a technique called fat saturation or 'fat sat' for short (see Figs 14.13E and 14.15D). This is an extremely useful technique, which also makes it possible to confirm that a structure is fat-containing (e.g. a lipoma) by obtaining images before and after fat saturation.

MRI is also routinely used to evaluate blood vessels (Fig. 14.8). These images can be generated without the use of intravenous contrast agents although contrast-enhanced studies are also used to acquire additional information. The latest and faster MRI sequences allow routine evaluation of the beating heart and are a valuable tool in complementing cardiac ultrasound and cardiac nuclear medicine studies. Magnetic resonance spectroscopy has the ability to evaluate the chemical composition of tissue and has shown promise in the diagnosis of cerebral tumors. MRI is also used to evaluate brain function, the so-called functional MRI.

Nuclear medicine

There are some fundamental differences between nuclear medicine and the other imaging modalities. Whereas the other modalities rely mainly on a change in anatomy caused by a pathological process, nuclear medicine is able to show images of changes in function or physiology as a result of pathological change. The energy source in nuclear medicine is a radionuclide that emits ionizing radiation in the form of gamma rays, which come from the same part of the electromagnetic spectrum as X-rays. The radionuclides are tagged with a biological compound that is used by a living tissue; this combination is called a radiopharmaceutical. Unlike the other forms of imaging, the radiopharmaceutical is placed inside the patient, usually by an intravenous route, and taken up by the organ/cells or pathological process of interest. During decay of the radionuclide, gamma rays are emitted and pass out of the body and are collected by a gamma camera to produce an image. The most common radionuclide used is technetium 99 m, and a common study is a bone scan in which the technetium is labeled with diphosphonate (Tc-MDP) (Fig. 14.11A and B). This is quickly taken up by bone, particularly in areas of bone remodeling, for example, fracture repair and most bone metastases. The camera is positioned over the area of interest and images obtained in a two-dimensional plane (the planar image) (Fig. 14.11C). As in CT, images can also be obtained by rotating the camera slowly around the patient

to obtain a cross-section or tomogram. This is referred to as SPECT (single photon emission tomography), and is used in, for example, SPECT bone imaging and thallium SPECT imaging of the heart.

The ability of nuclear medicine to show cellular function can be demonstrated by positron emission tomography or PET. In this technique, the radionuclide fluorine-18, in combination with glucose [18-flourodeoxyglucose (FDG)], is readily incorporated into cells allowing the utilization of glucose to be imaged; this is proving to be an extremely useful way to diagnose and monitor disease. For instance, it has been shown that FDG accumulates in most tumors to a greater amount than normal tissue, allowing recognition of the tumor (Fig. 14.11D). It is used to diagnose, stage and evaluate the treatment response of several tumors. This list is growing and includes lung, colon, breast, head and neck cancer, lymphoma and melanoma. Positron-emitting radionuclides also produce gamma rays but require a specially designed camera for imaging. With small lesions or complex anatomical areas, PET may not provide enough anatomical detail to accurately depict the exact site of the lesion. By performing a CT scan at the same time as the PET scan (PET/CT) and fusing the images, anatomical localization of the lesion is improved, and the two modalities used together have proved to be complementary, resulting in a more accurate diagnosis.

SCREENING, INTRAVENOUS CONTRAST AND SAFETY

Screening

Using imaging to screen for disease, particularly cancer, has been a desirable goal for many years; however, the development of an effective screening test has been elusive. Screening mammography is an exception. A review of eight randomized controlled trials demonstrated a 20% reduction in breast cancer mortality when women aged 40–74 years of age were invited for screening; this represents a significant reduction in mortality (Smith et al 2004). The National Cancer Institute, the American Cancer Society and the American College of Radiology recommend annual mammography screening for all women over 40 years of age. All mammography facilities in the US are regulated under the federal Mammography Quality Standards Act (MQSA). Despite these advances, it must be remembered that no perfect test has been found; breast cancer still remains the second most common cancer in women after lung cancer. The sensitivity and specificity of mammography screening is 83–95% and 90–98% respectively. Sensitivity is especially reduced in women with dense breasts. Breast self-examination and clinical examination remain essential for diagnosis.

The National Lung Screening Trial is evaluating the effectiveness of CT in screening for lung cancer. CT colonography is a new technique, which uses MPR and three-dimensional reconstruction to noninvasively view the colon, and is currently being evaluated as a possible screening tool for colorectal cancer. For these and other trials, including the effectiveness of imaging guided therapies such as RF tumor ablation, refer to the American College of Radiology Imaging Network website (www.acrin.org).

Issues related to intravenous contrast

Intravenous contrast agents are widely used and considered safe. However, adverse reactions can occur. For the most part, these are minor reactions that do not require treatment, including hives, nausea and facial swelling. More moderate reactions that require observation and/or treatment include hypotension, bronchospasm and bradycardia. Rarely, the reaction may be life-threatening requiring

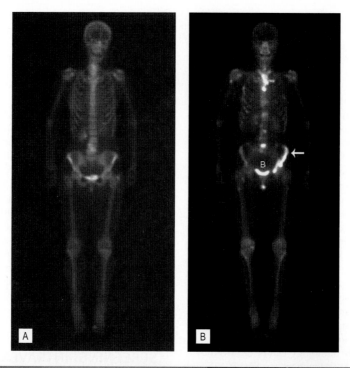

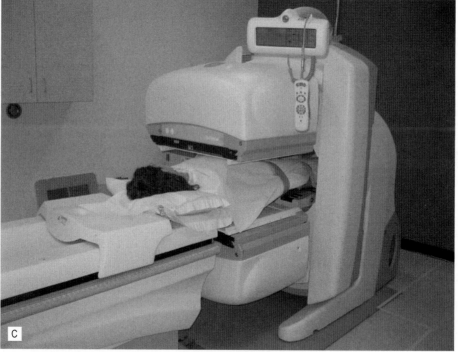

Figure 14.11 **Nuclear medicine whole body bone scan.** (A) Normal bone scan. This anterior view was obtained 4 h after the intravenous injection of the radionucleide – Tc 99 m MDP. The images show expected bone uptake in a 60-year-old female. The scan is routinely delayed to allow clearance of the radionuclide from the blood and soft tissues which would interfere with bone visualization. Note the symmetry of uptake. Increased activity at the shoulder and iliac wings in the pelvis is normal. Activity in the lower neck is due to normal thyroid cartilage activity. The tracer is cleared through the kidneys hence expected increased activity in the bladder and kidneys. Increased activity at L4/5 is due to degenerative disk and facet joint disease. (B) Bone metastases. Anterior view of a 65-year-old woman with metastatic bone disease from breast carcinoma. Increased activity is seen in the spine, left ilium (white arrow), sternum, the proximal right humerus and femur. The bone scan is used to diagnose the presence, extent and response of disease to treatment. (C) Nuclear medicine gamma camera. There are two gamma cameras (dual head), one above and one below the patient. This allows anterior and posterior images to be collected simultaneously, speeding up the examination. The cameras can be rotated around the patient to allow oblique and lateral projections.

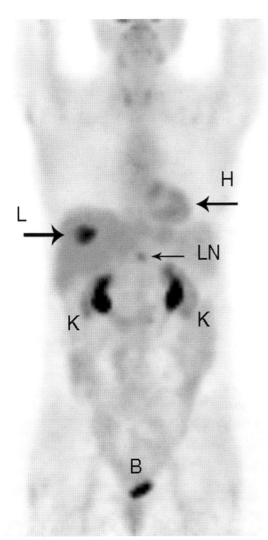

Figure 14.11 (D) **Positron emission tomography (PET).** Example of a PET scan with fluorodeoxyglucose (FDG). It was obtained to stage the colon cancer in this 60-year-old woman. Note the round area of increased activity in the liver (L arrow) from a single metastasis. This confirmed the CT findings. Increased activity in a small upper abdominal lymph node (LN) is also consistent with metastatic disease. This was not suspected on CT which relies on lymph node enlargement to make the diagnosis. FDG is excreted via the kidneys, hence the normal activity in the kidneys (K) and bladder. (B) Normal activity is also seen in the heart (H).

immediate treatment and usually hospitalization. With low osmolar iodinated contrast media, used with X-ray and CT, the incidence of a severe reaction is 1–2 per 10 000 examinations. Gadolinium chelates, which are used as intravenous contrast agents for MRI, are very well tolerated and have a much lower incidence of adverse reactions; severe reactions are extremely rare. Patients who have had a previous contrast reaction are more likely to do so again. Current practice is to pretreat these patients with corticosteroids at least 6 h prior to injection. An antihistamine, such as 50 mg of diphenhydramine, is also used and given 1 h before the contrast injection. This may prevent or minimize a minor or moderate contrast reaction but is unlikely to prevent a major life-threatening event.

Iodinated contrast-induced nephropathy is a risk, particularly in patients with preexisting renal failure (Box 14.1). It is usually transient, with renal function returning to the baseline within 10 days. Adequate

hydration prior to the examination is important. In patients with poor renal function or repeated severe contrast reactions, it is recommended that the study be undertaken without contrast or by using a different imaging modality.

According to the ACR manual on contrast media, version 5 (see Bibliography), gadolinium does not cause renal toxicity. Also patients with end-stage renal disease requiring regular dialysis can be given contrast agents. However, recent reports have indicated that a new and rare disease, nephrogenic systemic fibrosis (NSF), may occur in patients with moderate to end-stage renal disease following the administration of a gadolinium-based contrast agent. The US Food and Drug Administration (FDA) in December 2006 issued a public advisory along these lines and is evaluating these reports. For details go to the FDA website (see Bibliography). As this is a new and evolving problem, if you have patients with renal failure, particularly end-stage disease, who may require MRI, it is suggested that you also contact your MRI center for their current guidelines before ordering the test.

Patients using metformin to treat diabetes are at risk of developing lactic acidosis if the blood level of metformin is high. Metformin is excreted via the kidneys. Therefore, the development of renal failure following intravascular iodinated contrast in patients taking metformin is of added concern. Current recommendations are to stop metformin before administration of intravenous contrast and recommence after 48 h, once it is established that renal function has not been affected.

A word about radiation effects

X-rays used in radiography, fluoroscopy and CT, and gamma rays used in nuclear medicine, have enough energy to cause ionization of atoms within the body. This form of energy or radiation is called ionizing radiation, and it can result in damage to DNA and the induction of tumors, both benign and malignant. Bone marrow, gastrointestinal tract, mammary glands, gonads and lymphatic tissue are most susceptible, and children are more susceptible than adults. The latency period for solid tumors is 25+ years, whereas for leukemia it is 5–7 years. While the higher the exposure, the greater the likelihood of getting cancer, there is no demonstrable threshold at which this can occur. In contrast, a single high dose can cause immediate cell death and may cause cataracts, skin burns and hair loss.

Imaging studies are only one source of ionizing radiation. Everyone is exposed to natural background radiation, which, in the US, is

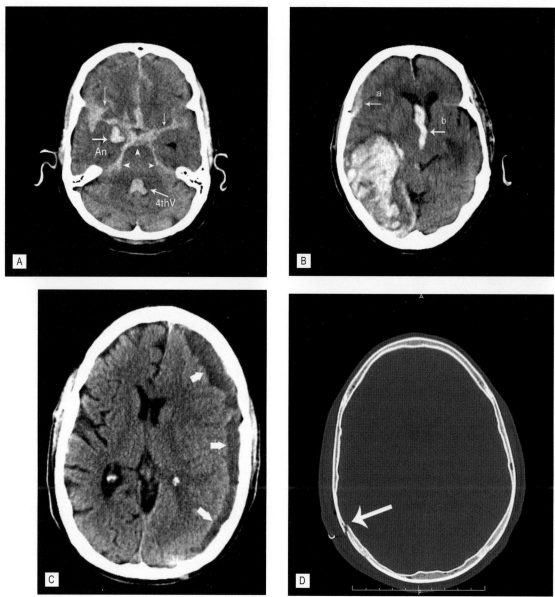

Figure 14.12 **Brain imaging.** MRI and CT are used to image the brain. Both have their strengths and weaknesses. Generally speaking, MRI is the modality of choice. However, when speed is of essence, such as in an emergency situation or with patients unable to lie still, CT is preferred. CT is used in patients with a pacemaker and in those who suffer from claustrophobia. In the acute setting, CT is usually the initial choice because of its availability, fast examination times and ability to identify acute intracranial blood, skull and facial fractures (A–D). (A) Subarachnoid hemorrhage in a 75-year-old female who presented with an acute severe headache behind the right eye. Acute blood is seen in the basal cisterns (arrow heads), Sylvian fissure (arrows) and 4th ventricle. Acute blood appears white on CT and is easily differentiated from the darker brain parenchyma. This was caused by a rupture of a right posterior communicating artery aneurysm (An). The 15 mm triangular white area to the right of the circle of Willis represents blood around and thrombus within the aneurysm. Treatment was surgical clipping. In the right candidate, such aneurysms can be treated by placing small metal coils into the aneurysm and sealing them off; this is achieved by threading small catheters up to the brain via arteries in the groin and using fluoroscopy to guide the placement. (B) Intracerebral hemorrhage in a 90-year-old patient who presented with acute collapse. There is a large cerebral hematoma with considerable mass affect on the adjacent brain. Blood has ruptured into the lateral and 3rd ventricle (arrow b) and there is a small subdural component (arrow a). Elderly hypertensives are at particular risk for intracerebral hemorrhage. (C) Chronic subdural hematoma. The small arrows show a rim of chronic hematoma between the brain and the inner table of the skull. In contrast with acute blood, chronic subdural blood appears gray or dark on CT. Note the mass effect on the adjacent brain with loss of the sulci (compare opposite side) and shift of midline structures to the right. Subdural hematomas result from tearing of cortical bridging veins following head trauma. With an obvious episode of trauma and alteration of mental status, the diagnosis is straightforward. However, the episode of trauma may be minor, particularly in patients on anticoagulants. In the elderly, subtle changes of behavior may be difficult to define and the patient may not remember the traumatic event, making clinical diagnosis difficult. Not surprisingly, most chronic subdurals occur in the elderly. Symptoms are headache followed by deteriorating neurological function. Treatment is surgical drainage. (D) Skull fractures. Easily appreciated on CT, as shown by the arrow. (Continued.)

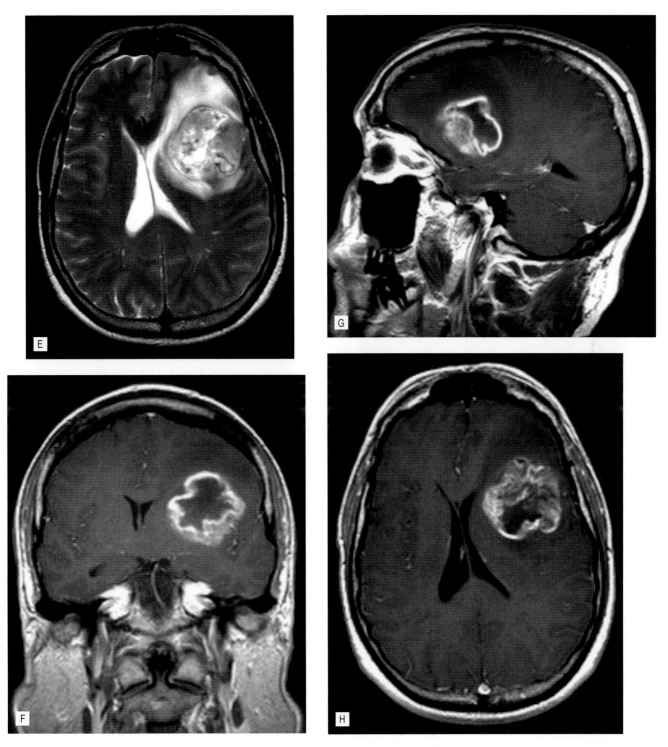

Figure 14.12 **Primary brain tumor** (gliobastoma multiform). This case demonstrates the ability of MRI to routinely display pathology in multiple planes and the superior soft tissue depiction. The brain tumor in the left frontal region is well defined on these sagittal, coronal and transverse images (E–H). The T1 weighted images (G and H) were obtained following intravenous gadolinium and show bright areas of enhancement in the periphery of the lesion. The bright area in the T2 weighted image (E) surrounding the tumor indicates associated edema. (H) The central part of the tumor is fluid containing, dark on T1 (C) and bright on T2 (E), and probably indicates cystic change or central necrosis. Mass effect on the adjacent structures is well appreciated.

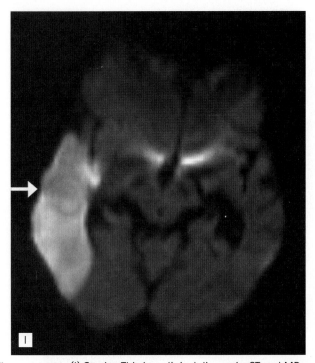

Figure 14.12 (I) **Stroke.** This is a clinical diagnosis. CT and MR are both used in patient evaluation. Although CT is usually used initially it may appear normal in the first few hours. Traditionally, its value is the assessment of stroke mimics, such as tumor and any associated hemorrhage. More recently, CT and MR have been used to assess perfusion of the brain and level of arterial vascular obstruction or stenosis with non-invasive vascular imaging (see Fig. 14.8). This figure is an example of diffusion-weighted MR (DWI) and acute brain infarct. This 85-year-old woman presented with acute onset of confusion, left-sided weakness and visual field defect. MRI is capable of measuring the motion of water through brain tissue. With acute infarction diffusion becomes restricted in those areas affected. This represents the bright area in the right temporal lobe (arrow). This is in the vascular territory supplied by the inferior division of the right middle cerebral artery. The change can be seen within minutes of the event and has revolutionized stroke diagnosis.

Table 14.1 Typical radiation doses

	Dose (mSV)
Natural background	3.0/year
Chest X-ray (marrow)	0.1
Mammogram (breast)	0.7
Nuclear medicine	2.0–10.0
CT scan: head	2.0
CT scan: abdomen	10.0

approximately 3 mSv/year. Table 14.1 lists some typical radiation doses. It is unknown exactly what the cancer risk is from diagnostic studies. It is assumed that there is a potential risk; however, the risk may be zero or very small. This is especially so with a chest X-ray where the dose is small and estimated to be equivalent to 10 days of background radiation. These factors must be weighed against the risk to the patient's health if the study is not performed.

From Table 14.1, it is clear that the examination resulting in the most patient exposure is a CT scan, which is of particular concern in children. If a patient needs a CT scan in order to improve their health and there is no other way of obtaining the information, then the choice is easy. However, until a clearer picture of the exact risks of diagnostic X-rays emerges, it is recommended that CT scans be used prudently.

Using the argument that the greater the dose, the greater the risk, strategies to reduce patient exposure are part of modern radiological practice. These include using the minimal amount of exposure to produce a study, modern equipment, trained personnel and considering alternative studies such as MRI or ultrasound, which do not use ionizingradiation.

MRI safety

MRI uses no ionizing radiation and is a safe procedure. No long-term biological effects from MRI have been described. However there are some caveats. MRI uses a strong static magnetic field and ferromagnetic objects can become airborne projectiles. These include stainless-steel surgical instruments, ferrous oxygen tanks and car keys and, therefore, such items are not allowed into the MRI room. Ferromagnetic implants may move with potential catastrophic consequences; certain cerebral aneurysm clips, especially the older type, are in this category. Newer magnetic resonance-safe clips are of no concern. If it is not possible to determine the type of clip used prior to the scan, the procedure is not undertaken. Implantable devices are assessed on a case-by-case basis. Generally cardiac valve replacements, annuloplasty rings, arterial stents and joint replacements are safe. However, these devices may cause image artifacts, which may limit the usefulness of the study. Other contraindications include cochlear implants and currently all cardiac pacemakers, although this is likely to be modified in the case of pacemakers. Metallic foreign bodies within the orbit are a contraindication and, if concern exists, a radiograph of the orbits is obtained prior to the study.

The magnetic field gradients used to produce a magnetic resonance image produce their own set of potential problems. These gradients can stimulate peripheral nerves but, at the Food and Drug Administration (FDA) limit for gradient field strength, this is not a practical problem. The loud knocking noises heard while in the scanner are produced by the changing field gradients. The noise has the potential to induce hearing loss and ear plugs or noise-abating headphones must be worn.

Because of the potential for the RF pulse to heat the body, the FDA has recommended RF exposure limits. Care must also be taken to prevent burns that may develop from electrical currents in materials that are capable of producing a conductive loop, such as electrocardiogram (EKG) leads. Technical staff receive specific and continuous safety training, and rigorous patient screening, including a detailed safety form, is completed prior to any study. Removable metallic objects including jewelry, car keys and hairpins are not permitted in the MRI room; this includes credit cards, which will become damaged. Only MRI-safe equipment is allowed in the suite and the patient is closely monitored during the scan.

WHICH IMAGING STUDY TO CHOOSE?

All of the imaging modalities have their strengths and weaknesses and none is perfect (Table 14.2). It is important to decide which test will answer the clinical problem with least risk and cost to the patient. New research and the march of technology mean that this will always be a moving target; what is the best test today may be old hat tomorrow. However, one of the most useful pieces of information for the imaging facility and interpreting radiologist is the clinical history. This

Table 14.2 Advantages and disadvantages of the various imaging modalities

	X-ray	CT	Nuclear medicine	MRI	Ultrasound
Ionizing radiation	Yes, but the dose is usually small	Yes; has the highest doses	Yes	No	No
Scan time	Fast	Fast	May need delayed images	30–60 min	10–30 min
Cross-sectional, multiplanar and three-dimensional images	No	Yes, but current technology requires additional time	Yes; shows function-limited anatomical detail	Yes; routine and no extra time for reconstruction	Yes; three-dimensional is new but likely to be used more
Mobility/bedside imaging	Yes	No	No	No	Yes
Cost	Inexpensive	Expensive	PET scanners are expensive	Most expensive	Relatively inexpensive
Claustrophobia	No	Uncommon	Rarely	Yes; 1–4%	No
Large patients	No weight limit; image quality reduced	Weight limit; image quality reduced	Generally no weight limit; image quality reduced	Weight limit; also, if patient too wide they will not fit in the magnet bore	Images for deep structures limited; superficial images OK
Strengths	Still the most widely used imaging modality; fast and inexpensive; lungs and bones well seen; good overall view of anatomy	Fast; maximum amount of information in a short time frame; excellent in emergencies, e.g. acute hemorrhage, intra-abdominal air, complicated fractures; lung, bone and vessels well seen	Unsurpassed functional imaging; excellent for diffuse bone metastases; PET good for diagnosis and treatment of cancer; thallium and sestamibi used in diagnosis of IHD	Best for soft tissue and bone marrow; imaging of choice for brain, spine and musculoskeletal; nonionizing; list of uses increasing	Fast, mobile, real time and nonionizing; first line in many situations especially superficial structures; used for abdomen, pelvis, heart, carotids and limb DVT

DVT, deep vein thrombosis; IHD, ischemic heart disease; PET, positron emission tomography.

information is critical in order to answer the clinical question and tailor the examination to ensure that the appropriate images are acquired.

In general, MRI with its superb tissue contrast and ability to image bone marrow with routine multiplanar imaging and nonionizing radiation is the method of choice for most brain, spine and musculoskeletal lesions (Figs 14.12E–I, 14.14A–G, 14.15A–D and 14.16A–C). It also has an increasing role to play in the evaluation of the abdomen and pelvis. Noninvasive imaging of the biliary and pancreatic ducts, so-called MRCP, is now a routine investigation.

Ultrasound is recommended as the initial modality for evaluating the abdomen, especially the gall bladder and bile ducts. Ultrasound is a good place to start when evaluating renal masses and possible renal obstruction as a cause for renal failure. It is the method of choice for initially evaluating uterine and ovarian masses. It allows excellent detail of superficial structures and is a reasonable place to start with superficial masses, for example thyroid masses. Joint and tendon pathology is usually evaluated with MRI but nonosseous problems, e.g. the rotator cuff, biceps and Achilles tendon tears, are well evaluated with ultrasound (Fig. 14.14C and 14.15E–F). For patients who are unable to undergo MRI, ultrasound or CT may be helpful.

In the case of trauma and emergency situations, X-ray and CT are the modalities of choice; they are readily available and quick to perform. Modern CT is very fast with a typical brain scan taking only a few seconds. CT is very accurate at demonstrating acute intracerebral hemorrhage (Fig. 14.12A–C). Acute chest and abdominal problems are routinely evaluated with CT (Figs 14.5 and 14.6). With stroke, CT is currently used in an initial evaluation; however, CT has a limited ability to diagnose this important condition in the first few critical hours when treatment options need to be decided. Its role is mainly in excluding intracranial hemorrhage and stroke mimics such as tumors (Fig. 14.12A–C). This situation is changing, and new sequences such as perfusion CT and MRI can evaluate areas in the brain with no perfusion or limited perfusion that are at risk for further infarct and which may benefit from intervention with intravenous or intra-arterial thrombolysis using tissue plasminogen activator (tPA). MRI is able to diagnose stroke within minutes of the event. A sequence called diffusion imaging has revolutionized the diagnosis of this acute problem (Fig. 14.12I) and is likely to play a major role along with perfusion imaging in acute stroke management.

Fractures are best evaluated by X-ray imaging. However, in the elderly, in whom bone density is reduced, undisplaced fractures may not be apparent (Fig. 14.13A and B). Limited mobility, as in patients with spine and complex fractures, may reduce the usefulness of standard

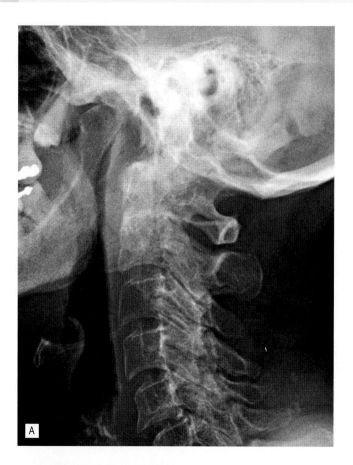

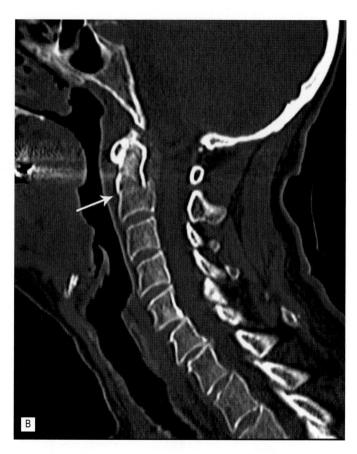

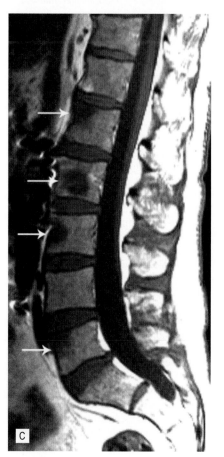

Figure 14.13   **Neck and back pain.** Neck and back pain are common clinical problems. The following four cases show how CT and MR can be used to evaluate spine pain. (A) and (B) Cervical spine injury in the elderly. Lateral radiograph and sagittal, multiplanar reconstructed computed tomogram (MPR/CT) of a 78-year-old woman with neck pain following a minor fall. (A) The radiograph shows mild swelling of the prevertebral soft tissues at C2 of concern for a bony injury but none definitely detected. (B) The CT clearly demonstrates an undisplaced fracture through the base of the odontoid. This case serves to illustrate several common clinical situations. Firstly both falls and neck pain are common in the elderly. Cervical spine fractures are also common in the elderly and odontoid fractures are disproportionately represented. Secondly fractures of the cervical spine often occur following minor trauma and may, initially, not be suspected. Osteopenic bones add to the difficulty of diagnosis. MPR/CT overcome many of the limitations of plain radiographs and can be useful when plain films do not fit the clinical picture or further detail is required of a known fracture (see Fig. 14.7A–D). Suspected cord injury is best evaluated with MRI. (C) **Vertebral metastasis.** Sagittal T1-weighted image of the lumbar spine in a 57-year-old with back pain and lung cancer. The changes are typical for metastatic vertebral disease. Multiple oval areas of low signal (arrows) are seen replacing the bone marrow at multiple levels. The spine is the most common site of skeletal metastases which are seen most frequently with breast, lung and prostate cancer. Whereas whole body nuclear medicine bone scanning is the preferred method for accessing total skeletal involvement (Fig. 14.11B), MR is the preferred method for evaluating the spine. Because of its superior imaging of bone marrow it can identify metastatic disease, to the spine, earlier than other techniques. In addition it is able to evaluate other causes of back pain and possible causes of neurological deficits including cord compression. (Continued.)

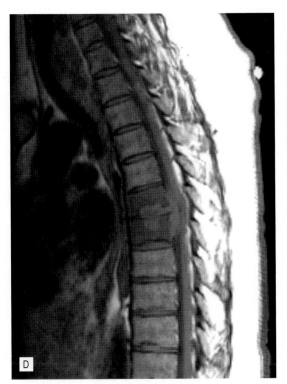
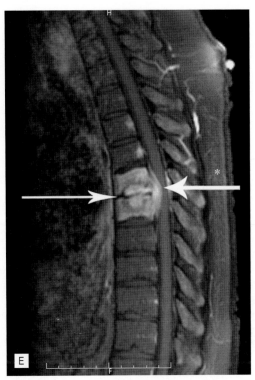

Figure 14.13 **Diskitis.** This is an infection of the intervertebral disk, which usually occurs via bloodborne bacteria which implant in the vertebral endplate and spread to the disk. It typically presents with focal back pain and tenderness. Elderly diabetics and the immunocompromised are particularly susceptible. MRI with excellent soft tissue and bone marrow detail has proven an accurate way to diagnose and monitor response following antibiotic treatment. (D) Sagittal T1-weighted image without intravenous gadolinium. (E) Sagittal T1 image following intravenous contrast. In this image, the bright fat signal has been removed (bright fat in D is now gray* in E) by a technique called fat saturation and allows dramatic appreciation of the increased enhancement (the bright area) across the disk and adjacent endplate (arrows) indicating infection. Note also involvement of the adjacent epidural space and compression of the spinal cord.

radiographs (Fig. 14.16). MRI, with its ability to display bone marrow edema, has proved useful in evaluating the presence of acute compression fractures, metastatic disease of the spine and suspected fractures, especially hip fractures, not detected on initial radiographs (Figs 14.13C, F–J and 14.16A and B). CT, with its multiplanar three-dimensional capabilities and superb bone detail, is well suited for the evaluation of complex and difficult-to-diagnose fractures (Figs 14.7, 14.12D, 14.13A and B, and 14.16D and E). Nuclear medicine bone scans are also used in this situation; however, in the elderly, it may take a few days for the nuclear medicine scan to become positive. For diffuse bone metastases, whole body nuclear bone scanning is best, whereas spine metastases are evaluated well with MRI (Figs 14.11B and 14.13C). Nuclear medicine still has a major role to play in the diagnosis of pulmonary embolus despite the move to CT. Acute cholecystitis, bile leaks, intestinal bleeding and infection are other diagnoses that can be made with nuclear medicine. FDG PET, as outlined above, has a major and increasing role to play in cancer imaging (Fig 14.11D). It also has a role in the diagnosis of brain disorders including Alzheimer's disease, Parkinson's disease and seizures. In the future, it will also likely be used in the evaluation of myocardial perfusion.

Diagnostic vascular imaging is now mainly performed noninvasively using ultrasound, CT and MRI. Long and deep vessels, e.g. the thoracic and abdominal aorta and entire lower limb arterial supply, are best seen with magnetic resonance arteriography (MRA) and computed tomography arteriography (CTA) (Fig. 14.8). Ultrasound with Doppler is very effective for short superficial vessels and is excellent

for evaluating carotid artery stenosis in the neck. It is also the best test for deep vein thrombosis in the upper and lower limb.

Infection of the foot, especially with diabetes, is a common problem. The foot is first evaluated with X-ray imaging. This provides a lot of basic information including the presence of arthritis and neuropathic changes. However, plain film changes of osteomyelitis are a late finding and soft-tissue infection and viability are poorly seen. On the contrary, MRI has proven very useful in evaluating foot and spine infection (Figs 14.13D and E, and 14.14F and G). For more information/updates go to the ACR website and navigate to Appropriateness Criteria (see Bibliography).

CONCLUSION

Medical imaging has come a long way in the past 100 years. The improvements have mirrored developments in technology. This has brought faster imaging times, improved anatomical detail and, more recently, molecular imaging. As a result, medical imaging is an important and integral part of modern medical practice. Future developments promise to build on these capabilities and help provide insight into the cause of disease, improved diagnosis, earlier detection and improved and targeted treatment regimes. With constant change in the capabilities of the various modalities, new knowledge of disease processes and each patient's unique set of problems, it is

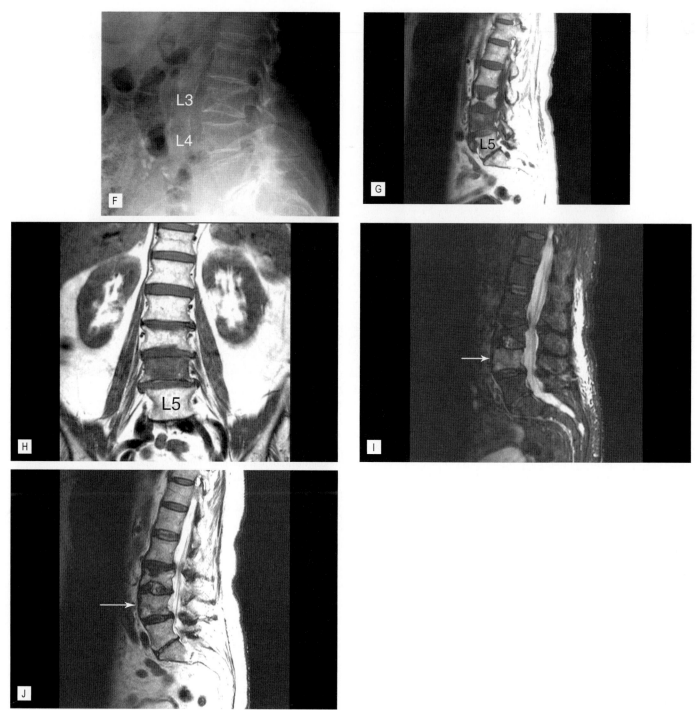

Figure 14.13 **(F–J) Vertebral compression fractures.** Vertebral fractures are a common cause of back pain in the elderly. This 70-year-old sustained a lumbar compression fracture, following a fall. The case illustrates how MR is used to determine if the fracture on X-ray is recent or old and diagnose occult fractures. The radiograph (F) shows a fracture at L3. MRI also shows the fracture. However, on the sagittal and coronal T1 images (G and H) the vertebra is bright, the same as all the other vertebrae with the exception of L4 which is dark. L4, however, is bright on the STIR or fluid-sensitive image (I). What does this mean? The radiograph certainly shows a fracture at L3. However, it is an old fracture that has healed. This is confirmed on the MR where the signal of this vertebra is normal. L4 represents the acute fracture as seen by the bone marrow edema – dark on T1, bright on STIR. The fracture has not resulted in any loss of height of the vertebra, making it hard to pinpoint on the radiograph. A sagittal T2-weighted image (J) shows the fracture line. This serves to illustrate a frequent problem. In older individuals, compression fractures, usually related to osteoporosis, are common. The radiograph is able to show the fracture, providing there is compression of the vertebra or a fracture line. However, unless a recent study is available for comparison, it is not able to tell if this is new or old, and, as in this case, it can underdiagnose injury. The MR by demonstrating the bone marrow edema is able to show that an acute fracture has occurred and that it occurred at L4, not L3 as suggested on the radiograph. It is important to know which vertebra is involved prior to treatment and MR is frequently used to sort out this common conundrum. (Continued.)

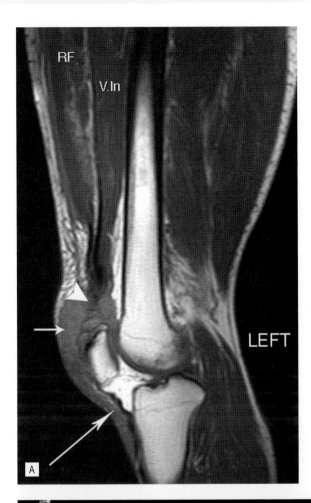

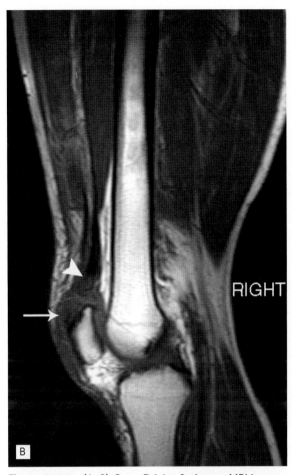

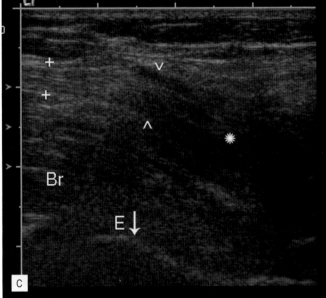

Figure 14.14   (A–G). **Superficial soft tissues.** MRI is very useful for evaluating superficial soft tissue pathology, particularly complex and acute problems. Lesions with calcium require X-ray. Ultrasound can be used for small or focal lesions. Radio-opaque foreign bodies need X-ray, whereas non-radio-opaque foreign bodies can be evaluated with ultrasound. (A and B) **Acute bilateral quadriceps rupture.** This 59-year-old male was unable to extend his knees after a fall. The sagittal T1-weighted image of both knees shows rupture of both quadriceps tendons at the attachment to the patella (arrow head). Loss of the normal dark signal of the tendon is seen. There is an associated hematoma on both sides (arrow), left > right. (V. In vastus intermedius, RF rectus femoris muscle). Note the crumpled patellar tendon and slight distal patellar displacement on the left side (long arrow). Quadriceps rupture is more common above the age of 40 and considered to be secondary to tendon degeneration. Bilateral rupture is unusual, however. MRI allows excellent depiction of this problem. The tendons were surgically reattached. (C) **Ultrasound of biceps tendon rupture.** This 71-year-old woman presented with anterior elbow and upper forearm pain and swelling following a fall. She tried to catch herself by grabbing the table with her hand while the elbow was flexed. This is a sagittal ultrasound of the lower end of the biceps tendon as it starts to dive towards its insertion onto the radial tuberosity, just below the elbow. The tendon is torn from the tuberosity. The normal linear fibers of the tendon (++) are interrupted and irregular (between the two arrows ><). The distal tendon is bulbous, representing degenerated torn tendon, fibrous tissue and surrounding edema (*). These findings were confirmed at surgery during reattachment of the tendon to the tuberosity. Brachialis muscle deep to the biceps tendon (Br). Anterior bony margin of the elbow (E). (Continued.)

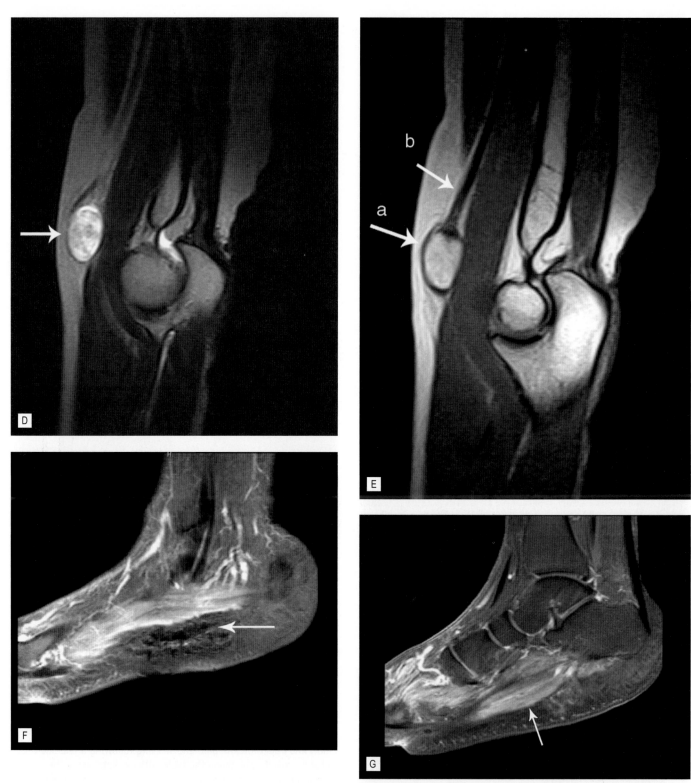

Figure 14.14   (D) **Nerve sheath tumor.** This 56-year-old female presented with hand numbness, upper extremity pain and soft tissue mass anterior to the elbow. The nerve sheath tumor is exquisitely demonstrated by MR. The nerve (arrow b) can be seen running into the tumor (arrow a). The MR findings are characteristic with the tumor bright on T2 (D) and enhancing with gadolinium on the T1 image (E). Surgical and pathological confirmation. (F and G) **Foot infection: cellulitis and osteomyelitis.** A combination of radiographs and nuclear medicine has traditionally been used to evaluate osteomyelitis in the foot. MR with its excellent soft tissue and bone marrow depiction is able to show both soft tissue and bone infection. This case shows an MRI of a 54-year-old diabetic with diffuse foot swelling and infected non-healing plantar ulcer. (F) and (G) are sagittal views of the foot. They are T1-weighted images with fat saturation obtained after intravenous injection of gadolinium chelate. There is increased enhancement of the plantar soft tissues (bright area and vertical arrow) indicating infection. The bright tubular structures are veins. The black area or signal void is due to gas in adjacent devitalized tissue (horizontal arrow). These findings were confirmed at surgery.

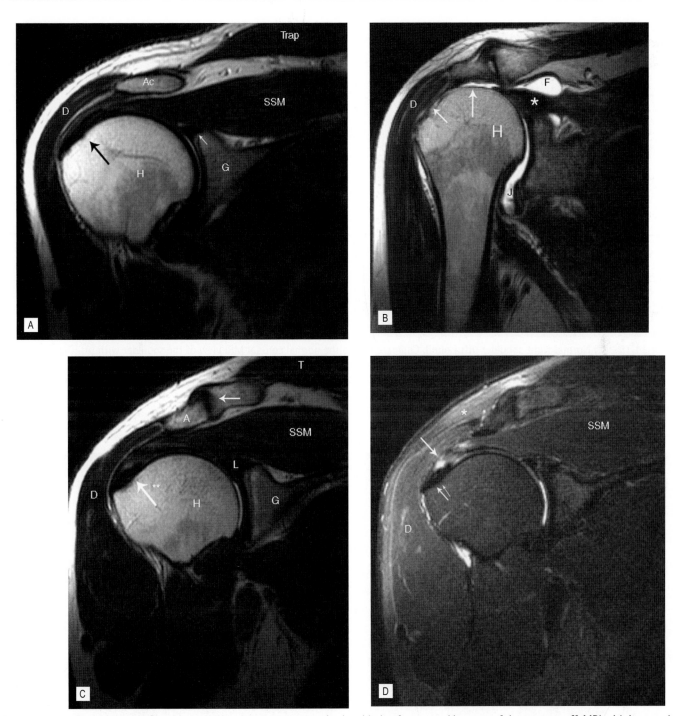

Figure 14.15   **Shoulder pain.** Shoulder pain is a common symptom in the elderly often caused by tears of the rotator cuff. MRI with its superb soft tissue contrast and multiplanar abilities is well suited for imaging the rotator cuff. In patients unable to undergo MRI, ultrasound with its ability to image superficial soft tissue structures is an excellent technique for evaluating the rotator cuff. (A) **Normal right shoulder MRI.** This is a coronal view using a T2 weighted imaging sequence (T2WI). This view is part of a MR assessment of the rotator cuff, a common source of tendon tears. The supraspinatus muscle (SSM), part of the rotator cuff, is well seen. The muscle arises from the supraspinous fossa of the scapula. It passes under the acromion to insert anteriorly on the greater tuberosity (black arrow) of the humerus (H) shown above. The lateral margin of the deltoid (D) is well seen in this view, arising from the lateral and upper margin of the acromion (Ac). Superior labrum (small white arrow), trapezius muscle (Trap). (B) **Full thickness tear of the supraspinatus tendon.** Compare normal shoulder in (A). This coronal MRI, T2WI shows that this patient has sustained a large full thickness tear of the supraspinatus tendon. Note how the greater tuberosity and superior humeral head (arrows) are now bare. The tendon is retracted medially almost to the superior margin of the glenoid. (*) The humeral head is displaced superiorly and abuts the under surface of the acromion. Fluid is seen in the subacromial bursa (F) and in the glenohumeral joint (J). (C and D) **Partial tear of the supraspinatus tendon.** (C) is a coronal MRI, T2W1, showing mild increase in signal in the bursal or superior fibers of the tendon (white arrow and two stars). Note the normal bright signal from the subcutaneous fat overlying the deltoid. Acromioclavicular joint (small white arrow), glenoid (G), labrum (L). (D) Same area using an additional fat saturation sequence to remove the fat signal. Note how the subcutaneous fat is now gray. (*) Note also the bright signal in the tendon caused by the tear is better appreciated (single arrow). (Double arrow, normal dark signal from unaffected lateral margin of tendon.)

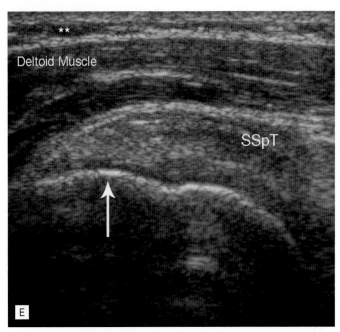

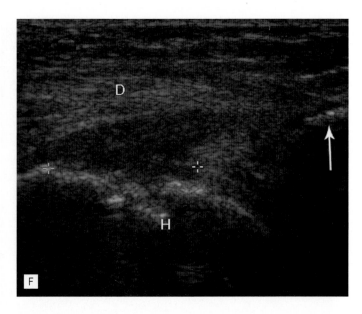

Figure 14.15 (E) **Normal right shoulder ultrasound.** Compare this to the normal coronal MRI view of the shoulder with (A). The supraspinatus tendon (SSpT) is well seen inserting into the greater tuberosity of the humerus (white arrow). (** subcutaneous fat overlying the deltoid). (F) **Right shoulder ultrasound. Full thickness tear.** Compare this to the MRI full thickness tear (B). The horizontal echogenic fibers of the tendon are separated by a distance of 1.7 cm(++). The space is filled with hypoechoic material representing fluid and granulation tissue. Acromion (arrow), deltoid muscle (D), greater tuberosity and head of humerus (H).

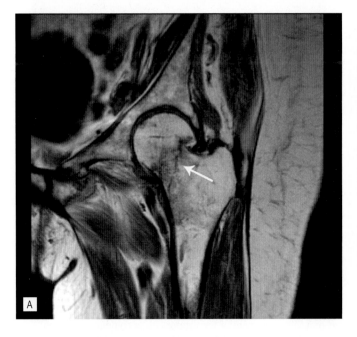

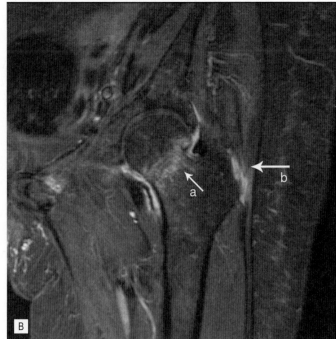

Figure 14.16 **Hip pain.** This 76-year-old woman experienced left hip pain following a fall. The hip radiograph was normal. (A) is a T1-weighted coronal image of the left hip. This shows the fracture line (arrow) and gray areas in the adjacent bone marrow representing edema. (B) is a fluid-sensitive coronal image showing a linear bright area representing edema at the level of the fracture (arrow a). While the radiograph was negative, the MR was able to confirm the clinical suspicion of a fracture and allow treatment in a timely manner. Note the associated partial tear of the gluteus medius at its insertion (B, arrow b) illustrating MRI's ability to show other causes of hip pain following trauma such as adjacent muscle strain or tears and pelvic fractures.

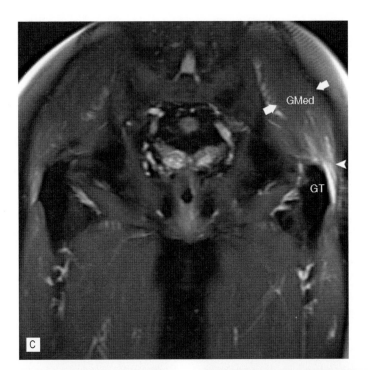

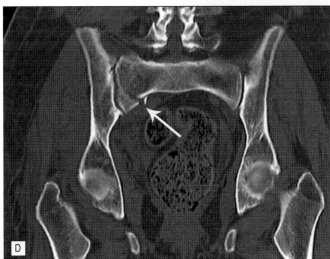

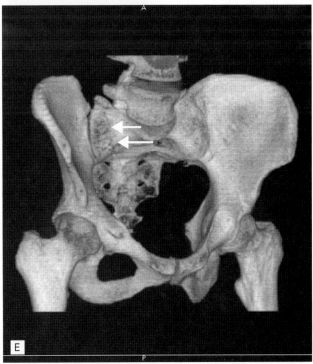

Figure 14.16   (C) **Tear of the gluteus medius muscle**. This is a coronal fluid-sensitive MRI (STIR) scan of the pelvis and both hips in a 76-year-old women with left trochanteric pain. This demonstrates a full thickness tear of the lateral fibers of the gluteus medius muscle (GMed, between arrows) at its insertion onto the greater trochanter of the left femur (arrow head). So-called trochanteric pain syndrome is more common in middle-aged and elderly women. This has often been ascribed to trochanteric bursitis. However with the advent of MRI it is now felt that this syndrome is more likely due to tendinopathy of the gluteus minimus and medius muscles, which both insert into the greater trochanter, and the bursitis is a secondary effect. The changes are analogous to tears of the rotator cuff of the shoulder. (D and E) **Hip pain**. This 56-year-old female experienced right hip and pelvic pain following a fall. The radiographs were normal. (D) is a coronal reconstructed CT image showing a fracture of the right sacrum (arrow). (E) is a 3D volume-rendered image elegantly demonstrating the fracture (arrows). The right hip was normal.

not possible to be dogmatic on which modality is best suited for a given situation. However, an understanding of the strengths and weaknesses of the current imaging modalities will be of benefit when deciding the appropriate study for addressing the patient's particular clinical problem.

Finally, despite all of the spectacular progress over the past 100 years, medical imaging remains but one tool in the clinical armamentarium and is still no substitute for a good clinical history and physical examination.

ACKNOWLEDGMENTS

I would like to thank the technical staff from the Radiology Department, Lancaster General Hospital and MRI Group, Lancaster, Pennsylvania. With special thanks to Chris Weir, Mark Houseman, Idriz Dizdarevic, Dean Hollenbacher, Kory Mollica, Kevin Barnhar, Doug Peterson, Corinne Daubenhauser. Jerry Kornfield for computer and graphics advice.

Note

Left and right sides are defined from the perspective of the radiologist looking at the patient from the foot of the bed. The patient's right side is opposite the radiologist's left. This is why in Fig. 14.12C the shift is to the patient's right although in the image it is to the left.

References

Smith RA et al 2004 The randomized trials of breast cancer screening: what have we learned? Radiol Clin North Am 42:793-806

Bibliography

Grainger & Allison's Diagnostic Radiology: A Text Book of Medical Imaging, 4th edn. This is a good general radiology text.
Radiologic Clinics of North America. Available: http://www.theclinics.com. Excellent up-to-date monographs published bimonthly.
Radiological Society of North America (RSNA) website. Available: http://rsna.org. While you need to be a member to gain access to all the information there are lots of free articles and information. Click on Patient information. Lots of information here including the Radiology in motion section with short, funny, video clips on various imaging modalities.
The American College of Radiology website. Available: http://www.acr.org. Again you need to be a member to gain full access but there is a lot of free information. For evidence-based guidelines on the most appropriate way to image patients, go to Quality and Patient Safety. From the pop-up menu choose Appropriateness Criteria. Also in this section is the Manual on Contrast Media and MR Safety.
The Food and Drug Administration (FDA) website. For updates on gadolinium contrast agents go to www.fda.gov/cder

UNIT **2**

Musculoskeletal disorders

UNIT CONTENTS

Chapter 15

Posture

Timothy L. Kauffman

INTRODUCTION

Posture is the alignment of body parts in relationship to one another at any given moment. Posture involves complex interactions between bones, joints, connective tissue, skeletal muscles and the nervous system, both central and peripheral. The complexity of these interactions is compounded when one considers the near infinitesimal variety of human balance, motor control, and movement in relation to gravity. Furthermore, with the passage of time, each organism undergoes change resulting from microtrauma and frank injuries to, and the effects of disease on, the connective tissues, muscles and neural control mechanisms, which results in the unique variations of aging posture.

Posture is commonly assessed using a grid or a plumb line, with the patient in a static standing position; however, within the aging population, this becomes more difficult because of the age-associated increase in postural sway (O'Brien et al 1997). This can be seen in the two photos of a 98-year-old man taken only moments apart (Fig. 15.1). The postural control mechanisms produce minor shifts in weight in order to avoid fatigue, excessive tissue compression and venous stasis (Soderberg 1986). Hence, a photographic assessment of posture represents a fixed instant of a postural set. Thus, posture is actually a relative condition requiring full body integration and both static and dynamic balance control, as shown in Fig. 15.2.

Multiple factors are involved in common age-related postural changes. These factors may be pathological, degenerative or traumatic, or may result from primary musculoskeletal changes, primary neurological changes or a combination of diminutions in the neuromusculoskeletal system.

Degenerative joint disease is a common age-related pathology involving bony and joint surface changes (see Chapters 20, 25 and 26). The osteophytes that result from arthritis may prevent normal joint motion, cause pain and possibly encroach on nerves with a subsequent radiculopathy that includes muscle weakness and imbalance. Postural adjustments may be the result of attempts to unload weight from an osteophyte in order to reduce pain or to accommodate a radiculopathy (Kauffman 1987).

AXIAL AND APPENDICULAR SKELETAL CHANGES

The common age-associated postural changes in the axial skeleton and their clinical implications are enumerated in Table 15.1 and may be seen in Figures 15.3 and 15.4. The idiosyncratic effects of 20 years of aging can be seen by comparing the images of the 78-year-old man in Figures 15.3B and 15.4B with the photographs in Figures 15.1 and 15.5, which were taken when the man was 98 years old. In the lateral view, note the large increases in trunk kyphosis and hip flexion. By comparing images of the posterior view at different ages (Fig. 15.4B and Fig. 15.5), the kyphoscoliosis with upper extremity extension, increased hip and knee flexion and loss of muscle mass in all four extremities and trunk are evident. A different individual, aged 93 years and shown in Figure 15.3C, also demonstrates extension of the upper extremities. The 98-year-old man's postural set (Figs 15.1 and 15.5) may be affected by his chief musculoskeletal complaints of right hip pain and decreased sensation and strength in the lower extremities. He lives in assisted living and uses a wheeled walker for most ambulation.

It is important to note that not all of these changes should be classified as being faulty or abnormal. Some of the adjustments may be normal compensatory changes resulting from other neuromusculoskeletal alterations in the spine, extremities or central control mechanisms. For example, the head-forward position, especially when there is an increased extension of the upper cervical spine, may be the result of the body's attempts to counter a dorsal kyphosis caused by wedged thoracic vertebrae.

The effect of osteoporosis in the vertebrae on posture and vice versa is profound, with an abundance of recognized fractures, silent

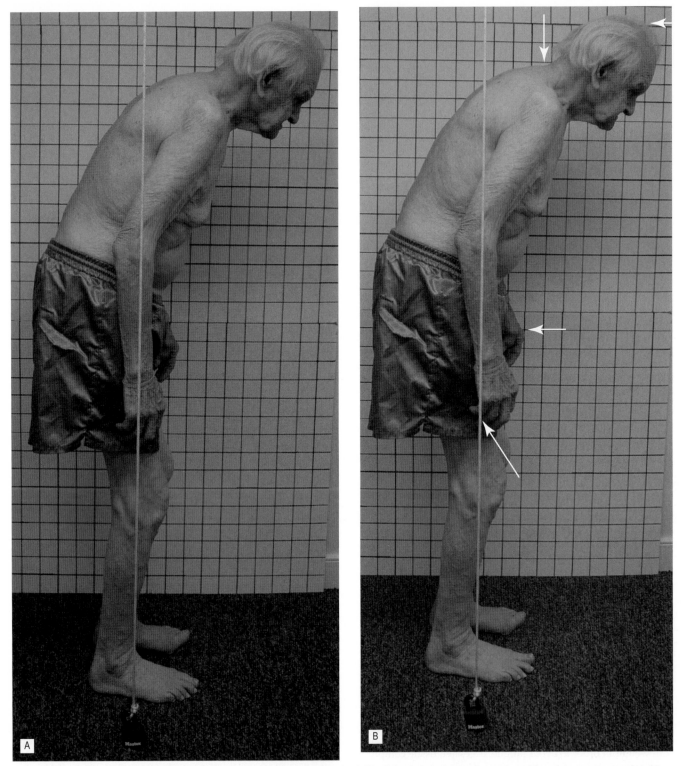

Figure 15.1 (A and B) This 98-year-old man's posture shows a subtle shift of the hands forward, trunk and head more erect and right great toe extension. The photos were taken less than 1 s apart.

or no-known-antecedent-event fractures and microfractures (see Chapters 19 and 62 for more detail).

Spinal spondylosis is found in the vast majority of people by the age of 55 (Badley 1987). This may include deterioration of the spinal facet joints, loss of vertebral height, narrowing of the spinal canal or neural foramina, loss of intervertebral disk space, anterior lipping, formation of bony bridges and calcification of the periarticular connective tissue. Clinically, these changes may cause pain and reduction

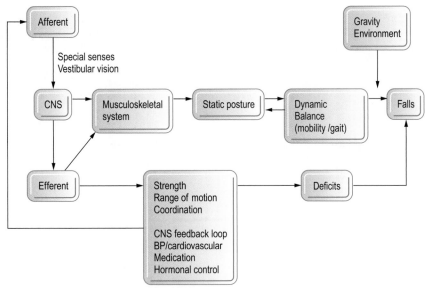

Figure 15.2   Factors affecting posture and falls. Multiple interactive forces govern static posture and dynamic balance. CNS, central nervous system; BP, blood pressure. From Kauffman 1990, with permission.

Table 15.1   Age-associated postural axial skeletal changes and their clinical implications

Axial skeletal changes	Clinical implications
Head forward	Shifts center of mass forward; may increase dizziness because of a compromised basilar artery
Dorsal kyphosis	Reduces trunk motions for breathing and motor responses; encourages scapular protraction; may provoke shoulder pathologies
Flat lumbar spine	Reduces trunk/hip extension for gait strides
Occasional kyphosis of lumbar spine	Results from compression of vertebral bodies; not reversible
Increased lordosis (least common)	Results in tightness of trunk/hip extensors; weakened abdominals
Posterior pelvic tilt	Results from prolonged sitting; reduces trunk/hip extension for gait strides
Scoliosis	May alter balance, breathing and extremity motions

in spinal motions, especially the subtle rotation motions involved in segmental rolling and the normal reciprocal pattern of the extremities in normal gait. The sit-to-stand motion may be more difficult because of the loss of coordinated spine flexion and extension.

In the appendicular skeleton, numerous combinations of changes occur as a result of a lifetime of wear and tear, habit, trauma and pathology in the neuromusculoskeletal system. These changes result in the unique postural features of aging individuals. The common

age-associated extremity changes and clinical implications are enumerated in Table 15.2 and may be seen in Figures 15.3 and 15.4.

SOFT TISSUE

Postural changes caused by soft-tissue alterations may be a result of previous injuries that have lengthened or tightened tendons, ligaments and joint capsules. Collagen is a major component of skin, tendons, cartilage and connective tissue and it may become increasingly stiff because of cross-linkage between collagen fibers. Elastin is another major fibrous component of connective tissue that is found in the skin, ligaments, blood vessels and lungs. With increasing age, elastin is supplanted by pseudoelastin, which is a partially degraded collagen or faulty elastin protein (Hall 1985).

Additional soft-tissue changes that may lead to postural alterations can be found in the muscle. The muscle length may be increased or decreased. There is a loss of muscle fibers, which is likely to result in reduced strength. The type I and type II muscle fiber relationship may be altered, which can influence postural control responses and mechanisms. In addition, there is an increase in non-contractile tissue because of the deposition of fat and collagen, which causes the muscle to become increasingly stiff. Muscle tone may increase, decrease or vary because of changes in nervous system control. A more extensive discussion of these nervous system changes may be found in Chapter 5.

CLINICAL CONSIDERATIONS

In the geriatric population, posture should be assessed not only in the standing and sitting positions but also in bed, especially in a patient who is confined to bed because of an injury or illness. It is particularly important to prevent pressure areas, and special care

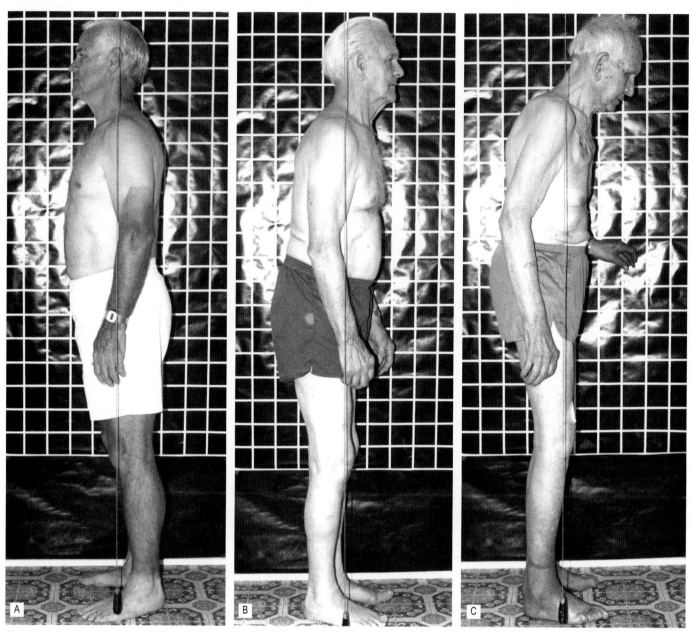

Figure 15.3   Lateral posture of (A) a 60-year-old man; (B) a 78-year-old man; and (C) a 93-year-old man.

should be taken to avoid muscle imbalances resulting from pro- longed positioning. Areas of particular importance are the triceps surae, hip and knee flexors, and hip abductors and adductors, espe- cially after hip surgery. It is common for the patient to assume a supine but side-bent posture that may lead to muscle imbalance. The patient who side-bends toward the operative side will suffer a contralateral hip abductor lengthening and an ipsilateral hip abduc- tor shortening. The converse is true for the patient who side-bends away from the operative side. These muscle imbalances will become significant during rehabilitation when the patient attempts to regain independent ambulation and they may contribute to a Trendelenburg gait (see Chapter 16 for further discussion of muscle lengthening and the concept of stretch-weakness changes).

Ryan and Fried (1997) studied the relationship between moderate to severe kyphosis and physical performance in 231 community

dwellers between the ages of 59 and 89. Kyphosis was associated with slower speeds of gait and stair climbing and difficulties with reaching or heavy lifting. Sinaki et al (2005) reported that commu- nity dwelling females with osteoporotic-related kyphosis had reduced anteroposterior displacement and velocity and increased mediolateral displacement and velocity on a balance force platform when compared with slightly younger healthy control subjects. The kyphotic subjects also had greater balance abnormalities when measured on posturography.

Hyperkyphosis measured in the supine position in 1578 older community dwelling males and females was significantly associated in a stepwise manner with declining self-reported function for bend- ing, walking, climbing and rising from a chair. Grip strength was also significantly associated with this postural change; the greater the kyphosis, the less the strength. Based on their technique of

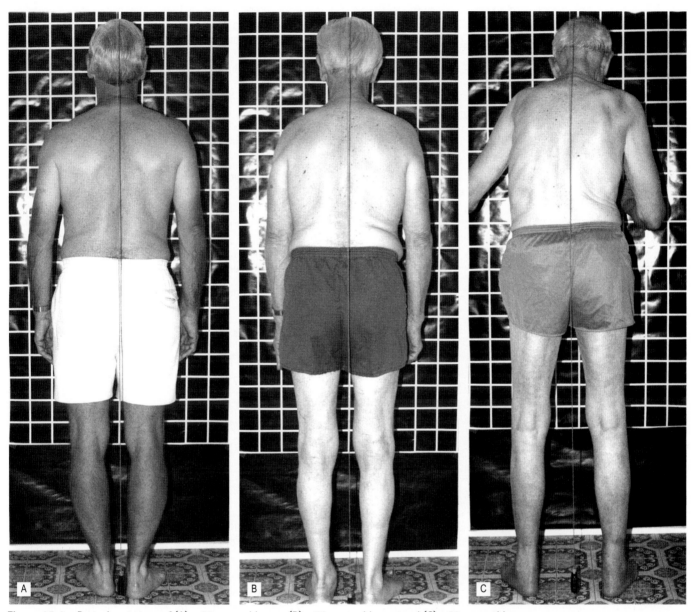

Figure 15.4   Posterior posture of (A) a 60-year-old man; (B) a 78-year-old man; and (C) a 93-year-old man.

measuring kyphosis, by placing blocks behind the head to achieve a neutral position, they found that males were approximately twice as likely to be classified as hyperkyphotic than females (Kado et al 2005).

Brown et al (1995) demonstrated the important relationship between the strength of postural muscles in the lower extremities and functional tasks including walking, stair climbing and getting up from a chair. Weakness of calf muscles coupled with insufficient strength of the scapulothoracic stabilizers can contribute to increased kyphotic posture and loss of balance, especially when reaching forward with the upper extremities.

Menz and Munteanu (2005) established the validity of the foot posture index in older people (mean age 78.6 years). The index involves postural assessment in the relaxed bipedal stance position of the following eight criteria: talar head, malleolar position, Helbing's sign (the angle of the Achilles tendon insertion to the calcaneus), frontal plane of the calcaneus, position of the talonavicular joint, the medial longitudinal arch, lateral border of the foot and abduction/adduction of the rear or forefoot. Menz et al (2005) reported significant associations between the foot posture index and walking speed and balance impairments.

Clinical intervention should be undertaken in the case of postural changes if they cause pain, impair function or are likely to lead to future impairment. Typical interventions are listed in Box 15.1. These clinical interventions are not listed in order of importance. One or all of the interventions may be appropriate, depending upon the clinical assessment and the individual patient's condition and prognosis.

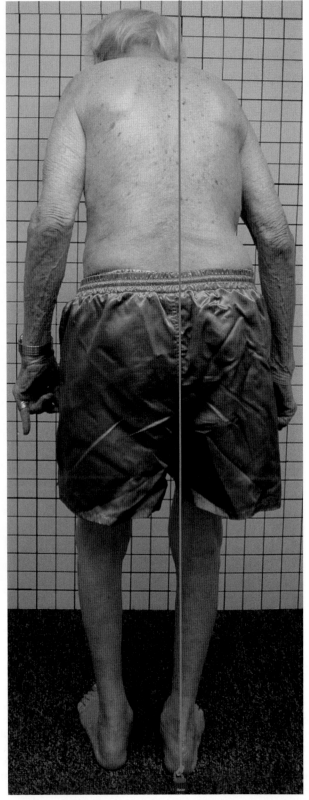

Figure 15.5   Postural changes are quite evident in this 98-year-old man when compared with his posture 20 years earlier (Fig. 15.4B). This degree of change is unique to this individual but is common in aging individuals. Note the kyphoscoliosis with extension of the upper extremities, increased hip and knee flexion and loss of muscle mass in all four extremities and trunk.

Table 15.2   Age-associated postural extremity changes and their clinical implications

Extremity skeletal changes	Clinical implications
Scapular protraction or abduction	Alters normal scapulohumeral rhythm, leading to painful shoulder conditions
Tightness/contractures in elbow flexion, wrist ulnar deviation, finger flexion	Reduces reach and hand function
Hip flexion contractures (loss of hip extension to neutral or 0°)	Reduces stride length; may increase energy cost of mobility and may increase postural control requirements, especially if change is unilateral
Knee flexion contractures (loss of knee extension to neutral or 0°)	Reduces stride length and gait push-off; may increase energy cost of mobility and may increase postural control requirements, especially if change is unilateral
Varus/valgus changes at hip, knee, ankle	Reduces stride length and gait push-off; may increase energy cost of mobility and may increase postural control requirements especially if change is unilateral. Usually is a cause of pain because of mechanical deformation and strain on musculoskeletal tissues

Box 15.1   Clinical interventions for postural changes causing pain or dysfunction

1. Brace, support, immobilize, protect
2. Heat, cold, electrical stimulation
3. Therapeutic exercise to enhance functional muscle strength, tone, length, coordination, and balance between agonist and antagonist
4. Medications
5. Surgery

CONCLUSION

It is crucial to note that postural changes occur with increasing age and their characteristics are unique to each individual. Although not present in a young healthy adult, the new traits are not necessarily faulty. As noted above, they may indicate normal compensation for a degradation in the neuromusculoskeletal alignment or a loss of control of any of its component parts. Many of these changes have taken place slowly over decades and may not be ameliorated easily, if at all.

References

Badley E 1987 Epidemiological aspects of the aging spine. In: Hukins D, Nelson M (eds) The Ageing Spine. Manchester University Press, Manchester, UK, p 1–17

Brown M, Sinacore D, Host H 1995 The relationship of strength to function in the older adult. J Gerontol Ser A 50A:55–59

Hall D 1985 Biology of aging: structural and metabolic aspects. In: Brockelhurst J (ed.) Textbook of Geriatric Medicine and Gerontology. Churchill Livingstone, New York, p 46–61

Kado D, Huang M, Barrett-Connor E et al 2005 Hyperkyphotic posture and poor physical functional ability in older community-dwelling men and women: the Rancho Bernardo Study. J Gerontol Med Sci 60A(5):633–637

Kauffman T 1987 Posture and age. Top Geriatr Rehabil 2:1328

Kauffman T 1990 Impact of aging-related musculoskeletal and postural changes on falls. Top Geriatr Rehabil 5:34–43

O'Brien K, Culham E, Pickles B 1997 Balance and skeletal alignment in a group of elderly female fallers and nonfallers. J Gerontol Biol Sci 52A:B221–B226

Menz H, Munteanu S 2005 Validity of 3 clinical techniques for the measurement of static foot posture in older people. J Orthop Sports Phys Ther 35:479–486

Menz H, Morris M, Lord S 2005 Foot and ankle characteristics associated with impaired balance and functional ability in older people. J Gerontol Med Sci 60A(12):1546–1552

Ryan S, Fried L 1997 The impact of kyphosis on daily functioning. J Am Geriatr Soc 45:1479–1486

Sinaki M, Brey R, Hughes C et al 2005 Balance disorder and increased risk of falls in osteoporosis and kyphosis: significance of kyphotic posture and muscle strength. Osteoporosis Int 16:1004–1010

Soderberg G 1986 Kinesiology: Application to Pathological Motion. Williams & Wilkins, Baltimore, MD, p 309–336

Chapter 16

Muscle weakness and therapeutic exercise

Timothy L. Kauffman and Michelle Bolton

INTRODUCTION

The term 'sarcopenia' has been coined to describe the less than normal strength of muscle and diminished muscle mass that is associated with aging. Weakness has long been connected with aging; however, the role of muscle involves more than just providing strength. Muscle is involved with movement, which is crucial for joint nutrition as well as for cardiopulmonary health. Also, muscle is related to the circulatory system, as smooth muscle supports the walls of arteries and skeletal muscle is involved in the return of venous blood. Muscle is also involved in bone health and density. It also provides impetus to the nervous system, as primary sensory fibers of the muscle spindle respond to muscle stretching. A principal source of body heat comes from muscle and, additionally, it provides a cushion of compressible tissue that helps to absorb impact in the event of trauma (Wagner & Kauffman 2001).

DEFINITIONS

Muscle is principally noted for its roles in strength and movement. Strength may be defined as the tension that is generated by contracting muscle and is best expressed as a force. Torque, a result of angular displacement, is the product of force and the perpendicular distance from the line of the force's action to the axis of rotation. Time is also a consideration for the tension that is generated and thus should be considered muscle power.

The generation of muscle tension is determined largely by the cross-sectional area of the muscle and the recruitment of motor units (Fiatarone-Singh 2004). Other biomechanical factors, such as muscle length and angle of displacement, and physiological factors, such as metabolism and muscle fiber type, also influence strength. Insufficient strength to perform a functional motor task should be considered weakness.

There are various types of muscle contractions. When there is no change in muscle length, a static contraction occurs, which is also referred to as isometric (same length). Dynamic contractions are a lengthening or shortening of a muscle, also called eccentric and concentric contractions respectively. Isotonic (same tone) contractions involve movement of a constant weight through a motion. Normally, raising a weight is a concentric contraction and lowering it is an eccentric contraction. When a mechanical device resists the tension generated by the contracting muscle, thereby controlling the speed of the limb's movement, an isokinetic (same speed) contraction occurs. Isokinetic devices are essential for assessing torque at various speeds, which is clinically important because of the age-related loss of fast-twitch type II muscle fibers. This loss is one of several factors that probably contribute to the increasing inability to recover from a stumble, which results in an increased risk of injury.

ASSESSMENT

Assessment of muscle strength can be performed using a manual muscle test (MMT). Although the MMT is an ordinal scale measurement, it is invaluable because it can be performed in nearly every treatment setting. When using the MMT, it is crucial to specify the type of contraction being performed. The original MMT was designed to be an assessment of strength throughout the available range of motion (ROM), but it has been modified in many circumstances to a 'make' test, in which the patient performs an isometric contraction at a specific joint position. Modification of the MMT may be especially necessary for aging patients (Jan et al 2005) and others who have painful arcs or restrictions in motion (Kauffman 1982). When measuring plantar flexor strength in the weight-bearing position on one leg, Jan et al (2005) found that men and women between 61 and 80 years of age were able to heel raise a mean of 4.1 and 2.7 times respectively. Men and women aged between 21 and 40 years were able to perform 22.1 and 16.1 repetitions respectively. Clarity in documentation is enhanced when these specifics (type of test and position) are recorded.

In contrast, a 'break' test is used when the patient is asked to hold the joint in a specific position and the evaluator attempts to break the tension that is generated. This changes it from an isometric to an eccentric contraction. It should be noted that in healthy muscle, the highest tension is generated with an eccentric contraction followed by an isometric contraction, and the least tension is generated with an isotonic contraction. As noted above, lowering a weight is an isotonic eccentric contraction and may be a helpful technique for strength-training patients. For example, lowering a flexed upper extremity that is weight-loaded may be effective for increasing the strength of the lower trapezius, rhomboids and deltoids.

Caution should be used when attempting to measure strength with the MMT in aging individuals because of the frequent necessity of modifying the test positions. In the aging patient, the test positions as enumerated in the standard manuals may have to be modified because of injury or disease. Also, a more functional position may be necessary because areas of weakness may be found only in certain positions of the joint's ROM. These areas of weakness may be the result of joint-surface irregularities or changes in periarticular connective tissue and muscle length.

Hand-held and isokinetic dynamometers are very useful for assessing strength. Caution must be used to avoid pain in and injury to swollen areas and ulcerated or atrophied skin; the verbal extolling that frequently accompanies this testing may have to be restrained. Also, a greater risk of joint injury because of age-related changes in periarticular connective tissue (see Chapters 4 and 63) should be considered when dynamometers are being used (Wagner & Kauffman 2001).

Another strength-assessment technique that is gaining popularity is the 1 RM or 10 RM technique. The 'RM' stands for repetition maximum: a 1 RM test measures the maximal weight (dynamic and isotonic) that can be moved through the ROM once, and 10 RM is the maximal weight that can be moved 10 times. Some guessing must be involved in determining the starting test weight, which may be too heavy or too light, and weight adjustments must be made accordingly. These techniques are safe for older patients but caution must be used during testing. Preexisting joint pathologies or limitations should be considered and the Valsalva maneuver should be avoided (Di Fabio 2001). Manor et al (2006) reported another method of assessing strength (and really power and endurance) by using elastic bands and recording the number of complete repetitions of the joint motion that can be achieved in 30 seconds. They found that the elastic band technique was significantly correlated with a 30-second test using dumb-bells and with maximal isokinetic torque.

Perhaps more important than a frank measurement of the force of a muscle contraction is a functional assessment of motor performance, such as the ability to ascend and descend a flight of steps or to raise a 1-kg (2-lb) can of food onto the second shelf of a cupboard. Noting that a patient was able to ascend six steps before catching a toe or failing to elevate the lower extremity would be a functional parameter of muscle performance. Endurance is an important consideration, too, especially as it relates to functional outcomes. It is one factor in the 10 RM test and is frequently measured with isokinetic devices. In activities of daily living, endurance is always a consideration; for example, carrying a full 1-gallon jug [8 lb (3.6 kg)] of water from the refrigerator to the kitchen table requires muscular strength and endurance (Wagner & Kauffman 2001).

STRENGTH TRAINING

Strength-training research since the early 1980s has shown that the potential to increase strength is maintained in older people (Kauffman 1985). The benefits of strength training with isometric, isotonic and isokinetic routines have been shown (Wagner & Kauffman 2001, Dodd et al 2004). Simple calisthenics without the use of

machines are efficacious (Fiatarone-Singh 2002). Hypertrophy occurs even in individuals aged 90 years and above, although hypertrophy itself is not necessarily a primary objective of care; however, as noted above, muscle mass does act as a shock absorber. Functional outcomes are related to strength and motor performance and should be the objective of rehabilitation.

Newman and associates (2006) reported that grip strength and isokinetic quadriceps strength were strongly related to mortality in the Health, Aging and Body Composition Study but that muscle size was not. Exactly how strength and mortality are associated is unclear but these researchers suggested that the assessment of strength may measure other important aspects of the aging process. It is possible that hormonal factors related to strength, such as testosterone and insulin-like growth factor (IGF), may contribute to the strength–mortality association (see comments below under Special considerations post-stroke) (Vaynman & Gomez-Pinilla 2005).

For excellent reviews of the benefits of therapeutic exercise on diseases, disability, performance and longevity see Barry and Carson (2004) and Fiatarone-Singh (2002, 2004).

Modifying strength training

When planning a strength-training routine for geriatric patients, it is crucial to consider the need to modify the training regimen in order to accommodate pathology in the cardiopulmonary and cardiovascular systems as well as in the neuromusculoskeletal system. Guidelines for exercise in patients with heart disease are presented in Chapter 41. The aging individual is more susceptible to skin tears as well as injuries to muscles, joints and ligaments; however, injuries can be minimized with the use of individualized and sound exercise techniques (Dodd et al 2004). Fatigue, poor physical work capacity and deconditioning are important considerations, especially in the frail elderly who have multiple diagnoses. The Valsalva maneuver must be avoided. Isometric exercises are safe, provided that the hold time is no more than 5–10 s, the standard isometric contraction. Blood pressure has been shown to be adversely affected by isometric contractions longer than 30 s in duration.

Aging patients who need an exercise program benefit from individualized instruction that is tailored to meet functional goals. Some individuals are fully cognitive and capable of engaging in standard strengthening and fitness exercises. Others do not have the same physical, cognitive or communicative abilities and, to be effective, the exercise program must be modified.

Monitoring response to exercise is requisite. This is achieved by observing and recording pulse rate, respiratory rate, perceived exertion and quality of movement. For example, asynchronous muscle contractions or obtaining full ROM for only the first six repetitions and not all 10 would be indicative of low quality of movement.

Blood pressure should be taken before, during and after exercise, especially in patients with known or suspected cardiovascular, cardiopulmonary or cerebrovascular disease. However, the repeated measurements with the use of a sphygmomanometer can become cumbersome in busy outpatient clinics and in home healthcare. An oxygen pulsimeter is used to measure oxygen levels and may be helpful for establishing safe exercise parameters. Clinically, the talk test is beneficial (Hourigan 2004). This is a simple safeguard that avoids overloading patients beyond capability by talking with them during the exercise routine. When overexercised, the patient will become dyspneic and be unable to talk in two- to three-word sentences.

Postexercise hypotension is a concern in patients who experience lightheadedness or near-syncope, especially after endurance training. In these cases, further workup is necessary to rule out cardiac, cardiopulmonary or other potential causes of the problem. These symptoms may result from carotid sinus hypersensitivity when the pulse is taken at the carotid artery. Compression at the carotid sinus may send impulses to the vasomotor and cardioinhibitory centers in the medulla resulting in hypotension (Ziegelstein 2004).

Training considerations

The overload principle is necessary but care must be taken to avoid excessive overload (*Merck Manual of Geriatrics* 2000, Hourigan 2004). Some patients with cognitive or communicative difficulties may benefit from gestures or ROM exercises, including passive, active assistive, active and resistive exercises, as well as proprioceptive neuromuscular facilitation. Physical contact may assist not only in attaining a desired movement but also in establishing a trusting rapport between patient and care provider. Also, the benefit of sensory stimulation to muscle activation has been recognized, especially in work with children and individuals with neurological conditions.

With a weight-training technique, it is common to start the therapeutic exercise routine with five to six contractions, using only 50% of the maximal voluntary contraction (MVC). Successive sets of five to six repetitions are performed using 60%, 70% and 80% of the MVC. The same technique of progressive resistive exercise may be done after a strength assessment with a hand-held dynamometer.

Functional activities done repeatedly, such as sit-to-stand 10 times, will not only strengthen muscles but also enhance coordination, endurance and motor learning (Hourigan 2004). Neural adaptations will occur in the motor cortex and in the spinal level that facilitates activation of individual muscles and coordinates groups of muscles (Barry & Carson 2004). Practice is important for skill acquisition (see Chapter 5).

Some patients have pathologies, for example chronic obstructive pulmonary disease, or are too deconditioned to effectively undergo typical exercise routines (*Merck Manual of Geriatrics* 2000) such as progressive resistive exercise and standard weight-loading programs; however, they may benefit from a graded circuit routine using a combination of chair exercises and, if possible, ambulatory activities. For example, with supervision, a patient may perform bilateral shoulder flexion 10 times followed by 10 repetitions of long-arc quads, two repetitions of sit-to-stand and 10 repetitions of hip flexion. Pulse rate should be monitored before and after exercise, and the talk test may also be employed. The speed and number of repetitions of these simple exercises can be increased or decreased according to the patient's response to exercise. Walking exercises can also be added. Some individuals may only be able to exercise for 1 min with this type of circuit routine, whereas others may be able to advance to 3–4 min. A rest of 1–5 min should be taken before repeating the routine. It is safe to start the routine again when the pulse rate has returned to the pre-exercise level. Sample circuit exercises are provided in Box 16.1.

Exercise machines clearly have benefits for some patients (*Merck Manual of Geriatrics* 2000). Weight-training units, bicycles, stair-steppers and rowing machines are all beneficial. As mentioned above, simple calisthenics and walking are mainstays in the exercise armamentarium for aging patients. Use of low weights at the ankles and wrists can increase the physical work carried out during simple walking exercises. Aquatic exercise is excellent for strengthening, conditioning and balance retraining especially after joint replacement, back surgery or in those with painful arthritic joints (see Chapter 73).

Special considerations post stroke

In a study performed by Mount et al (2005), it was found that individuals older than 50 years of age who had had a stroke more

> ### Box 16.1 Sample circuit exercises for the severely deconditioned or chairbound patient
>
> 1. Check pre-exercise pulse, respiratory rate or pulse oximetry.
> 2. Raise both arms over head 10 times.
> 3. Straighten each knee 10 times (alternate sides).
> 4. Abduct both arms 10 times.
> 5. Flex each hip 10 times.
> 6. Repeat above routine or expand to additional exercises, if possible, such as wheelchair push-ups; elbow flexion/extension; sit-to-stand; shoulder shrugs; gluteal squeezes; deep inspiration and forced exhalation; resistive exercise with or without elastic tubing; and walking. Length of exercise should vary based on the patient's ability and limitations. These more exertional exercises are best performed after the easier warm-up exercises in 2 to 5.
> 7. Check postexercise pulse, respiration rate or pulse oximetry.
> 8. Rest until heart rate returns to approximately pre-exercise rate, then repeat the routine, if appropriate.

than 6 months previously could make improvements by undertaking balance and functional activities. This case study consisted of four subjects who underwent a balance intervention twice a week for eight weeks. Activities varied from a warm-up, including stretches and yoga-like poses, to dynamic gait and Theraball™ exercises. Each class lasted approximately 1 h. All subjects were assessed using the Berg Balance Scale (BBS) and Performance Oriented Mobility Assessment (POMA), before and after intervention. All four subjects made gains in their functional balance as measured by these two assessment tools. This study illustrates that gains can be made after a traditional course of therapy. Further research is needed to determine the effect of this class in improving functional balance and decreasing the risk/incidence of falls.

Vaynman and Gomez-Pinilla (2005) reported that exercise has beneficial effects on the central nervous system by increasing regional blood supply and by the actions of trophic factors like IGF and brain-derived neurotrophic factor (BDNF). These factors promote neuronal and synaptic plasticity especially in the hippocampus which is crucially involved in learning and memory. Exercise three or more times weekly has been shown to delay the onset of dementia and to demonstrate benefits in physical performance and cognition (Larson et al 2006).

Cancer

Galvao and Newton (2005) reviewed 26 published studies of exercise interventions for patients with breast, stomach, prostate, colorectal, Hodgkin's and non-Hodgkin's cancers. Exercises included cardiovascular, resistance and flexibility activities. The benefits were dose dependent, but overall improvements were found in strength, oxygen consumption, flexibility, fatigue and psychological well-being.

WHEN STRENGTH TRAINING IS NOT EFFECTIVE

When an aging patient is undergoing a strength-training routine but there is no marked improvement in strength, a number of factors may be involved in reducing the patient's potential to improve muscular performance. First, adequate nutrition is critical. Sufficient calorie and protein intake is necessary if any exercise routine is to be performed. However, malnutrition is common among the elderly; frequently, ill health precedes it. Decreased physical activity may also contribute to malnutrition, and bereavement, depression, dementia and living alone are all factors that can result in a decreased appetite. Changes in the gastrointestinal tract (see Chapter 8) and medications may also diminish food and fluid intake. Vitamin D deficiency is a factor in osteoporosis that can contribute to back pain and subsequent weakness.

Second, dehydration is an important consideration when conducting exercises with patients, especially in the home-health setting. Adequate hydration is a concern not only during hot humid months but also during cold dry periods. Dehydration can alter mental status and thus decrease receptiveness to exercise. Lightheadedness, syncope and orthostatic hypotension may also present as findings in the dehydrated elderly patient.

The use of statins for hypercholesterolemia may cause muscle complaints such as weakness, myalgia, myositis and even rhabdomyolysis. The last two conditions can be very serious and rhabdomyolysis can even be fatal (Thompson et al 2003). Other factors that may limit muscle responses to exercise include poorly oxygenated blood resulting from chronic lung disease and faulty or reduced cardiac responses. Beta blockers and pacemakers often reduce the ability of the heart to respond to the increased demands from exercise, thereby circumscribing the effects of exercise (see Chapters 6, 7, 41 and 45 for more complete details).

Blood chemistry imbalances

Iron deficiency anemia is not likely to occur in aging individuals with a sensible, balanced diet; however, it may be found in those with neoplasms and gastrointestinal bleeding. This may manifest as decreased hemoglobin or hematocrit levels in the blood chemistry, and the patient may present with fatigue and weakness.

Magnesium is a mineral that is important for normal muscle contraction, and a deficiency is commonly found with low serum levels of calcium, potassium and phosphate. Hypomagnesemia is associated with muscle excitability, hyperreflexia, tetany, seizures, ataxia, tremors and weakness (*Merck Manual of Geriatrics* 2000).

Faulty calcium regulation may also contribute to changes in muscle performance. Hypercalcemia is often associated with primary hyperparathyroidism but may also be found after immobilization in patients with Paget's disease or with malignancies with bone metastases. The elevated calcium levels depress nervous system responses and muscle actions become sluggish and weak (*Merck Manual of Geriatrics* 2000). Hypocalcemia is caused by low serum calcium or low extracellular fluid concentration of calcium ions. It is associated with hypoparathyroidism, renal disease and vitamin D deficiency (Anderson & Xu 2005). This may increase the excitability of the neuronal membrane leading to spontaneous discharging and tetany contractions, possibly manifesting as carpopedal spasm. Trousseau's sign is an evaluative procedure used to determine the presence of tetany from hypocalcemia by inducing carpopedal spasm 3–4 min after reducing blood flow to the hand with the use of a tourniquet or blood pressure cuff on the arm (Urbano 2000). Carpopedal spasm is a condition usually found in confused, aging individuals. It manifests as hyperflexion at the wrist and the metacarpal phalangeal and proximal interphalangeal joints on the third to the fifth fingers (Fig. 16.1). The distal interphalangeal joints of these three fingers are commonly hyperextended as they come into contact with the palm. The thumb and the index finger are usually in opposition and pointing. This

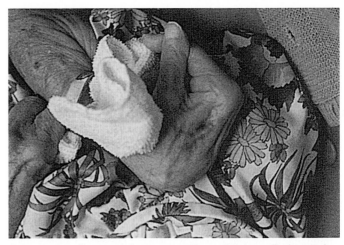

Figure 16.1   Carpopedal spasm manifests with hyperflexion at the wrist and at the metacarpal phalangeal and proximal joints of the third to fifth fingers.

condition can lead to tissue maceration and ulceration of the palm and the hands.

Reversal of Trousseau's sign is simple but treatment of longstanding carpopedal spasm is frustrating and often not effective. The goal is to prevent further injury. ROM exercises, in or out of water, may be helpful. Use of padding, washcloths or finger spreaders may be tried. Splinting and electrical stimulation to the wrist and finger extensors may be considered.

Hypokalemic myopathy results from decreased serum potassium, which is often secondary to the chronic use of diuretics. Muscle weakness develops slowly over days to weeks and may be the result of hyperpolarization of nerves and muscles, or tetany.

Hypophosphatemia is a low serum phosphate level. Phosphate is normally stored in bone as hydroxyapatite and contributes to energy metabolism and cell membrane function and regulation. Phosphate loss may lead to muscle weakness.

Hyponatremia is decreased serum sodium and excess water relative to the sodium. It is common in patients suffering from diarrhea, vomiting or suctioning. Use of diuretics may also contribute to this condition. Hyponatremia may present with fatigue, muscle cramps and depressed deep-tendon reflexes. Hypernatremia is an increased serum sodium; it may present with symptoms of weakness, lethargy and orthostatic hypotension (*Merck Manual of Geriatrics* 2000).

Hormonal imbalances

Hyperthyroidism can cause acute myopathy in elderly patients (Anderson & Xu 2005). It may also cause myokymia, which is a continuous quivering or undulating muscle movement. Proximal limb muscle weakness and muscle fatigue may be present.

Hypothyroidism may present with impaired energy metabolism within muscles and decreased contractile force (Anderson & Xu 2005). Fatigue, muscle weakness and muscle cramps may be seen, resulting from impaired calcium uptake by the sarcoplasmic reticulum.

Prolonged use of corticosteroids in chemotherapy or in conditions such as myasthenia gravis or Cushing's disease may cause a corticosteroid myopathy. Muscle atrophy may be present and may involve most skeletal muscles, but weakness usually occurs first in the hip and quadriceps muscles. Mild aching in the muscles is not uncommon (*Merck Manual of Geriatrics* 2000).

Asthenia

Asthenia is an ill-defined condition characterized by generalized weakness and usually involving mental and physical fatigue. The patient undergoing radiation therapy or chemotherapy may suffer from asthenia and thus may not tolerate the rigors of rehabilitation as defined by the Medicare system (twice-a-day treatments as inpatients in rehabilitation units or a minimum of three times a week in the home or outpatient setting). Other factors that may contribute to asthenia include anemia, malnutrition, infection, metabolic disorders and the use of medications such as methyldopa (Aldomet), Bactrim, Cardizem (Diltiazem), dexamethasone (Decadron), Donnatal, amitriptyline (Elavil), propranolol (Inderal), digoxin (Lanoxin), metoprolol (Lopressor), Novahistine, promethazine (Phenergan), Relafen (Nabumetone), co-careldopa (Sinemet) and alprazolam (Xanax). Asthenia is a factor in the rehabilitation of many frail patients.

Frailty is an emerging syndrome indicating decreased resilience and attenuated reserves. It involves multiple systems and causes a negative energy balance, sarcopenia, weakness and reduced tolerance to exertion. Frailty also features exhaustion, weight loss, weak grip strength, slow walking speed and low energy expenditure (Bandeen-Roche et al 2006). It represents multiple and aggregate diminutions in molecular, cellular and physiological systems.

STRETCH WEAKNESS

Stretch weakness is a theoretical construct for the clinical problem that results when a muscle remains in one position for a prolonged time (Kendall & McCreary 1983). This is in contrast to the increased tension that is generated by brief quick stretches, such as those that occur with manual stretches or polymetrics. It is thought that weakness manifests as the muscle remains elongated beyond its neutral physiological resting length (Gossman et al 1982). The exact physiology and morphology are not clearly known and the concept is not universally accepted; however, it remains a tenable theory.

Stretch weakness is caused by a combination of factors including change in sarcomere length and number, length of noncontractile musculotendinous structures, muscle spindle bias, joint structure and ROM, neural input including excitability of spinal motoneuronal pools (Barry & Carson 2004), habitual postures, gravity and pain. Often, a muscle imbalance between agonist and antagonist results. It is unclear how long it takes for these changes to occur in aging individuals but it is most likely gradual over months and years unless paralysis or surgery is involved. Rassier et al (1999) reported that, in laboratory animals (rabbits), significant increases in sarcomere numbers, which altered the shape of the length–tension curve, were found only 8 weeks after surgical release. A newer hypothesis is that the muscle weakness may be due to damage resulting from the stretching of muscles during contraction or from prolonged physical activity such as walking downhill for 2 h. The stretch-induced damage to muscle is more severe in aged animals and may contribute to the decline in muscle function in aging humans. The weakness in stretch-damaged muscle may be partially a result of altered function of the sarcoplasmic reticulum (Allen et al 2005). In addition, the intersarcomere dynamics and, especially, the passive viscoelastic element (which contributes to overall tension generation) may be altered (Telley et al 2003).

In humans, applying the classical length–tension curve concept is difficult because of the changing joint movements and the line of action of the muscle. It is important to recognize that force–length properties can and will adapt to the functional requirements imposed on the muscle (Rassier et al 1999).

The chronically shortened muscle will lose sarcomeres over time, which will decrease muscle resting length. The shortened muscle will have a leftward shift on the length–tension curve. On the other hand, the chronically lengthened, or elongated, muscle will have an increase in the number of sarcomeres. This will increase the resting length of muscle, and shift the length–tension curve to the right (Gossman et al 1982). These shifts indicate that, in the shortened muscle, the tension generated is greater in the shortened range and in the elongated muscle, tension is greater in the longer range, which may be beyond normal postural alignment.

Stretch weakness is commonly seen in postural malalignment and is often associated with arthritic and osteoporotic changes, as can be seen in Table 16.1. As noted by Gossman et al (1982), the habitually or posturally elongated muscle may test stronger at its new lengthened position but weaker in its more normal resting or postural position.

Table 16.1 Common areas of stretch weakness

Muscles involved	Contributing factors and manifestations	Related conditions
Scapular retractors or adductors	Prolonged sitting; dorsal kyphosis and head forward	Shoulder dysfunction, DJD, vertebral collapse, rib fracture
Gluteus maximus	Prolonged sitting; flat or kyphotic lumbar spine, loss of erect bipedal posture	Spinal DJD, vertebral collapse, hip DJD
Trunk extensors	Prolonged sitting; loss of erect posture, dorsal kyphosis	Faulty postural control, vertebral collapse
Knee extensors	Prolonged sitting; loss of erect posture, extensor lag at full knee extension	DJD
Gluteus medius	Hip fracture; trunk side-bent in bed, compensated or uncompensated gluteus medius limp	Scoliosis, leg-length shortening, hip DJD
Ankle dorsiflexors	Prolonged sitting or bedrest with feet resting in plantar flexion position; no heel strike or poor clearance of toes during swing phase of gait	Heel-cord shortening, gait/balance disturbance

DJD, degenerative joint disease.

The risk of prolonged sitting

An example of stretch weakness is seen in the patient who spends an excessive amount of time sitting in a chair, possibly even sleeping in the chair at night. This posture, involving hip, knee and trunk flexion, is likely to lead to increased resting-muscle length of the trunk extensors, knee vastus muscles and the hip extensors. Additionally, periarticular connective tissue may shorten anteriorly at the hip and posteriorly at the knee. Bony and cartilaginous changes may also occur at these joints and in the connective tissue. Full joint ROM is needed in order for proper nutrition to occur and, therefore, a person's inability to move through full ROM decreases joint nutrition.

Typically, a patient in this circumstance stands with hips and knees flexed, a position that has a higher energy cost than normal erect posture with a 0° extension at the hips and knees. When tested in the seated position for hip extension, strength on the MMT is likely to register in the good (4 out of 5) range. However, if the patient is placed prone, the standard test position, the stretch-weakened hip extensors are in a shortened position and are likely to grade in the fair (3 out of 5) range. The same may be found in knee extension: that is, good strength in the midrange and fair strength at terminal extension. An extensor lag may be present. Some patients are capable of performing a locking isometric muscle contraction, which grades as good (4 out of 5) or even normal (5 out of 5), but dynamic contraction in the terminal range may reveal less than good strength.

The risk of flexed posture

A flexed posture frequently occurs in aging individuals, showing the characteristic thoracic kyphosis, forward head and hip/knee flexion in more severe cases. Individuals with the flexed posture generally display muscle imbalances of spine extensors, ankle plantar flexors and dorsiflexors. These muscles along with the pectoralis major/minor and the hip flexors are also involved in more severe cases of flexed posture. The change in strength and ROM can lead to further disturbances with gait such as decreased velocity, increased base of support and reduced stride length and cadence. Abnormal loading of these joints can also lead to articular degeneration (Balzini et al 2003). Compression fractures of thoracic vertebrae also have a negative effect on respiratory capacity as noted in Chapter 19 (also see Chapters 15 and 62).

Treatment considerations for stretch weakness

Treatment should be directed toward (i) improving muscle strength throughout the joint's ROM, especially working the stretch-weakened muscles in the functionally appropriate physiological range; (ii) creating greater physiological balance between agonists and antagonists; (iii) achieving closer to normal postural alignment, both resting and active; (iv) preventing further losses in strength and function; (v) improving balance and gait performance; and (vi) using neurophysiological techniques to enhance motor control. Resistance training itself will not only enhance strength but will also cause favorable neural adaptations with improvements in motor unit recruitment, coordination of synergistic muscles and less agonist–antagonist co-activation (Barry & Carson 2004).

Use of modalities such as moist heat, deep heat and electrical stimulation may be helpful in relieving pain and facilitating the stretching of shortened musculoskeletal structures. Positioning and use of splints and braces should be considered to encourage normal resting length of the muscles and to prevent further stretching/lengthening of muscles and connective tissues. Emphasis should be placed on motor and postural control and active muscle actions of the agonist as well as on stretching of tightened antagonists and soft tissue. Caregivers and families must be taught about the dangers of prolonged sitting and immobility. Simple sit-to-stand and ROM exercises, especially in the antigravity muscles, are valuable.

In the above case of the prolonged sitting posture, terminal knee extension and the fully erect posture may be gained by working on static quad sets, static weight loading with weights at 0° of knee extension, extensor thrust exercises, bilateral and unilateral toe raises (plantar flexion) and gentle knee bends emphasizing return to full knee extension. Passive ROM may be needed to attain full extension; trunk extension strengthening exercises are also likely to be beneficial. These exercises should be considered not only for the additional ROM and strengthening that they produce but also for their proprioceptive and kinesthetic input into the postural control mechanism and their ability to teach the patient the necessary motion. By gaining good to normal (4 or 5 out of 5) strength in terminal hip and knee extension, a fully erect and energy-efficient posture may be attained; however, this is not always the case as the automatic postural control mechanism of this postural set may not be reprogrammable and one must consider that hip/trunk extension may aggravate spinal stenosis.

CONCLUSION

The loss of muscle strength and muscle tissue (sarcopenia) in aging individuals is an important but reversible condition that influences health, function and quality of life. Humane rehabilitative care requires paying attention to medical diagnoses, nutrition and blood chemistry as well as to the typical muscular evaluation. Recognizing the potential limitations of the muscular system when exercising allows realistic treatment goals and outcomes to be established.

Stretch weakness is a clinical condition that has yet to be fully investigated and defined. It clearly involves more than the length of the muscle and thus should be considered a neuromusculoskeletal problem. These neuromusculoskeletal changes may have a negative effect on posture, mobility and quality of life and should be considered when evaluating the aging patient. Amelioration is possible in some, albeit not all, cases.

References

Allen DG, Whitehead P, Yeung EW 2005 Mechanisms of stretch-induced muscle damage in normal and dystrophic muscle: role of ionic changes. J Physiol 567:723–735

Anderson W, Xu L 2005 Endocrine myopathies. eMedicine from WEBMD. Available: http://www.emedicine.com/neuro/topic125.htm. Accessed 21 April 2006

Balzini L, Vannucchi L, Benvenuti F et al 2003 Clinical characteristics of flexed posture in elderly women. J Am Geriatr Soc 51:1419–1426

Bandeen-Roche K, Xue Q, Ferrucci L et al 2006 Phenotype of frailty: characterization in the women's health and aging studies. J Gerontol Biol Sci 61A:262–266

Barry B, Carson R 2004 The consequences of resistance training for movement control in older adults. J Gerontol Biol Sci 59A:730–754

Di Fabio R 2001 One repetition maximum for older persons: is it safe? J Ortho Sports Phys Ther 31:2–3

Dodd K, Taylor N, Bradley S 2004 Strength training for older people. In: Morris M, Schoo A (eds) Optimizing Exercise and Physical Activity in Older People. Butterworth-Heinemann, Edinburgh, p 125–157

Fiatarone-Singh M 2002 Exercise to prevent and treat functional disability. Clin Geriatr Med 18:431–462

Fiatarone-Singh M 2004 Exercise and aging. Clin Geriatr Med 20:201–221

Galvao D, Newton R 2005 Review of exercise intervention studies in cancer patients. J Clin Oncol 23:899–909

Gossman M, Sahrmann S, Rose S 1982 Review of length-associated changes in muscle. Phys Ther 62:1799–1808

Hourign S 2004 Exercise prescription in residential aged care facilities. In: Nitz J, Hourigan S (eds) Physiotherapy Practice in Residential Aged Care. Butterworth-Heinemann, Edinburgh, p 209–238

Jan M, Chai H, Lin Y et al 2005 Effects of age and sex on the results of an ankle plantar-flexor manual muscle test. J Am Phys Ther Assoc 85:1078–1084

Kauffman T 1982 Association between hip extensor strength and stand-up ability in geriatric patients. Phys Occup Ther Geriatr 1(3):39–45

Kauffman T 1985 Strength training effect in young and aged women. Arch Phys Med Rehabil 66:223–226

Kendall F, McCreary E 1983 Muscles: Testing and Function, 3rd edn. Williams & Wilkins, Baltimore, MD

Larson E, Wang L, Brown J et al 2006 Exercise is associated with reduced risk for incident dementia among persons 65 years old and older. Ann Intern Med 144(2):73–81

Manor B, Topp R, Page P 2006 Validity and reliability of measurements of elbow flexion strength obtained from older adults using elastic bands. J Geriatr Phys Ther 29:16–19

Merck Manual of Geriatrics 2000. Merck Research Laboratories, Whitehouse Station, NJ

Mount J, Bolton M, Cesari M et al 2005 Group balance skills class for people with chronic stroke: a case series. J Neurol Phys Ther 29(1):24–33

Newman A, Kupelian V, Visser M et al 2006 Strength, but not muscle mass, is associated with mortality in the Health, Aging and Body Composition Study cohort. J Gerontol Med Sci 61A:72–77

Rassier DE, MacIntosh BR, Herzog W 1999 Length dependence of active force production in skeletal muscle. J Appl Physiol 86:1445–1457

Telley IA, Denoth J, Ranatunga KW 2003 Inter-sarcomere dynamics in muscle fibres. A neglected subject? Adv Exp Med Biol 538:481–500

Thompson P, Clarkson P, Karas R 2003 Statin-associated myopathy. J Am Med Assoc 289:1681–1690

Urbano F 2000 Signs of hypocalcemia: Chvostek's and Trousseau's signs. Hosp Physician 36:43–45

Vaynman S, Gomez-Pinilla F 2005 License to run: exercise impacts functional plasticity in the intact and injured central nervous system by using neurotrophins. Neurorehabil Neural Repair 19:283–295

Wagner M, Kauffman T 2001 Mobility. In: Bonder B, Wagner M (eds) Functional Performance in Older Adults, 2nd edn. FA Davis, Philadelphia, PA, p 61–85

Ziegelstein R 2004 Near-syncope after exercise. J Am Med Assoc 292:1221–1226

Chapter **17**

Contractures

Wade S. Gamber and Reenie Euhardy

INTRODUCTION

Contractures are defined as the lack of full passive range of motion (ROM) of a joint resulting from structural changes of non-bony tissues, such as muscles, tendons, ligaments, joint capsules and/or skin. Contractures develop when normal elastic connective tissues are replaced with inelastic fibrous tissue. There are many causes of contractures including chronic inflammation (rheumatoid arthritis), deformity (osteoarthritis, scoliosis), immobility (after fracture or surgery), injury (burns, stroke), disease (Parkinson's disease), or a combination of these factors. Joint flexibility is inversely related to aging. Generally, there is a systemic decrease in active and passive motion of all joints with age, with the decline becoming more pronounced during the ninth decade. However, not all elderly individuals experience a decline in joint flexibility as they age. Significant increases in ROM can be achieved with exercise, activity and good stretching programs (Hoffman et al 2005).

MECHANISMS OF CONTRACTURE

Usually, several factors combine to play a role in limiting full passive joint ROM in the elderly. The normal effects of aging, a decline in physical activity and, often, disease, injury(s) and/or pathology, at times occurring simultaneously, contribute to joint contracture. With the prevalence of fractures and surgeries in the older population, immobility is the most frequent cause of contracture.

Contractures can be divided into three categories according to the anatomical location of the pathological changes: (i) arthrogenic, including intra-articular adhesions; (ii) periarticular, including connective tissue and joint capsule stiffness; and (iii) myogenic, including shortened skeletal muscles of which there are two types, myostatic and pseudomyostatic. Other classification systems for identifying restricted joint motion involve intra-articular, periarticular and extra articular structures.

Myostatic contractures represent structural adaptation of muscle in response to changes in the position of the corresponding joint. Muscles with myostatic contracture are shorter than their normal physiological length and show a reduction in the number of sarcomere units but no decrease in individual sarcomere length, as is found with pseudomyostatic contracture (Henry 1995). Myostatic contracture can be the result of bracing, casting, immobilization or any restriction of joint movement, voluntarily (pain) or not, such as limited activity or bedrest.

Pseudomyostatic contracture is the loss of myofibril extensibility secondary to a decrease in individual sarcomere length; it is not accompanied by structural changes in the sarcomeres. Pseudomyostatic shortening may follow a tetanic muscle contraction such as a spasm or cramp. Myofascial trigger points may be local areas in muscle where actin and myosin filaments remain chemically locked.

NORMAL EFFECTS OF AGING

Normal age-related changes that affect joint flexibility include increases in the viscosity of the synovium, calcification of articular cartilages, muscular weakness or deconditioning, stiffness of capsular and ligamentous tissues and the reduction of elasticity of skin. Stiffness is measured by the stress–strain relationship of fibers. As the force (stress) on tissue is increased, the length (strain) of the tissue increases in a linear relationship once the slack is taken out, until the length at which the tissue ruptures is reached (Neuman 1993).

Other factors associated with contracture formation that may be age-related include previous injury, illness or abnormal postural patterns (see Chapters 15 and 63). Repetitive- motion stresses resulting from occupational or leisure activities may predispose to tenosynovitis or osteophyte formation and the remodeling of the joint surfaces, which limits joint flexibility related to contractures.

Activity level

The interaction between aging and activity level and joint contracture is not well understood. Why some individuals do not experience even slight reductions in joint ROM as they age is an important question that has not been answered; however, a decline in physical activity is typically related to joint contracture. Three components related to physical activity that play a role in the development of contracture are limb position, duration of immobilization and habitual movement patterns. The type and amount of physical activity that people engage in changes with age. Older adults often do not move their joints to the same extent or as frequently as younger individuals. Bedridden and extremely inactive or frail elderly people are particularly prone to the development of contractures (Kauffman 1987). Some degree of muscular shortening is present in sedentary people even if they are healthy, especially in muscles that cross multiple joints.

PATHOLOGY

Arthrogenic contractures are usually the result of chronic inflammation (rheumatoid arthritis), infection, degenerative joint disease or repeated trauma. Pain resulting from synovial effusion, which is associated with inflammation and/or arthritis, often culminates in voluntary and involuntary joint splinting and immobility. As joint movement is curtailed, contractures may develop. Osteoarthritic disease resulting in the deformity and remodeling of joint surfaces, and rheumatic processes resulting in the scarring of the synovium, contribute not only to intra-articular but also to periarticular joint contractures. Burns frequently restrict skin movement around a joint subsequently leading to joint contractures.

Neuromuscular dysfunction appears to be the most common cause of extra-articular physiological joint restriction, probably the consequence of spinal segment and supraspinal inputs that result in a shortening of the muscle fibers' resting length. Muscle spindle bias may be a factor. Pathology such as stroke, multi-infarct dementia and diseases that cause changes in neurotransmission, such as Parkinson's disease, may cause spastic posturing. Spastic posturing presents with a dynamic imbalance of muscle control in the involved extremities and results in myogenic contracture. Medications with extrapyramidal side effects such as antipsychotics may also contribute to contractures.

FUNCTION WITH CONTRACTURE

The functional significance of reduced joint ROM is determined by the amount of limitation, the overall physical condition and activity level of the individual and the location of the involved joint. It has been suggested that a 30° knee flexion contracture is associated with a loss of ambulatory ability. Hip flexion contractures affect gait by reducing pelvic rotation, shortening stride and increasing the energy cost of mobility. Loss of dorsiflexion ROM directly affects opposite leg stride length and cadence of the gait pattern and encourages a substitution pattern for balance and stability. The ability to negotiate curbs and steps may also be impaired. No guidelines have been established to determine what degree of shoulder contracture has a significant impact on function; however, activities of daily living (ADLs) are certainly more difficult with a contracture condition like adhesive capsulitis.

INCIDENCE

With aging, the upper extremity joints remain more flexible than the lower extremity joints; this parallels the change in strength seen with age, with the lower extremities becoming weaker sooner than the upper extremities, and may result from daily use. Men tend to lose ROM more rapidly than women. Hip abduction is the lower extremity motion most commonly limited with age. Limited full hip extension

(10° hyperextension beyond 0°, or neutral) is also common in the elderly, directly affecting gait and mobility. It is postulated that prolonged sitting is related to hip and knee flexion contracture (Kauffman 1987). Hip flexion declines the least, with significant reduction becoming apparent only after the age of 85. A recent study of rat soleus muscle has demonstrated changes in sarcomere length (shortening) after only one week of immobilization with contracture increasing with the duration of immobilization (Okita et al 2004). In addition, changes in collagen fibril arrangement occurred and may cause advanced contracture in later stages of immobilization.

TREATMENT

Prevention

Maintaining an active lifestyle and following a regular routine stretching exercise program that encourages full multijoint ROM are keys to preventing joint contractures in the elderly. Positioning and posture are critical for the prevention of contracture in patients who have limited mobility. In the supine position, the feet may need to be positioned in neutral dorsiflexion. The lower extremities should rest in neutral rotation with the hips and knees extended. Shoulders should be in neutral protraction–retraction. Elbows, wrists and fingers should also be extended, while allowing flexion to maintain grip and grasp and ADL functioning. Considerations relating to joint position and tissue length are crucial when placing patients in seated and sidelong positions. Muscles and joints should be stretched to their optimal ROM, ideally on a daily basis.

Thermal agents and passive stretching

Contractures can often be reduced by selectively heating the fibrous tissues that limit motion. Passive motion and/or stretching should be performed during or immediately following application of thermal agents such as heating pads, ultrasound or diathermy. Ultrasound may be the modality of choice for selectively heating contracted tissues because ultrasound affords deeper penetration of tissue (up to 3–5 cm) (Michlovitz 1986). Moist heat may be utilized for generalized superficial heating, to assist in muscle relaxation. The temperature of muscle tendon tissue can be raised to 104–109°F (40–43°C), which influences the viscous properties of connective tissues and maximizes the effects of stretching (Gersten 1955). Smaller joints may be heated by immersion in paraffin wax.

Before application of thermal agents, a careful clinical evaluation of the patient must be performed to rule out any persisting acute or subacute process or degenerative joint disease, and to determine whether joint limitation results from bone spurs. The use of selective heating in conjunction with stretching, ROM exercises or other joint mobilization techniques may aggravate persistent inflammatory reactions and is ineffective in the presence of bone spurs.

Massage and stretching

Soft-tissue techniques that can reduce connective tissue and myogenic contractures include massage and stretching. Massage can produce gains in length when pseudomyostatic shortening of a muscle has occurred. When contracture develops following prolonged immobilization, muscle and connective tissues lose up to 80% of their tensile strength. Care must be taken not to use abrupt or vigorous stretching forces; prolonged, low-load stretching is required. Guidelines for prolonged, low-load stretching include positioning the joint in its most extended position while applying heat and a light static weight to cause tension on the distal part of the joint lever arm for 5–10 min. Active exercise of the antagonist muscles should be encouraged, especially in the terminal range.

Soft-tissue mobilization, a type of deep massage, employs forceful passive movement of the musculofascial elements, beginning with superficial layers and progressing to deeper tissues. Massage can restore independent mobility of muscle, fascia and skin in the areas of fascial thickening and binding that occur in response to chronic postural deformity. The individual subjective response can serve as an indicator to gauge the appropriate amount of pressure to be applied. The technique is frequently described as a 'good hurt' when applied correctly. The use of too much force is revealed by involuntary muscle contracture, voluntary withdrawal or reports of pain.

Deep friction massage

Deep friction massage or cross-friction massage is another type of soft-tissue technique involving the application of concentrated, repetitive stroking that is directed perpendic-ular to the fiber orientation in a localized area of tendon, muscle, fascia or ligament at the site of contracture. Clinically, it is used to restore mobility between otherwise freely moving structures; however, research substantiating the effectiveness of transverse friction massage is limited. Deep friction massage can be a potentially harmful treatment for acute and chronic stages of rheumatoid arthritis or for joints with active or acute inflammation and should be employed cautiously.

Myofascial release

Myofascial release (MFR) applies firm mechanical forces in the direction of restricted motion to break up abnormal cross-linkages and restore independent mobility to fascial compartments. MFR techniques involve the application of traction or elongation combined with some element of simultaneous shearing, twisting and, often, compression. All soft-tissue techniques must be applied judiciously because of the skin and circulatory changes that are present in older people which increase the risk of injury.

Neuromuscular techniques

Neuromuscular techniques promote muscle relaxation preceding passive stretching, which facilitates effective reduction of myostatic contractures. Therapeutic approaches include muscle energy, hold–relax and contract–relax proprioceptive neuromuscular facilitation (PNF) and postisometric relaxation. Muscle relaxation and passive stretching are components of many of these techniques. Passive stretching is distinct from passive range of motion (PROM) in that the latter stops at the first feel of a barrier to further movement, whereas passive stretching, or overstretching, is a process in which additional load is applied slowly and consistently in order to elongate the tissues.

Manually resisted exercise in the available range preceding stretching or joint mobilization can enhance the effectiveness of treatment. When it is possible to use them, submaximal contractions against resistance that are performed through the available ROM are effective through several mechanisms: (i) they warm tissues; (ii) they increase afferent stimuli and thus reduce muscle guarding; and (iii) they fatigue the muscle, which limits resistance to passive stretching. Active contraction and passive stretching performed in tandem are thought to enhance muscle lengthening. A strong voluntary contraction is followed by a brief refractory period in which the muscle cannot contract, providing a moment when the muscle can be elongated.

Optimal passive stretching (overstretching) can occur only with muscle relaxation, so the participation of the patient is necessary to enhance treatment effectiveness. With cognitively impaired patients, relaxation as well as voluntary muscle contractions are often difficult to achieve; therefore, neuromuscular stretching techniques may not be useful.

Reporting on the results of a systematic literature review, Decoster et al (2005) found that a variety of stretching techniques including PNF and varying stretching positions and durations of stretch were effective in increasing hamstring length and ROM. It should be noted, however, that individuals over 60 years of age were not studied.

Joint mobilization

A loss of accessory or joint-play movement, the movement normally present in the joint but not under voluntary control, is often found with arthrogenic contractures. Particular techniques of joint mobilization that will affect joint dysfunction vary from one school of practice to another. Regardless of the particular technique used, the end result is to aid in restoring joint mobility by normalizing accessory movements. Oscillations, traction and distractions with glide may all be used. Cleland et al (2005) reported benefits of manual therapy, traction and strengthening exercises in middle-aged people with cervical radiculopathy. However, little research has been conducted with older individuals (over the age of 75); therefore, great care must be taken when applying these techniques in the elderly because of the osseous and soft-tissue changes that have occurred in addition to any underlying pathology a patient may have.

Splinting, casting and bracing

Splinting, casting or bracing techniques are applied to provide a constant passive stretch to the joint. Several studies have demonstrated improvements in contractures with the use of these devices in conjunction with traditional therapeutic intervention (Mackey-Lyons 1989, Jansen et al 1996). Serial casting is especially helpful for stretching plantar flexors, biceps, wrist flexors and hamstrings; these are muscle groups that commonly contract in older individ-uals with neurological pathology. However, neither splinting nor casting has been shown to be helpful in permanently reducing spasticity or posturing. Customized adjustable orthoses or bracing molded to the individual's limb can be changed at intervals to promote further slow stretching and may be more easily removed for skin monitoring and adjustments before reapplying. Use of commercially available splints, braces or continuous passive range of motion machines (CPMs) have been reported to successfully reduce knee, ankle, elbow and finger contractures in some cases.

CONCLUSION

The identification of the underlying cause and the structures implicated in a contracture determine the type and amount of treatment employed. Because several factors typically contribute to contracture formation, a variety of approaches to treatment may have to be used either individually or simultaneously to improve ROM. In general, the earlier the treatment for a contracture begins, the better and sooner a positive outcome may be achieved and prevention enacted. Caution must always be exercised when using these techniques, especially with elderly patients. Therapists must be sensitive to the frailty of aged tissues and should be cognizant of the coexisting pathologies that elderly patients commonly exhibit as they can affect outcomes.

References

Cleland J, Whitman J, Fritz J et al 2005 Manual therapy, cervical traction, and strengthening exercises in patients with cervical radiculopathy: a case series. J Orthop Sports Phys Ther 35:802–811

Decoster L, Cleland J, Altieri C et al 2005 The effects of hamstring stretching on range of motion: a systemic literature review. J Orthop Sports Phys Ther 35:377–387

Gersten JW 1955 Effects of ultrasound on tendon extensibility. Am J Phys Med 34:362–369

Henry JA 1995 Manual therapy of the shoulder. In: Kelley M, Clark WA (eds) Orthopedic Therapy of the Shoulder. Lippincott, Philadelphia, PA, p 285

Hoffman AJ, Jensen M, Abresch R et al 2005 Chronic pain and neuromuscular disease. Phys Med Rehabil Clin North Am 16:1099–1112

Jansen CM, Windau JE, Boutti PM et al 1996 Treatment of a knee contracture using a knee orthosis incorporating stress-relaxation techniques. Phys Ther 76:182–186

Kauffman T 1987 Posture and aging. Top Geriatr Rehabil 2:13–28

Mackay-Lyons 1989 Low-load, prolonged stretch in treatment of elbow flexion contractures secondary to head trauma. Phys Ther 69:292–296

Michlovitz S 1986 Thermal Agents in Rehabilitation. FA Davis, Philadelphia, PA, pp 144 and 151

Neumann DA 1993 Arthrokinesiologic considerations in the aged adult. In: Guccione AA (ed) Geriatric Physical Therapy. CB Mosby, St Louis, MO, p 47

Okita M, Yoshimura T, Nakano J et al 2004 Effects of reduced joint mobility on sarcomere length, collagen fibril arrangement in the endomysium and hyaluronan in rat soleus muscle. J Muscle Res Cell Motil 25(2):159–166

Chapter 18

Postpolio syndrome

Marilyn E. Miller

Postpolio syndrome (PPS) is defined as aging with poliomyelitis. As they age, the issues of PPS in long-term survivors continue to present challenges to them as well as to the rehabilitation professionals who serve them. The more than one million PPS survivors in the US, many of whom are in their later retirement years, find that their needs are increasing as they acquire other disabilities which accompany the natural changes of aging. To help these survivors avoid complications, rehabilitation professionals need to be sensitive to some of the special issues of PPS (Bartels & Omura 2005). Researchers estimate that 33–80% of polio survivors anywhere in the world will acquire PPS (Elrod et al 2005, Ragonese et al 2005). PPS is reported to be the most prevalent progressive neuromuscular disease in North America (Elrod et al 2005), with a significantly higher rate in women than in men (Ragonese et al 2005). The higher the age of initial onset of polio, the lower the rate of PPS.

The main clinical features of PPS are persistent new weakness, muscular fatigue, general fatigue and pain (Box 18.1) (Rush 1999). The cause of PPS onset is unknown but contributing factors may be the aging motor neuron, muscle overuse and disuse, chronic physical stress and the impact of socioeconomic conditions (Ragonese et al 2005, Trojan & Cashman 2005). Attention to an overall healthy lifestyle and prompt identification and treatment of secondary conditions before they progress to greater impairment and/or disability are important to preserve function and maintain quality of life in PPS patients (Stuifbergen 2005).

A systematic review of research to date indicates that conclusions cannot be drawn from the literature with regard to the functional course or prognostic factors in late-onset PPS; in fact, prognostic factors have not been identified (Stolwijk-Swuste et al 2005). Weakness of muscle itself defines the functional consequences experienced by individuals with PPS. There is little evidence that the fatigue common in PPS (and other diagnoses that involve spinal motor neuron death) is related to an increase in intrinsic fatigability of muscle fibers (Thomas & Zijdewind 2006). Thus, this PPS fatigue must be accounted for by other sources, as yet unidentified, perhaps similar to the fatigue reported by multiple sclerosis patients.

University of Michigan researchers (Kalpakjian et al 2005) have developed and validated an Index of Post-Polio Sequelae (IPPS), which offers clinicians a standardized scale to assess the severity of PPS. PPS is usually slowly progressive, with no specific interventions identified. However, an interdisciplinary management program is useful in controlling PPS symptoms (Trojan & Cashman 2005). Bartels & Omura (2005) have also recommended an interdisciplinary management program that may include (i) pharmacological interventions, limited to some anticholinergic agents, dopaminergic agents or amantadine; (ii) appropriate exercises, bracing and support; and (iii) the use of speech therapy and respiratory support when bulbar or

---

Box 18.1 Common complaints of individuals with postpolio sequelae

- Fatigue
- Weakness
- Muscle pain
- Joint pain
- Increased falling
- General instability
- Feeling 'brain dead'
- Muscle cramps
- Muscle fasciculations
- Sleep disorders
- Respiratory distress
- Dysphagia/choking
- Diminished endurance
- Hypersensitivity to cold
- Delayed strength recovery after exhaustion
- Psychosocial problems
- General medical problems

From Rush S, Geriatric Rehabilitation Manual 1999, with thanks.

---

respiratory symptoms are indicated. Brehm et al (2006) recommend maintaining function in individuals with PPS, focusing on stabilizing or decreasing the energy demands of physical activities with exercise programs and/or improvements in assistive devices for walking.

Of particular interest are the current findings related to gait, a significant functional determinant of personal independence. A study by Horemans et al (2005), which investigated the relationship between walking tests, walking activity in daily life and perceived mobility problems in a PPS population in the Netherlands, documented that PPS patients do not necessarily match their activity pattern to their perceived mobility problems. This study reported that PPS patients with the lowest test performance walked less in daily life. This same study also found no significant correlation between perceived mobility problems and walking activities. These researchers further reported that walking in daily life may be more demanding than walking under standardized conditions, an important finding to consider in future research.

Grabljevec et al (2005) studied isometric maximal voluntary contraction (MVC) torque and endurance of knee extensors in three matched groups of people including: (i) a group with new symptoms of PPS, (ii) a group with no new symptoms of PPS, and (iii) a healthy control group. The MCV torque was determined using a Biodex dynamometer at a 60° knee angle. This study found no significant differences in MCV torque and endurance between the two groups with PPS. However, the endurance of 'normal' strength knee extensor muscles in PPS subjects was generally lower than that of healthy subjects, regardless of the implication of normal strength and subjective observations of the PPS subjects.

In their study of gait, Hebert & Liggins (2005) used a knee–ankle–foot orthosis (KAFO) to compare the locked-knee joint versus the automatic stance-control knee joint in a 61-year-old male subject with PPS. This case indicated that a stance-control KAFO appears to improve gait biomechanics and improve energy efficiency compared with a locked-knee KAFO.

The study by Brehm et al (2006) compared the energy demands of walking in adults with PPS with those of matched healthy control subjects; this was achieved by assessing muscle strength and strength asymmetry. The findings indicated a significant difference between the groups for all walking parameters. Walking speed was 28% lower and energy consumption and energy cost were higher in PPS subjects than in healthy subjects. Further, the walking parameter measures were more variable for the PPS subjects than the healthy subjects. Reduced walking efficiency was strongly associated with the degree of lower extremity muscle weakness, correlated with comfortable walking speed, and accounted for 59% of the variance. This study also reported that the energy cost of walking was associated with muscle strength asymmetry. The physical strain of performing submaximal activities in relation to the severity of the polio paresis appeared to

be a determinant of the change of physical functioning over time. As noted above, these researchers recommend maintaining function in individuals with PPS by stabilizing or decreasing the energy demands of physical activities.

The almost complete eradication of polio in the industrialized nations has been an important achievement in world health policy. UNICEF (UNICEF 2006) formed the Global Polio Eradication Initiative in 1988 and has since made dramatic strides toward its goal. A disease once identified in 125 nations is now endemic in only four: Afghanistan, India, Nigeria and Pakistan. Increased transmission has been reported in Nigeria and other countries, where the disease is threatening to spread to neighboring regions because of budget shortfalls preventing the immunization programs (Bartels & Omura 2005, UNICEF 2006). The lessons learned now from PPS survivors may serve to improve care for future PPS survivors. Rehabilitation professionals and counselors must be knowledgeable about PPS and its possible impact on employment. The physical symptoms can be severe enough to significantly alter work function, impose lifestyle changes and decrease quality of life (Elrod et al 2005).

The existence of PPS questions the concept of polio as a static disease; this poses a challenge not only to patients and health professionals but also to policy makers charged with allocating resources. A study from the University of Spain reviewed the PPS research and developed some recommendations for policy decision making (Bouza et al 2005). The current research into PPS from diverse nations indicates the pervasiveness of these issues in the aging world population. This PPS global challenge of poliomyelitis is far from over.

References

Bartels MN, Omura A 2005 Aging in polio. Phys Med Rehabil Clin North Am 16(1):197–218

Bouza C, Munoz A, Amate JM 2005 Postpolio syndrome: a challenge to the health-care system. Health Policy 71(1):97–106

Brehm MA, Nollet F, Harlaar J 2006 Energy demands of walking in persons with postpoliomyelitis syndrome: relationship with muscle strength and reproducibility. Arch Phys Med Rehabil 87(1):136–140

Elrod LM, Jabben M, Oswald G et al 2005 Vocational implications of post-polio syndrome. Work 25(2):155–161

Grabljevec K, Burger H, Kersevan K et al 2005 Strength and endurance of knee extensors in subjects after paralytic poliomyelitis. Disability Rehabil 27(14):791–799

Hebert JS, Liggins AB 2005 Gait evaluation of an automatic stance-control knee orthosis in a patient with postpoliomyelitis. Arch Phys Med Rehabil 86(8):1676–1680

Horemans HL, Bussmann JB, Beelen A et al 2005 Walking in postpoliomyelitis syndrome: the relationships between time-scored tests, walking in daily life and perceived mobility problems. J Rehabil Med 37(3):142–146

Kalpakjian CZ, Toussaint LL, Klipp DA, Forchheimer MB 2005 Development and factor analysis of an index of post-polio sequelae. Disability Rehabil 27(20):1225–1233

Ragonese P, Fierro B, Salemi G et al 2005 Prevalence and risk factors of post-polio syndrome in a cohort of polio survivors. J Neurol Sci 236(1–2):31–35

Rush S 1999 Postpolio syndrome. In: Kauffman T (ed) Geriatric Rehabilitation Manual. Churchill Livingston, Philadelphia, PA p 81–82

Stolwijk-Swuste JM, Beelen A, Lankhorst GJ et al 2005 The course of functional status and muscle strength in patient with late-onset sequelae of poliomyelitis: a systematic review. Arch Phys Med Rehabil 86(8):1693–1701

Stuifbergen AK 2005 Secondary conditions and life satisfaction among polio survivors. Rehabil Nurs 30(5):173–179

Thomas CK, Zijdewind I 2006 Fatigue or muscles weakened by death of motoneurons. Muscle Nerve 33(1):21–41

Trojan DA, Cashman NR 2005 Post-poliomyelitis syndrome. Muscle Nerve 31(1):97–106

UNICEF 2006 Immunization plus. Available: http://www.unicef.org/immuniztion/index_polio.html. Accessed 02 April 2006

Chapter 19

Osteoporosis

Stephen Brunton, Blaine Carmichael, Deborah Gold, Barry Hull,
Timothy L. Kauffman, Alexandra Papaioannou, Randolph Rasch,
Hilmar H.G. Stracke and Eeric Truumees

CHAPTER CONTENTS

Osteoporotic vertebral compression fractures (VCFs) represent a significant challenge for primary care physicians (PCPs) in their diagnosis and management, and they are likely to become an increasingly important health issue for many patients as the population ages (Rao & Singrakhia 2003). Individuals with a VCF experience a decreased quality of life (QOL) and also show increases in digestive and respiratory morbidities, anxiety, depression and death (Cooper et al 1993, Ismail et al 2001, Papaioannou et al 2002, Gold 2003, Tosi et al 2004, Yamaguchi et al 2005). Most importantly, these patients have as much as a fivefold increased risk of another fracture within 1 year of the initial fracture (Lindsay et al 2001). Up to two-thirds of VCFs are undiagnosed (Papaioannou et al 2003a, Old & Calvert 2004,) and, even if diagnosed, many patients are treated only acutely; few (18% in one study) are managed long-term for the prevention of fractures (Nevitt et al 1998, Gehlbach et al 2000, Oleksik et al 2000, Andrade et al 2003, Papaioannou et al 2003a, Tosi et al 2004).

According to the National Osteoporosis Foundation (Health Issues Survey 2005), PCPs need to take a proactive role in assessing the risk for or presence of VCFs and in maintaining or improving general bone health: many patients consider back pain a normal part of aging and do not discuss it with their physician. Further, the PCP needs to act as the central point of care for a patient with a VCF, working with an orthopedist, physical therapist, clinical social worker, pharmacist and dietician to provide optimal management. This publication's recommendations stem from a review of the literature and panel members' clinical experience. Highlighted below are the impact of VCFs on overall QOL, risk factors for VCFs and a discussion of management options for patients with VCFs.

KEY POINTS AND RECOMMENDATIONS

- VCFs are common but often silent consequences of osteoporosis (strength of recommendation (SOR): A).
- The risk of death is increased several-fold during the year following a VCF (SOR: B).
- Calcium and vitamin D supplementation, antiresorptive and anabolic agents, and weight-bearing exercises are helpful in preventing secondary VCFs (SOR: A).
- The incidence of fractures can be reduced by 40–60% with pharmacological therapies (SOR: A).
- Magnetic resonance imaging of the spine is probably the single most useful test for evaluating a fracture (SOR: C).
- Vertebroplasty or kyphoplasty should be considered for patients in whom a progressive kyphotic deformity or intractable pain develops (SOR: A).

SOR: A – consistent and good quality evidence. SOR: B – inconsistent or limited quality evidence. SOR C: – consensus, usual practice, opinion, disease-oriented evidence.

PREVALENCE OF VCFs

Mild to severe VCFs are the most common consequence of osteoporosis. Of the 1.5 million fractures that occur each year in the US, 700 000 are spinal fractures (US Department of Health and Human Services 2005). One in two women and one in four men aged 50 years and older will have an osteoporosis-related fracture in their remaining lifetime (Hodgson et al 2001, National Osteoporosis Foundation: Prevention 2005). The incidence of VCF increases progressively with age throughout later life and, in one study, prevalence was roughly the same in men (21.5%) and women (23.5%), as measured using radiological evidence (Jackson et al 2000).

CLINICAL CONSEQUENCES OF VCFs

Active efforts to diagnose VCFs are critical because only about one-third of radiographically diagnosed VCFs cause symptoms (Black et al 1996), often just moderate back pain (Jackson et al 2000). Still, vertebral and other osteoporotic fractures produce cumulative and often irreversible damage (Papaioannou et al 2002, Tosi et al 2004), fracture-related medical problems (Andrade et al 2003) and increased risk of death. For example, lung function is reduced significantly in patients with a thoracic or lumbar fracture: one thoracic compression fracture may cause a 9% loss of the forced vital capacity (FVC) (Leech et al 1990). A fourfold higher prevalence of severe VCFs has been reported in patients with chronic obstructive pulmonary disease than in matched controls, as well as impaired lung function as measured by the percentage decrease in FVC (Papaioannou et al 2003a).

Multiple VCFs cause height loss, thoracic hyperkyphosis, loss of lumbar lordosis and subsequent compression of the internal organs as the spine no longer holds the body upright (Raisz 2005, Yamaguchi et al 2005). The rib cage presses on the pelvis, reducing the thoracic and abdominal space; with severe disease, this space may measure less than two finger widths.

Box 19.1 provides some examples of the other effects of VCFs on a patient's life (Papaioannou et al 2001, 2002, 2003a, Yamaguchi et al 2005).

Box 19.1   Clinical consequences of VCFs

- Protuberant abdomen
- Difficulty fitting clothes because of kyphosis, protuberant abdomen
- Back pain (acute and chronic)
- Height loss
- Reflux
- Early satiety
- Weight loss
- Reduced lung function
- Shortness of breath
- Impaired physical functioning
- Fear of fracture and falling
- Impaired activities of daily living (e.g. bathing, dressing)
- Depression
- Sleep disturbance
- Difficulty bending, lifting, descending stairs, cooking
- Increased length of fracture-related hospital stay by 2.0 days
- Increased mortality

From Papioannou et al 2001, 2002, 2003a and Yamaguchi 2005.

ASSESSMENT AND DIAGNOSIS

Symptomatic VCFs usually present as acute thoracic or lumbar back pain (Rao & Singrakhia 2003). Importantly, little correlation exists between the degree of vertebral body collapse and pain level. Evaluating the patient's risk, taking a history, conducting a physical examination and ordering radiological studies are essential parts of the assessment and diagnosis of a suspected VCF (Fig. 19.1).

Risk factors

Low bone mineral density

Bone mineral density (BMD) is a better predictor of osteoporotic fracture than cholesterol is for coronary heart disease or blood pressure is for stroke (Rao & Singrakhia 2003, Tosi et al 2004). The PCP should determine if the patient has had a workup for or diagnosis of osteoporosis; in the absence of a previous diagnosis of osteoporosis, the patient should be retested. Many VCFs occur in women with normal or osteopenic BMD scores suggesting the presence of contributing risk factors, which include long-term corticosteroid use.

Medical conditions and agents

Corticosteroids interrupt healthy bone metabolism in males and females of all ages and require therapy to slow or prevent progression

of osteoporosis (American College of Rheumatology 2001). Celiac disease, common in premenopausal women with idiopathic osteoporosis, may also be a risk factor (Armagon et al 2005). Other diseases or treatments that may affect risk include cancer and calcium malabsorption (diarrhea, gastrointestinal diseases, recent immobilization).

Patient history

Previous fracture

A history of a VCF and other fractures, for example of the wrist, are also strong predictors of a subsequent VCF (Burger et al 1994, Lindsay et al 2001).

Onset and duration of pain

The patient's activities at pain onset may help determine the cause. A recent event resulting in acute pain suggests a compression fracture. Pain lasting for months or years may stem from age-related spinal disorders. Leg pain or weakness indicates that there may be a neurological deficit and may warrant an immediate referral to a surgeon.

Diagnosis

Physical examination

The physical examination should be performed with the patient standing so that signs of osteoporosis, for example kyphoscoliosis, are more apparent. Otherwise, the patient should lie on one side. The recommended procedure is as follows. Beginning at the top and working down, depress the thumb on or over the spinous processes to examine the spine. Although VCFs can occur from the occiput to the sacrum, they most often occur in the midthoracic region (T7–T8) and at the thoracolumbar junction (Nevitt et al 1999). Ask the patient to indicate the presence of pain; repeat the spine examination as necessary to pinpoint the actual pain location. Pain associated with spinal palpation may indicate a compression fracture. Often, there is an accentuation of the normal spinal contour at the level of injury with associated prominence of the spinous processes in the painful area. The presence of a spinal deformity by itself does not indicate the cause or timing of the fracture. If there is no identifiable sharp pain, suspect other age-related spine problems. Have the patient flex and extend the spine; these movements often exacerbate pain resulting from VCFs. Moderate muscle spasm or splinting may occur as the antigravity muscles of the spine attempt to unload the pressure on the wedged anterior vertebral body. A neurol-ogical examination should also be performed. In rare cases, osteomyelitis mimics symptoms of a VCF.

Other findings associated with an increased risk of osteoporosis or spinal fracture are listed in Box 19.2 (Green et al 2004).

Radiology

During the physical examination, a radio-opaque marker may be applied to the skin next to the most painful region; this may, however, obscure evidence of neoplasm or endplate erosions suggestive of osteomyelitis. Standing posteroanterior and lateral radiographic studies may be ordered, with instructions to the radiologist that the objective is to rule out a VCF. A symptomatic VCF does not always show collapse on the initial radiograph.

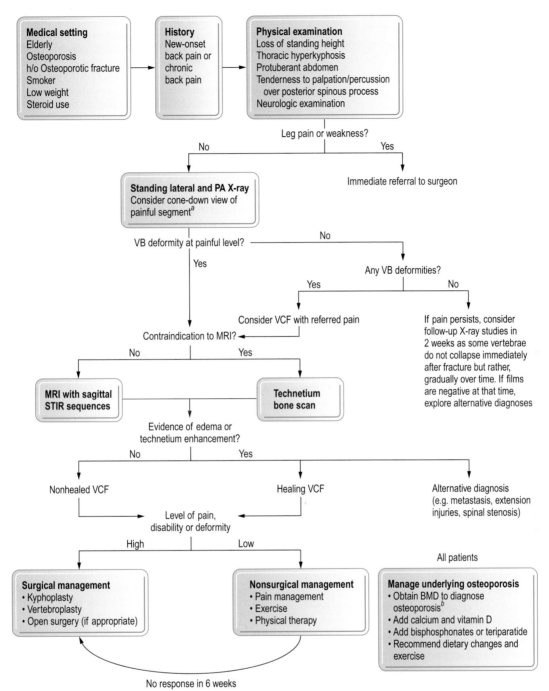

Figure 19.1 Management algorithm for acute painful VCFs. [a]Subtle T11–L1 fractures may be missed because they are at the lower end of a T spine and the top of an L spine film. Moreover, parallax obscures anatomical detail at the edges of an X-ray film. [b]If no osteoporosis, consider malignancy or other trauma as causes. BMD, bone mineral density; MRI, magnetic resonance imaging; PA, posteroanterior; STIR, short tau inversion recovery; VB, vertebral body; VCF, vertebral compression fracture.

Magnetic resonance imaging

If the source of pain remains undetermined, magnetic resonance imaging (MRI) may rule out a malignant tumor, identify the presence of a fracture and help identify appropriate treatment (Rao & Singrakhia 2003). A T1 sequence of an acute fracture will be darker than other vertebral bodies; a T2 sequence will be brighter. A short tau inversion recovery (STIR) sequence is ideal because it is very sensitive for osseous edema following a VCF. Routine imaging of the entire spine is probably not appropriate because of the expense. If the MRI does not reveal edema, the fracture has most likely healed and is not the cause of the pain. When an MRI is contraindicated, a technetium bone scan may be carried out instead.

Box 19.2   Findings on physical examination suggestive of multiple osteoporotic vertebral body compression fractures

- Rib–pelvis distance: <two finger-breadths between the inferior margin of the ribs and the superior surface of the pelvis in the midaxillary line
- Self-report of humped back
- Tooth count less than 20 teeth
- Wall–occiput distance: inability to touch occiput to the wall when standing with back and heels to the wall
- Weight less than 51 kg (women)

From Green et al 2004, with permission. Copyright© 2004 American Medical Association. All rights reserved.

PRIMARY CARE MANAGEMENT OF VCFs

For patients with or at risk of a VCF, PCPs should seek to prevent or rehabilitate fractures with nonpharmacological and pharmacological therapies as well as with lifestyle changes and other practices that protect bone (Box 19.3) (Health Professional's Guide 2003). Organizations have developed management guidelines (Hodgson et al 2001, Brown & Josse 2002, National Osteoporosis Foundation

---

Box 19.3   Rehabilitation of chronic back pain in patients with VCFs

- Practice good body mechanics
- Avoid activities such as forward bending that increase compression on vertebrae
- Prescribe an appropriate therapeutic exercise program:
  Strengthening exercises for the trunk, pelvis, thighs and lower extremities.
  Emphasis should be on trunk extension and avoidance of trunk flexion and rotation.
  T'ai Chi activities have been shown to be beneficial at increasing strength, balance and posture.
  Gentle aerobic activity, including walking, even with the use of a wheeled walker with hand brakes, may improve mobility.
  Exercises should be done for a minimum of 30 min at least three times weekly.
- Use appropriate medications for pain control and bone enhancement
- Assess and treat as needed any psychosocial issues
- Use modalities for pain control and as adjuncts to exercises
- Utilize community support to supplement patient knowledge and understanding of disease

Adapted from Health Professional's Guide to Rehabilitation of the Patient with Osteoporosis 2003.

Consider complementary and alternative treatment approaches such as acupuncture, guided visualization, relaxation techniques or biofeedback.

2005) that focus on (i) decreasing pain; (ii) preserving or increasing function; (iii) preventing additional fractures; and (iv) restoring spine alignment (Phillips 2003), if possible (Table 19.1) (American College of Rheumatology 2001, Hodgson et al 2001, Papaioannou et al 2001, South-Paul 2001, Woolf & Akesson 2003, Old & Calvert 2004, National Osteoporosis Foundation 2005).

In the past, conventional treatment included bedrest, opioid analgesics and back bracing to reduce the pain. Unfortunately, prolonged bedrest can contribute to further bone loss, thereby increasing the risk of subsequent fractures (Cooper et al 1992). Opioid analgesics should be used cautiously as their central nervous system effects may increase the risk of falling.

Nonpharmacological prevention strategies

Many nonpharmacological therapies for osteoporosis also help prevent secondary VCFs, as described below. Additionally, a home assessment may help reduce environmental factors that increase risk (Woolf & Akesson 2003).

Exercise

Weight-bearing and resistance exercises may maintain or increase BMD and promote mobility, agility and muscle strength, which may help prevent falls (National Osteoporosis Foundation 2005). There has been interest in high impact exercises including bouncing, vibrating and jumping activities (Stanford et al 2005), but such exercises should be supervised as they may aggravate arthritis in weight-bearing joints. If a fracture has been diagnosed, care should be taken to avoid further fracture, especially until BMD has improved. Long-term participation in an exercise program increases patients' QOL with respect to symptoms, emotion, leisure time and social activity. Further, as energy levels are increased, pain levels are reduced (Papaioannou et al 2003b).

Diet

Adequate daily intake of dietary or supplementary vitamin D and calcium is essential. In one meta-analysis, 700–800 IU/day of the cholecalciferol form of vitamin D was associated with a 26% reduction in the risk of hip fracture and a 23% reduction in the risk of nonvertebral fracture compared with calcium or placebo (Bischoff-Ferrari et al 2005). Strong evidence shows that alcohol consumption in excess of two drinks per day is a major risk factor for osteoporosis. Cigarette smokers undergo earlier menopause, have increased catabolism of endogenous estrogen and experience more hip fractures than do nonsmokers (Hodgson et al 2001).

Patient education and counseling

Because compliance with an exercise program or pharmacological regimen declines as early as 1 year after initiation (Papaioannou et al 2003b), especially in those who believe that their BMD test did not indicate osteoporosis (Tosteson et al 2003), patient education is essential. Referral to a clinical social worker may be useful to identify premorbid anxiety and depression.

Physical therapy

A physical therapy program helps prevent deformity by strengthening antigravity muscles and promoting postural retraining. Breathing exercises to encourage thoracic expansion and improve pulmonary function reduce the risk of pulmonary compromise.

Table 19.1 Medical management of a VCF

	Management
Who to screen Patient type	Women >65 years with no other risk; adult women with a previous history of fracture; women and men on corticosteroids >3 months
What to look for BMD finding	Within 1 SD of the mean: diagnosis normal; between 1 and 2.5 SD below the mean: diagnosis osteopenia; at least 2.5 SD below the mean: diagnosis osteoporosis.[a] The risk of fracture increases with age and with each SD below the mean. A minimum of 2 years may be needed to reliably measure a change in BMD, but a longer interval may be adequate for repeated screening to identify new cases of osteoporosis
Other prominent risk factors (also see Box 19.1)	Previous fracture, low body weight, persistent back pain
What to do All patients	Advocate 1500 mg calcium with 800 IU vitamin D daily and weight-bearing exercise; educate on importance of good exercise and calcium intake; prescribe and encourage compliance with a medication that increases BMD; refer to physical therapy if help is needed to promote an osteoporosis exercise program; identify any coexisting medical conditions that cause or contribute to bone loss (Cushing's syndrome, diabetes mellitus, inflammatory bowel syndrome, multiple myeloma, end-stage renal disease, chronic metabolic acidosis) by ordering initial lab workup that includes: complete blood count; spinal films; chemistry profile (calcium, total protein, albumin, LFTs, creatinine, electrolytes); 24-h urine calcium; vitamin D levels (25-hydroxy vitamin D, dihydroxyvitamin D-25 levels); thyroid-stimulating hormone; erythrocyte sedimentation rate; alkaline phosphatase; phosphorus
Acute treatment	Bedrest (prolonged bedrest can lead to further bone loss); analgesics (NSAIDs may inhibit repair of the bone fracture, whereas opioids may cause constipation); braces; pharmacological treatment of osteoporosis; for patients with persistent back pain, refer to a spine specialist for workup for vertebroplasty or kyphoplasty
Long-term management	Patient may require home care for an assessment of risk of falls at home; be aware that VCF may cause loss of physical functioning and depression in our patients; be prepared for a consultation to assess social and physical functioning
Prevention strategies	Physical therapy: gait and back strengthening, education on proper lifting etc, appropriate use of walker or cane; patient education: smoking cessation, calcium and vitamin D supplements, medication, importance of BMD results, exercise; environmental assessment: lighting, carpeting, living on one floor vs multilevel

From American College of Rheumatology 2001; Hodgson et al 2001; Papaioannou et al 2001; South-Paul 2001; Woolf & Akesson 2003; Old & Calvert 2004; and National Osteoporosis Foundation: Prevention (2005).
[a]Young adult mean.
BMD, bone mineral density; LFTs, liver function tests; NSAIDS, nonsteroidal antiinflammatory drugs; SD, standard deviation; VCF, vertebral compression fracture.

Bracing

To allow early physical therapy and control pain, use of a limited contact brace may be warranted. However, long-term bracing is discouraged. Compliance with bracing is low, especially with the rigid body jackets or the Knight–Taylor orthoses. Lightweight thoracolumbar braces (easier to put on and take off) may improve compliance. For lumbar fractures, a chairback brace is recommended, whereas cruciform anterior spinal hyperextension (CASH) or Jewett braces are appropriate for thoracic fractures. Lumbar corsets are not recommended as they place additional stress on fractures at the thoracolumbar junction (Patrick 1999). Standard braces can be obtained at some rehabilitation facilities or orthopedic and physical therapy clinics. Braces may need to be adjusted for individual patients by an orthotist or therapist; customized braces can also be ordered from orthotic facilities. An increasingly popular brace is the lightweight moldable Spinomed® (Medi-Bayreuth, Germany). Weighing approximately 0.5 kg (1 lb), the brace runs from the shoulders to the pelvis and is worn like a backpack. It has been shown to improve trunk strength, decrease kyphosis, decrease postural sway, improve forced expiratory volume and reduce pain (Pfeifer et al 2004).

Pharmacological therapy

Pharmacological therapy is an important component of care for patients with a VCF. Other than the acute management of pain, the role of pharmacological therapy is to maintain or increase BMD and reduce the risk of future fractures (French et al 2002, Campbell et al 2003, Cronholm & Barr 2003). There are a number of available agents including estrogen, selective estrogen receptor modulators, calcitonin and bisphosphonates (Health Professional's Guide 2003). The choice of a specific drug may be dependent on the patient's fracture risk, tolerance and the drug side effects, but drugs should always be used in combination with calcium and vitamin D.

SURGICAL MANAGEMENT OF VCFs

Kyphoplasty and vertebroplasty, two minimally invasive procedures, stabilize a VCF, reduce pain, increase spinal function and restore normal daily function (Predey et al 2002, Health Professional's Guide 2003, Rao & Singrakhia 2003). Open surgical treatment can address deformity but is reserved for cases of neurological deficit. In many cases, poor bone strength precludes the use of orthopedic screws or other open surgical treatment. Although kyphoplasty and vertebroplasty are performed by orthopedic spine surgeons, neurosurgical spine surgeons and interventional radiologists, PCPs should consider referral for these procedures as appropriate (see www.spine-health.com and www.spineuniverse.com for a list of spine specialists). Both procedures involve an incision site of less than 1 cm and can be performed on an inpatient or outpatient basis under local or general anesthesia. Kyphoplasty restores spinal alignment, theoretically reducing the risk of subsequent fractures.

Kyphoplasty: an overview

Kyphoplasty involves the stabilization of the fracture using bone cement (polymethylmethacrylate [PMMA]). The procedure is initiated by inserting a balloon tamp into the vertebral body under fluoroscopic guidance. The balloon is inflated, restoring vertebral height and moving the weightbearing axis posteriorly to reduce spinal deformity (Fig. 19.2). The size of the void created by the balloon is determined, the balloon is removed and the void is filled with a precise amount of cement at low pressure to minimize extravasation (Phillips 2003). Pain reduction occurs in 60–97% of patients with rapid improvement in daily activity levels and QOL; benefits are sustained for at least 2 years (Garfin et al 2001, Lieberman et al 2001, Coumans et al 2003, Ledlie & Renfro 2003). Physical functioning shows significant improvement with an increase from 12 to 47 in the physical functioning subscale score of the Short Form 36 (SF-36) (Liebermann et al 2001), a survey assessing health status in eight different areas including physical functioning, bodily pain and general mental health.

The extent of fracture deformity correction has been expressed variously in different studies as the angular correction (i.e. Cobb angle), the amount of correction or the degree to which the vertebral body returns to the expected height. Overall, a mean 50% of the lost height

is restored. Acute or 'readily reducible' fractures are typically corrected to 90% of their prefracture height (Garfin et al 2001, Liebermann et al 2001, Theodorou et al 2002, Phillips et al 2003, Crandall et al 2004, Grohs & Krepler 2004). Early referral of appropriate patients is important because the likelihood of height restoration decreases with time after the injury. However, the age of the fracture is irrelevant if the fracture is painful and STIR-sequence MRI reveals edema at the culprit vertebrae. Procedure-related complication rates range from 0.2% to 0.7% and include extravasation, embolism and nerve root injury.

Vertebroplasty: an overview

Initially used to treat symptomatic hemangiomas of the vertebral body, vertebroplasty is now used more frequently in the management of painful osteoporotic VCFs. Unlike kyphoplasty, a balloon tamp is not involved in vertebroplasty and so this procedure does not restore height or reduce spinal deformity. Bone cement is injected under fluoroscopic guidance into the vertebral body to stabilize the fracture in its current position. Pain relief is achieved in 63–100% of patients; most maintain a benefit for 1 year or more (Gangi et al 1994, Barr et al 2000). One study showed a reduction in the mean pain rating from 7.7 before the procedure to 2.8 after 1 day (McKiernan et al 2004). In another report, 90% were able to return to their normal activities without opioid use (Garfin et al 2001). Unfortunately the spinal deformity remains as the fracture is cemented in place. The failure and complication rates are low, but extravasation of the cement leading to local tissue or nerve injury or embolism is possible.

Insurance coverage for kyphoplasty and vertebroplasty varies from state to state. Payment for kyphoplasty is sometimes limited to two vertebral levels.

Following either procedure, it is important that calcium, vitamin D and other pharmacological and nonpharmacological measures be implemented to prevent a secondary VCF.

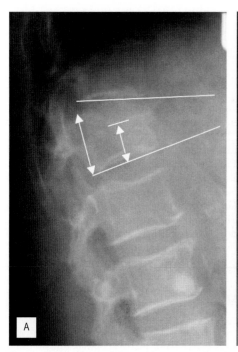 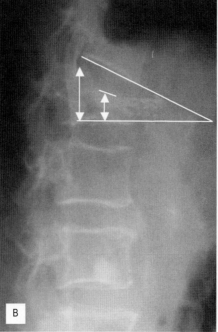 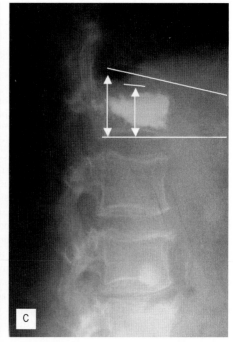

Figure 19.2   Kyphoplasty: effect on vertebral height and reduction of spinal deformity. (A) Immediately post fracture, kyphosis = 16°; (B) post fracture + 4 days, kyphosis = 25°; (C) post kyphoplasty, kyphosis = 10°. Reproduced with the permission of Dr Isador Lieberman.

Case study A KYPHOPLASTY

A 69-year-old woman experiences excruciating and immediate back pain after slipping on ice. X-ray studies demonstrate marked collapse of the L2 vertebra. Nonoperative management with bracing, nasal miacalcin, opioids, relative rest and physical therapy fail to control pain. Patient is nonambulatory. MRI STIR sequences demonstrate intense uptake in the L2 vertebral body, whereas the T1 marrow signal is decreased. Subsequent radiographs demonstrate further collapse of the vertebra. Because of progressive deformity and intense pain, a kyphoplasty is performed, with balloons inserted into the L2 vertebral body under local anesthesia. Serial inflation of the balloons allows restoration of lost vertebral body height; the fracture is stabilized with PMMA. A postoperative computed tomography (CT) scan reveals excellent restoration of the vertebral morphology without cement leak. Long-term therapy with a bisphosphonate, vitamin D and calcium are also instituted.

Case study B VERTEBROPLASTY

A 74-year-old woman with primary osteoporosis complains of 4 weeks of gradually increasing low back pain after having picked up a potted plant. Radiographs reveal a mild superior endplate fracture of L3. Initial management (brace, physical therapy and pain medications) fails to relieve pain. The patient's pacemaker precludes an MRI scan. A bone scan and CT scan demonstrate intensely increased uptake suggestive of an acute fracture without evidence of lytic lesion or canal compromise. To relieve intractable pain, a vertebroplasty is performed under local anesthesia. The patient notes immediate relief of her pain. Postoperative plain radiographs and a CT scan demonstrate an appropriate cement mantle with only mild intravascular leakage. Long-term therapy with a bisphosphonate, vitamin D and calcium are also instituted.

CONCLUSION

VCF is a relatively common but often unrecognized consequence of osteoporosis. Back pain is the typical presenting symptom; patients older than 50 years with acute back pain should undergo a clinical workup for a VCF. Primary care clinicians have important roles as educators about bone health and as providers of pharmacological therapies. Additionally, they are critical in coordinating the multidisciplinary care of a patient with a VCF. Kyphoplasty and vertebroplasty stabilize a VCF, increase spinal function and restore normal daily function. Both may be performed as an inpatient or outpatient procedure, as determined by medical necessity. They provide rapid pain improvement with a low complication rate. Restoration of the vertebral height is an added benefit of kyphoplasty.

ACKNOWLEDGMENT

Modified from Brunton S et al 2005 Vertebral compression fractures in primary care: recommendations from a consensus panel. J Fam Pract 54:781–788, with permission.

References

American College of Rheumatology 2001 Ad hoc committee on glucocorticoid-induced osteoporosis. Recommendations for the prevention and treatment of glucocorticoid-induced osteoporosis: 2001 update. Arthritis Rheum 44:1496–1503

Andrade SE, Majumdar SR, Chan KA et al 2003 Low frequency of treatment of osteoporosis among postmenopausal women following a fracture. Arch Intern Med 163:2052–2057

Armagon O, Uz T, Tascioglu F et al 2005 Serological screening for celiac disease in premenopausal women with idiopathic osteoporosis. Clin Rheumatol 24:239–243

Barr JD, Barr MS, Lemley TJ, McCann RM 2000 Percutaneous vertebroplasty for pain relief and spinal stabilization. Spine 25:923–928

Bischoff-Ferrari HA, Willett WC, Wong JB et al 2005 Fracture prevention with vitamin D supplementation: a meta-analysis of randomized controlled trials. JAMA 293:2257–2264

Black DM, Cummings SR, Karpf DB et al 1996 Randomised trial of effect of alendronate on risk of fracture in women with existing vertebral fractures. Fracture Intervention Trial Research Group. Lancet 348:1535–1541

Brown JP, Josse RG 2002 Clinical practice guidelines for the diagnosis and management of osteoporosis in Canada. Can Med Assoc J 167(suppl):S1–34

Burger H, van Daele PL, Algra D et al 1994 Vertebral deformities as predictors of non-vertebral fractures. Br Med J 309:991–992

Campbell BG, Ketchell D, Gunning K 2003 Clinical inquiries. Do calcium supplements prevent postmenopausal osteoporotic fractures? J Fam Pract 52:234–237

Cooper C, Atkinson EJ, O'Fallon WM, Melton LJ III 1992 Incidence of clinically diagnosed vertebral fractures: a population-based study in Rochester, Minnesota, 1985–1989. J Bone Miner Res 7:221–227

Cooper C, Atkinson EJ, Jacobsen SJ et al 1993 Population based study of survival after osteoporotic fractures. Am J Epidemiol 137:1001–1005

Coumans JV, Reinhardt MK, Lieberman IH 2003 Kyphoplasty for vertebral compression fractures: 1-year clinical outcomes from a prospective study. J Neurosurg Spine 99:44–50

Crandall D, Slaughter D, Hankins PJ et al 2004 Acute versus chronic vertebral compression fractures treated with kyphoplasty: early results. Spine J 4:418–424

Cronholm PF, Barr W 2003 Densitometry identifies women in whom treatment will reduce fracture risk. J Fam Pract 52:114–117

French L, Smith M, Shrimp L 2002 Prevention and treatment of osteoporosis in postmenopausal women. J Fam Pract 51:875–882

Gangi A, Kastler BA, Dietemann JL 1994 Percutaneous vertebroplasty guided by a combination of CT and fluoroscopy. AJNR Am J Neuroradiol 15:83–86

Garfin SR, Yuan HA, Reiley MA 2001 New technologies in spine: kyphoplasty and vertebroplasty for the treatment of painful osteoporotic compression fractures. Spine 26:1511–1515

Gehlbach SH, Bigelow C, Heimisdottir M et al 2000 Recognition of vertebral fracture in a clinical setting. Osteoporos Int 11:577–582

Gold DT 2003 Osteoporosis and quality of life, psychosocial outcomes and interventions for individual patients. Clin Geriatr Med 19:271–280

Green AD, Colon-Emeric CS, Bastian L et al 2004 Does this woman have osteoporosis? JAMA 292:2890–2900

Grohs JG, Krepler P 2004 Minimal invasive stabilization of osteoporotic vertebral compression fractures. Methods and preinterventional diagnostics [in German]. Radiologie 44:254–259

Health Professional's Guide to Rehabilitation of the Patient with Osteoporosis 2003. National Osteoporosis Foundation, Washington, DC, 20037.29

Hodgson SF, Watts NB, Bilezikian JP et al 2001 American Association of Clinical Endocrinologists. Medical guidelines for clinical practice for the prevention and management of postmenopausal osteoporosis. Endocr Pract 7:293–312

Ismail AA, Cockerill W, Cooper C et al 2001 Prevalent vertebral deformity predicts incident hip though not distal forearm fracture: results from the European Prospective Osteoporosis Study. Osteoporos Int 12:85–90

Jackson SA, Tenenhouse A, Robertson L 2000 Vertebral fracture definition from population-based data: preliminary results from the Canadian Multicenter Osteoporosis Study (CaMos). Osteoporos Int 11:680–687

Ledlie JT, Renfro M 2003 Balloon kyphoplasty: one-year outcomes in vertebral body height restoration, chronic pain, and activity levels. J Neurosurg Spine 98:36–42

Leech JA, Dulberg C, Kellie S et al 1990 Relationship of lung function to severity of osteoporosis in women. Am Rev Respir Dis 14:68–71

Lieberman IH, Dudeney S, Reinhardt MK, Bell G 2001 Initial outcome and efficacy of 'kyphoplasty' in the treatment of painful osteoporotic vertebral compression fractures. Spine 26:1631–1638

Lindsay R, Silverman SL, Cooper C et al 2001 Risk of new vertebral fracture in the year following a fracture. JAMA 285:320–323

McKiernan F, Faciszewski T, Jensen R 2004 Quality of life following vertebroplasty. J Bone Joint Surg Am 86A:2600–2606

National Osteoporosis Foundation. Health issues survey: attitudes and actions regarding osteoporosis. Available: www.nof.org/news/pressreleases/2004_health_issues_survey.htm. Accessed July 26 2005

National Osteoporosis Foundation. Prevention. Available: www.nof.org/prevention/ index.htm. Accessed April 26 2005

Nevitt MC, Ettinger B, Black DM et al 1998 The association of radiographically detected vertebral fractures with back pain and function: a prospective study. Ann Intern Med 128:793–800

Nevitt MC, Ross PD, Palermo L et al 1999 Association of prevalent vertebral fractures, bone density, and alendronate treatment with incident vertebral fractures: effect of number and spinal location of fractures. The Fracture Intervention Trial Research Group. Bone 25:613–619

Old JL, Calvert M 2004 Vertebral compression fractures in the elderly. Am Fam Physician 69:111–116

Oleksik A, Lips P, Dawson A et al 2000 Health-related quality of life in postmenopausal women with low BMD with or without prevalent vertebral fractures. J Bone Miner Res 15:1384–1392

Papaioannou A, Adachi JD, Parkinson W et al 2001 Lengthy hospitalization associated with vertebral fractures despite control for comorbid conditions. Osteoporos Int 12:870–874

Papaioannou A, Watts NB, Kendler DL et al 2002 Diagnosis and management of vertebral fractures in elderly adults. Am J Med 113:220–228

Papaioannou A, Parkinson W, Ferko N et al 2003a Prevalence of vertebral fractures among patients with chronic obstructive pulmonary disease in Canada. Osteoporos Int 14:913–917

Papaioannou A, Adachi JD, Winegard K et al 2003b Efficacy of home-based exercise for improving quality of life among elderly women with symptomatic osteoporosis related vertebral fractures. Osteoporos Int 14:677–682

Patrick D 1999 Orthotics. In: Kauffman TL (ed) Geriatric Rehabilitation Manual. Churchill Livingstone, Philadelphia, PA

Pfeifer M, Begerow B, Minne HW 2004 Effects of a new spinal orthosis on posture, trunk strength, and quality of life in women with postmenopausal osteoporosis: a randomized trial. Am J Phys Med Rehabil 83:177–186

Phillips FM 2003 Minimally invasive treatments of osteoporotic vertebral compression fractures. Spine 28(suppl):S45–53

Phillips FM, Ho E, Campbell-Hupp M et al 2003 Early radiographic and clinical results of balloon kyphoplasty for the treatment of osteoporotic vertebral compression fractures. Spine 28:2260–2265

Predey TA, Sewall LE, Smith SJ 2002 Percutaneous vertebroplasty: new treatment for vertebral compression fractures. Am Fam Physician 66:611–615

Raisz LG 2005 Clinical practice. Screening for osteoporosis. N Engl J Med 353:164–171

Rao RD, Singrakhia MD 2003. Painful osteoporotic vertebral fracture. Pathogenesis, evaluation, and roles of vertebroplasty and kyphoplasty in its management. J Bone Joint Surg Am 85A:2010–2022

South-Paul JE 2001 Osteoporosis: part II. Nonpharmacologic and pharmacologic treatment. Am Fam Physician 63:1121–1128

Stanford VA, Houtkooper LB, Day SH et al 2005 The BEST exercise program for osteoporosis prevention. Paper presented at the Sixth International Symposium on Osteoporosis: Current Status and Future Directions. April 6–10, Washington, DC

Theodorou DJ, Theodorou SJ, Duncan TD et al 2002 Percutaneous balloon kyphoplasty for the correction of spinal deformity in painful vertebral body compression fractures. Clin Imaging 26:1–5

Tosi LL, Bouxsein ML, Johnell O 2004 Commentary on the AAOS position statement: recommendations for enhancing the care for patients with fragility fractures. Techniques Orthopediques 19:121–125

Tosteson AN, Grove MR, Hammond CS et al 2003 Early discontinuation of treatment for osteoporosis. Am J Med 115:209–216

US Department of Health and Human Services. Bone health and osteoporosis: a report of the Surgeon General. Available: www.surgeongeneral.gov/library/ bonehealth. Accessed July 26 2005

Woolf AD, Akesson K 2003 Preventing fractures in elderly people. Br Med J 327:89–95

Yamaguchi T, Sugimoto T, Yamauchi M et al 2005 Multiple vertebral fractures are associated with refractory reflux esophagitis in postmenopausal women. J Bone Miner Metab 23:36–40

Chapter 20

Rheumatic conditions

June E. Hanks and David Levine

INTRODUCTION

The impact of arthritis is highly significant and is expected to affect one-quarter of the US population by the year 2030 (National Health Interview Survey and US Census Bureau 2002). Worldwide it is estimated that over 50% of chronic conditions in people over the age of 65 years are attributed to joint diseases. To increase attention to this human problem, the World Health Organization, the World Bank and the United Nations designated the years from 2000 to 2010 as the Bone and Joint Decade. The initiative is a campaign to enhance awareness, understanding and research of musculoskeletal disorders with the goal of improving quality of life (Lidgren 2003, www.bone-jointdecade.org). A diagnosis of arthritis may be established following careful attention to clinical manifestations, laboratory tests, radio-graphic and imaging studies and responses to drug therapy. Although arthritis can affect anyone, certain types of arthritis are commonly associated with aging. The pathophysiology, medical management and recommended therapy for the following rheumatic conditions: osteoarthritis, rheumatoid arthritis, systemic lupus erythematosus, gout, pseudogout, polymyalgia rheumatica, bursitis and tendonitis are discussed below.

OSTEOARTHRITIS

Osteoarthritis (OA), also called osteoarthrosis or degenerative joint disease, is the most common joint disorder and one of the leading causes of disability in the elderly. The condition involves cartilage degeneration, the remodeling of subchondral bone and overgrowth of bone at joint margins. Joint effusion and thickening of the synovium and capsule may also occur. Osteoarthritis affects women more than men; however, both genders are affected with severity increasing with age. The most affected joints are the weight-bearing synovial joints of the lower extremity, the spine and the carpometacarpal and distal interphalangeal joints of the hand (Hannan 2001).

Osteoarthritis occurring without a predisposing condition is called 'primary OA' whereas 'secondary OA' results from a local or systemic factor, such as trauma, developmental deformity or infection, or following cartilage damage as a result of another disease or form of arthritis. The disease process of OA affects the entire joint including the articular cartilage, synovium, subchondral bone and surrounding supportive connective tissues. The most marked changes in OA involve the articular cartilage. In an unaffected joint, the articular cartilage provides a smooth, almost frictionless weight-bearing joint surface that spreads and minimizes local loads. Repeated excessive loading of normal cartilage and subchondral bone or normal loading of biologically deficient cartilage and subchondral bone may lead to microcracks and uneven distribution of chondrocytes. The degenerating, thinning cartilage is less able to redistribute forces, leading to greater force transference to the subchondral bone (Klippel 2001). This results in subchondral bone hardening and the formation of osteophytes (bone spurs) at joint margins. As the joint surface deteriorates, the joint capsule may become lax, leading to joint instability. OA can be detected on radiographs by decreased joint space, osteophyte formation, subchondral sclerosis and subchondral trabecular fractures. Radiographic evidence of OA is present in the majority of older individuals although not all are symptomatic. Generally, however, a positive correlation exists between clinical and radiographic findings. Factors contributing to OA include aging, excess body weight, occupational or sport joint injury and metabolic or endocrine disorders.

Clinical characteristics include joint pain, stiffness, tenderness, instability and enlargement. Periarticular muscle atrophy and weakness occur, contributing to disability. Early in the disease course, pain is worsened by activity and relieved by rest. With disease progression, pain is often present even at rest and may lead to significant functional impairment. Articular cartilage is devoid of nerve endings, thus the pain associated with OA arises from innervated intra-articular and periarticular structures. In the spine, bony overgrowth may encroach on emerging nerve roots, causing pain. Stiffness, usually occurring in the mornings and following periods of rest, is relieved by movement. Motion limitation may be caused by irregular joint surface movement because of cartilage degeneration, muscle spasms due to pain, muscle weakness due to disuse and osteophyte formation. Crepitus, a clicking or crackling sound, may occur as the joint is moved. Joints may enlarge because of synovitis, joint effusion, connective tissue overgrowth or osteophyte formation. Joint deformity may occur, as forces are inappropriately distributed between joint structures.

Inflammation is not a typical characteristic of OA but may occur as the irritated synovium contributes to the activation of chondrocytes causing production of a wide range of inflammatory mediators that release cartilage–damaging products. The imbalance between chondrocyte synthesis and degradation stimulates further production of proinflammatory mediators and proteinases. The naturally occurring tissue inhibitors become overwhelmed and crystals may be deposited in the degenerating cartilage, sometimes breaking off into the joint and creating acute or chronic inflammation (Walker & Helewa 2004).

The aim of therapeutic intervention is to relieve symptoms, maintain and improve function and limit the degree of functional impairment. Typical therapeutic interventions for OA include education, rest, pharmacological agents, exercise, weight reduction and possibly surgery. Patients should be instructed in joint protection and energy conservation techniques to help prevent acute flare-ups and to help minimize joint stress and pain. Regularly administered pharmacological agents include analgesics and nonsteroidal antiinflammatory agents (NSAIAs). Intra-articular corticosteroid injections may benefit acute joint inflammation.

Rehabilitation should include appropriate weight-bearing and nonweight-bearing exercise. The evidence-based clinical practice guidelines of the Ottawa Panel recommend therapeutic exercise for managing pain and functional impairment of OA (Ottawa Panel 2005), particularly strengthening and general activity, with or without manual therapy. Individualized programs should include strengthening, range of motion and cardiovascular fitness. To minimize stress on the joints, the design of the strengthening program should include the use of low weights and high repetitions. Exercise in water is an excellent activity because buoyancy in water reduces the effect of gravity and the loading effect on joints. Resistive exercise that produces increased joint pain during or following exercise probably indicates too much resistance is being used, stress is being placed at an inappropriate part of the range of motion or the exercise is being incorrectly performed. Stretching exercises incorporating a low load, such as prolonged stretch performed three or more times a day, will lead to a more appropriate length–tension relationship for the muscles surrounding the affected joints and may lead to decreased stress in the intra-articular and periarticular joint structures. Home exercise programs must be carefully planned and monitored. Heat may decrease pain and stiffness and cold may decrease pain and inflammation. Splints, braces and gait devices, such as crutches, a walker or a rolling walker, may be helpful in decreasing joint stress. Weight loss may prevent the onset of symptoms or alleviate symptoms when present.

Surgical interventions such as arthroscopy, arthroplasty and angulation osteotomy may provide symptomatic relief, improved motion and improved joint biomechanics. The most common major orthopedic procedure performed in the elderly is hip surgery, the indications for this being fracture or pain resulting from OA. A large percentage of hip and knee replacements are for OA (see Chapters 22 and 23). Although elderly patients are at higher risk for complications than younger patients, most have a satisfactory outcome and significant relief of pain. Experimental surgical techniques to stimulate cartilage repair or transplant cartilage are generally not successful although select patient populations with focal defects may benefit (Buckwalter & Mankin 1998).

RHEUMATOID ARTHRITIS

Rheumatoid arthritis (RA), one of the most common of the rheumatic diseases, is a chronic systemic inflammatory autoimmune disorder. Clinical features vary among individuals and within the same individual over the course of the disease. The hallmark feature of RA is chronic inflammation of the synovium, peripheral articular cartilage and subchondral marrow spaces. In response to the inflammation, granulation tissue (pannus) forms leading to the erosion of articular cartilage. Early in the disease process, the synovitis may be clinically detected as warmth and swelling in joints. As the disease progresses, joint immobility and reduced vascularity of the synovium makes the degree of inflammation more difficult to detect. Inflammation in tendon sheaths may lead to tendon fray or rupture. The clinical manifestation of synovial inflammation is morning stiffness related to immobilization which lasts for more than 2 h after rising. As a systemic connective tissue disease, RA may result in systemic and extra-articular pathological changes and these are the predominant feature of the disease process in some people. Systemic and extra-articular manifestations include muscle fibrosis and atrophy, vasculitis, pericarditis, fatigue, weight loss, generalized stiffness, fever, anemia, pleural effusion, interstitial lung disease, keratoconjunctivitis, increased susceptibility to infection, and neurological compromise leading to sensory and/or motor loss. Subcutaneous nontender nodules may occur on the extensor surface of the forearm or other pressure areas. The effect of RA is broad, ranging from mild symptoms resulting in only occasional pain and discomfort and only slight decreases in function to severe symptoms with significant pain, decreased function and joint deformity.

The prevalence of RA increases with age, is 2.5 times higher in women than men and has a peak incidence between the fourth and sixth decades (Klippel 2001). The onset of RA may be acute but is usually insidious. The clinical course of RA is variable and unpredictable. In the initial stages, joint pain and stiffness are prevalent, especially in the mornings. With disease progression, motion becomes more limited and ankylosis may develop. Radiographic evidence of the disease becomes apparent over time. Treatment effectiveness may be difficult to determine because of spontaneous exacerbations and remissions. Testimonials of 'cures' with unproven remedies are common, as certain treatment approaches may have been initiated during the initial stages of a spontaneous remission.

The etiology of RA is unknown. Evidence exists for a genetic predisposition for the disease, which may be triggered by bacteria or viruses. The pathogenesis of RA is better understood than the etiology. The characteristic chronic inflammatory process begins with synovitis, developing as microvascular endothelial cells become swollen and congested. As the disease advances, the synovium becomes progressively thickened and edematous, with projections of synovial tissue invading the joint cavity. Pannus, tumor-like thickened layers of granulation tissue, infiltrates the joints destroying periarticular bone and cartilage. Fibrotic ankylosis may eventually occur, with bony malalignment, visible deformities, muscle atrophy and subluxation of joints. In advanced RA, bony ankylosis and significant disability may occur.

A definitive diagnosis is based on a combination of clinical manifestations and laboratory findings, as there is no laboratory test specific for RA. Frequent laboratory findings in people with RA include decreased red blood cell count, increased erythrocyte sedimentation rates and positive rheumatoid factor (RF). A positive test of RF is not diagnostic as RF is found in a small percentage of normal individuals. However, RF is found in the serum of most adults with RA and may indicate increased severity (Braun et al 2007).

Joint manifestations occur bilaterally, principally affecting the small joints of the hands and feet, ankles, knees, wrists, elbows, hips and shoulders. Typically, the metacarpophalangeal and proximal interphalangeal joints of the hand are affected, with sparing of the distal interphalangeal joints. In axial involvement, the upper cervical spine is most affected. Tenosynovitis of the transverse ligament of the first cervical vertebra and disease of the cervical apophyseal joints may lead to instability and cord compression. A thorough neurological examination should be conducted to determine involvement. Most of the joints ultimately affected by RA will be involved during the first year of the disease.

Joint deformities result from synovitis, pannus formation, cartilage destruction and voluntary joint immobilization because of pain. The change in joint mechanics from cartilage degeneration and the erosive effect of chronic synovitis may lead to ligament laxity. The changed mechanics result in abnormal lines of pull from tendons, leading to joint deformity. Additionally, tenosynovitis may occur, causing an obstruction of tendon movement within the tendon sheath and/or tendon rupture. Nodular thickening may occur, leading to a 'locking' sensation or rupture of the tendon. Synovitis can lead to compression of nerves, particularly in the carpal tunnel and, less commonly, the tarsal tunnel. The ulnar nerve may be compressed at the elbow or in the hand.

Common deformities of the hand include radial deviation of the wrist, ulnar deviation at the metacarpophalangeal joints and deformities in the fingers. Flexion deformity of the elbow and loss of shoulder motion is common. Because of the weight-bearing nature of the lower extremity, major disability can result, particularly in the toes and ankles. Cock-up deformities of the toes and subluxation of the metatarsal heads with concurrent migration of the metatarsophalangeal fat pad result in significant pain in walking.

Effective treatment of RA attempts to reduce the inflammation, provide pain relief, maintain and restore joint function and decrease the development of joint deformity. Medications include NSAIAs, corticosteroids, slow-acting antirheumatic drugs and disease-modifying antirheumatic drugs. Patients must balance activity and rest. Fatigue may be decreased with appropriate rest, which may include 8–10 h of sleep at night and an afternoon nap. Energy should be conserved for daily activities. Prolonged bedrest has not proven to be beneficial. Therapeutic exercise cannot alter the course of the disease but can help prevent deformity and loss of motion and muscle strength. Clinical practice guidelines developed by the Ottawa Panel emphasize shoulder, hand, knee and whole body functional strengthening at low intensities (Ottawa Panel 2004a). Active and passive range of motion exercise, pain-free isometrics and proper positioning and posture should be performed regularly to achieve functional goals. Joint-stressing activities should be avoided. Water is an excellent medium for active individual or group structured exercise, although the water temperatures for patients with RA may need to be higher than usual. Splints and assistive devices should be used as needed to protect the joints. During active inflammatory periods, exercise should be performed carefully, with special care taken to protect the joints. Heavy resistive exercise should be avoided as the joint compression that occurs with this exercise could increase pain and contribute to joint damage. Because the limitation of motion is due to distended joint capsules and not to adhesions, forceful stretching should be avoided. During times of remission, non- or low-impact aerobic conditioning such as swimming or stationary bicycling can be performed within the patient's tolerance. Gentle stretching can be performed. Relaxation exercises often help to decrease muscle tension and stress.

Strong clinical evidence exists for the inclusion of low-level laser therapy, therapeutic ultrasound, thermotherapy and transcutaneous electrical stimulation in the management of RA. Convincing evidence is lacking on the benefit of electrical stimulation for treating RA

(Ottawa Panel 2004b). Surgical procedures may be performed with the goal being to reduce pain, improve function and correct instability or deformity. Common surgical procedures include tenosynovectomy, tendon repair, synovectomy, arthrodesis and arthroplasty.

SYSTEMIC LUPUS ERYTHEMATOSUS

Systemic lupus erythematosus (SLE) is an autoimmune disease primarily affecting young women. The peak incidence of SLE occurs between the ages of 15 and 40, but it may affect both younger and older people, with a female to male ratio of approximately 10:1. The disease course varies widely from a relatively benign to a life-threatening illness (Robbins 2001). Mortality rates increase with age and are higher among people of lower socioeconomic status (Ward et al 1995).

The etiology of SLE is unknown but may involve immunological, environmental, hormonal and genetic factors. The prime causative mechanism is thought to be autoimmunity in which tissues are damaged as antibodies are produced against many body components such as blood vessels, red blood cells, lymphocytes and various organs. Antibodies directed against components of the cell nucleus, antinuclear antibodies (ANA), are found in most SLE patients.

Two ANA molecules, ANA-DNA and ANA-Sm, are unique to SLE and are used as diagnostic criteria. The diagnosis of SLE is based on clinical manifestations supported by laboratory tests. Clinical criteria developed by the American College of Rheumatology for classification of SLE include skin rash, renal dysfunction, blood disorders, arthritis, cardiopulmonary dysfunction, neurological/psychiatric problems and abnormal immunological tests (Hochberg 1997). Clinically apparent nephritis develops in many cases and biopsies may be used to assess the degree of kidney damage. Photosensitive skin disorders are common, especially an acute inflammatory rash on the malar regions of the face, known as 'butterfly rash', or on the upper extremities or trunk. Subacute symmetrical and widespread lesions or chronic disk-shaped scaly lesions may appear. Pleurisy, pericarditis, chronic interstitial lung inflammation, heart valve abnormalities and thromboses are common with varying degrees of severity. Neurological and psychiatric manifestations include seizures and psychosis. Gastrointestinal manifestations include diffuse abdominal pain, nausea and vomiting, and anorexia. The arthritis associated with SLE may be symmetrical or nonsymmetrical and typically affects the small joints of the hands, wrists and knees. Typically, the arthritis is nonerosive but deforming arthropathy, particularly of the hands, can develop as a consequence of recurrent inflammation.

Although the short-term prognosis has improved in recent years, the long-term outlook for patients with SLE is generally poor, with complications resulting from either the disease itself or as a consequence of treatment. Late complications of SLE include end-stage renal disease, athero-sclerosis, pulmonary emboli, venous syndromes, avascular necrosis and neuropsychological dysfunction (Robbins 2001).

Treatment of SLE is determined by disease activity and severity. Drugs that suppress inflammation and interfere with immune system functioning are commonly prescribed. NSAIAs may be used to treat musculoskeletal complications. Skin lesions may be treated with corticosteroids and antimalarial agents. Corticosteroids are used in the treatment of systemic symptoms of SLE such as pericarditis, nephritis, vasculitis and central nervous system involvement. In some patients, cytotoxic drugs such as methotrexate, azathioprine and cyclophosphamide are prescribed. Patients must be monitored closely for side effects.

Patient education is paramount in the treatment of SLE. The patient must understand that periods of remission and exacerbation are typical. Many SLE patients are photosensitive and must be reminded to avoid or reduce sun exposure when possible. SLE patients are at an increased risk of infection and should be informed of the importance of the prompt evaluation of unexplained fever. The patient should be urged to get adequate rest. Physical rehabilitation may be helpful to increase strength and motion and to splint affected joints. Heat may be used to relieve joint pain and stiffness. Regular active exercise may prevent contractures.

GOUT

Gout is a metabolic disease characterized by the deposition of monosodium urate crystals in connective tissues, resulting in painful arthritis. The hyperuricemia associated with gout may result from a variety of factors including a genetic defect in purine metabolism, which leads to an overproduction and/or undersecretion of uric acid. Other associated factors include obesity, diet, lifestyle, renal dysfunction and hemoglobin levels. Diuretics can lead to an underexcretion of uric acid and may play a role in the pathogenesis of gout (Choi et al 2005). Primary gout typically occurs in men, with a peak incidence in the fifth decade, and commonly causes short-term disability. Gout may also occur in postmenopausal women especially when diuretics are used. Secondary gout occurs primarily in the elderly and results from the hyperuricemia associated with diseases such as diabetes mellitus and hypertension. The mechanisms are not fully defined but are probably due to diminished renal function, dehydration, decreased tissue perfusion and the effect of certain drugs leading to uric acid overproduction or underexcretion. Gout is relatively common in organ transplant recipients because of the use of ciclosporin and due to reduced renal function, regardless of the organ transplanted.

The clinical course of gout typically follows four stages: asymptomatic, acute, intercritical and chronic. An asymptomatic period of urate crystal deposition in connective tissue often appears before the first episode of gouty arthritis. The initial episode of gout is typically sudden, often occurring during the night. The patient awakes with severe unexplained joint pain and swelling. The first metatarsophalangeal joint is commonly affected. The ankle, tarsal joints and knee may also be involved. Acute attacks may be precipitated by trauma, alcohol, drugs or acute medical illness. The intercritical stage is characterized by symptom-free periods which may last from months to years. The presence of crystal deposition persists during these asymptomatic periods and aspiration of the joints may confirm the diagnosis. The chronic stage of gout is characterized by tophi, large masses of urates within the subarticular bone or surrounding soft tissues. Less commonly, tophi form in the internal organs. Tophi deposits precipitate joint erosion and tendon rupture. The arthritic clinical manifestation of chronic gout may resemble RA, although gout is usually more asymmetrical and can involve any joint.

Not all individuals with hyperuricemia will develop gout. The presence of monosodium urate crystals in synovial fluid is generally considered necessary to establish a definitive diagnosis. Even during asymptomatic periods, monosodium urate crystals may be demonstrated in synovial fluid aspirated from previously involved joints as well as from joints that have never been involved. Serum uric acid levels are less helpful in definitive diagnosis, especially in the acute phase, but levels will eventually become elevated.

Treatment of gout is aimed at terminating acute attacks, reducing hyperuricemia, preventing recurrence and preventing erosive joint damage and kidney complications. During acute attacks, NSAIAs or colchicines may be used to relieve symptoms. Corticosteroids and adrenocorticotrophic hormone may be used when colchicines and NSAIAs are ineffective or contraindicated (Robbins 2001). Included

in the treatment regime are bedrest, joint immobilization and local cold application to inflamed joints. Attack frequency may be decreased by certain dietary and lifestyle changes. Recom-mended dietary modifications include the avoidance of alcohol and a restriction of purine-rich foods, such as liver, kidneys, shellfish, salmon, peas, beans and spinach. Weight loss and the avoidance of repetitive trauma are helpful prophylactic measures that may enable drug therapy to be avoided during intercritical periods. Infected or ulcerated tophi may require excision.

Practical considerations include the use of a bed cradle to keep bed covers off inflamed joints, the intake of plenty of fluids to prevent the formation of kidney stones, prompt treatment of acute attacks and rapid attention to the side effects of drug therapies. Assistive devices may also be used to decrease stress on inflamed joints.

PSEUDOGOUT

Pseudogout (PG), a chronic recurrent arthritis similar to gout, results from calcium pyrophosphate dihydrate (CPPD) crystal deposition in articular and periarticular structures. The presence of CPPD crystals in joint tissue is common in the elderly, and there is only a weak correlation with joint pain. The risk of CPPD-associated disease increases with age but occurs half as commonly as gout, with a near equal occurrence in men and women. The pattern of joint involvement is symmetrical, although possibly more advanced on one side. Acute PG is characterized by self-limiting attacks of acute joint pain and swelling. Any synovial joint may be affected but the knee is the most common. The pain associated with PG is less severe than with gout. Calcification from CPPD crystal deposits will characteristically be demonstrated on well-exposed radiographs of the knees and wrists. Acute attacks may be provoked by surgery, trauma or severe illness. Joint inflammation and destruction may occur simultaneously or independently, thus resembling other rheumatic diseases. Definitive diagnosis is made through the demonstration of CPPD crystals. Acute attacks are managed through joint aspiration to relieve pressure, injection of steroids, administration of analgesics and NSAIAs, as well as the use of oral or intravenous colchicines.

Individuals with PG may experience multiple joint involvement, with low-grade inflammation lasting for weeks or months. The morning stiffness, fatigue, synovial thickening and flexion contractures associated with PG may lead to a misdiagnosis of RA. The pattern of joint degeneration in PG is distinctive from OA in that symmetrical involvement is most typical. Rehabilitation of individuals with pseudogout should focus on joint protection during acute attacks, maintenance of range of motion and energy conservation practices.

POLYMYALGIA RHEUMATICA

Polymyalgia rheumatica (PMR) is a common systemic inflammatory disorder in the elderly and is characterized by the gradual development of persistent pain, weakness and stiffness in proximal muscles, combined with fever, weight loss and high erythrocyte sedimentation rates. More common in women than men, PMR occurs mostly in those over 50 years of age, with a peak incidence in the sixth to eighth decades. PMR affects the white population more than other ethnic groups and particularly those in the northern areas of the US (Ramesh 2003). Symptoms are usually symmetrical and onset may be abrupt. Stiffness is typically worse in the morning. Tenderness and stiffness is most common in the muscles of the shoulder and pelvic girdles and neck but may be present in the knees, wrists and hands. Differential diagnosis of PMR from hypothyroidism, malignancies, RA, SLE and infectious diseases is critical. Giant cell arteritis (GCA), also known as temporal arteritis, is a systemic inflammatory disorder affecting large and medium-sized blood vessels. The pain presentation may be similar to that in PMR and the conditions may coexist in some people. The vasculitis associated with GCA may lead to severe occlusive disease and result in stroke and blindness. Symptoms include headache, visual disturbance, scalp tenderness and abnormalities in the temporal arteries. The coexistence of PMR and GCA is common in the elderly (Kennedy-Malone & Enevold 2001) and GCA results in blindness more often in men than in women (Nir-Paz et al 2002).

The diagnosis of PMR is based on clinical manifestation supported by laboratory tests such as high erythrocyte sedimentation rates and C-reactive protein levels. Results of muscle enzyme tests and biopsies, and plain film radiographs, do not contribute to differential diagnosis. PMR responds dramatically to prednisone therapy; thus, the response is used in diagnosis as well as treatment. The optimal dose is the lowest dose that will control symptoms and long-term side effects such as osteoporosis, diabetes, hypertension and gastrointestinal problems should be monitored and treated. The disease is typically self-limiting, lasting 2–7 years. Patients should be warned of the signs and symptoms of GCA. Later in the course of the disease, stretching and strengthening exercises may be helpful. Modalities such as ice and electrical stimulation may be used to decrease pain. The use of assistive devices may decrease the risk of falls.

BURSITIS

Bursas are small sacs with a synovial-like membrane that contain a fluid that is indistinguishable from synovial fluid. Located in areas of potential friction, bursas are commonly located between bones and ligaments, skin or muscles. An example is the ischial bursa, which lies between the ischial tuberosity and the gluteus maximus. Bursitis is defined as inflammation of the bursa and may occur in the superficial bursas of the shoulder, greater trochanter, knee or elbow, or in deeper bursas of the ischial tuberosity, iliopsoas and popliteal areas. As a response to the stimulus of inflammation, the lining membrane may produce excess fluid, causing distension of the bursa.

Bursitis may be caused by an acute trauma, such as a direct blow to the area, for example when trochanteric bursitis develops as a result of a fall on the greater trochanter. Chronic trauma may be causative, as is seen with overuse syndromes such as olecranon bursitis, which results from leaning on the elbow for extended time periods. Septic bursitis may occur secondary to the entry of bacteria from a puncture wound or fissuring of the bursal sac, such as may occur with other disease processes such as RA, gout, tuberculosis and syphilis. The bursal fluid may be aspirated and cultured to determine if infection is present.

Clinical characteristics may include joint distension (effusion), pain, redness, increased temperature and loss of function at the involved joint. Pain is usually worsened by activity at the involved joint and relieved by rest; however, pain may continue to be present at rest but with a lesser severity. The pain is typically described as a deep aching discomfort. Both active range of motion (AROM) and passive range of motion (PROM) are usually normal, with increased pain at the end of the range in the direction of stress to the bursa (e.g. elbow flexion with olecranon bursitis). Range of motion may be limited because of pain if the condition is very acute or the bursa becomes pinched during the movement, as with shoulder flexion or abduction causing the subacromial bursa to be pinched under the acromion process. Resistive testing is usually negative as the bursa is a noncontractile tissue, but discomfort may be caused from the contraction of neighboring muscles encroaching on the swollen bursa. Palpation directly over the area is typically painful.

Therapeutic interventions for acute bursitis include protecting and resting the area, icing, antiinflammatory medications, iontophoresis and phonophoresis. Relieving the cause of the bursitis by altering postures or modifying environmental factors is helpful. An example is padding wheelchair armrests or wearing protective elbow pads to reduce trauma to the olecranon bursa. Another example is discontinuing work performed overhead, a position that may further aggravate an inflamed subdeltoid bursa. Oral NSAIAs or local corticosteroid injections may be beneficial in reducing the inflammation and pain. As the acute inflammation subsides, pain-free AROM is encouraged to help to increase metabolism in the area and decrease swelling. In cases of chronic bursitis, determining the cause of the problem becomes the most important factor in successful treatment. A patient with chronic trochanteric bursitis may benefit from stretching of a tight iliotibial band. Surgical intervention is uncommon and depends on the extent of the disease process. Surgery usually has the goal of creating more area for structures to move, such as an acromioplasty or removal of osteophytes from the undersurface of the acromion process and acromioclavicular joint.

TENDONITIS

Tendonitis is defined as inflammation of a tendon; tenosynovitis is defined as inflammation of a tendon and tendon sheath. The tendon may become inflamed in many areas, as a result of several mechanisms. Inflammation may occur within the tendon itself, at the area where the tendon fuses with the muscle (musculotendinous junction) or where the tendon attaches to bone (tenoperiostial junction). Determining the exact location of the lesion is extremely important, as successful treatment needs to be directed at the exact lesion site. Tenosynovitis may occur from overuse, unaccustomed activity or puncture wounds. In the absence of a precipitating trauma, the presence of tenosynovitis may indicate a systemic inflammatory process.

A common cause of tendonitis is anatomical or biomechanical constraint to the tendon, such as supraspinatus tendon impingement by the coracoacromial arch. Other common mechanisms include microtrauma because of repeated overload, such as the flexor tendons of the hand undergoing repeated contractions in a keyboard operator, and macrotrauma to a tendon. Calcific tendonitis occurs when calcium deposits form in the tendon, resulting in decreased blood supply to the tendon. Commonly affected tendons are the Achilles, rotator cuff, bicipital, patellar, posterior tibial and the common extensor group of the wrist. In the geriatric population, pain from Achilles or posterior tibial tendonitis must be differentiated from pain of vascular origin, such as thrombosis or thrombophlebitis. Calf deep vein thrombosis may be identified by the clinical Homan's sign test or by Doppler ultrasonography.

Clinical characteristics of tendonitis include pain, edema, redness, increased temperature and loss of function at the involved joint. Symptoms are typically worsened by use of the involved tendon, especially with eccentric loading of the tendon, for example when going downstairs with patellar tendonitis. Use of the tendon in a range of motion in which it is likely to be impinged (painful arc) will also reproduce the patient's pain. An example is the painful arc produced by overhead abduction with supraspinatus tendonitis. Although commonly relieved by rest, if acute, pain may be present even at rest. Active motion may be painful with muscle contraction of associated tendons. Passive motion may be painful, especially that resulting in full elongation of the tendon such as full shoulder extension, elbow extension and pronation with bicipital tendonitis. Resistive testing is the key clinical diagnostic test with the tendon being strong and painful upon resistance. Palpation directly over the tendon is typically painful. In the case of a partial tear of the tendon, the resisted motion will characteristically present as weak and painful.

Typical therapeutic interventions for acute tendonitis include protection and rest of the area and the use of ice and antiinflammatory medications. Also essential is the relief of any possible causes of the tendonitis by altering or modifying work and/or environmental factors that may be contributing to the problem, such as an office worker with extensor carpi ulnaris tendonitis who may further aggravate the condition by continuing to type. Corticosteroid injections into the tendon or tendon sheath may be beneficial in acute cases but are not indicated for chronic lesions (Speed 2001).

As the acute inflammation subsides, pain-free active motion is encouraged to help provide nutrition to the area and decrease swelling. In cases of chronic tendonitis, determining the cause of the problem becomes the most important factor in successful treatment. If a patient has a chronic supraspinatus tendonitis, the cause, for example weak shoulder external rotators or a bone spur on the inferior side of the acromion, needs to be identified. Chronic tendonitis is usually the result of poor blood flow to the injured area combined with a continued stress that does not allow for adequate maturation of the healing tissue. Transverse friction massage may be used in chronic tendonitis to increase the mobility of the scar and stimulate healing of the scar tissue with normal fiber alignment. Surgical intervention is only performed when conservative measures have not improved the condition. These procedures usually have the goal of creating more area for structures to move, such as an acromioplasty or removal of osteophytes from the undersurface of the acromion process and acromioclavicular joint in impingement syndrome.

CONCLUSION

Considering the increasing prevalence of rheumatic conditions, especially in the aging population, therapists should be aware of the signs and symptoms, current research, medical management and therapeutic interventions. It is important to note that there are more than 100 types of arthritis and many people live with chronic joint symptoms but have not yet been diagnosed with a disease. The clinician should engage in prevention and self-management education, make appropriate referrals to other healthcare providers and advocate for access to advances in medical care, surgery and physical rehabilitation.

References

Braun CA, Anderson CM 2007 Pathophysiology: Functional Alterations in Human Health. Lippincott Williams & Wilkins, Philadelphia, PA, p 56

Buckwalter JA, Mankin HJ 1998 Articular cartilage repair and transplantation. Arthritis Rheum 41(8):1331–1342

Choi HK, Atkinson K, Karlson EW et al 2005 Obesity, weight change, hypertension, diuretic use, and risk of gout in men: the health professionals follow-up study. Arch Intern Med 165(7):742–748

Hannan MT 2001 Epidemiology of rheumatic diseases. In: Robbins L (ed) Clinical Care in the Rheumatic Diseases, 2nd edn. American College of Rheumatology, Atlanta, GA, p 9

Hochberg MC 1997 Updating the American College of Rheumatology revised criteria for the classification of systemic lupus erythematosus. Arthritis Rheum 40(9):1725

Kennedy-Malone LM, Enevold GL 2001 Assessment and management of polymyalgia rheumatica in older adults. Geriatr Nurs 22(3):152–155

Klippel JH 2001 Primer on the Rheumatic Diseases, 12th edn. Arthritis Foundation, Atlanta, GA, p 209–287

Lidgren L 2003 Editorial. Bull WHO 81(9):629

National Health Interview Survey and US Census Bureau 2002. Available: http://www.cdc.gov/arthritis/data_statistics/national_data_nhis.htm#future

Nir-Paz R, Gross A, Chajek-Shaul T 2002 Sex differences in giant cell arteritis. J Rheumatol 29(6):1219–1223

Ottawa Panel 2004a Evidence-based clinical practice guidelines for therapeutic exercises in the management of rheumatoid arthritis in adults. Phys Ther 84(10):934–972

Ottawa Panel 2004b Evidence-based clinical practice guidelines for electrotherapy and thermotherapy interventions in management of rheumatoid arthritis in adults. Phys Ther 84(11):1016–1043

Ottawa Panel 2005 Evidence-based clinical practice guidelines for therapeutic exercises and manual therapy in the management of osteoarthritis. Phys Ther 85(9):907–971

Ramesh K 2003 Polymyalgia rheumatica and temporal arteritis. In: Koopman WJ, Boulware DW, Heudebert GR (eds) Clinical Primer of Rheumatology. Lippincott Williams & Wilkins, Philadelphia, PA, p 206

Robbins L 2001 Clinical Care in the Rheumatic Diseases. American College of Rheumatology, Atlanta, GA, p 97–98, 131

Speed CA 2001 Fortnightly review: corticosteroid injections in tendon lesions. Br Med J 323:382–386

Walker JM, Helewa A 2004 Physical Rehabilitation in Arthritis, 2nd edn. Saunders, St Louis, MO, p 67

Ward MM, Pyun E, Studenski S 1995 Long-term survival in systemic lupus erythematosus: patient characteristics associated with poorer outcome. Arthritis Rheum 38:274–283

www.bonejointdecade.org

Chapter 21

The shoulder

Edmund M. Kosmahl

INTRODUCTION

Shoulder pain and dysfunction are common complaints for elderly individuals. The prevalence of impairments of the shoulder increases steadily with age, affecting about 20% of those aged 70 years and older (Makela et al 1999, Vogt et al 2003). Shoulder disorders in the elderly can lead to significant disability. Functional limitation is correlated with shoulder impairment, especially loss of range of motion (ROM) (Chakravarty & Webley 1993). Important activities such as feeding, dressing and personal hygiene can be compromised. Impairment combined with intermittent or constant pain can diminish the quality of life.

Because shoulder impairment and pain can produce functional limitation, tests and measures of pain, impairment and functional limitation should always be incorporated into the examination and evaluation of the aging shoulder. Visual analogue scales have been shown to be valid and reliable measures of pain (Bergh et al 2000). The Shoulder Pain and Disability Index (Roach et al 1991) and the simple Shoulder Test (Beaton & Richards 1996) are measures of shoulder function for which validity and reliability have been established. Other shoulder function measures are available, and they will be discussed later in this chapter. The purpose of this chapter is to review rehabilitation concepts for the following shoulder problems that may affect the elderly: (i) degenerative rotator cuff; (ii) fracture of the proximal humerus; (iii) shoulder arthroplasty; and (iv) shoulder pain with hemiplegia.

DEGENERATIVE ROTATOR CUFF

Rotator cuff pathology is the most common affliction of the shoulder (Akpinar et al 2003). The rotator cuff is composed of the musculotendinous insertions of the supraspinatus, infraspinatus, teres minor and subscapularis muscles. These structures are important for nearly all shoulder functions, especially activities that require overhead arm function.

Advancing age is correlated with pathology of the rotator cuff (Feng et al 2003). A lifetime of activity can lead to degeneration of the rotator cuff in association with osteoarthritis of the glenohumeral and acromioclavicular joints. Degeneration can cause partial or full thickness tears in the cuff.

Degeneration of the rotator cuff can be associated with subacromial impingement syndrome. It is important to evaluate the postures of the thoracic spine and scapulae when evaluating the patient with degenerative rotator cuff disease. Subacromial impingement can be induced by excessive thoracic kyphosis and protracted scapulae. These postural misalignments place the glenoid and acromion in a downward and forward position, which encourages subacromial impingement when the arm is elevated (Fig. 21.1). When these postural malalignments are present, interventions should include exercises aimed at establishing a more upright postural alignment. Exercises for degenerative rotator cuff should be designed to avoid worsening a subacute inflammatory process. The therapist should incorporate exercises to avoid positions that cause subacromial

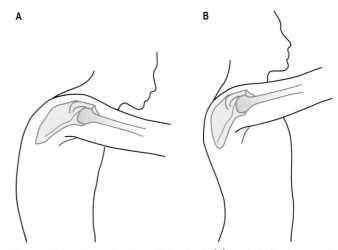

Figure 21.1 Excessive thoracic kyphosis (A) leads to impingement in the subacromial space during elevation of the arm. Upright posture (B) allows arm elevation without impingement.

impingement and pain. Table 21.1 summarizes rehabilitation interventions for degenerative rotator cuff without tear.

When tear of the degenerative rotator cuff is present, the history and presentation are typical. The patient usually does not report trauma. A common scenario involves the sudden inability to raise the arm overhead during a functional activity. Pain may or may not be reported. Examination shows that the patient cannot hold the arm in the 90° abducted position (failure of the drop-arm test). Because of the poor condition of the degenerative tissues, operative repair for tears of the rotator cuff is rarely considered for older individuals. The metaphor of 'trying to anastomose cooked spaghetti' is sometimes helpful to conceptualize the rationale for nonoperative management of degenerative rotator cuff tear.

The success of nonoperative management of rotator cuff tear is associated with the initial amount of ROM and strength (Itoi & Tabata 1992). For this reason, it is unreasonable to expect full functional return for the degenerative rotator cuff tear patient who cannot actively raise the arm above the head at initial evaluation. Management should be aimed at decreasing inflammation and pain (when present), maintaining full passive ROM and maximizing strength and functional ability. The interventions summarized in Table 21.1 are appropriate for the

patient with degenerative rotator cuff tear. Because the restoration of full active overhead mobility is unlikely, assisted ROM exercises must often be continued indefinitely. This is important to prevent additional pathology such as adhesive capsulitis.

FRACTURE OF THE PROXIMAL HUMERUS

Nondisplaced fracture of the proximal humerus is a common injury in older individuals. A fall on the outstretched arm is often the mechanism of injury. These fractures are sometimes labeled as pathological; this is because generalized osteoporosis has weakened the bone enough that relatively minor trauma is sufficient to cause a fracture (McKinnis 1997). Metastatic bone disease can also lead to pathological fracture.

Nondisplaced or minimally displaced fractures account for approximately 85% of fractures of the proximal humerus (Skinner et al 1995). There is generally no need for operative fixation of these fractures. Management involves a period of sling immobilization followed by early ROM exercises. The sling continues to be worn when not exercising. There is no clear consensus regarding the length of time for immobilization before the initiation of exercise. Initial formation of bone callus takes about 3 weeks, and some recommend that movement should be avoided during this period to stabilize the fracture fragments (Malone et al 1995). Others suggest that exercises should begin within 7–14 days of injury (Basti et al 1994, Koval et al 1997). One should expect loss of function of the joint capsule and muscles about the shoulder during the period of immobilization. This is primarily a function of the development of fibrous adhesions in response to bleeding in the capsule.

When callous formation allows, active–assistive motion exercise should begin. It is unwise to apply passive stretching until there is radiographic evidence of fracture union (usually about 6 weeks). External resistance exercises should also be avoided during this period. Isometric exercises may be considered from the time of injury, provided there is no risk of displacement of the fracture fragments by muscular contraction. This is a concern whenever the fracture involves the greater or lesser tuberosities. Submaximal isometric exercise may be appropriate to encourage muscle contractility without risking displacement of fracture fragments. An outline of general exercise interventions for nonoperative proximal humeral fractures appears in Table 21.2.

About 15% of fractures of the proximal humerus involve displacement of fragments by more than 1 cm, or angulation of fragments by more than 45°. The four important fracture fragments are: (i) humeral head; (ii) greater tuberosity; (iii) lesser tuberosity; and (iv) humeral

---

Table 21.1 Interventions for degenerative rotator cuff

Problem	Intervention
Pain and inflammation	Rest, modalities (ice, heat, ultrasound, electrical stimulation)
Excessive thoracic kyphosis	Thoracic spinal extension exercises
Protracted scapulae	Scapular retraction exercises
Maintain or improve ROM	Passive and assisted ROM exercises (assistance from noninvolved upper extremity, overhead pulley, wand)
Maintain or improve strength	Isometrics, side-lying isotonics for internal and external rotators, assisted eccentric lowering of arm from overhead
Maximize function	Gradual introduction: touch top of head, back of neck, low back. Adapt activities of daily living to functional capabilities

---

Table 21.2 Exercise interventions for proximal humeral fracture (nonoperative)

Problem	Exercise	Timeline
Maintain or improve ROM	Assisted ROM (wand, wall climbing, pendulum) Passive ROM, stretching (overhead pulley)	7–14 days or radiographic evidence of callus (usually 3 weeks) Radiographic evidence of union, usually 6 weeks
Maintain or improve strength	Submaximal isometrics Full active ROM against gravity External resistance isotonics	Usually immediately; no risk of fragment displacement Radiographic evidence of union, usually 6 weeks Ability to perform full active ROM against gravity; radiographic evidence of union, usually 6 weeks
Maximize function	Touch top of head, back of neck, low back	Assisted: radiographic evidence of callus, usually 3 weeks. Unassisted: radiographic evidence of union, usually 6 weeks

shaft. These fractures usually require operative reduction and internal fixation (ORIF) to allow fracture healing and return of function. More serious fractures can interrupt the blood supply to the humeral head. This interruption can lead to necrosis, which may require hemiarthroplasty.

Rehabilitation following ORIF varies depending on the classification of the injury and stability of fixation. Close communication with the surgeon can facilitate proper progression of the rehabilitation program without risking a delay in healing or reinjury. Some older patients may not be candidates for ORIF because they cannot reasonably be expected to tolerate (or survive) anesthesia. In other cases, osteoporosis may reduce bone stock to the point at which hardware fixation cannot be achieved. Complete restoration of function may be an unrealistic goal for these patients. Still, every attempt should be made to maximize functional outcomes (e.g. dressing and grooming).

In 1970, Neer described five categories for classification of proximal humeral fractures. Category I involves one part and is non or minimally displaced. Category II is a two part fracture with one part displaced more than 1 cm or angulated greater than 45°. A category III is a three-part fracture involving two parts displaced and/or angulated from each other and from the remaining part. A category IV fracture is described as four parts displaced and/or angulated from each other. A category V is a fracture dislocation with displacement of the humeral head from joint space with fracture.

SHOULDER ARTHROPLASTY

Arthroplasty at the shoulder can be categorized as hemiarthroplasty or total shoulder arthroplasty (TSA). Hemiarthroplasty replaces only the humeral head, whereas total shoulder arthroplasty replaces both the humeral head and the scapular glenoid surface. Hemiarthroplasty is often the procedure of choice for older individuals who have suffered three- or four-part fractures, especially if there has been substantial damage to the articular surface of the humerus or when there is substantial osteoporosis (Hartsock et al 1998). The primary indication for TSA is severe, chronic and progressive pain related to osteoarthritis of the glenohumeral joint (Fenlin & Frieman 1998). Hemiarthroplasty is favored over TSA when rotator cuff deficiency coexists with arthritis (Smith & Matsen 1998). Approximately 85% of TSA surgery is performed for patients with osteoarthritis or rheumatoid arthritis, with secondary arthritis accounting for the remaining 15% of TSA surgeries (Cuomo & Checroun 1998). TSA can be further subdivided into nonconstrained, constrained and semi- or partially constrained. Stability of the nonconstrained TSA relies on several factors, including surgical reconstruction of the soft tissues surrounding the joint and anatomical alignment and fit of the components. Today, nonconstrained is the most common type of TSA. Semiconstrained TSA uses the architecture of the device (usually a 'hooded' glenoid component) to minimize instability in one direction (i.e. superior migration of the humeral component). The glenoid component of a constrained TSA completely engulfs the humeral head component in a 'ball and socket' arrangement so that unwanted motion is controlled by the components. This type of TSA is rarely used today. Modern humeral arthroplasty components are often modular, which means that different balls can be sized to different stems. Modularity is thought to promote optimal anatomical sizing and fit. Humeral and glenoid components may or may not be cemented in place.

It can be appreciated from the preceding discussion that there are a myriad of surgical variables that may influence the course of postoperative rehabilitation. It is imperative that the therapist communicate carefully with the surgeon to ensure an adequate understanding of the particulars of each patient's case. Realizing a successful functional outcome following shoulder arthroplasty requires a well-coordinated and consistent effort by patient, surgeon and therapist (Brown & Friedman 1998). Often, the patient may consider the outcome successful if pain has been reduced enough to allow an uninterrupted night of sleep. Significant functional loss preoperatively, especially that related to coexisting degenerative rotator cuff disease, may necessarily limit expectations for functional outcomes (Iannotti & Williams 1995). Expected outcomes for ROM have been reported by Brown and Friedman (1998) (see Table 21.3). At a minimum, pain-free performances of feeding, dressing and personal hygiene activities are desirable. Failure rates for this procedure range from 9.6% to 25% (Wirth & Rochwood 1994). Because of the relatively high potential for complications, the rehabilitation program should be carefully designed to advance the patient through progressive stages of tissue healing, joint mobilization and muscle strengthening (Brems 1994). The focus of the rehabilitation program should be on ROM and strengthening exercises, and the restoration of functional capabilities. Thermal, electrical and acoustical modalities should play an adjunctive role only.

Ideally, the therapist should meet with the patient and primary caregivers preoperatively. Impairments of ROM and strength and functional disability should be measured and documented. Several systems have been developed for the assessment of pain, disability and dysfunction (Kuhn & Blasier 1998). Validity and reliability have been established for some of these systems. One system, the American Shoulder and Elbow Surgeons Standardized Shoulder Assessment and Shoulder Score Index, includes subjective (patient self-evaluation) and objective (measurement of impairments) components. A numerical score (maximum 100 points) can be derived from this assessment.

The results of the preoperative evaluation, along with postoperative exercises, precautions and activities should be demonstrated and discussed with the patient and caregivers. The patient should understand that pain and stiffness are to be expected but that they will resolve with diligent performance of the postoperative program. The patient should begin practicing the exercise program immediately to promote ease of performance postoperatively. The therapist should discuss preoperative findings with the surgeon. This preoperative consultation provides the opportunity to establish specific interventions that may be required on a case-by-case basis.

The postoperative program can begin as early as the day of surgery when surgical anesthesia and postoperative analgesics may minimize pain and facilitate movement. It is unwise to delay initiation of the program longer than 48 h. Initially, the patient typically wears a sling when not exercising to protect the shoulder in a position of internal rotation, a few degrees of flexion and a few degrees of abduction. Pillows may be used to assist in maintaining this protected position and ice may be applied to minimize swelling and pain.

Table 21.3 Expected passive range of motion at 12 months after shoulder arthroplasty

Motion	Intact rotator cuff	Tissue-deficient
Elevation	160°	90°
External rotation	75°	30–40°
Internal rotation	80°	45–50°

After Brown DD & Friedman RJ 1998, with permission.

Table 21.4 Timeline for progression of postoperative rehabilitation program

Phase	Exercise examples
Protective (weeks 0–4)	Passive and assisted shoulder elevation, external rotation; pendulum; active elbow, wrist and hand movements
Early strengthening (weeks 4–6)	Isometric shoulder movements; stretch shoulder internal rotation; scapular strengthening; resisted elbow, wrist and hand movements
Moderate strengthening (weeks 6–10)	Active shoulder elevation; resisted shoulder internal and external rotation
Maximal strengthening (week 12 to 6 months)	Resisted shoulder movements; functional specificity

After Brown DD & Friedman RJ 1998, with permission.

Brown and Friedman (1998) have suggested a timeline strategy for the postoperative rehabilitation program (see Table 21.4). Timeline strategies use known principles of soft-tissue healing to direct progression of the rehabilitation program. The patient's ability to attain functional milestones should also be incorporated in the decision-making process regarding progression of the rehabilitation program. Considering the patient's ability to attain functional milestones while respecting soft-tissue healing principles can ensure a customized and safe postoperative rehabilitation program.

Initial postoperative intervention begins with three or four assisted ROM exercise sessions per day. These sessions should be short (about 5 min) and can be preceded by the application of modalities or analgesics. Assisted ROM exercises should include: pendulum, supine elevation, supine external rotation with wand for assistance, overhead pulley elevation and supine abduction with external rotation (hands clasped behind neck). Exercises should be designed so that the patient can assist with the unaffected upper extremity. Gentle passive motion can be applied by the therapist to ensure attainment of maximum available ROM. Each exercise should be held in the position of maximum available ROM for 15 seconds, and should be repeated three or four times.

If all has gone well, ROM should improve to about 120° elevation and 40° external rotation by the time sutures are removed (10–14 days postoperatively). Exercise frequency may be decreased to twice daily, and duration of exercise can be increased to 10 minutes. Each exercise should be held in the position of maximum available ROM for 30 seconds and should be repeated three or four times. An assisted internal rotation ROM exercise (hands behind back, uninvolved hand pulls involved hand up the back) can be added to the program; the assisted external rotation exercise can be progressed so the patient stands and uses a doorway for assistance; and the assisted elevation exercise can be advanced to the standing position using a wand or the doorway for assistance. Active strengthening exercises should be initiated at this time (see below).

Once the elevation range reaches 160° and the external rotation range reaches 60° (usually within 3–6 weeks postoperatively), elevation, external rotation and internal rotation stretching exercises should increase in vigor. Stretching into the direction of horizontal adduction should be added. All exercises should be held in the position of maximal available stretch for 60 seconds and repeated two or

three times. Elevation, external and internal rotation, and horizontal adduction stretching exercises should be continued indefinitely.

Active strengthening exercises should normally be initiated 10–14 days after surgery. The strengthening exercise program should consist of 10 repetitions of each exercise, twice daily. Depending on the initial level of strength, easier exercises may be unnecessary. In the case of associated rotator cuff repair, the surgeon should be consulted before beginning gravity-resisted exercises.

Supine elevation is initiated as follows: (i) the patient should lie supine with the arm at the side and the elbow flexed to 90°; (ii) the patient reaches for the ceiling by flexing the shoulder and simultaneously extending the elbow; if this cannot be accomplished actively, the patient assists with the uninvolved upper extremity; (iii) the patient lowers the elbow toward the supporting surface causing an eccentric contraction of the shoulder flexors as the elbow simultaneously flexes; there should be no assistance for this eccentric exercise. Once the patient can do 10 unassisted repetitions both concentrically and eccentrically, a 0.5-lb weight should be added to the wrist or hand. When the patient can do 10 repetitions, the weight should be increased in 0.5-lb increments until 5 lbs (2.3 kg) can be lifted 10 times.

When 10 repetitions of supine elevation can be completed with a 5-lb weight, upright eccentric elevation is begun: (i) the patient should sit in a sturdy chair and use the uninvolved upper extremity to elevate the operative extremity as far above the head as possible; (ii) the patient should balance the arm above the head without assistance, then *slowly* lower the arm while simultaneously flexing the elbow. When this can be completed 10 times, a 0.5-lb weight should be added to the hand or wrist. The weight should be increased in 0.5-lb increments each time 10 repetitions can be completed until the patient can do 10 repetitions with 5 lbs.

When the patient can complete 10 repetitions of the upright eccentric elevation exercise using 5 lbs of resistance, exercises using elastic tubing should be instituted. Exercises for shoulder flexion, extension, abduction, and internal and external rotation should be used. These are best done with the patient sitting in a sturdy chair. Flexion, extension and rotation exercises are accomplished by looping the tubing around a nearby doorknob and positioning the patient appropriately. The abduction exercise is done by holding the tubing in both hands and stretching the operative arm away from the uninvolved arm. The patient should pull the tubing as far as possible, hold for 5 seconds and then slowly return to the starting position. The patient should do 10 repetitions twice daily. These exercises should be continued indefinitely. Some patients may also require strengthening exercises aimed specifically at improving function of the scapulothoracic musculature.

Arthroplasty patients may exhibit excessive thoracic kyphosis and protracted scapulae (see Fig. 21.1). These postural misalignments put the glenoid fossa in a downward and forward position, which can complicate the postoperative restoration of shoulder elevation ROM. For these patients, the exercise program should include spinal extension and scapular retraction exercises. These exercises are accomplished most easily in the sitting position. The exercise program should also include exercises to maintain or improve the ROM and strength of elbow, wrist and hand.

SHOULDER PAIN WITH HEMIPLEGIA

In the preface to his 1980 book, Cailliet stated that, 'The hemiplegic patient can improve his ambulation, communication, balance, and self-care through treatment, but in the overall picture of functional return, the shoulder remains an enigma' (Cailliet 1980). Unfortunately, the intervening years have added little in the way of understanding the

Table 21.5 Factors associated with shoulder pain in hemiplegia

Factor	Statistically significant
Prolonged hospital stay[a]	+
Poor return of function[a]	+
Glenohumeral subluxation[a]	+
Complex regional pain syndrome[a]	+
Capsulitis	−
Rotator cuff degeneration and tears	−
Tendonitis	−
Bursitis	−
Spasticity	−
Flaccidity	−
Loss of external rotation ROM[a,b]	+
Severity of CVA	−
Time since onset of hemiplegia[b]	+

+ , yes; −, no.
[a]From Roy et al 1994.
[b]From Bohannon et al 1986.

causes and effective interventions for the patient with shoulder pain and hemiplegia. The purpose of this section is to review the incidence, suspected causes and reported interventions for shoulder pain with hemiplegia.

Van Ouwenaller et al (1986) stated that, 'Shoulder pain is probably the most frequent complication of hemiplegia'. In spite of this statement, the incidence of this problem has been reported to vary from 5% to 84% (Turner-Stokes & Jackson 2002, Ratnasabapathy et al 2003). Operational definitions used for patient selection may account for these differences. For example, 'pain', 'tenderness', 'mild shoulder discomfort' and 'adhesive capsulitis' are all terms that have been used to identify patients with hemiplegia and shoulder pain. Perhaps the definitive frequency study was conducted by Van Ouwenaller and colleagues (1986). They followed 219 patients with cerebrovascular accident (CVA) for 1 year and found that 72% of patients had at least one incidence of shoulder pain during the recovery period. This figure agrees exactly with later reports by Roy et al (1994) and Bohannon et al (1986). Roy and colleagues followed 76 patients for a period of 12 weeks after the onset of CVA. They found the greatest incidence of shoulder pain (24% at rest and 58% with movement) at 10 weeks post-onset. The smallest incidence (12% at rest and 35% with movement) occurred during the first week post-onset.

The causes of shoulder pain with hemiplegia are poorly understood. A combination of factors may be at fault (Gilmore et al 2004). Some associated factors are listed in Table 21.5; unfortunately, there is little empirical evidence to support or refute causality for any of these factors. Still, it appears that there is a statistically significant relationship between shoulder pain with hemiplegia and the following associated factors: loss of external rotation ROM (Bohannon 1986, Roy et al 1994), time since onset of hemiplegia (Bohannon 1986), prolonged hospital stay (Roy et al 1994), poor return of function (Roy et al 1994), glenohumeral subluxation (Roy et al 1994) and complex regional pain syndrome (Roy et al 1994). It is important to note that 'a statistically significant relationship' does not imply causality. Whether therapeutic interventions aimed at decreasing

these suggested causes will reduce the incidence of shoulder pain with hemiplegia remains to be proven.

In the absence of a clear understanding of the causes of shoulder pain with hemiplegia, intervention should be directed by clinical observations. Evaluation and reevaluation of signs, symptoms and responses to interventions must continually be used to reformulate the intervention plan. Patients should be evaluated for signs of musculoskeletal problems (capsulitis, rotator cuff degeneration and tears, tendonitis, bursitis, etc). Interventions for such problems should be similar to intervention regimens in patients without hemiplegia who exhibit musculoskeletal shoulder problems. Preventing the loss of external rotation ROM as a result of capsulitis appears to be a particularly important therapeutic goal. The intelligent use of exercise and modalities should have a beneficial effect on musculoskeletal causes of shoulder pain with hemiplegia.

Glenohumeral subluxation as an etiology for shoulder pain with hemiplegia is a multidimensional problem. Theoretically, inferior subluxation places abnormal stresses on periarticular structures and leads to pain. The tension created by inferior subluxation can lead to ischemia, which is thought to cause inflammation and pain. One approach suggests the use of various types of slings to reduce the glenohumeral subluxation. Although a sling can accomplish reduction, it may also delay the return of voluntary muscular control. Because flaccidity is also a suspected cause of shoulder pain with hemiplegia, the anticipated gains afforded by reduction of the subluxation may be derailed by a delay in return of voluntary muscular control. Some slings are designed to reduce the subluxation while simultaneously allowing functional use of the extremity. These are preferable to slings that prevent voluntary use.

Another approach to the glenohumeral subluxation problem focuses on return of voluntary muscular control. The muscles that upwardly rotate the scapula (trapezius and serratus anterior) and elevate the humeral head (supraspinatus and deltoid) are the targets of this approach. The scapular muscles are important for maintaining a vertical position of the glenoid fossa. The humeral elevators can maintain the humeral head in the glenoid fossa as long as the fossa is not rotated downwards. The requisite synergy between these muscle groups dictates that if any of these muscles is dysfunctional (flaccid or spastic), subluxation is likely to occur. Therapeutic interventions for this problem include exercise, electromyographic biofeedback and functional electrical stimulation. Interventions should be designed to restore normal voluntary control of these muscles. Renzenbrink and Ijzerman (2004) have shown that percutaneous electrical stimulation can produce statistically significant improvements in pain, subluxation, pain-free range of external rotation and Fugl-Myer motor test scores at 18 weeks postintervention. They used indwelling electrodes in the supraspinatus, upper trapezius and posterior and middle deltoid to deliver biphasic balanced pulses (20 mA, 12 Hz, 10–200 μs, 10 s on/10 s off), 6 h daily for 6 weeks. By contrast, Yelnik and colleagues (2003) demonstrated the effectiveness of botulinum toxin injection in spastic subscapular muscles to reduce shoulder pain and increase ROM. The success of these apparently dichotomous approaches underscores the need to carefully evaluate the signs and symptoms for each person as recovery progresses. Clearly, patients with flaccid paralysis must be cared for differently compared with patients with spastic paralysis.

Another issue to consider is that of poor positioning and handling of the affected upper extremity. Although not established empirically, many feel that poor handling produces trauma and causes pain. This is thought to be more of a problem for patients with flaccid paralysis. Until proven otherwise, prudence dictates that caregivers should use the utmost care when positioning and handling the affected upper extremity. The affected upper extremity should be positioned so that the scapula is protracted, the glenohumeral joint slightly flexed and abducted, and wrist and fingers slightly extended (Turner-Stokes & Jackson 2002). Pillows, lapboards and slings may be incorporated into positioning interventions. Caregivers should not use the patient's affected upper extremity when assisting in transfer or ambulation. The rapid restoration of voluntary motor control should be high on the list of therapeutic goals for the patient with flaccid paralysis.

Shoulder pain with hemiplegia is poorly understood. Possible interventions are variable because of the lack of understanding of causes. Patients with hemiplegia and shoulder pain should be evaluated for the presence of all of the suspected possible causes. Intervention should be directed at reducing possible causes that can be identified on a case-by-case basis.

References

Akpinar S, Ozkoc G, Cesur N 2003 Anatomy, biomechanics, and physiopathology of the rotator cuff. Acta Orthop Traumatol Turc 37(suppl1):4–12

Basti JJ, Dionysian E, Sherman PW, Bigliani LU 1994 Management of proximal humeral fractures. J Hand Ther 7:111–121

Beaton DE, Richards RR 1996 Measuring function of the shoulder. A cross-sectional comparison of five questionnaires. J Bone Joint Surg Am 78(6):882–890

Bergh I, Sjostrom B, Oden A, Steen B 2000 An application of pain rating scales in geriatric patients. Aging (Milano) 12(5):380–387

Bohannon RW, Larkin PA, Smith MB et al 1986 Shoulder pain in hemiplegia: statistical relationship with five variables. Arch Phys Med Rehabil 67(8):514–516

Brems JJ 1994 Rehabilitation following total shoulder arthroplasty. Clin Orthop 307:70–85

Brown DD, Friedman RJ 1998 Postoperative rehabilitation following total shoulder arthroplasty. Orthop Clin North Am 29(3):535–547

Cailliet R 1980 The Shoulder in Hemiplegia. FA Davis, Philadelphia, PA

Chakravarty K, Webley M 1993 Shoulder joint movement and its relationship to disability in the elderly. J Rheumatol 20(8):1359–1361

Cuomo F, Checroun A 1998 Avoiding pitfalls and complications in total shoulder arthroplasty. Orthop Clin North Am 29(3):507–518

Feng S, Guo S, Nobuhara K et al 2003 Prognostic indicators for outcome following rotator cuff tear repair. J Orthop Surg 11(2):110–116

Fenlin JM, Frieman BG 1998 Indications, technique and results of total shoulder arthroplasty in osteoarthritis. Orthop Clin North Am 29(3):423–434

Gilmore PE, Spaulding SJ, Vandervoort AA 2004 Hemiplegic shoulder pain: implications for occupational therapy treatment. Can J Occup Ther 71(1):36–46

Hartsock LA, Estes WJ, Murray CA, Friedman RJ 1998 Shoulder hemiarthroplasty for proximal humeral fractures. Orthop Clin North Am 29(3):467–475

Iannotti JP, Williams GR 1995 Diagnostic tests and surgical techniques. In: Kelley MJ, Clark WA (eds) Orthopedic Therapy of the Shoulder. JB Lippincott, Philadelphia, PA, p 185

Itoi T, Tabata S 1992 Conservative treatment of rotator cuff tears. Clin Orthop 275:165–173

Koval KJ, Gallagher MA, Marsicano JG et al 1997 Functional outcome after minimally displaced fractures of the proximal part of the humerus. J Bone Joint Surg Am 79(2):203–207

Kuhn JE, Blasier R 1998 Assessment of outcomes in shoulder arthroplasty. Orthop Clin North Am 29(3):549–563

Makela M, Heliovaara M, Sainio P et al 1999 Shoulder joint impairment among Finns aged 30 years or over: prevalence, risk factor and co-morbidity. Rheumatology 38:656–662

Malone TR, Waser-Richmond G, Frick JL 1995 Shoulder pathology. In: Kelley MJ, Clark WA (eds) Orthopedic Therapy of the Shoulder. JB Lippincott, Philadelphia, PA, p 104

McKinnis L (ed.) 1997 The shoulder joint complex. In: Fundamentals of Orthopedic Radiology. FA Davis, Philadelphia, PA, p 325

Neer CS II 1970 Displaced proximal humeral fractures. I. Classification and evaluation. J Bone Joint Surg Am 52A:1077

Ratnasabapathy Y, Broad J, Baskett J et al 2003 Shoulder pain in people with a stroke: a population-based study. Clin Rehabil 17(3):304–311

Renzenbrink GJ, Ijzerman MJ 2004 Percutaneous neuromuscular electrical stimulation (P-NMES) for treating shoulder pain in chronic hemiplegia. Effects on shoulder pain and quality of life. Clin Rehabil 18(4):359–365

Roach KE, Budiman-Mak E, Songsiridej N, Lertratanajul Y 1991 Development of a shoulder pain and disability index. Arthritis Care Res 4(4):143–149

Roy CW, Sands MR, Hill LD 1994 Shoulder pain in acutely admitted hemiplegics. Clin Rehabil 8(4):334–340

Skinner HB, Diao E, Gosselin R et al 1995 Musculoskeletal trauma surgery. In: Skinner HB (ed.) Current Diagnosis and Treatment in Orthopedics. Appleton & Lange, East Norwalk, CT, p 51

Smith KL, Matsen FA III 1998 Total shoulder arthroplasty versus hemiarthroplasty: current trends. Orthop Clin North Am 29(3):491–506

Turner-Stokes L, Jackson D 2002 Shoulder pain after stroke: a review of the evidence base to inform the development of an integrated care pathway. Clin Rehabil 16:276–298

Van Ouwenaller C, Laplace PM, Chantraine A 1986 Painful shoulder in hemiplegia. Arch Phys Med Rehabil 67(1):23–26

Vogt M, Simonsick E, Harris T et al 2003 Neck and shoulder pain in 70- to 79-year-old men and women: findings from the Health, Aging and Body Composition Study. Spine J 3(6):435–441

Wirth MA, Rochwood CA 1994 Complications of shoulder arthroplasty. Clin Orthop 307:47–69

Yelnik AP, Colle FM, Bonan IV 2003 Treatment of pain and limited movement of the shoulder in hemiplegic patients with botulinum toxin a in the subscapular muscle. Eur Neurol 50(2):91–93

Chapter 22

Total hip arthroplasty

Mark A. Brimer

INTRODUCTION

The total hip arthroplasty (THA) is an orthopedic procedure that is performed more than 120 000 times annually in the US. International data indicate that 60–100 hip arthroplasty procedures (including replacement, partial replacement and revision procedures) per 100 000 inhabitants were carried out in the late 1990s (Merx et al 2003). The presence of severe and continuing pain and disability and the inability to perform one's job or participate in social and leisure activities generally make the decision to undergo surgery easier for the patient and surgeon.

INDICATIONS FOR THA

The primary indications for a total hip replacement are:

- severe osteoarthritis;
- rheumatoid arthritis;
- avascular necrosis;
- traumatic arthritis;
- hip fractures;
- benign and malignant bone tumors;
- arthritis associated with Paget's disease;
- ankylosing spondylitis;
- juvenile rheumatoid arthritis.

There are relatively few contraindications to the total hip arthroplasty procedure other than active local or systemic infection and other medical conditions (e.g. diabetes mellitus, peripheral vascular disease) that increase the risk of perioperative complications or death (Barrett et al 2005). Hemiarthroplasty, or partial reconstruction of the hip, is performed when the acetabular cartilage is intact and joint pathology is limited to the femoral side of the joint (Dalury 2005).

Previously, obesity had been considered a contraindication to surgery because of a reported high mechanical failure rate in heavier patients. The prospect of long-term reduction in pain and disability for heavier patients may, however, offset the risk associated with potential mechanical failure (Phillips et al 2003).

Data indicate that 62% of all THA procedures that are performed in the USA are in women, with two-thirds of these procedures performed in individuals older than 65 years of age. The highest age-specific rate of THA in men is between the ages of 65 and 74 years. For women, the highest age-specific rate is between 75 and 84 years.

If patients want to undergo bilateral hip replacement sequentially, it is recommended that they wait at least 6 weeks between operations to avoid the increased risk of complications from the presence of an occult venous thrombus from the first procedure. Otherwise, the bilateral procedure poses no increase in frequency of postoperative complications.

Historically, aseptic loosening of implanted components was identified as a major problem with THA. This problem was especially prevalent in younger and more active patients and in those who had undergone revision surgery. In the past two decades, however, the number of complications involving mechanical loosening has declined significantly, as a result of improved fixation techniques, to the point where more than 90% of the total number of joints are never revised.

SURGICAL APPROACHES FOR THA

The primary surgical approaches used for THA are the anterolateral and the posterior approaches. The choice of surgical approach often depends upon the surgical training of the physician. Many of the difficulties associated with using the anterolateral approach are related to the anterior third of the gluteus medius muscle, which partially obstructs the insertion of the stem of the component into the femur. This has become a more critical element with the introduction of cementless technology. The anterolateral approach does, however, provide excellent exposure of the acetabulum, which is why some surgeons prefer this approach.

Regardless of the approach taken, difficulties are occasionally encountered. When using the posterior approach, there is a tendency to place the femoral component in less than normal anteversion, thereby leading to less postoperative external rotation because of the presence of an intact anterior capsule. A patient who undergoes the anterolateral approach commonly demonstrates less internal rotation postoperatively and a weaker hip abductor, which is associated with surgical interference with the function of the abductor muscle.

Table 22.1 THA gait training and ROM guidelines

| | Arthroplasty | | | |
	Conventional (cemented THA)	Bipolar osteonics ingrowth	Porous coated	Trochanteric osteotomy[a]
Mobilize (out of bed)	Postoperative day (POD) 1–2	POD 2	POD 2	POD 2–5
Ambulation, weight–bearing	Partial weight-bearing (PWB) to weight-bearing as tolerated at discharge	(Porous coated stem, bipolar head) PWB 40–50 lbs	PWB 40–50 lbs	PWB
Range of motion of hip flexion	Same criteria for all: POD 2, up to 30° POD 4–6, up to 60° POD 6–10, up to 90°			
Precautions	Applies to all: avoid dislocation forces at hip, which are a combination of hip flexion, adduction and internal rotation; no hip flexion greater than 90°			
				No resisted abduction of hip; initially walk with a slightly abducted gait

From K Lawrence, orthopedic team supervisor of Physical Therapy Department, Medical College of Virginia, Richmond, VA, with permission.
[a]No active abduction.

Recently, there have been reports about the effectiveness of the minimally invasive approach to THA. This approach was designed to transect less muscle and tendon and, therefore, was expected to reduce the length of hospital stay, reduce pain levels, promote a quicker recovery and yield an improved cosmetic appearance (Berger 2004). Total blood loss utilizing the minimally invasive procedure has been determined to be less than that with conventional arthroplasty (Higuchi et al 2003). Preliminary studies indicate that the use of this procedure has not been found to increase the rate of postoperative dislocation (Siguier 2004).

The cement and noncement techniques

There are two surgical mechanisms available that can be used to properly secure the acetabular and femoral stem components. The cement technique adheres one or both of the replacement components to the surface of the bone with polymethylmethacrylate bone cement. The cementless technique relies upon bone growth into porous or onto roughened surfaces for fixation.

The choice of which component to use with a particular patient may be based upon the individual's level of strenuous physical activity, age, health and well-being and bone density. Surgical revision of both component types, as evaluated by the use of modern techniques, has been reported to be less than 5% for the cemented femoral component over a 10-year period, and approximately 2% for the uncemented acetabular component over a 7-year follow-up period.

Of primary concern in the cementless implants is the importance of the precise mechanism of load transfer to the bone. If the fit in the proximal femur is too loose and the distal end is too tight, then the proximal part of the component will be stress-shielded, which could cause increased porosity or bone loss. If the proximal segment fits well but the distal end underfills the medullary cavity, then the patient may exhibit distal toggling while under load, which causes persistent thigh pain.

REHABILITATION

Inpatient postoperative rehabilitation considerations

The primary concern following THA is to encourage the patient to begin to walk. Patients with uncomplicated THAs are generally encouraged to ambulate, beginning on the first day postoperatively (Wright 2004). Although ambulation may be brief in duration, the role of the therapist is to encourage mobility, self-care and proper weight-bearing and gait, and to teach the patient how to get into and out of bed in the proper manner [see Table 22.1 for gait training and range-of-motion (ROM) guidelines].

In the initial stages, most orthopedic surgeons recommend that the patient does not exceed 90° of hip flexion after surgery. It is important to instruct the patient to avoid internal rotation and adduction of the hip, especially if the posterior approach has been used. Any of these motions, singularly or in combination, may produce a dislocation of the replacement. The complication of hip dislocation is more likely to occur in a patient who presents with a neurological disorder or is mentally confused. A common mechanism to prevent dislocation is the use of an abduction pillow. As a general rule, abduction pillows are used for a 1-month period (Box 22.1).

The hospital rehabilitation department that is preparing the patient for home or a skilled-nursing placement should address the environment in which the patient will be placed. For example, a patient returning home should be thoroughly informed about the proper use of an elevated toilet seat, how to negotiate steps or stairs, and how to deal with carpeted surfaces and the surfaces encountered outside the home. It is particularly important that a patient understands the proper positions for sleeping and what types of chairs are considered too low for comfortable and safe seating. A patient who plans return visits to the physician in the office must be instructed on how to properly enter, sit in and exit from a car, to avoid excessive hip flexion.

Activities of daily living should be discussed with the patient and immediate caregivers. Because a large majority of THA procedures are performed in the geriatric population, special consideration should be given to visual, balance and endurance losses that may have occurred. A patient should be encouraged to use safe ambulation procedures until outpatient rehabilitation gait-training needs can be addressed (Jagmin 1998).

Outpatient and home–healthcare rehabilitation considerations

In the outpatient or home-healthcare environment, the focus is on restoring normal activities of daily living and safe walking techniques

Box 22.1   THA postoperative concerns

Therapists are advised to individualize these programs by adding or subtracting exercises depending on the patient's postoperative condition. Additional preoperative instructions to the patient may address the following immediate postoperative concerns:

1. Most THA procedures require the presence of an abduction pillow or wedge placed between the legs when the patient is in bed or in a wheelchair.
2. Patients are cautioned not to exceed 90° of flexion of the operative hip.
3. Passive or forcible movement of the hip that causes pain is contraindicated.
4. Internal rotation and adduction are contraindicated.
5. The patient is encouraged to perform active ankle exercises (rhythmic active dorsal and plantar flexion) frequently during the first few days postoperatively to prevent thrombophlebitis.
6. No weight-bearing or standing should take place unless under the direct supervision of the physical therapist.
7. Transfers and log-rolling should be performed away from the operative side, with the leg supported by a staff member.

From Echternach J 1990 Physical Therapy of the Hip. Churchill Livingstone, New York, with permission.

Box 22.2   Homecare instructions for THA patients

First 6 weeks postoperatively

Do not

- sit in low chairs or sofas
- cross your legs
- force your operated leg to flex (bend) or rotate at the hip
- sit down on the floor of a bath tub
- lean forward or raise your knee higher than your hip
- discard the walking assistive device until instructed to do so
- drive until permitted
- force hip abduction, external rotation or extension if your doctor has performed an anterolateral surgical approach

Do

- use help for putting on shoes and stockings
- use your compression stockings
- exercise as instructed
- sleep on your back
- place a pillow between your knees when sitting or sleeping
- use caution when sitting and reaching towards the floor or towards the phone/table on operative side. These motions encourage hip flexion and adduction, which are motions to be protected on the operative side
- use caution getting into and out of bed and on and off a toilet seat. Avoid hip adduction, internal rotation and flexion approach beyond 90° if your doctor has performed a posterolateral approach

(Box 22.2). In the initial stages (0–6 weeks), the patient should be advised to follow all dislocation precautions. These include the avoidance of excessive hip flexion and, in the case of the posterior approach, adduction and internal rotation. The patient should continue to use elevated chairs and toilet seats until cleared by the surgeon to do otherwise.

In the 6 weeks following surgery, rehabilitation should focus on hip abduction (presuming no contraindications exist) and mild hip flexor and extensor strengthening. The patient may progress to standing with full weight-bearing, as permitted by the surgeon. A patient who has undergone the cementless technique may be required to maintain limited weight-bearing until sufficient new bone growth can be seen by the physician on a radiograph. A falls risk assessment should be part of the continuous reexamination process during rehabilitation.

Desired rehabilitation outcomes for the THA patient

Most patients who undergo THA require limited outpatient physical therapy once a normal gait pattern can be resumed. The use of home programs as well as general conditioning exercises allows the patient to resume normal activities quickly. Gait may progress from using a walker to using a cane and then to using no assistive devices, as tolerated by the patient. Differences in leg length should be assessed and a shoe insert recommended if gait abnormalities persist. Once component stability has been obtained and dislocation potential has lessened, many surgeons encourage their patients to gain additional range of motion in the hip. Patients are generally encouraged to resume physical activities in moderation, for example golf, tennis, bicycle riding and walking.

The self-administered hip-rating questionnaire shown in Form 22.1 has been used to assess patients' perspectives on outcomes after THA. As can be seen in Figure 22.1, most benefits were obtained in the first 6 months, and some favorable changes took place after 6 months. Functional improvements can be expected in many areas, including stair climbing and reduced support while ambulating.

CONCLUSION

When rehabilitating a patient who has received a THA, it is important to understand the specific procedures and to implement properly the specific guidelines for mobility, weight-bearing and range of motion. Normal recovery timelines and progressions must be followed, with special attention paid to the recommendations of the physician. Favorable functional outcomes are expected in 6–12 months (Katz et al 2003).

Form 22.1 Self-administered hip-rating questionnaire

Question	Score
1. Please describe any pain in your hip:	
A. No pain	44
B. Slight pain or occasional pain	40
C. Mild, no effect on ordinary activity, pain after unusual activity, uses aspirin or similar medication	30
D. Moderate pain that requires pain medicine stronger than aspirin/similar medications. I'm active but have had to make modifications and/or give up some activities because of pain	20
E. Marked or severe pain that limits activity and requires pain medicine frequently	10
F. Totally disabled-wheelchair or bed ridden	0
2. Amount and type of support used:	
A. None	11
B. Cane for long walks	7
C. Cane all the time	5
D. 2 canes	2
E. 1 crutch	3
F. 2 crutches or walker	0
G. Unable to walk	0
3. Limp. This should be judged at the end of a long walk using the *type* of support chosen in question 2.	
A. None	11
B. Slight	8
C. Moderate	5
D. Severe	0
4. Distance that you can walk. This should be judged with the aid of a support if you use one.	
A. Unlimited	11
B. 5–6 blocks	8
C. 1–4 blocks	5
D. In the house only	2
E. Unable to walk	0
5. Climbing stairs:	
A. Normally	4
B. Need a banister or cane or cratch	2
C. Must put both feet on each step/severe trouble climbing stairs	1
D. Unable to climb stairs	5
6. Shoes and socks:	
A. Can put on socks and tie a shoe easily	4
B. Can put on socks and tie a shoe with difficulty	2
C. Cannot put on socks and shoes	0
7. Sitting:	
A. Comfortable in any chair	5
B. Comfortable only in high chair, or can sit comfortably for only 0.5 hour	3
C. Cannot sit for 0.5 hour because of pain	0

From Mahomed N et al 2001 The Harris Hip Score: comparison of patient self-report with surgeon assessment. J Arthroplasty 16:575–580, with permission from Elsevier.

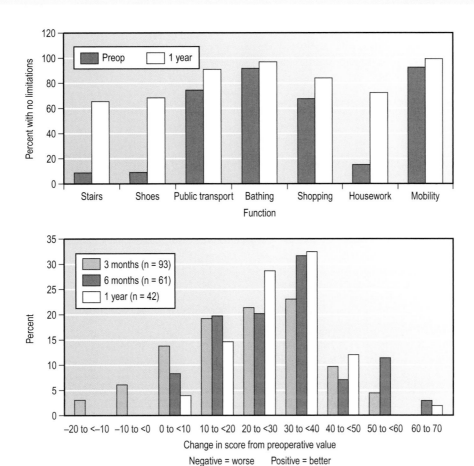

Figure 22.1   Change in function following total hip arthroplasty. Top graph shows changes in activities of daily living. Bottom graph shows changes in functional scores at 3, 6 and 12 months postoperatively.
(From Johanson NA, Charlson ME, Szatrowski TP et al 1992 A self-administered hip-rating questionnaire for the assessment of outcome after total hip replacement. J Bone Joint Surg Am 74A:587–597, with permission from Elsevier.)

References

Barrett J, Losina E, Baron JA et al 2005 Survival following total hip replacement. J Bone Joint Surg Am 87:1965–1971

Berger RA 2004 Mini-incision total hip replacement using an anterolateral approach: technique and results. Orthop Clin North Am 35:143–151

Dalury DF 2005 The technique of cemented total hip replacement. Orthopedics 28:s853–856

Merx H, Dreinhofer K, Schrader P et al 2003 International variation in hip replacement rates. Ann Rheum Dis 62:222–226

Higuchi F, Gotoh M, Yamaguchi N et al 2003 Minimally invasive uncemented total hip arthroplasty through an anterolateral approach with a shorter skin incision. J Orthop Sci 6:812–817

Jagmin MG 1998 Postoperative mental status in elderly hip surgery patients. Orthop Nurs 17:32–42

Katz JN, Phillips CB, Baron JA et al 2003 Association of hospital and surgeon volume of total hip replacement with functional status and satisfaction three years following surgery. Arthritis Rheumatol 48:560–568

Phillips CB, Barrett JA, Losina E et al 2003 Incidence rates of dislocation, pulmonary embolism, and deep infection during the first six months after elective total hip replacement. J Bone Joint Surg Am 85A:20–26

Siguier T 2004 Mini-incision anterior approach does not increase dislocation rate: a study of 1037 total hip replacements. Clin Orthop Related Res 426:164–173

Wright JM 2004 Mini-incision for total hip arthroplasty: a prospective, controlled investigation with 5-year follow-up evaluation. J Arthroplasty 5:538–545

Chapter **23**

Total knee arthroplasty

Mark A. Brimer

INTRODUCTION

Total knee replacement (TKR), also referred to as total knee arthroplasty (TKA), is one of the most common surgical procedures performed for patients with advanced arthritis of the knee (Mahomed et al 2005). There are well over 150 brand-name implants currently on the market, which may be divided into three categories: the linked prosthesis, the resurfacing implant and the conforming implant.

THE THREE CATEGORIES OF IMPLANTS

In the linked prosthesis, the femoral and tibial components are physically fastened together at the time of manufacture or at some point during the surgical procedure. The linked prosthesis may be fully constrained, thereby permitting only flexion and extension, or it may permit flexion, extension and limited axial rotation. Used primarily in the 1970s, the linked prosthesis is no longer commonly used because of the loosening of components that occurs when stresses are applied to the tibial side of the joint. However, they may be appropriate for patients who have markedly unstable knees or after failure of one or more previous arthroplasties.

A resurfacing implant has a flat polyethylene tibial surface that articulates with the metallic femoral condylar component. A resurfacing implant requires proper balancing of the collateral and cruciate ligaments and, therefore, is not indicated in a case in which either the cruciate or the collateral ligament is absent or deficient. Because a large number of patients with advanced arthritis have a missing or attenuated cruciate ligament and compromised soft-tissue balancing, which is necessary for the procedure to succeed, resurfacing implants are not the primary choice of many surgeons.

A conforming implant consists of a metallic femoral condylar component and a polyethylene tibial component. Designed to resist some of the translatory and shear stresses, they are currently used in 95% of all TKR procedures (Heck et al 1998). The design of the conforming implant requires surgical sacrifice of the anterior cruciate ligament and, in some cases, depending upon the design of the particular implant, also the posterior cruciate ligament. The posterior cruciate is almost always removed in cases in which the patient presents with a fixed varus or valgus contracture of 15–20° and the associated fixed flexion deformity.

FIXATION OF THE IMPLANT

Surgical fixation of all of the knee components is accomplished through one of two methods. The first involves the use of polymethylmethacrylate bone cement; one or both of the components is cemented to the bone surface. In the second method, the implants are inserted and one or both of the components are attached in a cementless manner. Although cemented knee components are still utilized, the preferred mechanism for attachment is cementless. Some of the problems that have been identified with the use of cemented components include the following:

1. The polymethylmethacrylate bone cement is known to be brittle. If the cement fragments in the joint, it can become trapped between components, which results in excessive component wear.

2. As the polymethylmethacrylate hardens, it is known to become thermotoxic to adjacent bony cells. It has also been known to decrease leukotaxis (attraction of leukocytes) and thereby increase the risk of infection at the implant site.

3. The use of bone cement is known to make surgical revision more difficult.

The cementless technique relies upon bone growth onto porous or roughened surfaces for firm fixation. Proper and precise surgical placement of cementless components is essential if firm component attachment is to be obtained. Studies indicate that bone will not grow across gaps greater than 1–2 mm.

The choice of component may be based upon the patient's level of strenuous physical activity, age, health and well-being, and bone density. The primary contraindication to the use of a cementless component is severe osteoporosis.

Monitoring for potential infection is particularly important in TKA because a large amount of foreign material is implanted in a superficial joint. Although a TKA is a relatively safe orthopedic procedure, wound-healing difficulties can occasionally be seen, including problems such as marginal wound necrosis, skin sloughing, sinus tract formation and hematoma formation (Norton et al 1998). The presence of any of these complications may adversely affect the outcome. This is especially true with regard to range of motion (ROM), in cases in which therapy must be stopped until the problem can be resolved. The use of the minimally invasive total knee replacement may, however, reduce the potential for postoperative complications (Bonutti et al 2004).

REHABILITATION

Inpatient postoperative rehabilitation considerations

The primary concern after a TKA is to ensure that the patient begins to walk (Katz et al 2004). A patient with an uncomplicated TKA is generally encouraged to walk on the first day postoperatively, even if ambulation time is brief. The role of the therapist is to encourage mobility, self-care, proper weight-bearing and gait, and getting into and out of bed in the proper manner (Kane et al 2005).

During the first few days after surgery, many surgeons ask their patients to use a continuous passive motion (CPM) device to maximize ROM results. These devices are used two or three times a day in conjunction with physical therapy exercises and ROM and gait-training sessions. Patients are often encouraged to remain in the CPM device unless attending a physical therapy session or resting.

When a hospital rehabilitation department is preparing a patient to go home or to a skilled-nursing facility, staff members should consider the environment into which the patient is being discharged. For example, a patient returning home should be thoroughly trained in how to negotiate steps and flights of stairs, carpeted surfaces and surfaces that might be encountered outside the home. It is particularly important that the patient understands the proper positioning of the knee during sleep in order to prevent unwanted contractures.

The performance of the activities of daily living should be discussed with the patient and the immediate caregivers. Because a large majority of TKA procedures are performed in members of the geriatric population, special attention should be paid to any impairments of vision, balance or endurance that may have occurred. A falls risk assessment should be performed and documented. Patients should be encouraged to monitor the integrity of the wound site on a daily basis and to use safe ambulation procedures until outpatient gait-training needs can be addressed.

Outpatient and home–healthcare rehabilitation considerations

In the outpatient or home-healthcare rehabilitation environment, the focus is on restoring the ability to perform normal activities of daily living, restoring ROM of the knee and teaching safe ambulation. In the initial stages (0–4 weeks), it is vital to maximize ROM. Functional ROM is considered to be between 110 and 120° of flexion and full extension. Patients should be actively involved in home programs that focus upon the prevention of flexion or extension contractures of the knee.

In the period between 0 and 4 weeks after surgery, rehabilitation should focus upon strength gains in the quadriceps, hamstring, hip flexor and hip extensor muscles. The patient may be allowed to progress to walking with full weight-bearing, as indicated by the physician. A patient who has undergone the cementless technique may be required to maintain limited weight-bearing for a period of 4–6 weeks or until sufficient new bone growth can be seen by the physician using radiography.

Desired rehabilitation outcomes for the TKA patient

Patients who undergo TKA commonly require extensive outpatient physical therapy for a period of approximately 6 weeks in order to maximize ROM. Swelling may persist for several months until sufficient collateral circulation can develop. Persistent or excessive calf pain and swelling should not be ignored because asymptomatic deep vein thrombosis may occur in up to 40% of TKA patients, even up to 18 months after surgery (Schindler & Dalziel 2005). The use of home ROM programs as well as general conditioning exercises allows the patient to resume normal activities quickly. Strenuous exercise is to be avoided until approved of by the physician. A knee evaluation scale is shown in Table 23.1; it may be helpful in documenting post-surgical outcomes.

The patient may progress from using a walker to using a cane and then to ambulating with no assistive devices, as tolerated by the individual. Differences in leg length should be assessed and a shoe insert may be recommended if gait abnormalities persist. After several months, patients are often encouraged to resume physical activities in moderation, for example golf, tennis, bicycle riding and walking (Lingard et al 2004).

Although TKA is very effective in relieving pain, it is important to note that functional activities of daily living, for example stair climbing, getting in and out of a bath, negotiating ramps and sitting in low chairs, may be compromised. It is worth bearing in mind that, in general, patients with better preoperative knee flexion have a better postoperative ROM, even though they lose more motion than patients who have a worse ROM going into surgery. In other words, those with considerably less ROM going into surgery tend to gain rather than lose ROM (Rowe et al 2005). Obesity, prior surgery and tightness of retained posterior cruciate ligaments are additional factors that may compromise knee flexion. The minimal amount of knee flexion necessary for most normal activities is 90°, with 67° needed for the swing phase of gait and 90° for climbing stairs. If sufficient flexion is not attained, a manipulation under anesthesia may be performed (Chiu et al 2002). Underlying causes of persistent knee pain and limited flexion include arthrofibrosis, infrapatellar spur, impinging hypertrophic synovitis, impinging posterior cruciate ligament and prosthetic wear or loosening. These diagnoses were made after arthroscopies of problematic knees with improvements noted postoperatively (Klinger et al 2005).

CONCLUSION

TKA is a surgical procedure commonly used in cases of advanced knee arthritis. There are many brand-name implants, which can be divided into three categories: linked prostheses, resurfacing implants and conforming implants. The components of the knee replacement may be surgically fixed with bone cement or a cementless technique can be used. Rehabilitation is similar after the use of both of these methods, but a patient who has had the cementless procedure may be limited in weight-bearing for 4–6 weeks. Following discharge from the inpatient setting, continued rehabilitation should increase functional activities, restore normal ROM (110–120° of flexion and full extension are desirable) and ensure safe walking. Normal physical activities can be resumed several months after the operation.

Table 23.1   Knee Society clinical rating system

Patient category

A. Unilateral or bilateral (opposite knee successfully replaced)
B. Unilateral, other knee symptomatic
C. Multiple arthritis or medical infirmity

Pain	Points	Function	Points
None	50	Walking	
Mild or occasional	45	Unlimited	50
Stairs only	40	>10 blocks	40
Walking and stairs	30	5–10 blocks	30
		<5 blocks	20
Moderate		Housebound	10
Occasional	20	Unable	0
Continual	10		
		Stairs	
Severe	0	Normal up and down	50
Range of motion	25	Normal up; down with rail	40
(5 degrees = 1 point)		Up and down with rail	30
Stability (maximum		Up with rail; unable down	15
movement in		Unable	0
any position)		Subtotal	
Anteroposterior		Deduction (minus)	
<5 mm	10	Cane	5
5–10 mm	5	Two canes	10
10 mm	0	Crutches or walker	20
Mediolateral		Total deductions	
<5 degrees	15	Function score	
6–9 degrees	10		
10–14 degrees	5		
15 degrees	0		
Subtotal			
Deductions (minus)			
Flexion contracture			
5–10 degrees	2		
10–15 degrees	5		
16–20 degrees	10		
>20 degrees	15		
Extension lag			
<10 degrees	5		
10–20 degrees	10		
>20 degrees	15		
Alignment			
5–10 degrees	0		
0–4 degrees (3 points each degree)	15		
11–15 degrees (3 points each degree)	15		
Other	20		
Total deductions			
Knee score (if total is a minus number, score is 0)			

From Insall JN, Dorr LD, Scott RD et al 1989 Rationale of the knee society clinical rating system. Clin Orthop 248:13–14.

References

Bonutti PM, Mont MA, McMahon M et al 2004 Minimally invasive total knee arthroplasty. J Bone Joint Surg Am 86A:26–32

Chiu K, Ng TP, Tang WM et al 2002 Review article: knee flexion after total knee arthroplasty. J Orthop Surg 10:194–202

Heck DA, Melfi CA, Mamlin LA et al 1998 Revision rates after knee replacement in the United States. Med Care 26:661–669

Kane RL, Saleh KJ, Wilt TJ et al 2005 The functional outcomes of total knee arthroplasty. J Bone Joint Surg Am 87:1719–1724

Katz JN, Barrett J, Mahomed NN et al 2004 Association between hospital and surgeon procedure volume and the outcomes of total knee replacement. J Bone Joint Surg Am 86A:1909–1916

Klinger H, Baums MH, Spahn G et al 2005 A study of effectiveness of knee arthroscopy after knee arthroplasty. Arthroscopy 21:731–738

Lingard EA, Katz JN, Wright EA et al 2004 Predicting the outcomes of total knee arthroplasty. J Bone Joint Surg Am 86A:2179–2186

Mahomed NN, Barrett J, Katz JN et al 2005 Epidemiology of total knee replacement in the United States Medicare population. J Bone Joint Surg Am 87:1222–1228

Norton EC, Garfinkel SA, McQuay LJ et al 1998 The effect of hospital volume on the in-patient complication rate in knee replacement patients. Health Serv Res 33:1191–1210

Rowe PJ, Myles CM, Nutton R et al 2005 The effect of total knee arthroplasty on joint movement during functional activities and joint range of motion with particular regard to higher flexion users. J Orthop Surg 13:131–138

Schindler OS, Dalziel R 2005 Post-thrombotic syndrome after total hip or knee arthroplasty: incidence in patients with asymptomatic deep venous thrombosis. Orthop Surg (Hong Kong) 13:113–119

Chapter **24**

The aging bony thorax

Steven Pheasant and Jane K. Schroeder

INTRODUCTION

The bony thorax has the primary function of protecting the organs of circulation and respiration. Some protection is also given to the liver and stomach. In addition, the muscles of respiration attach to the bony thorax and the ribs are mechanically involved in the mechanism of respiration. These elements are shown in Figure 24.1. The bony thorax also serves as the foundation from which the shoulder complex functions, therefore influencing the efficiency of the upper extremities.

The thorax is composed of 12 thoracic vertebrae posteriorly, the sternum anteriorly and 12 pairs of ribs, which encircle the thorax. The first 10 pairs of ribs are true ribs, with joints that attach the thoracic vertebra to the sternum. The last two pairs do not attach to the sternum anteriorly and are referred to as floating ribs. These bony relationships are shown in Figures 24.2 and 24.3.

The sternum is composed of three parts – the manubrium, the body and the xiphoid process – that are connected by fibrocartilage. The manubrium is the most superior and has notches for the clavicles. The body is a thin flexible bone and is the part used for closed cardiac compression. The xiphoid process is attached to the distal part of the body.

Each rib has a small head at the posterior end that presents upper and lower facets divided by a crest. Each facet articulates with the adjacent vertebral body. The next part of the rib, the tubercle, articulates with the transverse process of the corresponding vertebra. The shaft of the rib curves gently from the neck to a sudden sharp bend called the angle of the rib. Each rib is separated from the others by an intercostal space that houses the intercostal muscles. On the lower border of each rib there is a costal groove. This groove provides protection for the costal nerve and blood vessels (Rosse & Gaddum-Rosse 1997).

KINESIOLOGY

Mechanics of the ribs

There are two kinds of rib movements. The pump-handle type is noted at the upper ribs, where movement is limited by joint articulations anteriorly and posteriorly. When these upper ribs move upward, as a result of the costosternal joints, the sternum is thrust forward and glides upward. This movement increases the anteroposterior diameter and depth of the thorax.

The lower ribs swing outward and upward during inspir-ation, each pushing against the rib above. This movement increases the transverse diameter of the thoracic cage. The movement is similar to a bucket-handle movement and is given this name. These two movements greatly increase the volume of the thorax, which creates the negative pressure responsible for air exchange during inhalation (Moll & Wright 1972, Wilson et al 1987, Burgos-Vargas et al 1993).

Muscles of the thorax

The primary muscle of respiration is the large dome-shaped diaphragm that separates the thoracic and abdominal cavities. The two halves of the diaphragm each have attachments to the sternum at the posterior aspect of the xiphoid process.

The costal parts of the diaphragm arise from the inner surfaces of the lower ribs and lower six costal cartilages. These interdigitate and transverse the abdomen to insert into a central tendon. There is also a lumbar part that arises from the bodies of the upper lumbar vertebrae and extends upward to the central tendon.

The intercostal muscles arise from the tubercles of the ribs and travel above, down and forward to the costochondral junction of the ribs below, where they become continuous with the anterior intercostal membrane. The membrane then extends forward to the sternum. These 11 external and 11 internal intercostals, along with the erector spinae, rectus abdominus, internal oblique abdominals and transverse abdominals, also contribute to respiration. The specific muscles and their innervations and functions are listed in Table 24.1 (Loring & Woodbridge 1991, Oatis 2004).

Postural stresses on the thoracic spine

The thoracic spine possesses a naturally occurring kyphosis. The kyphosis results, in part, from the wedge shape of the thoracic verte-bral bodies (taller dorsally and shorter ventrally). The magnitude of the thoracic kyphosis and the resultant postural stresses imposed on

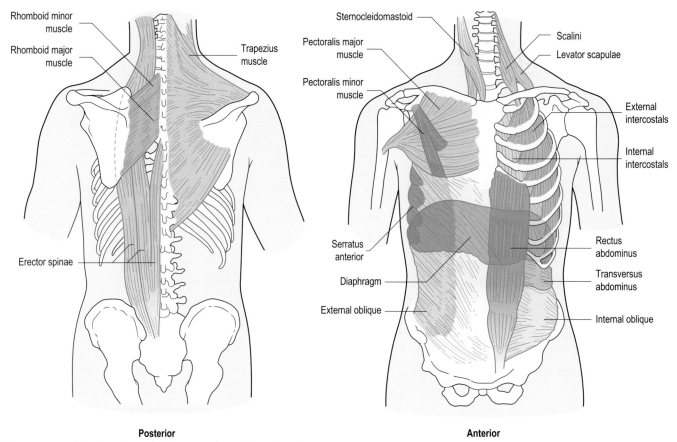

Figure 24.1   Muscles of ventilation, posterior and anterior views.
(From Starr JA 1995 Pulmonary system. In: Sgarlat-Myers R (ed.) Saunders Manual of Physical Therapy Practice. WB Saunders, Philadelphia, PA, p 259, with permission.)

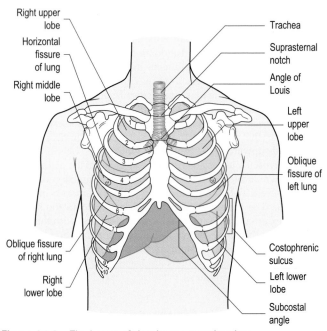

Figure 24.2   The bones of the thorax, anterior view.
(From Starr JA 1995 Pulmonary system. In: Sgarlat-Myers R (ed.) Saunders Manual of Physical Therapy Practice. WB Saunders, Philadelphia, PA, p 254, with permission.)

the vertebral bodies both increase substantially with a forward-thrust head posture. Increased postural stresses render the thoracic vertebral bodies vulnerable to compression fractures particularly in those who are osteoporotic. Compression fractures in the thoracic spine can lead to increased vertebral wedging, greater postural stresses and a progressive thoracic kyphosis, which further compound the impairment (White & Panjabi 1990, Oatis 2004). Information regarding vertebral compression fracture management and rehabilitation can be found in Chapters 26, 27, 62 and 70.

PATHOLOGIES INVOLVING THE BONY THORAX

Obstructive lung diseases

Obstructive lung diseases cause an overinflated state in the lungs. The thoracic cage tends to assume the inspiratory position and the diaphragm becomes low and flat. The anteroposterior (AP) and transverse diameters of the chest are increased and the ribs and sternum are always in a state of partial or complete expansion.

Restrictive lung diseases

In restrictive lung diseases, the lungs are prevented from fully expanding because of restrictions in the lung tissue, pleurae, muscles, ribs or sternum. The AP and transverse diameters of the chest should increase with inspiration but do not increase to normal levels

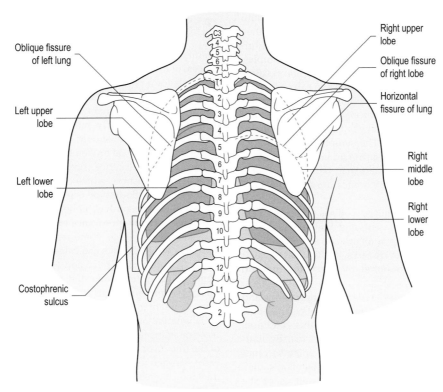

Figure 24.3   The bones of the thorax, posterior view.
(From Starr JA 1995 Pulmonary system. In: Sgarlat-Myers R (ed.) Saunders Manual of Physical Therapy Practice. WB Saunders, Philadelphia, PA, p 254, with permission.)

Table 24.1   Muscles of respiration innervation and function

Muscle (innervation)	Functions
Inspiratory muscles	
Diaphragm (C3–5)	Expands thorax vertically and horizontally; essential for normal vital capacity and effective cough
Intercostals (T1–12)	Anterior and lateral expansion of upper and lower chest
Sternocleidomastoids (cranial nerve XI and C1–4)	When head is fixed, elevates sternum to expand chest superiorly and anteriorly
Scalenes (C3–8)	When neck is fixed, elevates first two ribs to expand chest superiorly
Serratus anterior (C5–7)	When scapulae are fixed, elevates first 8–9 ribs to provide posterior expansion of thorax
Pectoralis major (C5–T1)	When arms are fixed, elevates true ribs to expand chest anteriorly
Pectoralis minor (C6–8)	When scapulae are fixed, elevates third, fourth and fifth ribs to expand chest laterally
Trapezius (cranial nerve XI and C3–4)	Stabilizes scapulae to assist the serratus anterior and pectoralis minor in elevating the ribs
Erector spinae (C1 down)	Extends the vertebral column to allow further rib elevation
Expiratory muscles	
Abdominals (T5–12)	Helps force diaphragm back to resting position and depress and compress lower thorax leading to higher intrathoracic pressure, which is essential for effective cough
Internal intercostals (T1–12)	Depresses third, fourth and fifth ribs to aid in forceful expiration

From Watchie 1995, with permission.

in these conditions. Interstitial fibrosis, sarcoidosis and pneumoconiosis are examples of disease processes that decrease elasticity (or compliance) of the lung tissue.

Abnormalities in the pleural tissue, such as pleurisy, pleuritis and pleural effusion, cause compression of the lungs. Also, any condition that elevates the diaphragm and prevents full excursion of this muscle diminishes the ability of the chest to expand. Examples of such conditions are ascites, obesity and abdominal tumors of any kind.

Numerous musculoskeletal conditions cause disturbed respiratory mechanics. The autoimmune (collagen) diseases can affect any joint in the body, including the costochondral and costovertebral joints. Additionally, these are systemic diseases and, therefore, they can also involve the pleural or lung tissue as well. Rheumatoid arthritis, systemic lupus erythematosus and scleroderma are examples. Other less severe forms of autoimmune disease such as fibromyalgia and dermatomyositis may affect the musculature and can cause pain and restriction of the myofascial structures and thereby limit chest expansion. Costochondritis (Tietze's syndrome) is an inflammatory condition of the costochondral tissue that can be viral or occur secondary to strain or unknown reasons. The symptom of chest pain can occur with this condition and be mistaken for myocardial infarction. An effusion of the costosternal joint may be mistaken for a painful breast lump during self-breast examination (Watchie 1995, Frownfelter & Dean 1996).

Orthopedic conditions such as kyphosis, scoliosis and kyphoscoliosis primarily affect the vertebral segments and costovertebral articulations. Even with mild changes of spine alignment, the mechanics of the ribs and sternum are altered. In severe cases, the lung tissue, heart and major vessels may be compromised by the deformity and altered mechanics.

Ankylosing spondylitis can be considered in the autoimmune and orthopedic categories. It is considered separately here because of the severe consequences it can have on the thorax. In this condition, there is gradual fusion of spinal zygapophyseal joints, usually starting in the sacroiliac joints. As more and more of the spine becomes involved, X-rays demonstrate a bamboo-like image (bamboo spine). There is calcification of the spinal segments as well as of the costovertebral joint, which causes severe restriction of chest expansion (Dutton 2004).

Accidental or surgical trauma can cause muscle splinting, which may restrict chest expansion or relaxation. After thoracic and cardiovascular surgery there is a tendency for the patient to breathe in a shallow, rapid and guarded manner, using accessory muscles such as the scalenes and sternocleidomastoids rather than the diaphragm. Even after healing, the posture of such patients has often changed and shows an increase in thoracic kyphosis, a marked forward-thrust head, protraction of the shoulder girdles and an adducted and internally rotated position of the shoulders. The acquired posture compromises not only spinal and respiratory function but also function of the upper extremities.

Another type of trauma to the thorax that is not often considered is an injury that occurs during a motor vehicle accident. If the person is using a seat belt/shoulder strap type of restraint at the time of the accident, the shoulder strap may cause damage to the thoracic fascial structures and muscles or sternum and ribs, as well as fractures. However, soft-tissue and joint injuries are often overlooked, even though they may contribute to painful postural and respiratory dysfunction.

Compression fractures in the thoracic spine are commonplace in the geriatric population. The increased mechanical stresses that result from the forward-thrust head, rounded shoulder, kyphotic posture that frequently follows a thoracic compression fracture, predispose the individual to further pain, reduced spinal motion and compromised function (Melton 1997, Old & Calvert 2004) (see Chapters 15, 26 and 27). Also, multiple compression fractures may lead to a protruding abdomen with reduced abdominal cavity space and subsequent difficulty with eating a normal meal. The floating ribs may rest upon the iliac crests leading to considerable pain (Brunton et al 2005).

When muscular, fascial, spinal, rib or sternal components are the cause of restriction of lung capacity, the patient may benefit from physical therapy, which can improve mechanics and lower the pain factor, thus improving quality of life in spite of the underlying disease process.

ASSESSMENT

History is very important. Understanding the underlying disease process or mechanism of trauma can help in defining the problem and the goals for a particular patient. Histories of the present illness as well as of past medical and surgical problems are vital to proper examination and treatment. Laboratory and radiographic data, medication lists, particularly pulmonary and cardiac drugs, and psychosocial information should be gathered.

Examination can be broken down into many components, starting with general appearance (Box 24.1). This consists of assessing the level of consciousness, which can indicate adequacy of oxygenation of brain tissues. Body type is evaluated as normal, obese or cachectic. An obese person has higher energy demands, even for simple activities. General appearance can also indicate whether the person is deconditioned. Also, some respiratory conditions are caused by excessive weight, which can cause restriction of the diaphragm. The cachectic patient may have had weight loss associated with a carcinoma or eating may take too much energy, meaning that caloric intake becomes insufficient.

In evaluating posture, the therapist should note any spinal malalignment or unusual postures. The extremities are observed for nicotine stains (which indicate a history of heavy smoking), clubbing of the fingers or toes (a sign of cardiopulmonary or small bowel disease), swollen joints, tremors and edema. Any of these parameters may indicate respiratory system impairment.

The color of the skin and face should be noted. A patient might show evidence of a bluish tinge to the mucous membranes or nail beds, indicating severe arterial oxygen desaturation. A plethoric facial color (red or ruddy) may indicate hypertension, whereas a cherry-red coloring may be a sign of carbon monoxide poisoning.

Posture should be noted initially, especially sitting and standing patterns. In a patient with chronic obstructive pulmonary disease (COPD) there is usually a forward-thrust head, increased kyphosis in the thoracic area and abduction and protraction of the shoulder girdles. If there is less than a two-finger space between the iliac crests and the lower ribs, osteoporosis should be suspected and further appropriate workup and care considered (Brunton et al 2005). There may also be elevation of the shoulder girdles if the accessory muscles of breathing are the primary respiratory muscles. With spinal curvature, there are changes in posture from the sagittal and frontal views. When trauma is the mechanism of dysfunction, any or all of the above can be seen as well as changes related to joint dysfunction and muscle involvement (Palmer & Epler 1998).

Vital signs, including blood pressure, heart rate and rhythm, and respiratory rate and rhythm, should be noted. It may be pertinent to assess these at rest and with exertion. Pulmonary function volumes and diseases are described in Chapters 7 and 47. Pulmonary function might have to be assessed by means of spirometry. Respiratory patterns include factors such as rate and rhythm and use of particular muscles for respiration. When accessory muscles are used, the upper chest and neck muscles are moving and strained. Bracing postures or any unusual postures taken to assist breathing increase the work of breathing. The depth of inspiration and whether expiration is either passive (as is normally expected at rest) or forced should be observed (Watchie 1995, Frownfelter & Dean 1996).

Chest wall excursion can be recorded taking circumferential measurements with a tape measure at the floor of the axillae, at the tip of the xiphoid and at the lower costal border at the midaxillary line of the 10th rib. These measurements should be taken for inspiration and expiration during quiet breathing, as well as for maximum inspiration and forced expiration. These landmarks (or others of the therapist's choice) should be consistent and reproducible (Harris et al 1997).

Auscultation, or listening to the breath sounds, is another important aspect of assessment. When possible, the patient should sit forward for this part of the examination. The anterior and middle lobes can best be auscultated at the front of the patient whereas the posterior lobes are best heard at the patient's back Figure 24.4. The patient should breathe in and out through an open mouth. A comparison of breath sounds in each segment of each lung should assess the intensity, pitch and quality. There is a system of nomenclature and it is helpful to use these standard terms. Quality is defined as absent, decreased, normal or bronchial. If abnormal sounds are heard, they can be further described as crackles, rales, wheezes or rhonchi. During vocalization, sounds can be normal, increased or decreased. All the above can help to define the area of the chest and lungs involved in the pathology. It is also possible to hear rubs from the pleura or the pericardium. Crunches may indicate air in the mediastinal space.

Range of motion (ROM) assessment, formal or functional, should include the head, neck, upper extremities, lower extremities and trunk. Emphasis on specific areas may change depending on the pathology. However, as the neck, upper back and shoulder girdles are consistently involved to a large degree, these areas must be accurately assessed on an ongoing basis (Palmer & Epler 1998). Flexibility is an important parameter to consider, especially that of the anterior chest muscles. The pectoralis major and minor, sternocleidomastoids and scalenes may all be shortened or overused. Unless a normal length can be regained in these muscles, normalization of posture cannot occur.

Strength may also be specifically or functionally tested. In most cases, testing of functional strength is all that is necessary. However, when working on postural correction, it may be important to specifically test the trapezius, rhomboids and rotator cuff muscles as well as neck and back extensors (Palmer & Epler 1998). Coordination among muscle groups should be examined.

It is extremely important to note functional abilities because it is these activities that most concern outcome measures. Basics such as bed mobility, transfers, feeding, bathing and toileting may be possible but higher level activities such as housekeeping, food preparation and shopping may be limited. Whatever the functional limitation, it is important to note them in measurable ways. Gait pattern, balance, endurance and need for assistive devices should be evaluated. The ability to traverse a specific distance in a measured time clarifies functional mobility. For example, the minimum walking velocity determined to allow safe street crossing according to Lerner-Frankiel (1986) is 30 m/min, a measure that is particularly important for community-dwelling individuals.

On palpation, skin, fascia and each layer should be pliable and extensible and each layer should be separated from adjacent layers. With the absence of any of these qualities, movement at any or all layers or planes may be restricted and painful, thus creating guarding or spasm, which may prevent normal joint kinematics and mobility.

Joint mobility can be restricted by surgical, traumatic or soft-tissue conditions. The costosternal and costovertebral joints may be involved, which limits general mobility of the ribs in their upward and downward movements. The sternum can also be prevented from gliding by soft-tissue restriction or dysfunction of the sternoclavicular joints and costosternal joints on one or both sides. Also important, but to a lesser extent, are the spinal joints of the cervical and thoracic areas. The scapulothoracic joints may also affect the mobility of the ribs and certainly affect posture.

The joints can be assessed by passive mobility testing involving AP and PA (posteroanterior) springs at the costosternal, costovertebral, cervical and thoracic segments. Monitoring the excursion of each rib anteriorly and/or laterally during inspiration and expiration demonstrates any dysfunctions. At the first rib, a distal spring at the midpoint of the supraclavicular space and AP and PA springs can be used to assess mobility. Glides of the scapula in all planes detect disturbances of the scapulothoracic joints. Particular care should be exercised when assessing passive joint mobility of the vertebral and costal structures in patients with osteoporosis.

Psychological factors can affect a patient's condition, goals, treatment plan and outcome measurements. The patient's family situation, the availability of a caregiver and the type of dwelling should be recorded. The patient's and the family's reactions to the disease process may affect the pathology and the outcome, so it is important to allow the patient to discuss problems and concerns. It is to be hoped that the patient's and family's goals are congruent with those of the medical providers.

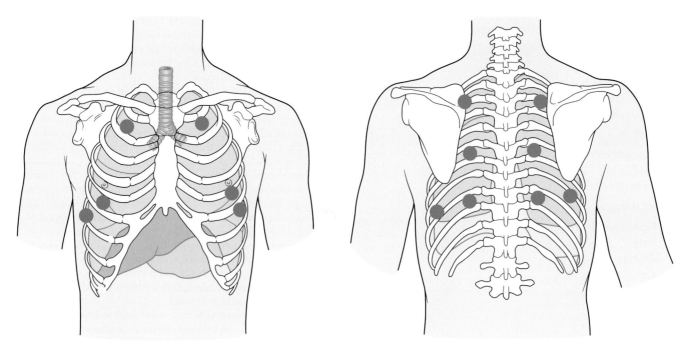

Figure 24.4   Anterior, lateral and posterior auscultation sites.
(From Starr JA 1995 Pulmonary system. In: Sgarlat-Myers R (ed.) Saunders Manual of Physical Therapy Practice. WB Saunders, Philadelphia, PA, p 270, with permission.)

REHABILITATION INTERVENTION

Optimal breathing, normal or forced, is performed by the diaphragm, with distal excursion on inspiration and return to baseline or elevation on expiration. This results in expansion of the lower chest and abdomen on inspiration and retraction of these areas on expiration. The person should be encouraged to inhale through the nose (to filter, warm and moisturize the air) and to exhale through pursed lips to ensure the emptying of the alveoli.

Lateral costal expansion can also be promoted as this requires rib movement in a bucket-handle fashion and may improve mobility. Use of tactile stimulation over the diaphragm or the lateral costal margins can facilitate the proper function. Resistance may also be performed by using weights on the diaphragm area or by resisting chest expansion with elastic exercise bands or tubing. When a specific area of the lungs is not expanding, segmental breathing exercises may be useful. Again, tactile stimulation may provide the sensory input that will promote increased expansion of the specific area.

In conjunction with proper breathing techniques, postural correction exercises can assist with more efficient breathing patterns. However, in the case of chronic cardiopulmonary diseases, postural changes may have occurred to assist air exchange and, if so, these corrections can be detrimental to the patient's overall condition. Each case must be considered on an individual basis.

In order to improve posture, several factors must be considered. Some muscles will have shortened whereas others will have overstretched and weakened. Joints may have lost passive mobility in one or several planes. Body awareness and proprioception may be impaired, so high patient motivation and a long-time commitment to exercise and awareness are necessary. ROM, strengthening and flexibility exercises are vital for postural changes, functional improvements and general well-being. All areas of the body should be considered, but practicality stresses exercises for the most severely involved areas. When pulmonary disease is present, the ability of the muscles to extract oxygen can be enhanced by strengthening exercises. This improved extraction of oxygen allows the patient to have increased efficiency and endurance during routine activities.

Strengthening exercises may include any or all of the following: active ROM, progressive resistive exercises with gradually increasing weight and repetition, and use of exercise equipment such as a bicycle ergometer, treadmill, rowing machine or ski machine. Proprioceptive neuromuscular facilitation exercises and closed-chain activities or functional activities with increasing time and difficulty can enhance strength and fitness.

For patients with musculoskeletal conditions in the thoracic or rib area, physical therapy modalities including heat, cold, ultrasound and electrical stimulation may be indicated.

If restriction of skin, fascia or muscle is identified during the evaluation, manual techniques may be used to regain tissue extensibility. Treatment techniques are identified by many different names but the goals of all such techniques are the same – to improve the extensibility of tissues and to allow one layer to move separately from adjacent layers.

Mobilization of the joints may be necessary in order to recover full ROM, full flexibility and correct posture. The first rib as well as the costosternal and costovertebral joints can be mobilized by AP and PA spring and distal glide mobilizations in grades 1–4, depending on the patient's condition and tolerance. Mobilization techniques used on the ribs can encourage elevation or depression.

CONCLUSION

The bony thorax is often overlooked in caring for an aging patient unless there is frank pathology. In addition to overt pathologies of the thorax, insidious age-related declines contribute to changes in structure and function that necessitate a thorough assessment. Breathing, posture, mobility and strengthening exercises are important rehabilitation interventions.

REFERENCES

Brunton S, Carmichael B, Gold D et al 2005 Vertebral compression fractures in primary care. J Fam Pract 54(9):781–788

Burgos-Vargas R, Castelazo-Duarte G, Orozco JA et al 1993 Chest expansion in healthy adolescents and patients with seronegative enthesopathy and arthropathy syndrome or juvenile ankylosing spondylitis. J Rheumatol 20:1957–1960

Dutton M 2004 Orthopedic Examination, Evaluation and Intervention. McGraw-Hill, New York, NY

Frownfelter D, Dean E 1996 Principles and Practice of Cardiopulmonary Physical Therapy, 3rd edn. Mosby, St Louis, MO

Harris J, Johansen J, Pederson S et al 1997 Site of measurement and subject position affect chest excursion measurements. Cardiopulmonary Phys Ther 8:12–17

Lerner-Frankiel 1986 Functional community ambulation: what are your criteria? Clin Manage 6:12

Loring SH, Woodbridge JA 1991 Intercostal muscle action inferred from finite-element analysis. J Appl Physiol 70:2712–2718

Melton LJI 1997 Epidemiology of spinal osteoporosis. Spine 22:2S–11S

Moll JM, Wright V 1972 An objective clinical study of chest expansion. Ann Rheumatol Dis 31:1–8

Oatis CA 2004 Kinesiology: The Mechanics and Pathomechanics of Human Movement. Lippincott Williams & Wilkins, Philadelphia, PA

Old JL, Calvert M 2004 Vertebral compression fractures in the elderly. Am Fam Physician 69(1):111–116

Palmer ML, Epler ME 1998 Fundamentals of Musculoskeletal Assessment Techniques, 2nd edn. Lippincott Williams & Wilkins, Philadelphia, PA

Rosse C, Gaddum-Rosse P (eds) 1997 Hollingshead's Textbook of Anatomy, 5th edn. Lippincott-Raven, Philadelphia, PA

Watchie J 1995 Cardiopulmonary Physical Therapy. WB Saunders, Philadelphia, PA

White AA, Panjabi MM 1990 Clinical Biomechanics of the Spine, 2nd edn. JB Lippincott, Philadelphia, PA

Wilson TA, Rehder K, Krayer S et al 1987 Geometry and respiratory displacement of human ribs. J Appl Physiol 62:1872–1877

Chapter 25

Conditions of the geriatric cervical spine

Jeff A. Martin, Zoran Maric, Robert R. Karpman and Timothy L. Kauffman

INTRODUCTION[DB1]

The aging process can be 'a pain in the neck', literally as well as figuratively. As early as 1932, Schmorl and Junghann (1932) reported that 90% of males over the age of 50 and 90% of females over the age of 60 have radiographic evidence of spinal degeneration. It is common for elderly individuals to experience neck symptoms, the majority of them related to cervical spondylosis or degenerative disease of the spine (Modic et al 1989). These conditions occur as a result of degeneration of the intervertebral disks, with loss of the water content within the disk and subsequent disk collapse. The most common clinical syndromes associated with degenerative disk disease include cervical spondylosis, radiculopathy and myelopathy.

COMMON CLINICAL SYNDROMES

Cervicalgia

Cervicalgia is defined as neck pain. The pain tends to be located posteriorly in the area of the paraspinous muscles. Patients often complain of occipital headaches as well as interscapular pain. The symptoms are exacerbated by neck motion and by abducting the arms in the over-the-shoulder position. Gore et al (1987) reported on a 10-year follow-up of patients with cervicalgia and noted that 79% of the patients had decreasing neck pain and 32% had only residual or moderate pain. The symptoms are relieved by various therapeutic modalities, including hot packs, ultrasound, electrical stimulation, traction and soft-tissue techniques such as massage. Immobilization with a cervical orthosis along with neck-strengthening exercises may be helpful. It should be noted, however, that older patients have difficulty wearing a soft collar because it tends to be too large and uncomfortable. Rigid supports should rarely be used.

Radiculopathy

Radiculopathy is defined as pain in a specific nerve root distribution. Radiculopathy is a result of herniation of a soft disk as opposed to constriction, where the nerve root exits the spinal foramina because of the presence of osteophytes. Clinically, it is characterized by pain and paresthesia both proximally and distally along the involved nerve root. It is not uncommon to find overlapping in multiple dermatomes. The interspace most commonly involved is the C5–6 interspace (Simeon & Rothman 1992).

Myelopathy

Myelopathy is often missed but is more commonly found in patients over 55 years of age. Radiographs of the spine show the typical osteophytes and narrowing of disk spaces. Compression of the spinal cord is likely if the spinal canal diameter is less than 10 mm (*Merck Manual of Geriatrics* 2000). Typical neurological findings include lower motor neuron and reflex changes at the level of the lesion and upper motor neuron involvement below the level of the lesion. Spastic gait or other gait abnormalities are the most common clinical concern (*Merck Manual of Geriatrics* 2000). The myelopathy tends to have an insidious onset and develops gradually over a long period of time.

HISTORY, PHYSICAL EXAMINATION AND IMAGING

When taking a history, it is extremely important to specify the type of pain and its anatomical distribution (Kesson & Atkins 2005). Complaints of deep aching pain and a burning sensation are suggestive of spinal cord involvement. Many patients lose hand dexterity. In patients who have been institutionalized for long periods, it may be difficult to assess an insidious myelopathy because many patients already have bladder incontinence. In these instances, a more careful neurological examination is necessary to determine the cause of the incontinence.

On physical examination, most patients present with decreased range of motion (ROM) of the neck and with paras-pinous muscle spasm. There may or may not be tenderness directly over the spinous process. The pain is typically exacerbated by moving the shoulders and it is common for pain to radiate either within a specific nerve distribution down the arm or proximately into the occiput. Particularly in cases of cervical myelopathy, both upper and lower neurological examination should be performed. Imaging modalities are extremely useful in differentiating various types of cervical disease. Probably the most useful test is computerized tomography (CT) with intrathecal contrast. This technique provides an excellent differential between bone and soft-tissue lesions and can accurately demonstrate canal size and foraminal narrowing. Magnetic resonance imaging (MRI) is also useful as a noninvasive way of evaluating the spinal cord, soft tissues and neural structures (Wilberger & Chedid 1988). Plain radiographs can demonstrate bony changes and obvious foraminal narrowing but tend to be more generalized (see Chapter 14).

Differential diagnosis

In generating a differential diagnosis when working with an older individual, other diseases should be considered (Buszek et al 1983, Harrington 1986). Neoplasms, the most common being metastatic tumors from carcinoma of the breast, prostate, kidney or thyroid, should be sought. Pain resulting from metastatic disease tends to be more intense at night and is often unremitting.

Sepsis of the skeleton occurs infrequently in the cervical spine but is commonly seen in the lumbosacral spine and can occur following urogenital procedures. In those over the age of 65, sepsis of skin, soft tissue and bone accounts for 4.4% of all patients hospitalized for sepsis (Martin et al 2006). Other inflammatory diseases can also lead to myelopathy; they include rheumatoid arthritis, ankylosing spondylitis, Reiter's syndrome and diffuse idiopathic skeletal hypertrophy (DISH). However, most patients with such diseases present with other joint symptoms before the cervical spine becomes involved (Clark 1988, Wilberger & Chedid 1988).

Cervical disk disease must be differentiated from primary shoulder disorders (Hawkins 1985). Rotator cuff tendonitis, subacromial bursitis and acromioclavicular joint problems can present with shoulder pain that radiates into the paraspinous muscle area. It is possible for a patient to have both primary shoulder disease and degenerative disk disease of the cervical spine. Selective injections, particularly into the subacromial space or the glenohumeral joint, can be helpful in differential diagnosis. Polymyalgia rheumatica should also be considered when an older patient presents specifically with significant proximal pain and stiffness in the morning. This can develop into an acute emergency if the patient develops temporal arteritis and visual difficulties. The treatment of polymyalgia includes high-dose steroids. A patient who presents with these symptoms should be referred to a physician immediately for evaluation and treatment.

Other neurological findings that may be confused with cervical radiculopathies include compressive neuropathies such as entrapment of the suprascapular nerve, with pain in the upper scapular region and atrophy of the rotator cuff musculature. Median and ulnar nerve compression and thoracic outlet syndrome also present with shoulder pain, along with paresthesia or weakness. Differentiation can be determined by nerve conduction studies or electromyelograms (see Chapters 34 and 35 for discussion of neuropathies).

The bilateral vertebral arteries pass through the foramen transversarium and join to form the basilar artery and supply the circle of Willis. Age-related degenerative changes in the cervical spine may compromise this circulation, especially when the neck is extended, and are a possible cause of tinnitus, dizziness or balance complaints (Kesson & Atkins 2005).

TREATMENT

The majority of cervical symptoms in the geriatric patient can be treated by means of physical therapy and careful monitoring. Surgery is indicated primarily in a patient with myelopathy, progressive compression of the spinal cord or significant nerve root encroachment that causes pain and progressive weakness in a specific nerve distribution. As mentioned previously, the remainder of musculoskeletal problems can be treated with heat, electrical stimulation, ultrasound, traction, soft-tissue massage, ROM exercises and muscle strengthening. Other manual techniques, such as mobilization and stretching, are often helpful but the vertebrobasilar system must be cleared (Kesson & Atkins 2005). Clinically, cervical spondylosis, and especially the vertebral artery compromise, may limit cervical spine ROM exercises and the use of the Hallpike maneuver. Immobilization should be used only if necessary because it may encourage further stiffness and muscle atrophy.

When comparing the outcomes of surgery, individualized physical therapy and cervical collar use in individuals with 3 or more months of cervicobrachial pain with evidence of spondylosis, Persson et al (1997) reported that the surgical group had the best pain relief after treatment but that functional improvements (measured on the Sickness Impact Profile) were the same for the surgical and the physical therapy groups. At 12 months, there was no difference among the groups.

Vigorous manipulation should not be used because of the risk of encroachment on the vertebral arteries and the possibility of stroke. Antiinflammatory medications are a useful adjunct; however, many patients experience gastrointestinal irritation and bleeding as a result of such medication, and acetaminophen seems to provide similar symptomatic relief without the undesirable side effects. Generally speaking, a patient should not be restricted to bedrest for a spinal abnormality unless it is absolutely necessary and, in those instances, careful monitoring is vital to avoid excessive pressure that could result in decubiti and to avoid pulmonary compromise and subsequent development of pneumonia.

CONCLUSION

Neck pain is common in individuals over the age of 50 and may become more so because of environmental considerations, for example the use of a computer, driving and physical inactivity. Degenerative changes, the cause of the majority of problems, may cause encroachment on the spinal cord or spinal nerves and present as myelopathy or radiculopathy. Differential diagnosis is crucial because other conditions can cause the same or similar symptoms. Treatment with antiinflammatory medications and physical therapy procedures and modalities may provide successful outcomes. Surgery is indicated for patients with myelopathy, progressive spinal cord compression or significant nerve root encroachment. Bedrest is not a primary treatment.

References

Buszek MC, Szymke TE, Honet JS et al 1983 Hemidiaphragmatic paralysis: an unusual complication of cervical spondylosis. Arch Phys Med Rehabil 64:601–603

Clark CR 1988 Cervical spondylotic myelopathy: history and physical findings. Spine 13:847–489

Gore DR, Sepic SB, Gardner GM, Murray MP 1987 Neck pain: a long-term follow-up of 205 patients. Spine 12:1–5

Harrington KD 1986 Metastatic disease of the spine. J Bone Joint Surg Am 68:1110–1115

Hawkins RJ 1985 Cervical spine and the shoulder. Instruct Course Lect 34:191–195

Kesson M, Atkins E 2005 Orthopaedic Medicine: A Practical Approach. Elsevier, Oxford, p 267–324

Martin G, Mannino D, Moss M 2006 The effect of age on the development and outcome of adult sepsis. Crit Care Med 34:15–21

Merck Manual of Geriatrics 2000 Merck Research Laboratories, Whitehouse Station, NJ, p 181–194, 487

Modic MT, Ross J, Masaryk T 1989 Imaging of degenerative disease of the cervical spine. Clin Orthop Relat Res 239:109–120

Persson L, Carlsson C, Carlsson J 1997 Long-lasting cervical radicular pain managed with surgery, physiotherapy, or a cervical collar. A prospective, randomized study. Spine 22:751–758

Schmorl G, Junghann S 1932 Die gesunde und Kranke Wirtel Saule im Rontgenbild. Georg Thieme, Leipzig, Germany

Simeon FA, Rothman RH 1992 Cervical disc disease. In: Rothman RH, Simeone FA (eds) The Spine. WB Saunders, Philadelphia, PA, p 440–476

Wilberger JE Jr, Chedid M 1988 Acute cervical spondylitic myelopathy. Neurosurgery 22:145–146

Chapter 26

Disorders of the geriatric thoracic and lumbosacral spine

Robert R. Karpman, Timothy L. Kauffman and Katie Lundon

INTRODUCTION

Clinically, the aging spine presents with a loss of height and mobility. Degenerative changes in disks and spondylosis of the zygapophyseal joints are common. It is estimated that, by the age of 45, approximately 75% of males and 60% of females have some lumbar disk degeneration at grades 1–4. The amount increases to over 90% and 80%, respectively, by the age of 65, with increased frequency of grade 3–4 degeneration (Badley 1987). In the thoracic spine, osteoarthritis and osteoporotic problems are more common than intervertebral disk disease (Kesson & Atkins 2005).

DISORDERS OF THE THORACIC SPINE

Unlike the disorders typical of cervical and lumbosacral areas, the disorder of the thoracic spine that is most commonly seen in geriatric patients results from metabolic disease, particularly osteoporosis (Lane 1997). As bone mass decreases in elderly individuals, the vertebral bodies are at particular risk for compression fractures. A patient with multiple compression fractures in the thoracic spine can develop a severe kyphosis ('dowager's hump') and severe deformities. Minimal trauma or none at all may create compression fractures in the geriatric population with low bone mineral density (see Chapters 19 and 62). Patients complain of acute pain in the midthoracic region, which is often incapacitating. Examination reveals significant tenderness with palpation of the spinous process and an obvious deformity when multiple vertebral bodies are involved. There is also significant paraspinous muscle spasm. The neurological examination generally remains intact. Plain radiographs demonstrate

the abnormality as well as diffuse loss of bone mass in the adjacent vertebral bodies (see Chapter 19).

Compression fractures, however, must be differentiated from malignancies. It is not uncommon for a patient with multiple myeloma or metastatic disease to present with a compression fracture. A bone scan, which may demonstrate lesions in other areas of the skeleton, is useful in differentiating a malignancy from a compression fracture resulting from osteoporosis.

Other thoracic spinal abnormalities include infections and degenerative disk disease. Diffuse idiopathic skeletal hyperostosis (DISH) is more commonly found in the thoracic spine, presenting as stiffness and local pain. When it occurs in the cervical spine it can cause dysphagia (*Merck Manual of Geriatrics* 2000). In addition, other visceral problems can present as acute back pain in older patients, particularly ruptured aneurysms, myocardial infarctions, mediastinal tumors, acute pneumonia and peptic ulcer disease (Harrison 1986). A careful physical examination and laboratory and diagnostic studies can differentiate viscerogenic from spinal disorders.

Treatment of compression fractures

The treatment of a compression fracture involves analgesics and bedrest for a short period of time, followed by gradual mobilization and weight-bearing with assistive devices, if required. Caution must be exercised because the biomechanics (long lever arm) of lifting a walker can actually provoke increased thoracic pain. A wheeled walker reduces biomechanical strain. Prolonged bedrest leads to further osteopenia caused by disuse and to other complications, including pneumonia and urinary incontinence. If analgesics are incapable of resolving these symptoms or if polypharmacy is a concern, a transcutaneous electrical nerve stimulation (TENS) unit may be helpful in relieving the paraspinous pain. External immobilization such as hyperextension braces are often of little use for these patients because they can be extremely uncomfortable and often cause chest compression and resultant difficulties in lung expansion and breathing. If necessary, a simple extended corset can be used for support. The Spinomed (Medi-Bayreuth, Germany) lightweight moldable brace has been shown to improve trunk strength, improve forced expiratory volume and decrease kyphosis, pain and postural sway (Pfeifer et al 2004). Within a period of 1–2 weeks, once the symptoms have resolved, extension exercises may be useful in preventing further deformity. Jewett extension braces or other rigid external supports are frequently found to have been placed in the drawer next to the patient rather than on the patient because of the discomfort involved in using them; therefore, unless the deformity is severe, immobilization is not customary.

If pain persists for longer than 2–3 months, surgical intervention with the newer procedures of kyphoplasty or vertebroplasty may be beneficial (see Chapter 19).

Edmonds et al (2005) reported that aging females with osteoporotic-related vertebral deformities had significant limitations in pushing or pulling a large object like a living room chair; however, the presence or absence of back pain, aching or stiffness was a greater factor in functional activities. Women with vertebral deformities and back symptoms had greater functional limitations than women who had a deformity and no back symptoms.

DISORDERS OF THE LUMBOSACRAL SPINE

As in the cervical spine, degenerative disorders of the lumbosacral spine are common in older individuals (Badley 1987). These disorders are more prominent at the L4, L5 and S1 levels and involve the nucleus. The changes include loss of the water content, which diminishes from nearly 90% at birth to 65–71% at 75 years. Reductions also occur in the proteoglycans and number and structure of collagens (Kesson & Atkins 2005), thereby diminishing the pliability of the intervertebral disk leading to disk collapse and, occasionally, disk protrusion. As disks collapse, instability in the adjacent vertebrae develops, often causing mechanical low back problems. In addition, significant arthritic change can lead to stenosis of the central spinal canal or the foramina of the nerve roots.

A patient with spinal stenosis tends to have a classic presentation. Typically, there is pain in the lower back or pain radiating down both legs, usually after walking for a brief time. The symptoms are relieved with rest or flexion of the spine. Once the patient resumes walking, the symptoms recur. This is similar to the experience of lower limb claudication as a result of vascular compromise. Examination of a patient with spinal stenosis often demonstrates a replication of the symptoms after hyperextension of the spine. Hyperextension leads to a narrowing of the spinal canal in the lumbosacral region and results in cord compression. The symptoms may also be aggravated by stenosis of the vertebral foramina, which often leads to radicular symptoms in addition to the claudication.

Treatment of spinal stenosis in severe cases is almost always surgical; however, age-related comorbidities may limit this option (Reeg 2001). A patient experiences acute relief of symptoms following decompression of the spinal canal. Often, multiple vertebrae require decompression and so fusion is necessary to prevent instability of the lumbosacral spine. This is often accompanied by spinal instrumentation to provide rigidity and stability of the spine until the vertebrae have fused. This also allows for earlier mobilization of the patient.

The results of decompressive spinal surgery for stenosis demonstrate that most patients get some pain relief although not total relief. Patients are also able to increase walking distances, which is very important for the quality of life. However, other degenerative changes in the spine can continue to limit a patient's walking capacity (Herno et al 1999, Amundsen et al 2000).

In mild cases, nonsteroidal antiinflammatories and, occasionally, epidural steroid blocks may be helpful in relieving the patient's symptoms. In addition to history and physical examination, the diagnosis of spinal stenosis can easily be made with the use of computerized tomography, with or without intrathecal contrast.

As in the thoracic spine, lumbosacral supports and corsets are often uncomfortable and provide little if any relief of symptoms for a patient with low back problems. Abdominal exercises and stretching provide the most relief to a patient suffering from mechanical low back pain. Occasionally, massage, hot packs and ultrasound are also

useful in resolving symptoms. Reduced weight-bearing walking exercises in an aquatic program or in a harness suspension on land have been shown to reduce symptoms and improve exercise tolerance (Fritz et al 1997, Simotas 2001). It is important to remember that the patient with spinal stenosis has concomitant degenerative changes and, thus, a therapeutic exercise program should be individualized. This program may include postural retraining and overall strengthening and conditioning (Bodack & Monteiro 2001).

History and differential diagnosis

A medical history is very important because back pain can result from pathologies in other structures such as the aorta (especially aneurysm), kidney, bowel, uterus or prostate (*Merck Manual of Geriatrics* 2000, Kesson & Atkins 2005). When a patient experiences an acute onset of low back pain, a compression fracture or neoplasm must be considered. Plain radiographs and laboratory tests should differentiate the two abnormalities.

Unexplained loss of weight and pain without cause may raise a suspicion of cancer. Multiple myeloma is a neoplastic disorder involving immature plasma cells in bone marrow. It often produces back or rib pain. Non-Hodgkin's lymphoma may also involve bone (*Merck Manual of Geriatrics* 2000). Metastatic bone disease from primary breast or prostate cancers is frequently found in the lumbar spine and may present in a variety of ways. Metastasis from colon cancer is less common but can occur (Lurie et al 2000). Neoplastic bone pain is usually a boring pain that often wakes the patient at night; rest does not relieve the pain. These symptoms are significant in a patient with a history of cancer (Kesson & Atkins 2005). Weakness and fatigue may also be reported.

Osteomyelitis, diskitis and other spinal infections must be ruled out, especially because radiographic evidence of degenerative changes is common in the aging spine, as noted previously (see Chapter 14). Lurie and associates (2000) presented the case of an 80-year-old man with noted arthritic changes in the spine and hip, including severe spinal stenosis. Treatment with rest and medications, including codeine, was ineffective. The patient had a decompressive laminectomy without relief of his symptoms. After further workup and sound clinical reasoning, the patient was started on intravenous antibiotics for a spine infection, which rendered a gradual improvement. It should be noted that spinal infections mimic back pain and radicular complaints but they do not always present with typical features of infection. Fortunately, spinal infections are not common, accounting for about 0.01% of cases in primary care (Lurie et al 2000).

OSTEOMALACIA

Osteomalacia is a bone disease that involves the failure of newly formed or remodeling bone to mineralize, which results in an excess of unmineralized bone matrix (osteoid). Osteomalacia refers to the adult form of this condition; rickets is the same disease process but it specifically targets the epiphysis in the growing skeleton (Pitt 1991). Osteomalacia results from inadequate or delayed mineralization of mature cortical and spongy bone; this occurs because of the loss, altered intake or altered metabolism of 1,25-dihydroxyvitamin D3 (vitamin D3) and phosphate (*Merck Manual of Geriatrics* 2000).

The gross histopathological and radiological abnormalities of osteomalacia are the common result of a number of different diseases. In general, osteomalacia is considered to be most commonly caused by altered metabolism of vitamin D3 or phosphate or both, a condition for which the elderly population is at particular risk.

Recent advances in the understanding of the biochemistry of vitamin D3 metabolism have provided new insight into this condition. In developed countries, elderly individuals, particularly the housebound or institutionalized, are vulnerable to osteomalacia.

In general, vitamin D3 deficiency occurs in those whose vitamin D3 intake is close to zero and who, in addition, have minimal or no exposure to ultraviolet radiation. Vitamin D3 deficiency may be caused by an inadequate intake of vitamin D3 or by defective intestinal absorption of vitamin D3, as is observed in malabsorption syndromes such as jejunoileal bypass. In addition, there may be an age-related diminished response of the intestine to vitamin D3. In normal individuals, the main source of vitamin D3 is dermal synthesis. There is an age-related decrease in the dermal synthesis of 7-dehydrocholesterol, the precursor of vitamin D3. A deficiency can also occur if there is a defect in vitamin D3 metabolism. Most diseases are not caused by simple vitamin D3 deficiency but involve abnormal production or regulation of its synthesis in the liver or kidneys. The ultimate consequence is the inability to produce sufficient quantities of this vitamin.

Renal disorders are the main cause of difficulty in metabolizing phosphate. When phosphate depletion is a causative factor for osteomalacia, the serum phosphorus is markedly depressed. In osteomalacic patients, it is common to find very low plasma phosphate levels. Alimentary phosphate deficiency is additionally aggravated by vitamin D3 deficiency. Vitamin D3 promotes jejunal phosphate absorption and renal phosphate reabsorption. Disorders that affect phosphate absorption in the intestines or reabsorption in the kidneys include certain conditions for which large amounts of phosphate-binding antacids have been administered. This is of particular importance considering that these agents may be employed to manage other age-related disorders such as osteoporosis (Pitt 1991, *Merck Manual of Geriatrics* 2000).

Patients may have vague generalized bone pain, multiple fractures, thoracic kyphosis and loss of height because of multiple vertebral compression fractures, and deformity of the lower limbs because of the malunion or bowing associated with pseudofractures. Osteomalacia can affect bone turnover to the extent that fractures occur in situations that otherwise might constitute only a minimal to moderate impact stress. Lumbar scoliosis may develop because of the altered biconcave shape of affected vertebral bodies. The patient may complain of generalized bone pain of a dull aching nature and muscle weakness, particularly in the proximal muscle groups in the lower extremities (also referred to as pelvic girdle myopathy) and back. This diffuse skeletal pain is typically exacerbated by physical activity and tenderness may be elicited by palpation. Muscle weakness is a common accompaniment to prolonged vitamin D3 deficiency, although the mechanism is unknown. A characteristic waddling gait manifests with this condition and generalized muscle atrophy may be evident. Functional activities such as climbing stairs and ambulation may become difficult, making requisite the use of gait aids for support. In the extreme case, the composite presentation of weakness and muscle atrophy, skeletal deformities and fracture incidence may even lead the affected individual to become wheelchair-bound or bedridden (Lyles et al 1995, *Merck Manual of Geriatrics* 2000).

In most cases, the stereotypical presentation of osteomalacia can be cured or at least improved with appropriate therapy for the specific underlying abnormality. Although there may be different underlying causes of this skeletal disorder, most signs and symptoms resolve with supplementation of vitamin D3, which aims to restore plasma calcium and phosphate levels to normal. Bone pain should disappear promptly. Concurrent with appropriate pharmacological therapy, physical management strategies should include postural and peripheral muscle strengthening exercises and gait retraining in order to attain maximal functional status. There are no apparent contraindications, but sound judgment should be used and proper precautions taken when treating a patient who has osteomalacia with ultrasound, electrical stimulation, heat or cold, or when loading the bone with weight-bearing and resistive exercises.

PAGET'S DISEASE OF THE BONE

Paget's disease, also known as osteitis deformans, is a common bone disorder among the elderly; it rarely affects people below the age of 40. Approximately 60% of those affected with this condition are male. Paget's disease is a chronic asymmetrical focal bone disease that features increased osteoclastic bone resorption and aberrant secondary osteoblastic bone formation.

Paget's disease is more prevalent in people with northern European ancestry; it is common in the United Kingdom as well as in western Europe, Australia and New Zealand, but is rare in Scandinavia, Asia and Africa. The incidence of Paget's disease in North America appears to be comparable to that of Europe, with prevalence ranging from 1% to 3% of adults over 40 years of age (Papapoulos 1997).

The overall structure of the bone demonstrates a mosaic pattern in which packets of bone are laid down subsequent to a phase of osteoclastic bone resorption. The bone that becomes enclosed in individual packets consists of true woven bone as well as lamellar bone. There is marked net bone formation, which is essentially normal. Bone biopsy remains important for the differentiation between malignancy and the pagetic bone (*Merck Manual of Geriatrics* 2000).

Unlike osteomalacia, radiographs and bone scans are definitive in revealing an active disease process in Paget's disease, so these methods are useful in making a diagnosis. The typically focal nature of Paget's disease and the extent of spread in individual bones makes the bone scan useful in differentiating Paget's disease from other bone diseases, including metastatic carcinoma. A bone scan demonstrates an increased uptake of isotopes at diseased sites, reflecting the activity of bone formation.

Specific patterns of radiographic changes are featured in Paget's disease. A typical presentation includes radiolucent areas of patchy arrangement that indicate increased bone resorption, as well as evidence of regional bone formation processes represented by cortical and cancellous thickening and sclerosis, and uneven widths of affected bones. Patchy areas of resorption typical of Paget's disease are referred to as osteoporosis circumscripta. In the pelvis, there may be evidence of sclerosis along the iliopectineal line. In the vertebrae, cortical thickening and expansion are characteristic but this appearance may be difficult to distinguish from osteoblastic metastasis, which occurs without cortical thickening. In pagetic bone, neoplastic changes occur in less than 1% of cases but osteosarcoma is associated with Paget's disease in the elderly. In addition, fibrosarcoma and chondrosarcoma may occur (*Merck Manual of Geriatrics* 2000).

Clinical presentation

Approximately 90% of individuals affected by Paget's disease are asymptomatic. Diagnosis is usually made by reports of bone pain or deformity, radiography or inadvertent detection of elevated serum alkaline phosphatase levels upon routine biochemical testing. The most common complaints reported are pain, skeletal deformity and changes in skin temperature. Other clinical manifestations include diminished mobility and unsteady gait; in more severe cases of Paget's disease, pathological fractures may manifest. The major clinical features are outlined in Table 26.1.

Bone pain is often nocturnal and is thought to be the result of increased pressure on the periosteum or associated hyperemia.

Table 26.1 Major clinical features of advanced Paget's disease

Bones	Clinical features
Skull	Headaches, deafness, expanded skull size, cranial palsies
Facial bones	Deformity, dental problems
Vertebrae	Root compression, cord compression
Long bones	Deformity determined by stresses to bone, e.g. bowing of tibia (anterior) or femur (lateral); secondary osteoarthritis; incremental fissure fractures; excessive operative bleeding
General	Bone pain; malaise; immobility; deformity; bone sarcoma; heat over affected bones; high-output cardiac failure

From Anderson & Richardson (1992), with permission.

Other causes of pain may be nerve root compression or nerve entrapment if the diseased bone involves a nerve foramen or canal. The deep-rooted pain of Paget's disease is often unresponsive to simple analgesics and is more likely to be experienced when at rest than during movement. The efficacy of physical modalities in treating pagetic pain is unclear and is best applied on an individual basis. Mixed sensorineural and conductive hearing loss is a common clinical manifestation of Paget's disease. Auditory nerve compression occurs when Paget's disease involves the petrous temporal bone, and encroachment on the internal auditory meatus may cause compression of cranial nerve VIII, leading to hearing loss. Conduction deafness may result from otosclerosis or indirect involvement of the cochlea or ossicles and is also a common finding in patients with Paget's disease. Other cranial nerves may be affected as well. It is rare to find an extensive enough narrowing of the spinal canal to compromise the spinal cord (Anderson & Richardson 1992).

Because of abnormal bone remodeling processes inherent in the progression of Paget's disease, bone architecture becomes distorted in patients in the advanced stages of disease. Deformity develops in a slow and progressive manner, depending on the bone site affected. It appears that weight-bearing exacerbates the development of deformities, and pathological fractures occur most commonly in the long weight-bearing bones of the lower extremities (in the femoral neck and the subtrochanteric and tibial regions). An increase in skull size, lateral bowing of the long bones (especially the tibia, femur and humerus) and dorsal kyphosis are typical deformities in the Paget's patient. Lyles et al (1995) showed that, when compared with age- and gender-matched controls, patients with Paget's disease of the bone involving the tibia, femur or acetabular portion of the ilium demonstrated clinically and statistically significant functional and mobility impairments determined by the time taken to walk 10 feet (3.05 m), the number of steps taken to complete a 360° turn and the distance walked in 6 min.

CONCLUSION

Common disorders of the thoracic and lumbosacral spine are the result of osteoporosis and degenerative changes. However, the cause of the patient's complaints must be investigated with appropriate laboratory and radiographic studies because other bone disorders as well as metastatic disease and visceral problems may present as acute back pain.

In most cases, it is extremely important that patients with any kind of spinal disorder be mobilized as quickly as possible, in order to prevent further osteopenia because of disuse. Attempts should be made to provide appropriate assistive devices so that patients can be ambulatory as soon as possible, and rehabilitation interventions must be individualized.

References

Amundsen T, Weber H, Nordal H et al 2000 Lumbar spinal stenosis: conservative or surgical management? A prospective 10-year study. Spine 25:1424–1436

Anderson DC, Richardson PC 1992 Paget's disease of bone. In: Brocklehurst JC, Tallis RC, Fillit UM (eds) Textbook of Geriatrics and Gerontology. Churchill Livingstone, New York, p 783–791

Badley E 1987 Epidemiological aspects of the ageing spine. In: Hulkins D, Nelson M (eds) The Ageing Spine. Manchester University Press, Manchester, UK, p 1–18

Bodack M, Monteiro M 2001 Therapeutic exercises in the treatment of patients with spinal stenosis. Clin Ortho 384:144–152

Edmonds S, Kiel D, Samelson E et al 2005 Vertebral deformity, back symptoms, and functional limitations among older women: the Framingham Study. Osteoporos Int 16:1086–1095

Fritz J, Erhard R, Vignovic M 1997 A nonsurgical treatment approach for patients with lumbar spinal stenosis. Phys Ther 77:962–973

Grasland A, Pouchot J, Mathieu A et al 1996 Sacral insufficiency fractures. Arch Intern Med 156:668–674

Harrison KA 1986 Metastatic disease of the spine. J Bone Joint Surg Am 68:1110–1115

Herno A, Partanen K, Talaslahti T et al 1999 Long-term clinical and magnetic resonance imaging follow-up assessment of patients with lumbar spinal stenosis after laminectomy. Spine 24:1533–1537

Kesson M, Atkins E 2005 Orthopaedic Medicine: A Practical Approach. Elsevier, Oxford, p 325–352, 515–576

Lane JM 1997 Osteoporosis: medical prevention and treatment. Spine 22(24S):325–375

Lurie J, Gerber P, Sox H 2000 A pain in the back. N Engl J Med 343:723–726

Lyles K, Lammers J, Shipp K et al 1995 Functional and mobility impairments associated with Paget's disease of bone. J Am Geriatr Soc 43:502–506

Merck Manual of Geriatrics 2000 Merck Research Laboratories, Whitehouse Station, NJ

Papapoulos WE 1997 Paget's disease of bone: clinical, pathogenetic and therapeutic aspects. Baillieres Clin Endocrinol Metab 11:117–143

Pfeifer D, Begerow B, Minnie H 2004 Effects of a new spinal orthosis on posture, trunk strength, and quality of life in women with postmenopausal osteoporosis: a randomized trial. Am J Phys Med Rehabil 83:177–186

Pitt M 1991 Rickets and osteomalacia are still around. Radiol Clin North Am 29:97–118

Reeg S 2001 A review of comorbidities and spinal surgery. Clin Orthop 384:101–109

Simotas A 2001 Nonoperative treatment for lumbar spinal stenosis. Clin Orthop 384:153–161

Chapter 27

Orthopedic trauma

P. Christopher Metzger, Mark Lombardi and E. Frederick Barrick

INTRODUCTION

As the number of elderly people continues to increase, musculoskeletal injuries can be expected to become more prevalent and have a profound effect on both society and its healthcare system. Today, more than ever, many geriatric patients lead active and productive lives. Unfortunately, such a lifestyle can be dramatically changed by an inadvertent slip or fall that causes an orthopedic injury. This chapter focuses on the rehabilitation of such orthopedic injuries in the geriatric population.

Rehabilitation may be defined as the restoration of normal form and function after an injury or an illness (Dirckx 2001). What is meant by 'normal form and function' varies from individual to individual. A reasonable goal in the injured patient is to return them to their preinjury activities.

The American Academy of Orthopedic Surgeons (2005) has suggested that, by the year 2050, there will be an estimated 650 000 hip fractures annually in the US. At a cost of US$26 912 per patient, these injuries represent a staggering economic burden. Only 25% of these patients will make a full recovery, 30% will require nursing-home care and 50% will need either a cane or a walker. Within approximately 1 year, 30% of these elderly patients will die (Moran & Wenn 2005). Data from Europe indicate that hip fractures are a similarly serious problem (Lippuner et al 2005). Such statistics point out the need for expert and efficient musculoskeletal care.

The goal of fracture care in this age group is early mobilization and restoration of function. Lengthy periods of inactivity increase the risk of deep vein thrombosis, pressure ulcers and pulmonary complications such as pneumonia. Surgical intervention, when necessary, is best carried out within the first 48 h after injury, providing the patient is medically stable. Both the orthopedic surgeon and the physical therapist must understand that there may be a decline in the capacity for healing in the geriatric population.

BASIC PRINCIPLES FOR REHABILITATION

The goals of rehabilitation are to: (i) control and reduce inflammation, (ii) restore motion, (iii) regain strength, (iv) develop motor control and coordination, and (v) restore function. The rehabilitation process in pelvic or lower extremity injuries is begun by mobilizing the patient. This consists of getting the individual out of bed into a chair and is followed by ambulation with external support (cane, crutches or walker). At the same time, joint mobility and flexibility must be restored. This is accomplished with both active and passive range-of-motion exercises for the joints involved. As both mobility and range of motion are regained, emphasis must be placed on reacquiring motor control and coordination.

It is desirable to start mobilization as soon as the patient's medical condition permits. Learning to ambulate with either crutches or a walker in a reduced weight-bearing fashion is a challenge to most people. The amount of energy required to perform limited weight-bearing is 30–50% greater than that required for normal ambulation. This added demand could be particularly taxing for elderly individuals, especially if they have a decreased cardiopulmonary reserve.

In upper extremity injuries, patient mobilization is usually not as difficult to attain. The only necessary instructions may be to keep the arm elevated and to educate the patient on how to get in and out of bed and chairs without putting pressure on the injured extremity. In general, severe injuries, or those with upper and lower extremity involvement, pose a greater obstacle to mobilization. In such instances, initial attention may have to be focused on simple transfers from bed to chair because ambulation may not be possible. The use of adaptive equipment, such as forearm supports on assistive devices, may prove to be necessary. The geriatric patient may already have some preexisting impairment of mobility that has to be taken into consideration. The goal of rehabilitation is to get the patient back to their preinjury status, if at all possible.

MOTION

One of the therapist's responsibilities is to instruct and assist the patient in the restoration of range of motion after injury. At all times, the physician should communicate with the therapist regarding any precautions or restrictions. Such communication should take place on a regular basis and must always be documented.

MOTOR CONTROL AND COORDINATION

Motor control is necessary before any active exercise can begin or progress. Sometimes, electrical stimulation is needed to activate muscles that demonstrate atrophy or painful muscle guarding. Coordination is crucial to motor control. It involves smooth and accurate movement of the joints in the kinetic chain. The timing and sequencing of the movement of ipsilateral and contralateral joints requires neural control and musculoskeletal integrity. For example, a humeral fracture that disrupts the coordinated movement of the involved arm also reduces the contralateral arm swing during normal reciprocal gait. Proper breathing, decreased muscular guarding and reduced abnormal flexor and adductor tones facilitate coordination.

STRENGTHENING

When some degree of comfortable motion and muscle control are obtained, strengthening can be started. Increased strength often results in increased motion. It has been shown that age is no barrier to regaining or even increasing strength.

An effective method of strengthening is progressive resistance exercise (PRE). One such technique exercises each muscle group with enough weight (resistance) to allow 20–30 repetitions. Once 30 repetitions can be achieved, the resistance is increased and the progression of repetitions from 20 to 30 is repeated. Another method involves the patient completing three sets of 10–15 repetitions, decreasing the weights with each set, or three sets using the same weight but decreasing the number of repetitions (from 20 to 15 to 10).

ADAPTATION

At some point during rehabilitation it may become evident that there will be some permanent functional limitation or disability. Changes in anatomy, and consequently in function, may force changes in the patent's lifestyle. In order to adapt to these changes, different training techniques or equipment may be needed. These needs may be apparent early in the rehabilitation period if, for instance, there has been a major amputation. In other cases, it may become evident later in the course of rehabilitation that permanent loss of joint motion or strength is inevitable and that compensation during work or play is required.

The ability to restore some form of useful activity in the involved extremity is one of the primary goals of rehabilitation, although it may not always be attainable. It may be that the patient will need to adjust to a more sedentary lifestyle or pursue activities that are less physically demanding. Learning to accept these limitations is part of regaining a meaningful life.

TREATMENT OF OSTEOPOROSIS

One of the major contributing factors to the occurrence of musculoskeletal injuries is osteoporosis. Osteoporosis is a systemic disorder that is characterized by decreased bone mass and an increased vulnerability to pathological fractures. Fractures in osteoporotic bone occur most frequently in the metaphyseal region. In total, 50% of women and 18% of men older than 50 will sustain an osteoporotic

fracture (Cornell 2003). Treatment of this problem must be part of comprehensive fracture care.

Bone mineral density testing should be performed on all patients over the age of 50 to rule out osteoporosis and, if necessary, an appropriate treatment regimen initiated to minimize further bone loss. Calcium supplementation and adequate vitamin D intake are necessary for all patients with osteoporosis. If possible, regular physical activity, including weight-bearing and resistance exercise, may also be helpful.

REHABILITATION AFTER SPECIFIC INJURIES

Fractures of the proximal humerus

A fall onto the outstretched hand is the most common mechanism of injury for fractures of the proximal humerus. This is a frequently encountered injury in the elderly population. Fortunately, the great majority of these fractures are either nondisplaced or minimally displaced and can be treated by sling and swathe immobilization for 10–14 days followed by gentle range of motion exercises. Elbow flexion and extension, forearm pronation and forearm supination can be started during the period of immobilization. Prior to initiating the exercise program for the shoulder, clinical continuity (the fracture moves as a single unit) must be present. If the fracture is unstable, as is often the case when there is considerable comminution and displacement, an open reduction with internal fixation may lead to better range of motion, improved strength and a superior functional outcome. A humeral head prosthesis is often indicated for displaced four-part fractures of the proximal humerus.

If there is stability at the fracture site, passive and active assisted range of motion is started very early. This consists of pendulum exercises (Codman) and supine external glenohumeral rotation with a stick. About 3–4 weeks after the fracture has occurred, active-assisted forward elevation, pulley exercise, extension and isometrics can be added. After this first phase has been completed, active and early resistive exercises become important. Therabands are often used to strengthen the shoulder rotators and deltoid muscle. A program that emphasizes further stretching and strengthening is appropriate 3 months after a fracture.

It is important in the early stages of fracture healing for the patient to avoid using the affected arm when getting into and out of bed or a chair. Such actions can displace the fracture even when there has been stable internal fixation. Displacement is more likely to occur in the patient with multiple injuries or with limited cognitive capabilities. Throughout the entire rehabilitation program, the therapist should be working with and assessing functional mobility of the neck, scapula, elbow, wrist and hand. Most patients with fractures of the proximal humerus do obtain satisfactory results; however, it must be understood that usually there is some resultant loss of motion and strength. Complications include malunion, nonunion, delayed union and loss of motion.

Fractures of the distal radius

Fractures of the distal radius account for up to 16% of all fractures in adults, with women seven times more likely to be affected than men (Newport 2000). The most common musculoskeletal injury of the upper extremity in the geriatric population is a displaced fracture of the distal radius. Such fractures usually occur after a fall on an outstretched hand. A Colles' fracture involves the distal radial metaphysis, which becomes dorsally angulated and displaced. Often, the fracture is comminuted and involves the articular surface. A Smith's fracture demonstrates volar angulation of the distal radius whereas a Barton's fracture is a shear fracture (dislocation with displacement of the rim of the distal radius).

Treatment options for these fractures include simple cast immobilization, closed reduction with casting or external fixation and open reduction with internal fixation. The possible complications that may result from this particular type of fracture include delayed union, nonunion, malunion, median nerve compression, tendon damage, arthritic flares and loss of motion.

Restoration of motion and strength, which leads to improved function, is of vital importance in the rehabilitation of wrist fractures. After appropriate consultation with the attending physician, range of motion and strengthening exercises for areas of the upper extremities that are not immobilized should be initiated immediately, if possible, to prevent residual stiffness in the shoulder, elbow and hand. Once immobilization is no longer necessary, active-assisted and active exercises are encouraged in all six directions – flexion, extension, radial and ulnar deviation, pronation and supination. Modalities such as hydrotherapy, electrical stimulation, heat, cold or ultrasound may be helpful. Depending upon the status of fracture healing and the amount of joint stiffness, the therapist may incorporate specific mobilization techniques to increase the range of motion. The initiation of muscle control and coordination may be difficult when motion is painful. In addition to addressing the inflammatory process, which causes pain and swelling, the therapist should attend to the head, neck and trunk posture, which may contribute to the patient's discomfort and limitations of movement. As range of motion in the wrist increases, strengthening activities using motion against resistance should be included in the treatment plan. The final goal should be to restore range of motion and strength of the injured hand and wrist to preinjury levels. Unfortunately, this is not always possible and some degree of impairment may remain.

Intertrochanteric fractures

An intertrochanteric fracture occurs along a line that is located between the greater and lesser trochanters. These fractures are seen most commonly in the elderly and are usually the result of a fall. The goal of treatment for this particular type of fracture should be to restore the patient to his or her preinjury status as quickly as possible. Whenever possible, operative treatment is indicated for rapid mobilization, ease of nursing care, shorter hospitalization, decreased mortality and restoration of function.

Open reduction with internal fixation using either a compression hip screw or an intramedullary device is the treatment of choice. Ideally, the surgery should be performed within the first 48 h following the fracture. The success of the surgical procedure largely depends upon: (i) bone quality, (ii) fracture pattern, (iii) accuracy of the reduction, and (iv) the adequacy of internal fixation.

The major goal of rehabilitation after an intertrochanteric fracture is to enable the patient to walk, especially if they were ambulatory prior to the injury. Mobilizing the patient is best begun immediately following surgery. Range of motion exercises are encouraged as soon as the initial pain subsides and the patient can safely cooperate with the physical therapist. Range of motion in all directions is advised, to prevent flexion or adduction contractures that can make ambulation more difficult. Getting the patient to a level where they can control the involved limb is essential to permit adequate mobility in bed and prevent the onset of pressure ulcers, and to allow for independent transfers into and out of bed. Balance and coordination instructions are given concurrently with all phases of ambulation.

Usually the patient should get out of bed and transfer to a chair on the day following surgery. With intertrochanteric fractures, protective weight-bearing is often necessary. The weight-bearing status is determined by the accuracy and stability of the reduction achieved at the time of surgery, bone quality, premorbid status and mental alertness. An alert patient can understand the concept of limited weight-bearing and thus behave appropriately. A patient who is not strong enough to manage partial weight-bearing or not coherent enough to understand the therapist's instructions may be limited to a wheelchair and/or pre-gait activities, such as sit-to-stand and static stance with weight shift, until they are stronger or until the fracture has healed sufficiently to permit unrestricted weight-bearing. Early assisted swing (slide) phase of gait of the involved leg may be helpful in facilitating proper weight-bearing and restoration of functional gait in the future. This is achieved with the patient standing in the parallel bars or with a walker and simply sliding the foot of the involved leg forward and backward or lifting the involved leg over a low obstacle (cane, cup or cone) that is placed on the floor in front of the patient.

Strengthening the hip abductors gradually reduces the Trendelenburg gait pattern commonly seen following a hip fracture. Progressive resistance exercises are used, starting with abduction while standing or the use of a sliding board while supine. As strength increases, the patient is instructed to perform the exercises while lying on the contralateral side, thus abducting against gravity. Coexisting musculoskeletal and cardiovascular conditions may necessitate modification of these positions. Once 20–30 repetitions can be performed, progressive resistance is added. Strengthening for flexors, extensors, rotators and adductors is also important.

After the fracture heals and rehabilitation is complete, occasional decreased mobility may be the end result. Patient adaptation may involve having to accept the permanent use of a cane or a walker to aid in balance, reduce the Trendelenburg deviation that is associated with weak abductors and increase both patient safety and mobility. The patient with an intertrochanteric fracture should be expected to transfer and ambulate independently before being discharged home. If this is not possible, placement in an assisted-living facility or a nursing home may be necessary.

Femoral neck fractures

Femoral neck fractures occur most commonly in the eighth decade of life as a result of bone that is weakened by either osteoporosis or osteomalacia. The most common mechanisms of injury are either a fall that causes a direct blow to the greater trochanter or forced lateral rotation of the lower extremity (Rockwood et al 1996). If a fracture is displaced, the arterial supply to the most proximal end of the femur may be disrupted allowing either a nonunion or avascular necrosis to develop. Thus, many orthopedic surgeons choose to treat displaced femoral neck fractures by performing a hemiarthroplasty (replacement of the femoral head and neck with a prosthesis).

If a posterior surgical approach is used when the hemiarthroplasty is performed, caution must be used for the first month to prevent hip dislocation. A dislocation may occur with the combination of excessive hip flexion, adduction and internal rotation. The avoidance of this position in the early postoperative period is imperative. Safety measures must also be taken when patients are putting on their stockings and shoes as well as when they are recumbent in bed or sitting upright. In cases in which the stability of the prosthesis is in question, an abduction pillow is extremely helpful. These patients should also be instructed to sit in a leanback chair so that the hip is flexed no more than 90°. In most cases, when a prosthesis is inserted, a graduated weight-bearing program is indicated.

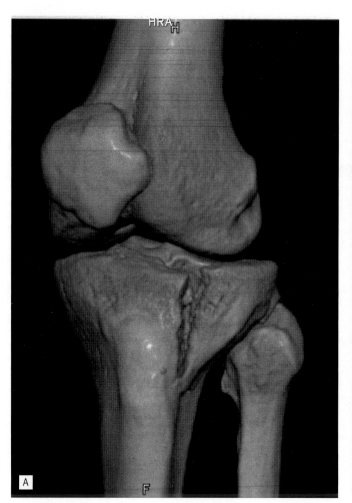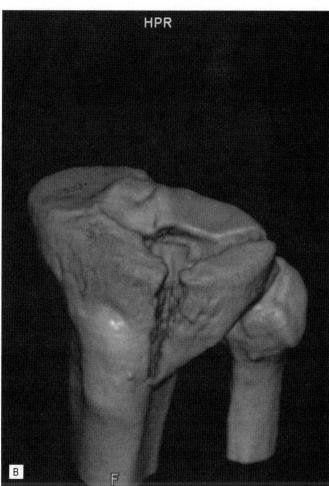

Figure 27.1   (A) Computerized tomography demonstrating the split component of a lateral tibial plateau fracture. (B) The same study showing significant depression of the lateral tibial plateau.

Supracondylar fractures of the distal femur

The supracondylar region of the distal femur is often weakened by osteoporosis and even low energy forces can create complex fracture patterns. The resulting fractures are often comminuted, displaced and intra-articular, making management quite difficult. Earlier forms of treatment consisted of traction and cast bracing, which often resulted in loss of joint motion. More recent internal fixation techniques often allow for an anatomical reconstruction of the osseous structures, more rigid internal fixation and earlier patient mobilization, allowing for improved range of motion and function.

If rigid internal fixation has been achieved at the time of surgery, the use of a continuous passive motion machine is advised. This encourages increased knee motion, less postoperative swelling and reduces the incidence of quadriceps adhesions. For the first 6 weeks, partial weight-bearing (up to 15 lbs (6.75 kg) of body weight) with a walker is allowed only if stable fixation is present. At the 6-week point, weight-bearing can be gradually increased if there is radiographic evidence of progressive fracture healing. Full weight-bearing with external support is often possible at 12 weeks. In instances in which stable fixation has not been achieved, supplemental support with a cast brace may be necessary.

The same principles that govern motor control, coordination, strengthening and adaptation in fractures of the proximal femur apply to fractures of the distal femur. In addition, attention to distal lower extremity pain, weakness and decreased range of motion will be required.

Fractures of the tibial plateau

The split depression is the most common fracture of the lateral tibial plateau in patients with osteoporosis (Cornell 2003) (Fig. 27.1). Such injuries result from a strong valgus force that is coupled with axial loading. Often, there may be an accompanying injury to the medial collateral ligament. The hallmarks of treatment for this particular type of intra-articular fracture are early range of motion and delayed weight-bearing.

In nondisplaced fractures or those with less than 5 mm of depression, nonoperative treatment is recommended (Cornell 2003). Initially, a hinged knee brace, locked in full extension, is applied. The brace is adjusted 2 weeks after injury to allow gentle range of motion exercises. Weight-bearing is delayed for 6–12 weeks, depending upon the amount of comminution and the rate of radiographic healing.

In fractures in which there is more than 5 mm of depression of the articular surface, an open reduction with internal fixation is indicated if the patient is medically stable. Often, supplemental bone grafting may be necessary in the face of a significant metaphyseal defect. When stable internal fixation has been achieved, the use of a continuous passive-motion exercise machine is indicated. As with nondisplaced fractures, weight-bearing is delayed by 6–12 weeks.

Complications of tibial plateau fractures include non-union, delayed union, malunion, post-traumatic arthritis and loss of motion. Rehabilitation should emphasize pain control, restoration of strength and range of motion and a return to preinjury status.

Compression fractures of the spine

As with other fractures in the elderly, osteoporosis plays a major role in compression fractures of the vertebral body. Compression fractures are more commonly seen in women than in men. Often compression fractures occur as a result of a fall on the buttocks; however, sometimes the patient does not give a history of trauma. Initial treatment generally consists of rest and mild analgesics. Once the pain begins to subside, the patient is encouraged to start moving. Physical therapy intervention should concentrate on increasing the patient's knowledge of safety, posture, transfers, performance of activities of daily living and ambulation. Great care is taken to avoid forceful flexion as this often duplicates the mechanism of injury. Gentle extension and exercises of the trunk are useful in attaining patient mobility. Postural exercises should include activities of the shoulder and scapulae to ensure overall strengthening and spinal stability. Occasionally, wearing either a lumbar or thoracolumbar support may be helpful.

CONCLUSION

The aging baby boomer population, together with the increased life expectancy seen today, will most certainly result in an increase in the number of musculoskeletal injuries. Excellent and efficient orthopedic care will become more important with the passing of time. Such care will enable patients to attain the highest possible level of function and satisfaction.

References

American Academy of Orthopedic Surgeons 2005 Falls and hip fractures. Available: http://www.orthoinfo.aaos.org/fact/thr_report.cfm?Thread_ID=77&topcategory=Hip. Accessed 16 Nov 2005

Cornell CH 2003 Internal fracture fixation in patients with osteoporosis. J Am Acad Orthop Surg 2(2):109–119

Dirckx JH (ed) 2001 Stedman's Concise Medical Dictionary for the Health Professions, 4th edn. Lippincott Williams & Wilkins, Philadelphia, PA

Lippuner K, Hauselmann HJ, Szucs TD 2005 A model of osteoporosis impact in Switzerland 2000–2020. Osteoporos Int 16(6):659–671

Moran CG, Wenn RT 2005 Early mortality after hip fracture: is delay before surgery important? J Bone Joint Surg Am 87(3):483–489

Newport ML 2000 Upper extremity disorders in women. Clin Orthop Related Res 372:85–94

Rockwood CA, Green DP, Bucholz RW, Heckman JD 1996 Rockwood & Green's Fractures in Adults, 4th edn. Lippincott-Raven, Philadelphia, PA

UNIT 3

Neuromuscular and neurological disorders

Chapter 28

Neurological trauma

Dennis W. Klima

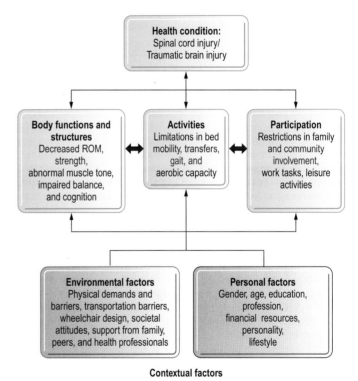

Figure 28.1 International Classification of Functioning, Disability, and Health: spinal cord injury and traumatic brain injury. ROM, range of motion.

INTRODUCTION

A key component of geriatric rehabilitation includes the management of older patients who have sustained neurological trauma to the brain or spinal cord. Therapists must consider the impact of these injuries along with adjacent neural changes that occur during the aging process. Management of older patients with both spinal cord and traumatic brain injuries requires the integration of musculoskeletal, neuromuscular and cognitive interventions to enable them to effectively progress towards established goals.

A thorough history must first be obtained from the patient or family to ascertain the previous level of function. A systems review will further corroborate any changes in physical status, affect and cognition that have occurred following the sustained injury. Selected tests and measures typically combine traditional examination activities along with instruments specifically geared towards patients with traumatic brain injury (TBI) or spinal cord injury (SCI). A summative evaluation will then be formulated, along with an appropriate rehabilitation diagnosis and prognosis. With both TBI and SCI patient populations, the rehabilitation diagnosis is influenced by a multitude of mitigating factors such as age-related changes in organ systems, as well as injury complications such as heterotopic ossificans and autonomic nervous system dysfunction.

The World Health Organization enablement model (ICFDH-2) illustrates how both TBI and SCI affect an older patient's ability to perform functional tasks and participate in community-related activities and employment (Fig. 28.1) (Australian Institute of Health and Welfare 2002). Strategic functional mobility interventions are implemented to address all established goals within the body structure/function, activity and participation domains. Outcomes may be measured through a variety of instruments including the Functional Independence Measure, or FIM, which has shown appropriate psychometric support for patients with both spinal cord and traumatic brain injury (Corrigan et al 1997).

TRAUMATIC BRAIN INJURY

Over one million people sustain a TBI each year in the USA and approximately 80 000–90 000 individuals will have a lifelong disability secondary to their injury (Thurman et al 1999). The leading cause of TBI for those aged 65 or older is a fall-related episode (Brain Injury Association of America 2005). TBI accounts for one-third of all injury-related deaths in the USA; individuals between the ages of 15 and 24 or those over 75 years of age demonstrate the greatest risk for a TBI (Thurman et al 1999, Brain Injury Association of Amercia 2005). TBI is the principal cause of seizure disorders worldwide, and the World Health Organization adapted criteria for head injury surveillance in 1993.

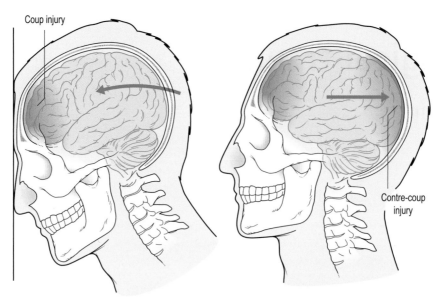

Figure 28.2   Coup and contre-coup injuries following traumatic brain injury.
Reprinted with permission from Klima D 2006, Clients with traumatic brain injury.
In: Umphred D, Carlson C (eds) Neurohabilitation for the Physical Therapist Assistant.
Slack, Thorofare, NJ. Illustration by Tim Phelps, CMI.

Head injury sequelae can be devastating for a geriatric client and affect nearly every component of the quality of life including self-care, employment and leisure activities. Poor recovery outcomes may warrant institutional placement if caregiving demands exceed available resources in the home environment. Fall prevention strategies for older clients are essential in preventing head injury. Geriatric individuals generally sustain falls secondary to either intrinsic or extrinsic causes. For example, intrinsic causes include sensory changes or vestibular pathology that impede effective balance modulation. Environmental barriers and obstacles resulting in trips and slips are included in the extrinsic category. Appropriate balance measures such as the Berg Balance Scale (Berg 1992) or performance-oriented mobility assessment (Tinetti 1986) can assist in identifying those clients most at risk for falling.

Head injuries may be characterized as either open or closed; open head injuries involve open penetration to the skull. The initial site of impact following a traumatic insult to the brain is known as the coup injury. A rebound effect often occurs in the cranium following the initial impact and causes a contre-coup injury (Fig. 28.2). Patients may also sustain additional complications because of skull fractures or hematomas. Skull fractures vary from relatively nonthreatening simple linear fractures to those with extensive comminuting fragments that require cranioplasty procedures (Fig. 28.3). Additionally, patients can incur complications such as internal organ damage or both spinal and extremity fractures. Patients may undergo extensive intensive care monitoring because of uncontrolled intracranial pressure or resultant seizure activity.

Initial trauma assessments are performed using the Glasgow Coma Scale. Composed of three divisions, this instrument assesses three areas of function in individuals following head injury: motor performance, eye opening and verbal response (Table 28.1) (Teasdale & Jennett 1974). Scores from 13 to 15 designate mild injury; from 9 to 12, moderate injury; and from 3 to 8, severe TBI. The rehabilitation team members should be aware of the initial Glasgow score and subsequent complications at the time of injury so that any examination or intervention activities can be adjusted. Patients who demonstrate a better medical prognosis include those with less loss of consciousness and post-traumatic amnesia immediately following their injury (Evans 1998).

Interventions for the geriatric client with a TBI include integrated strategies for both cognitive and neuromuscular impairments. Following recovery from a head injury, patients may be classified according to behavior associated with the Rancho Los Amigos Levels of Cognitive Function. Consisting of eight stages, this classification scheme illustrates progressive improvement from minimally responsive behavior to near full cognitive recovery (Table 28.2) (Hagen et al 1979).

Levels I–III: coma emergence

The initial stages depict coma emergent behavior. Patients may progress from initially exhibiting no response to demonstrating a variety of localized responses such as a hand squeeze or facial grimace. The rehabilitation team members may elect to track progress through a standardized coma emergence rating form such as the JFK Coma Recovery Scale–Revised or the Western Neuro Sensory Stimulation Profile (Duff 2001). Patients reaching maximum scores on these instruments may then have more advanced goals and intervention plans established. Patients emerging from minimally responsive states are progressively mobilized through tilt-table or standing-frame activities. Patients are started on a sitting schedule to gradually increase sitting time. A variety of sensory stimulation activities are utilized throughout functional tasks. Geriatric clients must be monitored carefully for vital sign fluctuations given premorbid medical conditions and adverse effects of bedrest acquired from extended intensive care unit (ICU) monitoring.

Level IV: the agitated client

Level IV depicts the agitated patient who cannot process the multitude of sensory experiences within the immediate environment. Individuals in this stage tend to exhibit disconcerted, agitated

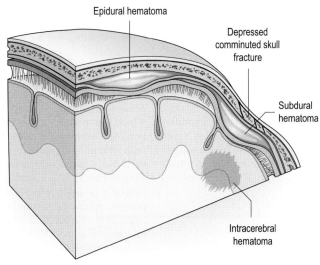

Figure 28.3   Hematoma and skull fracture complications following traumatic brain injury. Reprinted with permission from Klima D, 2006, Clients with traumatic brain injury. In: Umphred D, Calson C (eds) Neurohabilitation for the Physical Therapist Assistant. Slack, Thorofare, NJ. Illustration by Tim Phelps, CMI.

Table 28.1   Glasgow Coma Scale

	Response	Score
Eyes		
Open	Spontaneously	4
	To verbal command	3
	To pain	2
	No response	1
Best motor response		
To verbal stimulus	Obeys command	6
To painful stimulus	Localizes pain	5
	Flexion-withdrawal	4
	Flexion-abnormal (decorticate rigidity)	3
	Extension (decerebrate rigidity)	2
	No response	1
Best verbal response	Oriented and converses	5
	Disoriented and converses	4
	Inappropriate words	3
	Incomprehensible sounds	2
	No response	1
Total		3–15

Table 28.2   Rancho Los Amigos levels of cognitive function

I	No response
II	Generalized response
III	Localized response
IV	Confused–agitated
V	Confused–inappropriate
VI	Confused–appropriate
VII	Automatic–appropriate
VIII	Purposeful–appropriate

Levels V–VIII: progressive cognitive recovery

In levels V–VIII, cognitive recovery progresses from behavior that is confused and inappropriate to eventual appropriate and purposeful behavior. Unfortunately, older clients who sustain more severe injuries and complications may not achieve full recovery. In addition, both cognitive and neuromuscular recovery may not occur in tandem. The ultimate challenge in geriatric head trauma rehabilitation focuses on integrating both cognitive and functional training strategies to effectively guide the patient towards maximal functional independence. The added cognitive dimension of therapeutic interventions adds a level of complexity that necessitates specialized skills to facilitate psychomotor skill attainment and community re-entry.

Cognitive impairment following a traumatic brain injury may be substantial. Patients demonstrate slower processing and require increased time to optimize task performance. A diminished attention span may also be apparent and patients require ongoing redirection to the designated task. Learning of functional skills occurs at a diminished rate and suitable time allotment and cue sequences must be constructed within a treatment session to optimize skill acquisition.

behavior, which often escalates to bursts of hostility. Therapists must adjust treatment activities by scheduling shorter treatment sessions or holding sessions in quiet areas to avoid sensory overload. Therapists should also model calm behavior and allow agitated patients to feel that they have control over the immediate situation. Treatment sessions are structured accordingly to avoid or minimize painful or fearful activities. The Agitated Behavior Scale is an instrument that documents levels of agitation among patients with TBI (Corrigan & Bogner 1994).

Memory deficits continue to be problematic up to Rancho level VI. In addition, rehabilitation clinicians must be reminded that the issue of impaired judgment is still prominent in the final stages of the Rancho continuum. Patients at higher functional levels of mobility may still be unable to problem-solve in the event of an emergency situation.

Cognitive and functional interventions are merged in a variety of ways. For example, dual task activities are created to assess the patient's problem-solving ability during functional tasks. Patients can be challenged to react in the event of an emergency situation. In addition, elements of memory can be incorporated by observing and reinforcing safety strategies taught during previous sessions. At discharge, appropriate family training and instructions should be given to those family members who are caregivers for the older adult patient recovering from a TBI.

SPINAL CORD INJURY

SCI affects over 11 000 people in the US each year. According to the National Spinal Cord Injury Statistical Center (Institute on Disability and National Rehabilitation Research 2001), it is estimated that 180 000 individuals are currently living in the US with impairments and functional limitations sustained from their injury (American Spinal Injury Association 2000). This includes those individuals who are 65 years or older. Major causes of SCI worldwide include motor vehicle accidents, acts of violence and recreational activities. Injuries to the cervical spine often result in tetraplegia (also known as quadriplegia), with resultant impairments to all four extremities, the trunk and the pelvic organs. The term paraplegia indicates resultant lower extremity paralysis from a designated lesion occurring below the cervical spine and is associated with varying levels of trunk involvement in accordance with the lesion level. Functional outcomes parallel specific levels of function and benchmark muscles spared following an injury (Table 28.3). Geriatric clients may have similar causes of spinal cord pathology because of neoplasms or spinal stenosis conditions.

A comprehensive examination should be performed to address all resultant impairments (body structure/function), activity limitations and disabilities (participation) in the geriatric patient with SCI.

Table 28.3 Key muscles used to determine neurological classification of spinal cord injury (American Spinal Injury Association)

Level	Muscle groups associated with spinal level
C5	Elbow flexors (biceps brachii)
C6	Wrist extensors (extensor carpi radialis longus and brevis)
C7	Elbow extensors (triceps)
C8	Finger flexors (flexor digitorum profundus)
T1	Small finger abductors (abductor digiti minimi)
L2	Hip flexors (iliopsoas)
L3	Knee extensors (quadriceps)
L4	Ankle dorsiflexors (tibialis anterior)
L5	Long toe extensors (extensor hallucis longus)
S1	Ankle plantar flexors (gastrocnemius/soleus)

Sensory levels are utilized to determine C1–4, T2–L1 and S2–5 neurological levels.

Examination strategies are often aligned with major components of the American Spinal Injury Association (ASIA) assessment instrument, including key muscles indicative of important myotome levels. Residual muscle function and sensory integrity is linked to the ASIA Impairment Scale (Table 28.4) to discern complete or incomplete involvement (American Spinal Injury Association 2000). A thorough musculoskeletal assessment is performed to determine the presence or absence of available intact musculature and the extent to which key muscle groups will be able to assist in functional activities. Detailed range of motion (ROM) is examined to recognize pertinent joint integrity restrictions. Sensory testing should be completed to identify those dermatomal fields that are intact, impaired or absent. Finally, a full mobility examination identifies the patient's ability to perform important functional activities such as transfers, pressure relief, wheelchair propulsion and bed mobility tasks. Aerobic capacity is assessed through vital sign responses, pulse oximetry and tolerance to all activities performed; in addition, examination of the patient's respiratory function should include an assessment of the patient's breathing pattern, ventilatory muscle strength and overall cough quality.

Functional training

Of paramount importance to older individuals suffering from a SCI is the transition to wheelchair mobility. Following medical stabilization, patients in rehabilitation learn wheelchair propulsion techniques according to the level of damage to their spinal cord and residual muscle function. For example, patients with lesions below the C6 level learn to manually propel a wheelchair; however, higher lesions may necessitate the need for electric wheelchair operation. Endurance and strength impairments may prohibit the geriatric client from successfully navigating the home and community environments and goals may need to be adjusted.

Older adults with an SCI present a major challenge to rehabilitation clinicians. Often, patients are slower to achieve their target functional outcomes because of preexisting comorbidities. For example, patients with injuries at or below the C7 level should achieve independence in all bed mobility activities; however, the older client with insufficient upper extremity strength may be slower to achieve established outcomes. The use of bedrails and other adaptive equipment will assist patients in effectively transitioning from the supine position to sitting. Certain geriatric patients with respiratory pathology will be unable to assume or tolerate the prone position, thus

Table 28.4 ASIA Impairment Scale

A Complete	No motor or sensory function is preserved in S4–S5
B Incomplete	Sensory function is preserved below the neurological level and includes S4–S5
C Incomplete	Motor function is preserved below the neurological level. More than half of the key muscles below the neurological level are less than 3/5 muscle strength
D Incomplete	Motor function is preserved below the neurological level. At least half of the key muscles below the neurological level are 3/5 or above muscle strength
E Normal	Motor and sensory function is normal

requiring adaptations to therapeutic exercise programs and bed mobility maneuvers.

Two major priorities for the geriatric client with an SCI include pressure relief and continued strengthening exercise programs. Older adults are more susceptible to pressure ulcers following an SCI and ongoing pressure relief mechanisms should be emphasized (Chen et al 2005). For individuals with injuries above the C7 level, pressure relief will involve hooking the upper extremity onto the handgrip and incorporating a side-to-side lean. More dependent patients must utilize other modified positional leaning strategies or tilt maneuvers within the power chair. Patients with injuries at or below the C7 level will incorporate a full or modified push-up. Pressure relief strategies should be performed several times hourly to avoid pressure ulcer development.

Therapeutic exercise interventions for older adults with an SCI include both stretching and strengthening activities. Key muscle groups, such as the finger flexors in tetraplegia and trunk extensors in paraplegia, should remain tight. Hamstring flexibility, however, should be optimized to facilitate transfers and dressing activities. Shoulder girdle strength is maximized in rehabilitation to accomplish the task of ongoing wheelchair propulsion, given that the upper extremities may be striking the handrim as many as 3500 times per day (Boninger et al 2000). Recent evidence has identified that major shoulder muscles are involved with both the push and recovery phases of wheelchair propulsion among individuals with paraplegia and tetraplegia (Table 28.5) (Mulroy et al 2004). Unfortunately, repetitive trauma to the shoulder joint or pain syndromes can significantly hinder wheelchair propulsion in geriatric clients with longstanding injuries. Upper extremity therapeutic exercise programs have been effective in reducing the incidence of shoulder pain among individuals with SCI (Nash 2005).

In geriatric patients, the issue of ambulation following SCI is multifaceted. Patients must have the requisite strength, endurance and control to don and doff braces, arise to standing and ambulate with the appropriate gait devices. Older patients may lack sufficient requirements in any one of these areas. Patients with injuries between levels L3 and 5 will as a minimum require an ankle–foot orthosis and upper extremity assistive device for ambulation. Higher lesions require more extensive bracing. In a study of 41 patients with SCI who were 50 or older, patients who achieved ambulation were those with lower classifications (ASIA C and D) on follow-up after their injury (Alander et al 1997). Current studies with treadmill unweighting techniques continue to show promise in facilitating stepping and ambulation among individuals with incomplete spinal cord injury (Field-Fote et al 2005).

COMMON MANAGEMENT ISSUES FOR CLIENTS WITH TBI AND SCI

Upper motor neuron damage may result in extensive resultant spasticity among geriatric clients, and tone management becomes an essential priority. The modified Ashworth scale (Bohannon & Smith 1987) is utilized to grade hypertonic muscle groups and should be especially employed when implementing specific interventions to problematic muscle groups. Serial casting and splinting techniques are used to manage more severe spasticity, although therapists must use caution with older clients who have diabetes or compromised skin integrity. Medical management of hypertonicity may include the use of such centrally acting antispasmodics as baclofen or diazepam (Valium), or medications that act directly on muscle tissue itself such as dantrolene sodium (Dantrium).

Rehabilitation team members should be attentive to heterotopic ossificans, also known as myositis ossificans, following a TBI or SCI. Caused by ectopic bone formation, this condition can potentially result in significant joint ROM restrictions and pain. Therapists must acknowledge all abnormal joint end-feels when performing therapeutic exercise activities. Commonly affected joints include the hips, knees, shoulders and elbows. Diphosphates are used pharmacologically to inhibit the abnormal calcium metabolic process. Milder forms of heterotopic ossificans will not impose major functional limitations, although joints progressing to ankylosis will impede effective mobility activities such as transfers.

Management of both medical and autonomic complications of central nervous system trauma is a priority for all rehabilitation professionals. These conditions may become medical emergencies. For example, patients with spinal cord lesions above the T6 level may experience episodes of autonomic dysreflexia. Patients often experience such symptoms as a pounding headache, chills and profuse sweating in response to a noxious stimulus. Events triggering an episode of autonomic dysreflexia include restrictive clothing, a kinked catheter line and fecal impaction. Therapists should attempt to both recognize and eliminate the noxious stimulus if possible. Furthermore, the patient should be brought to a sitting position to alleviate dangerously elevated blood pressure.

Patients with both TBI and SCI should be monitored for episodes of orthostatic hypotension. Lower extremity paralysis and periods of prolonged bedrest are common predisposing factors. Geriatric patients are particularly at risk. Patients will require gradual postural changes when adjusting to the vertical position through use of a reclining wheelchair seating system and tilt-table activities. Ongoing skin inspections should occur for early detection of adverse swelling or deep vein thrombosis.

Neurological trauma sustained during injuries frequently includes trauma to the peripheral nervous system. Peripheral nerve damage can especially occur following a fall episode. For example, axillary nerve injury is a complication of humeral fractures, and sacral plexus damage and pelvic fractures often accompany high velocity injuries such as motor vehicle accidents. Additionally, brachial plexopathies can also arise from traumatic origins. Therapists must be vigilant during patient examinations to identify additional peripheral nerve damage not detected initially following medical management of the injuries sustained.

CONCLUSION

Comprehensive management of the geriatric client with neurological trauma requires strategic implementation of interventions designed to improve functional mobility limitations while, at the

---

Table 28.5 Shoulder muscle activation pattern in SCI during wheelchair propulsion

Push phase (following initial contact)	Recovery phase (return to handrim)
Anterior deltoid	Middle deltoid
Pectoralis major	Posterior deltoid
Supraspinatus	Supraspinatus
Subscapularis (tetraplegia)	Subscapularis (paraplegia)
Infraspinatus	Middle trapezuis
Serratus anterior	Triceps brachii
Biceps brachii	

same time, integrating the older patient's premorbid condition and limitations imposed by age-related changes in organ systems. Appropriate outcome measures are utilized to both track and prognosticate the patient's status in the continuum of recovery. Common complications in SCI and TBI, such as heterotrophic ossificans and hypertonicity, must be recognized and treatment activities altered accordingly. Effective management will both integrate and augment current evidence-based activities in the plan of care, as well as recognize the unique needs of the geriatric client who has sustained trauma to the brain or spinal cord.

References

Alander D, Parker J, Stauffer E 1997 Intermediate-term outcome of cervical spinal cord-injured patients older than 50 years of age. Spine 22(11):1189–1192

American Spinal Injury Association 2000 International Standards for Neurological and Functional Classification of Spinal Cord Injury. American Spinal Injury Association, Chicago, IL

Australian Institute of Health and Welfare 2002 The international classification of function, disability, and health 20:1–5

Berg K 1992 Measuring balance in the elderly: validation of an instrument. Can J Public Health 83:S9–11

Bohannon RW, Smith MB 1987 Interrater reliability of a modified Ashworth scale of muscle spasticity. Phys Ther 67:53–54

Boninger ML, Baldwin M, Cooper RA et al 2000 Manual wheelchair pushrim mechanics and axle position. Arch Phys Med Rehabil 81:608–613

Brain Injury Association of America 2005 CDC report shows prevalence of brain injury. Available: http://www.biausa.org/Pages/cdc_report.html

Chen Y, Devivo MJ, Jackson AB 2005 Pressure ulcer prevalence in people with spinal cord injury: age-period-duration effects. Arch Phys Med Rehabil 86(6):1208–1213

Corrigan JD, Bogner JA 1994 Factor structure of the Agitated Behavior Scale. J Clin Exp Neuropsychol 16:386–392

Corrigan JD, Smith-Knapp K, Granger CV 1997 Validity of the Functional Independence Measure for persons with traumatic brain injury. Arch Phys Med Rehabil 78:828–834

Duff D 2001 Review article: altered states of consciousness, theories of recovery, and assessment following a severe traumatic brain injury. Axone 23(1):18–23

Evans RW 1998 Predicting outcome following traumatic brain injury. Neurol Rep 22:144–148

Field-Fote EC, Lindley SD, Sherman AL 2005 Locomotor training approaches for individuals with spinal cord injury: a preliminary report of walking related outcomes. J Neurol Phys Ther 29(3):127–137

Hagen C, Malkmus D, Durham P 1979 Levels of cognitive functioning. In: Rehabilitation of the Head Injured Adult: Comprehensive Physical Management. Professional Staff Association of Rancho Los Amigos Hospital, Downey, CA

Mulroy BJ, Farrokhi S, Newsam CJ et al 2004 Effects of spinal cord injury level on the activity of shoulder muscles during wheelchair propulsion: an electromyographic study. Arch Phys Med Rehabil 85:925–934

Nash MS 2005 Exercise as a health-promoting activity following spinal cord injury. J Neurol Phys Ther 29:87–103

Teasdale G, Jennett B 1974 Assessment of coma and impaired consciousness: a practical scale. Lancet 2:81–84

The Institute on Disability and National Rehabilitation Research 2001 Spinal Cord Injury: Facts and Figures. The University of Alabama at Birmingham, Birmingham, AL

Thurman DJ, Alverson C, Dunn KA et al 1999 Traumatic brain injury in the United States: a public health perspective. J Head Trauma Rehabil 14:602–615

Tinetti M 1986 Performance-oriented assessment of mobility programs in elderly patients. J Am Geriatr Soc 34:119–126

Chapter **29**

Rehabilitation after stroke

Maureen Romanow Pascal and Susan Barker

OVERVIEW

A cerebrovascular accident (CVA), commonly referred to as a stroke, is the interruption of blood flow to brain tissue. The brain tissue that has been deprived of oxygen is damaged or dies. Strokes can be ischemic or hemorrhagic. Ischemic stroke is the most common type, accounting for 88% of CVAs. Ischemic strokes can be thrombotic, embolic or lacunar. Thrombotic CVA is caused by a thrombus that develops in an artery supplying part of the brain. Embolic CVA is caused by blood clots that form outside the brain and travel through the bloodstream to the brain. Lacunar infarcts result from disruption of blood flow at the ends of small penetrating vessels found in the basal ganglia, internal capsule and pons (Boissonnault & Goodman 1998). Hemorrhagic CVA usually results from trauma, vascular abnormality or hypertension (Jasmin 2004). Hemorrhagic CVA can be either intracerebral or subarachnoid. Intracerebral hemorrhage is the result of bleeding into brain tissue. Subarachnoid hemorrhage is the result of bleeding into the space between the arachnoid and pia mater.

The annual incidence of strokes worldwide is approximately 15 million (Mackay & Mensah 2004). In the USA, 700 000 people each year sustain strokes. In 2005, the estimated direct and indirect cost of stroke in the USA was US$56.8 billion. The disability-adjusted life years (number of years of healthy life lost) caused by stroke is expected to rise globally from approximately 38 million in 1990 to 61 million in 2020 (Mackay & Mensah 2004). Stroke is the leading cause of disability in the UK (Mackay & Mensah 2004) (Fig. 29.1).

RISK FACTORS

Some risk factors for stroke are nonmodifiable. These include age, gender, race, family history and history of prior stroke or heart attack.

The CVA risk doubles for every decade after the age of 55. CVA is more common in men than women, and African–Americans and Hispanics are at a greater risk for CVA than Caucasians. CVA risk increases if an immediate family member has had a CVA (Boissonnault & Goodman 1998).

Hypertension is the most important of the modifiable risk factors for CVA because, in most countries, about 30% of adults have hypertension (Mackay & Mensah 2004). Patients with atrial fibrillation have a five times greater risk of stroke but treatment with anticoagulants can reduce that risk by two-thirds. Physical inactivity increases stroke risk and even light physical activity can decrease that risk. Other modifiable risk factors include diabetes mellitus, hypercholesterolemia, cigarette smoking, drinking more than five alcoholic drinks per day and the combination of smoking and oral contraceptive use (Kwiatkowski et al 1999).

SIGNS AND SYMPTOMS

Signs and symptoms of a possible CVA include headache, vision changes (field cuts, blurriness), confusion, unilateral weakness or altered sensation of the face, arm and/or leg, dizziness and alterations in speech (Sullivan et al 2004). The development of most of these signs or symptoms should prompt the individual to seek medical attention. Stroke is sometimes called 'brain attack' to indicate that developing a stroke is an emergency. If the stroke is ischemic, blood supply may be restored through a thrombolytic agent such as tissue plasminogen activator; however, this treatment has been demonstrated to improve outcomes only if administered within the first 3 hours of the event (Hacke et al 1995, Clark et al 1999, Kwiatkowski et al 1999).

DIAGNOSIS

In developed countries, definitive diagnosis of stroke is most often made based on results of a computerized tomography (CT) or magnetic resonance imaging (MRI) scan. CT is used more commonly than MRI because it is generally more available and less expensive than MRI (Calautti & Jean-Claude 2003). Both CT and MRI can provide information about areas of infarction or hemorrhage. Some recent developments in MRI, such as weighted imaging (Keir & Wardlaw 2000, Bisdas et al 2004, Etgen et al 2004, Hermier & Nighoghossian 2004, Kidwell et al 2004) and fluid-attenuated inversion recovery (Bozzoa et al 2003, Xavier et al 2003), may make it

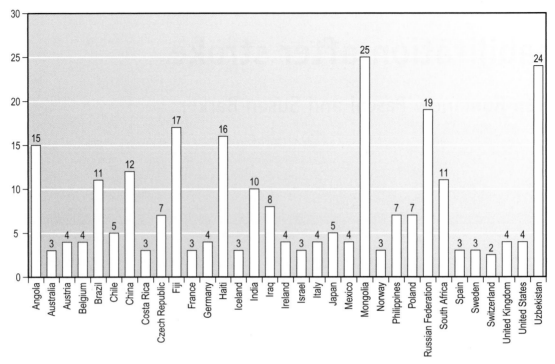

Figure 29.1   Disability-adjusted life years as a result of stroke in selected countries.

possible to diagnose infarction and hemorrhage earlier and with better specificity, helping to guide medical intervention. In addition to CT and MRI, echocardiography and ultrasound may be used to identify the location of the blood clot responsible for an ischemic event (Xavier et al 2003, Abdulla 2006).

PROGNOSIS

On CT, two signs have been correlated with prognosis: the hyperdense middle cerebral artery (HMCA) and the middle cerebral artery (MCA) 'dot' sign. The HMCA sign is positive when the MCA on one side appears denser than its counterpart and any other vascular structure (Barber et al 2001, 2004). It is associated with significant ischemia and infarction of the MCA, and with poorer outcomes. However, studies have shown that a positive HMCA sign alone is not a good prognostic indicator of poor function (Manelfe et al 1999). The MCA 'dot' sign is associated with occlusion of the distal branches of the MCA. On CT, it is seen as 'hyperdensity of an arterial structure (seen as a dot) in the sylvian fissure relative to the contralateral side or to other vessels within the sylvian fissure' (Barber et al 2001, 2004). Interestingly, the MCA 'dot' sign, in addition to the HMCA sign, is associated with a good prognosis.

Other imaging modalities that may be used to determine prognosis include positron emission tomography (PET), functional MRI (fMRI) and MRI spectroscopy (MRS). PET or fMRI can be utilized to evaluate the cortical activation pattern used to perform a functional movement. The pattern used by a patient after a stroke is well-correlated with the level of recovery and outcomes (Carey et al 2002, Ward et al 2003, Baron et al 2004, Ward & Cohen 2004). Patients who demonstrate activation maps similar to control subjects (i.e. they activate the left cortex for right-sided movements) have fewer residual impairments. Patients who demonstrate activation of the primary motor cortex ipsilateral to the lesion, plus bilateral activation of supplementary areas, generally have greater impairments and a poorer outcome (Ward & Cohen 2004). Because of the limited availability and costs associated with performing PET, fMRI and MRS, they are not currently in wide use.

In a study conducted in the Netherlands, Kwakkel et al (2000) found that, at 5 weeks post-stroke, physical and occupational therapists are able to accurately predict a patient's walking ability and manual dexterity at 6 months post-stroke. The severity of the stroke can play a role in prognosis. Patients who sustain a severe MCA stroke tend to have a poor prognosis for functional use of the affected upper extremity. The chance of recovery decreases if it takes longer for the patient to make functional gains or to regain active hand motion (Kwakkel et al 2000).

INTERVENTION

Several impairments and functional limitations may occur after a stroke. Hemiparesis involving the upper or lower extremity, or both, is one of the most common impairments that may need to be addressed by physical therapists. Patients may also experience sensory loss or altered sensation in the area of the body affected by the stroke. Other common impairments include decreased balance; sensory, visual and perceptual deficits; decreased coordination; increased tone and spasticity; and decreased motor control. Functional limitations often include decreased functional mobility in bed mobility, transfers, gait and activities of daily living (ADLs), especially those that are usually bimanual, for example dressing and bathing.

The paresis following a stroke appears to be related to several structural and physiological changes that occur after a stroke, including a decrease in the number of muscle fibers, a change in the types of muscle fibers and muscle recruitment patterns, and a decrease in peripheral nerve conduction velocity. The functional result is a decrease in the ability to produce adequate muscle force (Bourbonnais & Vanden Noven 1989, Patten et al 2004).

Improving physical function plays an important role in the quality of life after a stroke. A study by Duncan et al (2003) found that decreased physical abilities have the greatest effect on quality of life after stroke; loss of hand function is reported to be the most disabling.

One of the most commonly used treatment interventions for post-stroke rehabilitation is the Bobath approach, or neurodevelopmental treatment. This approach focuses on encouraging, or facilitating, normal movement and inhibiting abnormal movement patterns. The strengths of the Bobath approach are that many of the treatment techniques are designed to encourage increased functional mobility, and treatments are often performed in functional positions. Many experienced therapists who use the Bobath method apply motor learning principles and perform techniques during functional activities (Lennon & Ashburn 2000). The Bobath approach has been criticized for focusing too extensively on the reacquisition of normal movement instead of encouraging patients to use their existing strength and movement patterns to accomplish activities. Despite its wide use, there is currently no evidence that the Bobath approach is more effective than other methods used in stroke rehabilitation; however, there is also no evidence that it is an ineffective approach (Paci 2003). Because of the training involved and the variety of techniques that may be employed in the Bobath method, researchers have found it is difficult to perform controlled studies of this method.

Other common methods used in stroke intervention include Proprioceptive Neuromuscular Facilitation and intervention approaches developed by Brunnstrom, Rood, Johnstone and Ayres. Like the Bobath method, the effectiveness or ineffectiveness of these strategies has not been supported by controlled research studies (Van Peppen et al 2004).

Modalities that are frequently used in stroke rehabilitation include functional electrical stimulation (FES), neuromuscular electrical stimulation (NMES) and biofeedback. FES refers to the use of electrical stimulation specifically to improve a functional motion, such as walking ability. For the purposes of this chapter, NMES refers to electrical stimulation used to increase strength or range of motion (ROM), or specifically to cause change within the muscle. Studies indicate that there is limited evidence to support the use of FES to increase lower extremity strength and NMES to increase upper extremity strength. There is also insufficient evidence to support the use of biofeedback to improve upper extremity function, and no evidence to support biofeedback as an intervention to increase ankle ROM or increase gait speed. There is, however, strong evidence to support the use of NMES to both decrease inferior subluxation of the glenohumeral joint and to increase shoulder external rotation passive ROM (Van Peppen et al 2004).

A recent review of research found that the most effective methods of physical rehabilitation for patients with stroke were task-oriented, and that it is important to practice specific tasks that the patient must accomplish in daily life (Van Peppen et al 2004). The task-oriented approach is based on the concept that learning is goal oriented (Gordon 2000). Although the task-oriented approach does not preclude hands-on activity, it does imply that the patient should participate in some exploration of the task, including trial-and-error. One specific method based on the task-oriented approach is the Motor Relearning Programme. A recent Norwegian study demonstrated that this method can be effective in improving motor function and performance in ADLs in patients with acute stroke (Langhammer & Stanghalle 2000).

Because the paresis that results from stroke is related to functional limitations, strength training is an intervention that may be appropriate in post-stroke rehabilitation (Canning et al 2004, Morris et al 2004, Patten et al 2004). Although current evidence is limited, several studies have demonstrated functional improvements in patients who participated in both strength training and task-oriented functional training (Morris et al 2004, Patten et al 2004). There does not seem to be a link between strength training and increased spasticity (Patten et al 2004).

Some of the newer interventions that have been developed for rehabilitation of patients with stroke target specific impairments or functional limitations. One of these is constraint-induced therapy (CIT), which is also known as constraint-induced movement therapy and forced use. This intervention targets the hemiparetic upper extremity. A constraining device such as a sling or mitt is applied to the stronger upper extremity to promote increased use of the affected arm (Mark & Taub 2002). The current protocol requires 'massed practice with the more affected arm on functional activities, shaping tasks in the training exercises, and restraint of the less-affected arm for a target of 90% of waking hours' (Mark & Taub 2002). The protocol has been most successful with patients who have some ability to extend the affected wrist and fingers. It has been less successful in patients with little active movement, although improvement is still possible (Mark & Taub 2002).

An intervention that specifically targets walking ability is body-weight-supported treadmill training (BWS-TT). In this intervention, some of the patient's weight is suspended using a sling attached to an overhead harness. The patient is then assisted in performing gait training on a treadmill. Results from several randomized controlled trials indicate that BWS-TT can help to increase endurance for walking (Hesse 2004, Van Peppen et al 2004). Current evidence does not support using this method to improve walking ability or postural control (Van Peppen et al 2004). In contrast, gait training on a treadmill without body-weight support has been shown to improve walking ability (Van Peppen et al 2004).

Other interventions that are currently being studied to help reduce impairments and functional limitations after a stroke include the use of robotic training (Lum et al 2002, Stein et al 2004, Riener et al 2005) and virtual reality (Merians et al 2002, Weiss et al 2003, Deutsch et al 2004). As research in these areas continues, they may prove to be valuable adjuncts to current physical therapy practice.

CONCLUSION

Stroke is a global problem that can result in a multitude of impairments and functional limitations. Improvements in healthcare and public awareness of the importance of reducing risk factors may help to decrease the incidence and severity of this condition in the future. There are currently many types of physical therapy interventions used to improve the functional abilities of patients after a stroke. More randomized controlled clinical research is needed in this area to help therapists make informed decisions about which interventions are most appropriate for a particular patient.

References

Abdulla A 2006 Echocardiogram. ASM Systems Inc. Available: http://www.heartsite.com/html/echocardiogram.html. Accessed January 6 2006

Barber PA, Demchuk AM, Hudon ME et al 2001 Hyperdense sylvian fissure MCA 'dot' sign: a CT marker of acute ischemia. Stroke 32:84–88

Barber PA, Demchuk AM, Hill MD et al 2004 The probability of middle cerebral artery MRA flow signal abnormality with quantified CT ischaemic change: targets for future therapeutic studies. J Neurol Neurosurg Psychiatry 75:1426–1430

Baron JC, Cohen LG, Cramer SC et al 2004 First International Workshop on Neuroimaging and Stroke Recovery. Neuroimaging in stroke recovery: a position paper from the first international workshop on neuroimaging and stroke recovery. Cerebrovasc Dis 18:260–267

Bisdas S, Donnerstag F, Ahl B et al 2004 Comparison of perfusion computed tomography with diffusion-weighted magnetic resonance imaging in hyperacute ischemic stroke. J Comput Assist Tomogr 28(6):747–755

Boissonnault W, Goodman C 1998 Pathology: Implications for the Physical Therapist. WB Saunders, Philadelphia, PA

Bourbonnais D, Vanden Noven S 1989 Weakness in patients with hemiparesis. Am J Occup Ther 43(5):313–319

Bozzoa A, Floris R, Fabrizio F et al 2003 Cerebrospinal fluid changes after intravenous injection of gadolinium chelate: assessment by FLAIR MR imaging. Eur Radiol 13:592–597

Calautti C, Jean-Claude B 2003 Functional recovery after stroke in adults. Stroke 34:1553–1575

Canning CG, Ada L, Adams R et al 2004 Loss of strength contributes more to physical disability after a stroke than loss of dexterity. Clin Rehabil 18:300–308

Carey JR, Kimberley TJ, Lewis SM et al 2002 Analysis of fMRI and finger tracking training in subject with chronic stroke. Brain 125:773–778

Clark WM, Wissman S, Albers GW et al 1999 Recombinant tissue-type plasminogen activator (altepase) for ischemic stroke 3 to 5 hours after symptom onset. JAMA 282(21):2019–2026

Deutsch JE, Merians AS, Adamovich S et al 2004 Development and application of virtual reality technology to improve hand use and gait of individuals post-stroke. Restor Neurol Neurosci 22:371–386

Duncan PW, Bode RK, Min Lai S et al 2003 Rasch analysis of a new stroke-specific outcome scale: the Stroke Impact Scale. Arch Phys Med Rehabil 84(7):950–963

Etgen T, Grafin von Einsiedel H, Rottinger M et al 2004 Detection of acute brainstem infarction by using DWI/MRI. Eur Neurol 3(52):145–150

Gordon J 2000 Assumptions underlying physical therapy intervention: theoretical and historical perspectives. In: Carr J, Shepherd R (ed) Movement Science: Foundations for Physical Therapy in Rehabilitation. Aspen Publishers, Gaithersburg, MD

Hacke W, Kaste M, Fieschi C et al 1995 Intravenous thrombolysis with recombinant tissue plasminogen activator for acute hemispheric stroke. The European Cooperative Acute Stroke Study (ECASS). JAMA 274(13):1017–1025

Hermier M, Nighoghossian N 2004 Contribution of susceptibility-weighted imaging to acute stroke assessment. Stroke 35(8):1989–1994

Hesse S 2004 Recovery of gait and other motor functions after stroke: novel physical and pharmacological treatment strategies. Restor Neurol Neurosci 22:359–369

Jasmin L 2004 Intracerebral hemorrhage. Available: http://www.nlm. nih.gov/medlineplus/ency/article/000796.htm. Accessed October 14 2005

Keir SL, Wardlaw JM 2000 Systematic review of diffusion and perfusion imaging in acute ischemic stroke. Stroke 31(11):2723–2731

Kidwell CS, Chalela JA, Saver JL et al 2004 Comparison of MRI and CT for detection of acute intracerebral hemorrhage. JAMA 292(15):1823–1830

Kwakkel G, van Dijk GM, Wagenaar RC 2000 Accuracy of physical and occupational therapists' early predictions of recovery after severe middle cerebral artery stroke. Clin Rehabil 14:28–41

Kwiatkowski TG, Libman RB, Frankel M et al 1999 Effects of tissue plasminogen activator for acute ischemic stroke at one year. N Engl J Med 340:1781–1787

Langhammer B, Stanghalle JK 2000 Bobath or motor relearning programme? A comparison of two different approaches of physiotherapy in stroke rehabilitation: a randomized controlled study. Clin Rehabil 14:361–369

Lennon S, Ashburn A 2000 The Bobath concept in stroke rehabilitation: a focus group study of the experienced physiotherapists' perspective. Disabil Rehabil 22(15):665–674

Lum PS, Burgur CG, Shor PC et al 2002 Robot-assisted movement training compared with conventional therapy techniques for the rehabilitation of upper-limb motor function after stroke. Arch Phys Med Rehabil 83(7):952–959

Mackay J, Mensah G 2004 Atlas of Heart Disease and Stroke. WHO Press, Geneva, Switzerland

Manelfe C, Larrue V, von Kummer R et al 1999 Association of hyperdense middle cerebral artery sign with clinical outcome in patients treated with tissue plasminogen activator. Stroke 30:769–772

Mark VW, Taub E 2002 Constraint-induced movement therapy for chronic stroke hemiparesis and other disabilities. Restor Neurol Neurosci 22:317–336

Merians AS, Jack D, Boian R et al 2002 Virtual reality-augmented rehabilitation for patients following stroke. Phys Ther 82:898–915

Morris SL, Dodd KJ, Morris ME 2004 Outcomes of progressive resistance strength training following stroke: a systematic review. Clin Rehabil 18:27–39

Paci M 2003 Physiotherapy based on the Bobath concept for adults with post-stroke hemiplegia: a review of effectiveness studies. J Rehabil Med 35:2–7

Patten C, Lexell J, Brown HE 2004 Weakness and strength training in persons with poststroke hemiplegia: rationale, method and efficacy. J Rehabil Res Dev 41(3A):293–312

Riener R, Net T, Colombo G 2005 Robot-aided neurorehabilitation of the upper extremities. Med Biol Eng Comput 43:2–10

Stein J, Krebs HI, Frontera WR et al 2004 Comparison of two techniques of robot-aided upper limb exercise training. Am J Phys Med Rehabil 83(9):720–728

Sullivan KJ, Hershberg J, Howard R et al 2004 Neurological differential diagnosis for physical therapy. J Neuro Phys Ther 28(4):162–168

Van Peppen RPS, Kwakkel G, Wood-Dauphinee S et al 2004 The impact of physical therapy on functional outcomes after stroke: what's the evidence? Clin Rehabil 18:833–862

Ward NS, Cohen LG 2004 Mechanisms underlying recovery of motor function after stroke. Arch Neurol 61(12):1844–1848

Ward NS, Brown MM, Thompson AJ et al 2003 Neural correlates of outcome after stroke: a cross-sectional fMRI study. Brain 126:1430–1448

Weiss PL, Naveh Y, Katz N 2003 Design and testing of a virtual environment to train stroke patients with unilateral spatial neglect to cross a street safely. Occup Ther Internat 10(1):39–55

Xavier AR, Qureshi AI, Kirmani JF et al 2003 Neuroimaging of stroke: a review. South Med J 96(4):367–379

Chapter 30

Senile dementia and cognitive impairment

Osa Jackson Schulte

The rehabilitation goal for every patient with temporary or permanent cognitive impairment is to promote maximal involvement in self-care and satisfying life activities. Each individual defines the things that constitute meaningful life activities in a unique and personal way. The physical therapists who work with a patient with temporary or permanent cognitive impairment face the challenge of helping the patient, their significant others (family and friends) and caregivers to support their individuality and self-determination and to enhance their sense of safety. The caregivers must be recognized as key members of the team of providers and their needs must also be addressed (see Chapter 79). Overburdened caregivers may abuse the demented person. Educational interventions and comprehensive support, including respite care, have been shown to improve quality of care, delay institutionalization and reduce nursing home costs (Chow & MacLean 2001).

Care of the individual with dementia and cognitive impairment should be interdisciplinary, with physical and occupational therapists being key team members (Crooks & Geldmacher 2004). The physical therapy intervention can include, but is not limited to, consultation and training for caregivers and hands-on treatment for specific patient problems. Examples of this include adjusting wheelchairs or other chairs to maximize safe mobility and postural balance in sitting; problem-solving the height of the bed to maximize independence and safe transfers; functional evaluation and training in the performance of the activities of daily living (ADLs), for example bed mobility; neurological rehabilitation, focusing on facilitating procedural learning and the use of kinesthetic cuing to enhance participation in ADLs [using the smallest perceivable cues to increase the capacity for allowing active assistive range of motion (AAROM) of trunk diagonal motions in supine and to facilitate the capacity to stand and walk]; modification of communication (such as showing caregivers how sitting to one side and using light touch can enhance self-feeding); and environmental adaptation (such as setting up key environmental cues that enhance safety, for example curbs painted in bright colors for contrast). Also, rehabilitation specialists should be involved in off-setting the common declines in strength, mobility, conditioning and coordination as well as evaluating for injury risks and falls (Crooks & Geldmacher 2004).

Other members of the team include the physician who is responsible for the diagnosis and primary care, and for referral for other medical care. The nurse often provides care in the home, which may include monitoring the response to intervention and providing support for the caregiver. The social worker assists the patient and family in gaining access to support services such as respite care, crisis management, financial services and counseling. A nutritionist, lawyer and member of the clergy may also be helpful in meeting the nutritional, legal and spiritual needs of the patient and family (Crooks & Geldmacher 2004).

DEFINITION OF TERMS

The patient with cognitive limitations presents a unique set of needs because hands-on care and touch, rather than speech, eventually become the key tools for communication. The entire medical team is involved in making the diagnosis of dementia or cognitive impairment. Accuracy of diagnosis is a key factor as some temporary cognitive impairments can be reversed. Common examples of conditions in which impairment may be temporary include medication toxicity, depression, nutritional deficiency, anesthesia and allergic reaction (Jackson-Schulte et al 2006).

When working with dementia and cognitive impairment, a definition of terms is helpful.

1. Delirium: a decline in the level of cognitive function combined with drowsiness or agitation.

2. Dementia: a global decline in cognitive abilities in a person who is awake and aware of surroundings. The decline from previous status affects several kinds of cognitive tasks.

3. Alzheimer's disease: a degenerative disease of the brain of unknown cause. The onset is common in the early 60s and diagnosis is definitive with results from autopsy (*Merck Manual of Geriatrics* 2000).

4. Abstract thinking: this is commonly lost in dementia and cognitive impairment and involves an altered ability to relate to anything other than tangible reality – in dementia and Alzheimer's, this skill is predictably missing and is worse if the individual is afraid or anxious.

Alzheimer's disease

The most common symptoms of Alzheimer's disease include the following (some of these symptoms may also apply to other forms of dementia):

- recent memory loss affecting skills used in performing job or tasks;
- difficulty performing familiar tasks;
- problems with language;
- disorientation in terms of time and place;
- poor or decreased judgment;
- problems with abstract thinking;
- misplacing things;
- changes in mood or behavior;
- changes in personality;
- loss of initiative (Alzheimer's Association 1997).

At this time, Alzheimer's disease is a diagnosis that is made after ruling out the other major causes of cognitive impairment such as depression, cerebral infarct, thyroid dysfunction, normal-pressure hydrocephalus, tuberculosis, metal poisoning and Parkinson's disease (Mace et al 1989).

Progressive phases of Alzheimer's disease

In dementia/Alzheimer's, the behavior of the patient often progresses through three distinct phases, although each patient presents with unique minor variations in the progression of the disease. The common aspects of the three stages can be described as follows.

1. Between 2 and 4 years before diagnosis: common symptoms include low energy; emotional lability; slow reactions; picking up new information more slowly; showing less initiative and greater reluctance to try new things; sticking to familiar and predictable activities; taking longer to do routine chores; being unable to think of words, especially names of things; losing one's way to familiar places; having trouble with finances; and experiencing heightened anxiety.

2. Between 2 and 10 years after diagnosis: common symptoms include having trouble recognizing familiar people; finding it difficult to make decisions; making up stories to fill empty memory spaces; minimal content of speech or noticeably impoverished meaning; having trouble comprehending what is read; writing illegibly; becoming more self-absorbed; experiencing late afternoon restlessness (sundown syndrome); having difficulty with perceptual motor coordination; showing lability; acting impulsively; losing ADL skills; monitoring physical appearance inappropriately; repeating physical movements; experiencing delusions or hallucinations; overreacting to minor events; and gradually needing increasing supervision as the severity of symptoms increases.

3. Between 1 and 3 years before death (terminal phase): common symptoms include becoming apathetic and remote; being unable to recognize self or family; having poor short-term and long-term memory; losing orientation in familiar environments; becoming incontinent; losing the ability to communicate with words; gradually becoming unable to walk or get around; and possibly experiencing seizures or weight loss or the urge to put objects in the mouth. In the third phase, the person can still understand emotion and tone and can still participate in physical care. Patients can respond to physical therapy based on procedural learning (touch as a means of communication and teaching) (Ronch 1997, Willingham et al 1997).

REHABILITATION: EMPOWERING THE PATIENT

Contributions can be made by physical therapy intervention at any phase of the cognitive decline in order to enhance patient participation in ADLs and communication and minimize caregiver burnout. The key strategy is to build on the patient's intact skills, to explore new possibilities for communication and to create a sense of safety and enjoyment that includes modified ADL tasks for the patient. The clearest means of communication is to relate in ways that allow the person to feel emotionally safe and to build from an emotional tone that is perceived by the patient as being nurturing and positive.

Empowering the patient during interactions with caregivers and family means that individuality and a sense of safety and self-determination are the most important outcomes for each interaction. For staff and family, this means that there is a need to become aware of what works for the patient and what the patient can emotionally sense if the intention of the caregiver is to support their confidence and self-esteem.

The physical therapy interventions that are required for a person with dementia or cognitive impairment necessitate that the therapist be trained beyond the entry level. When a therapist or assistant is interested in working with older individuals with cognitive impairment, advanced training in kinesthetic contact, communication, procedural learning, neurological rehabilitation and handling skills is necessary. Emphasis on mastering neurological rehabilitation techniques to empower the patient through functional training and kinesthetic cuing is critical. The physical therapist works closely with caregivers to enhance the effectiveness of daily tasks that are important to the patient. Patients should always be seen for treatment in their own environment, if possible, and any new therapists should be introduced by someone who has a history of months of nurturing contact with the patient (Willingham et al 1997, Van Wynn 2001, Holtzer et al 2004).

Training of caregivers and significant others

As a therapist, assistant, caregiver or healthcare team member begins work with a person with cognitive impairment, it is critical that training includes an inventory of personal communication habits plus refinements so that communication with hands-on cuing is clearly reinforced by communication through posture, facial expression and breathing rate, for example. The primary approach to communicating with a person with cognitive impairment is to start with a single clear intention and then reinforce it with touch, gestures and body language that are perceived by the patient as being helpful (Drabben-Thiemann et al 2002).

Hands-on contact and touch can be a key strategy for communication that will enhance the life of a person with cognitive impairment. It is helpful to get input from family and caregivers about historical information and any special cultural or social significance of touch that are unique to the individual. A first step in a consultation is to help the family and caregivers to explore their awareness of their own quality of touch, of the cultural history related to touch and of their own body language. When words are not the main tool of communication, it becomes even more important to clarify the intention of each communication before initiating that communication. A place to start may be for the staff and family to develop a statement of philosophy concerning interaction with the patient (e.g. to agree that the most important thing to get across to the patient is that everyone supports that patient having the highest quality of life possible, as defined by the patient). The detailed definition of a philosophy provides the rationale for ongoing problem-solving and consultation, for example what behavioral cues are needed to support the philosophy and still get the patient out of another patient's room.

Key questions

Another way of empowering the patient is to use the patient's own perceptions as the guiding factors in all communication. As the consultant, the therapist guides staff members in identifying key questions for each individual patient. These can include, but are not limited to, the following:

1. What are the habits for nurturing or comforting at the present time?
2. Under what conditions does the patient enjoy being with other people?
3. What rituals appear to be important to the patient?
4. What are some of the patient's favorite activities?
5. How does this patient communicate enjoyment and displeasure?
6. What is the preferred rest/activity and eating/toileting cycle?
7. What activities, objects or people appear to anchor the patient into cognitive reality in the present?
8. What activities are known to produce agitation or discomfort?

It is hoped that this type of information can be collected by caregivers and family and incorporated into the care plan.

ENHANCING SELF-CARE

It is critical that all caregivers (family and healthcare personnel at all levels) have up-to-date information about the desires and abilities of each patient that they are caring for on a particular shift. Other specific issues for the elderly with dementia or cognitive impairment that can enhance patient self-care abilities include the following:

1. Establish a staffing pattern that allows the patient and the caregivers to gain familiarity and be comfortable with each other. A person with cognitive impairment does poorly in a constantly changing environment and develops better self-care habits in an environment in which there is a small familiar team of caregivers. It is important for the supervision of patients and the detection of new patient problems that the caregivers be familiar with the habits, likes and dislikes of each particular patient (Murray & Huelskotnner 1983).

2. Modify the pace of activity to the pace and abilities of each individual.

3. Provide options for one-to-one pleasant and nurturing contact several times each day.

4. Change the position of the non-ambulatory patient every hour as desired and allow rest for half an hour in bed, as needed; as a patient's abilities decline, it is important to allow the patient to rest in bed and to get up from bed as often as is desired.

5. Provide stable handrails in hallways and stable furniture in the environment so that patient can use it for balance and support during ambulation.

6. Encourage early introduction of rolling carts or walkers so that patients can remain safely mobile as long as possible.

7. Encourage caregivers to walk and talk with patients and provide nurturing contact such as offering the patient a hand or arm to hold.

8. Eat with patients in a normal social manner – one staff member joins two or three clients at a table and eats along with them, family style. When a client is unable to participate in this way, the staff member may eat with one client at a time; when the client

no longer wishes to eat, the staff member could simply sit and read, sing or talk to the patient in order to provide socially nurturing contact.

9. Encourage the patient to make choices as part of caregiving as long as the patient can be empowered by doing so. When this is not nurturing for the patient, then a predictable structure of events can help.

10. Help to perform ADLs so that the patient enjoys living. This could mean changing the style of clothing to avoid pulling clothing over the head, which may be irritating: a shirt with an opening at the front and a Velcro closure would avoid this. A shirt or jumpsuit that closes at the back can be helpful if the patient undresses during the day.

11. Perform functional cognitive assessments of the patient as part of daily caregiving. This means that caregivers must be trained as appropriate to their educational background in order to monitor gross changes in the cognitive and motor function of the patient.

Mini-Mental State Examination

The Mini-Mental State Examination can be a valuable resource and can be introduced to the majority of family members and caregivers (Mace et al 1989) (see Table 30.1). It is critical that those providing day-to-day care in the home or institutional setting be able to verify that cognitive abilities are present and unchanged from the previous day. The rationale is that the staff member or caregiver is the person who must modify the communication strategy if there are changes in the patient's abilities. The rationale for the daily review of cognitive status is that it forms the basis for clear and reasonable communication with the patient at the highest and most accurate level.

Supporting quality of life

The interventions necessary to support a good quality of life for each patient fall into the categories of treating excess disability, reducing patient stress and creating a supportive environment. Physical therapy consultation can be used by the healthcare team to maximize participation in ADLs in many areas of problem-solving. The ergonomic aspect involves creating a fit between the patient and the environment that encourages normalization of lifestyle. Common problems that are addressed include the selection, fitting and training to use canes, walkers, wheelchairs and beds. Bed height should be at chair height – approximately 16–18 inches (40.64–45.72 cm) from seat surface to floor – if an assistive device such as a sliding board is to be used to help with transfers. It is critical to understand the importance of sliding boards in the third phase of cognitive impairment in which the patient becomes less and less able to get in and out of bed. With a caregiver trained in the use of a sliding board, a patient can easily get up during the night to go to the toilet. The idea is that the patient is slid onto the board so that the caregiver may need to use only 40 lb (18.2 kg) of effort to help a 160-lb (72.7 kg) patient. Both the patient and caregiver benefit because the transfer takes less effort and is more pleasant. If beds are too high they appear to promote fear and falls in some patients, and two or more nurse's aides are required to help a 160-lb patient out of bed and into the bathroom (Alzheimer's Association 1997). Several resources are available for teaching sliding-board transfers from bed, chair, toilet and car (Buchwald 1979, Dick et al 2003).

The physical therapist can provide consultation for the caregiver when ADLs are no longer easy to perform. There are many functional profiles that can be used but it is important that a measure of how long tasks take to perform be included along with the amount of help

Table 30.1   A modified mini-mental state examination

	Maximum score
*Orientation**	
Name the day of the week, date, month, year, and season	5
Where are we located: town, street, state, home, facility?	5
Memory/registration	
The examiner names any three objects and asks the person to repeat all three; for example, "dog, book, shoe". The examiner may repeat three objects until the person has learned all three.	3
*Attention and calculation**	
Instruct the person to count backwards from 100 by 7s* or 3s (stop after five subtractions) or, spell "space" backwards	5
Memory II/recall	
Name the three objects from above	3
Language/commands	
Ask the person to repeat: "When it rains, it pours"	1
Ask the person to name two objects, such as a book and a watch	2
Ask the person to complete a three-stage command: "Take my pen in your left hand, pass it to your right hand, then set it on the table"	3
Follow the written command (shown in writing "shake my hand")	1
Ask the person to write a sentence	1
Ask the person to copy a written design such as two overlapping diamonds	1
Total possible score	30

Source: Adapted from *Journal of Psychiatric Research* (1975;12:196–197); *The summed scores of time orientation and the serial seven questions are good predictors of cognitive impairment and may be used for screening persons. The cut-off score for dementia is considered a score of 23 (Onishi et al 2007). The questions are modified, dependent upon the examination setting.

(physical assistance) and the assistive devices required. It is critical that the actual caregivers be present during physical therapy so that they can demonstrate solutions to the caregivers on other shifts. It is important that written instructions be left with caregivers after training is complete and the caregivers are able to perform independently. The physical therapy goals will be written in such a way that caregivers are trained to assist a patient to perform a particular task within a specific environment and time and with specific assistive devices. Functional evaluation for ADL problem-solving can be very helpful during the third phase of cognitive decline, when the patient will tend to want to spend an increasing amount of time in bed. For example, if there is only one caregiver and the patient needs to roll over but is a 'dead' weight, the caregiver with knowledge of basic handling skills can involve the patient to whatever degree possible and thus use less energy. Another key area of self-care that will need adaptation is bathing. Once the patient is fearful of standing, it may be necessary to give them a bed-bath instead of a tub-bath so that they are not afraid of the daily clean-up.

The physical therapist who has mastered a particular approach of neurofacilitation (such as the Bobath, Brunstromm or Feldenkrais methods) has a series of strategies available to them to help a person move or perform a specific task such as sitting up, standing up and walking that an untrained person does not have access to. It is important to acknowledge that evaluation and intervention is a complex process and that this is not a strategy that can be taught in 5 min to someone else. However, it is possible to teach a person how to reinforce the patient in using a particular technique by employing a specific kinesthetic cue.

Spaced repetition creates mastery of and strength in a new pattern of action enabling caregivers to provide valuable practice of new skills that the patient has mastered during a therapy session. The following example is used to clarify the teamwork that can exist between the caregiver and the physical therapist. When resting supine, the patient becomes rigid in the legs and is very hard to roll and help to a sitting position. The therapist explores and finds that placing a small towel roll (3" × 6") under the knees relaxes the hips and legs slightly. The therapist tries lightly stroking the feet one at a time for 3–4 min, and this appears to desensitize the feet. The therapist then explores various possibilities and finally finds that tapping the forefoot one at a time allows the legs to relax enough that support under the knees combined with rolling the leg out (externally rotating and abducting the hip) allows the knees to be bent one at a time and both legs to be brought to the standing position; thus, rolling the patient over becomes possible. The next step is to demonstrate this procedure to the caregiver so that they can feel the contact and points of leverage that create the ease of the movement response. Lastly, the caregiver explores and practices the process under the tutoring of the therapist until the procedure has been mastered.

Environmental adaptation to enhance independence is well described by Karlquist (1987). Organizing the furniture and rituals of caregiving to build on the patient's strengths is critical to enhance the sense of safety and enjoyment for the patient through each phase of the decline in cognitive function. Often, it is likely that environmental concerns will continue to need to be solved at regular intervals. The patient may find an extra blanket on the bed comforting but, 6 months later, that same extra blanket may be irritating. As a patient experiences cognitive changes, there will be periods when they may favor physical contact such as holding hands or walking arm-in-arm. Some patients may literally need someone to sit at the bedside for 5 min and sing in order to feel safe and be able to go to sleep.

The physical therapy consultation can involve a variety of detailed refinements. It is sometimes as simple as the fact that if you sit on the patient's hemiplegic side, the patient becomes agitated, but if you sit next to them on the unaffected side, the patient is calmed by your presence and goes to sleep. The key is to be available to support staff and caregivers so that they can accept patients as they are, for example to accept a show of affection even if it is not how an adult would be expected to act.

The family commonly needs referral to a family support group or to formal counseling so they can work through their emotional reactions (i.e. grief and anger). Counseling is often helpful to answer questions from grandchildren, who may not have been present to see the gradual decline but who are then introduced to a person who looks like grandmother but does not even recognize them. Children are often fine at accepting the limited abilities of a relative if they are given the right tools and support to enable them to be comfortable and feel safe in the situation.

Physical therapy: hands–on treatment and teaching caregivers

For a therapist or assistant trained in neurorehabilitation handling techniques, guided touch or hands-on facilitation can be a strategy to enhance communication, relaxation, balance, coordination and self-determination. When the therapist meets a patient, they are commonly found sitting in a primitive posture, for example with feet unsupported and hips flexed, head forward, hands resting unnaturally and showing overall tension and shallow breathing. Commonly, a therapist has been called in because bathing or some other basic task has become a source of great stress to the patient and has resulted in conflict between the caregiver and the patient. The first step is to create a sense of safety and comfort. It is helpful to know what has been comforting to the patient in the recent past. A dialogue between the therapist and the caregivers should occur so that there can be agreement from the beginning about the desired goals and the willingness of the caregiver to make minor but possibly key changes in the way a desired task is performed. There is an old statement that says, 'To keep doing the same thing and then being surprised that the results are the same is common when we are too stressed to see the obvious'. When the therapist meets the patient, a bond of trust must be established. This can involve any number of stimuli – a hot pack in the lap, a heating pad, a doll, some music to listen to or simply a hand to hold – and the ability to just sit and smile and wait for acceptance of the contact. The goals of therapy will vary but the component skills that create a positive therapeutic outcome are often the same.

Key physical changes

Key physical changes that may facilitate relaxation and thus the patient's involvement in assisted ADLs may include the following:

1. Evaluate the patient's breathing pattern for 1 min and take corrective actions if appropriate. Gentle tapping and touching procedures as described by Speads (1986) may enhance the ease of ventilation.

2. Place the patient in a supine position so that their legs can roll out slightly and the ankles are at or near neutral, not plantar flexed (use props as needed).

3. Allow active assistive and passive range of motion in each leg, as needed, to assist with dressing. This can be achieved by very slowly and gently abducting each lower extremity one at a time.

4. Position the patient in a seated posture with the feet relaxed, flat on the floor and hip-width apart, and covered with comfortable footwear for skin protection.

5. Use a correctly fitted ergonomically appropriate firm seat, especially for a wheelchair or a chair that is used frequently. This will enhance the sit-to-stand pattern of action (Jackson-Wyatt 1994).

6. Place the patient's hands on arm rests or on a pillow in their lap, with the wrists at a neutral position; avoid flexion of the wrists.

7. Use a functional lumbar support as needed for comfort, especially if the patient will be sitting for more than 15 min.

The importance of touch

During the therapist's process of exploration to discover what will enhance self-determination in the patient and minimize stress for the caregiver, touch can have many effects. Touch can be used simply to relax and to comfort, as in light massage, and the relaxation response will occur if that is what the patient needs. Touch can also be used to create awareness, for example helping patients prepare to stand by having them touch one foot to the top of the other or by rubbing their feet against each other in a gentle fashion. Touch can also be used to suggest change, to create a distraction and to help redirect a person. If a patient is focused on getting something that the caregiver cannot provide and then a new stimulus is offered, the first object is forgotten. Touch can also be used to actually initiate change, as in a directional movement to assist in communicating the need to stand up or sit down. In this application, the touch is usually clearly visible to the patient and the caregiver and involves more pressure than in other applications. The techniques of neurofacilitation use a repetitive or gradually increasing or decreasing touch to stimulate or erase a reflex response, which can then be used to reinforce improvement in functional activities.

For individuals with cognitive impairment, the use of touch to enhance functional abilities and participation in ADLs starts at the point of their awareness of their habitual response to what the caregiver is doing. In hands-on treatment, the habitual response of the patient to a particular input can often be changed from an undesirable response to a desirable response simply by making very minor changes in the stimulus – slowing down, using more or less pressure, using two fingers of contact rather than one or using a flat hand rather than the fingertips. Patients with cognitive impairment have the ability to know clearly what they need and can make precise distinctions in methods of handling, which, to the outsider watching, are not at all obvious. The patient with cognitive impairment is often sensitive to contact and touch and can respond to physical therapy by showing improved participation in life. The big question is whether the caregiver and the therapist are willing to acknowledge the tiny distinctions (such as flat-hand versus fingertip pressure) desired by patients and modify input so that patients can comfortably participate in life on their own terms and feel empowered rather than having to submit to others' terms.

Exercise and cognitive impairment

The role of exercise in the care of individuals with cognitive impairment has not been adequately addressed by research. However, clinically it may be seen that patients with social disengagement and little or no appropriate stimulation are often withdrawn, confused, physically aggressive and depressed. Almost 20%, and possibly as much as 86%, of patients with dementia are depressed (Teri & Wagner 1992); however, with social and physical activity (walking 15–20 min daily), behavior and cognition may be more appropriate (*Merck Manual of Geriatrics* 2000). Depression is a treatable condition that is common in demented patients; this is important because physical performance is more likely to decline in depressed individuals (Chow & MacLean 2001). As advocated by Crooks & Geldmacher (2004), physical therapy is indicated to curtail loss in physical performance.

Teri et al (2003) conducted a randomized controlled study of 153 community-dwelling patients with a diagnosis of Alzheimer's disease. Their intervention was caregiver training for behavior management and exercise assistance and encouragement. At 3 months, the exercise group, who carried out 60 min/week of aerobic, strength, balance and flexibility activities, scored significantly better on physical performance and depression tests when compared with control subjects who received routine medical care. At 2 years, they again significantly outscored the routine-care group on physical performance scores and showed a decrease of 19–50% in the rate of institutionalization for behavioral problems.

As the world ages, the findings of three recent papers merit further consideration and investigation. Exercising for three or more times a week (Larson et al 2006) and programs in which women walked for at least 1.5 h a week (Weuve et al 2004) were significantly associated with better physical performance, cognition and delayed onset of dementia. Men who walked less than 0.25 miles daily showed a 1.8-fold excess risk for dementia compared with those who walked more than 2 miles daily (Abbott et al 2004).

CONCLUSION

Recognizing that cognitive impairments caused by temporary conditions can be reversed is an important step. If the cognitive deficits are progressive, as in Alzheimer's disease, the stage to which it has progressed affects the intervention. The involvement of the family and caregivers is crucial and so educating them is a priority. Every change that enhances the treatment of the patient and facilitates their participation in self-care is of great value. Working with cognitively impaired patients can be deeply rewarding; however, it requires a willingness to explore the fine distinctions that can appear meaningless to the caregiver but which make the difference between creating a pleasant workable life for the patient or a 'living hell'.

References

Abbott R, White L, Ross G et al 2004 Walking and dementia in physically capable elderly men. J Am Med Assoc 292:1447–1453

Alzheimer's Association 1997 Is it Alzheimer's? Ten Warning Signs. Detroit Area Chapter. Alzheimer's Association – National Office, Chicago, IL

Buchwald LE 1979 Activities of Daily Living: A New Form. New York University Medical Center, Institute of Rehabilitation Medicine, New York

Chow TW, MacLean CH 2001 Quality indicators for dementia in vulnerable community-dwelling and hospitalized elders. Ann Intern Med 135:668–676

Crooks EA, Geldmacher DS 2004 Interdisciplinary approaches to Alzheimer's disease management. Clin Geriatr Med 20:121–139

Dick MB, Hsieh S, Bricker J et al 2003 Facilitating acquisition and transfer of a continuous motor task in healthy older adults and patients with Alzheimer's disease. Neuropsychology 2:202–212

Drabben-Thiemann G, Hedwig D, Kenklies M et al 2002 The effects of Brain Gym® on the cognitive performance of Alzheimer's patients. Brain Gym J 16(1)

Holtzer R, Stern Y, Rakitin BC 2004 Age related differences in executive control of working memory. Mem Cognit 8:1333–1345

Jackson-Schulte O, Stephens J, Marsh J 2006 Aging, the brain and dementia. In: Umphred DA (ed.) Neurological Rehabilitation, 5th edn. CV Mosby, St Louis, MO

Jackson-Wyatt O 1994 Natural Ease for Daily Living: Can You Move to Get the Job Done? Physical Therapy Center, Rochester, MI

Karlquist L 1987 Environmental assessment: adaptations for maximal independence. In: Jackson-Wyatt O (ed) Therapeutic Considerations for the Elderly. Churchill Livingstone, New York

Larson E, Wang L, Bowen J et al 2006 Exercise is associated with reduced risk for incident dementia among persons 65 years of age and older. Ann Intern Med 144(2):73–81

Mace N, Hardy SR, Rabins P 1989 Alzheimer's disease and the confused patient. In: Jackson-Wyatt O (ed) Physical Therapy of the Geriatric Patient, 2nd edn. Churchill Livingstone, New York

Merck Manual of Geriatrics 2000 Merck Research Laboratories, Whitehouse Station, NJ, p 357–377

Murray R, Huelskotnner M 1983 Psychiatric Mental Health Nursing: Giving Emotional Care. Prentice-Hall, Englewood Cliffs, NJ

Onishi J, Suzuki Y, Umegaki et al 2007 Which two questions of Mini-Mental State Examination (MMSE) should we start from? Arch Gerontol Ger 44:43–48

Ronch J 1997 Alzheimer's Disease: A Practical Guide for Families and Other Caregivers. Alzheimer's Association, Detroit Area Chapter

Speads C 1986 Ways to Better Breathing, 2nd edn. Felix Morrow, Great Neck, NY

Teri L, Wagner A 1992 Alzheimer's disease and depression. J Consult Clin Psychol 60:379–391

Teri L, Gibbons L, McCurry S et al 2003 Exercise plus behavioral management in patients with alzheimer disease. JAMA 290:2015–2022

Van Wynn EA 2001 A key to successful aging: learning-style patterns of older adults. J Gerontol Nurs 9:6–15

Weuve J, Kang J, Manson J et al 2004 Physical activity, including walking, and cognitive function in older women. JAMA 292:1454–1461

Willingham DB, Peterson EW, Manning C, Brashear R 1997 Patients with Alzheimer's disease who cannot perform some motor skills show normal learning of other motor skills. Neuropsychology 11(2):262–271

Chapter 31

Multiple sclerosis

Anita Alonte Roma

INTRODUCTION

As the life expectancy of the general population has increased, so has the life expectancy of the subpopulation of older adults with disabilities. In particular, individuals with multiple sclerosis (MS) have a relatively normal life expectancy (Cottrell et al 1999, Stern 2005). Aging is associated with numerous physiological changes. There are special considerations that need to be addressed in individuals who are aging with a disability; aging with MS presents unique challenges for the clinician and patient alike. In particular, issues that pertain to minimizing disability and morbidity, promoting functional independence and maintaining a positive quality of life need to be identified (Cruise & Lee 2005, Stern 2005).

Although there are data relating to all of the sequelae of MS, much of the earlier research on this disease involved younger subjects. Recent research is now beginning to examine the effects of aging on populations with MS. Many of the physiological changes of aging are similar to the effects of MS. These similarities include muscle atrophy, decreased cardiopulmonary reserve, impaired temperature regulation and depression (Stern 2005).

This chapter will highlight the signs and symptoms associated with MS and identify the issues that should be addressed in the rehabilitation of the aging patient who presents with this disease.

OVERVIEW

MS frequently begins in young adulthood and, although there are several predisposing factors that can lead to this condition, its actual cause is still unknown. It is the most common neurological disability seen in young adults; symptoms usually emerge between the ages of 20 and 40 (Goodman & Snyder 2000, Stern 2005). Onset is rare in children and in adults over the age of 50. Women are affected twice as often as men and a family history of MS increases the risk by 10-fold. MS may be the result of a genetic predisposition or it may be triggered by a virus or environmental factor. Environmental factors may affect the onset of symptoms; MS is five times more prevalent in the colder climates of North America and Europe than in tropical areas (Goodman & Snyder 2000). Life expectancy for individuals with all forms of MS is relatively normal, although it varies according to different studies; the general consensus is that, at most, lifespan may be reduced by 6–14 years (Cottrell et al 1999, Stern 2005).

MS is an autoimmune disease characterized by central nervous system (CNS) inflammation and demyelination. Demyelination leads to scarring or gliosis, which, in turn, forms plaques. The plaques or lesions are scattered throughout the white matter of the CNS and can lead to a wide array of brain and spinal cord syndromes (Goodman & Snyder 2000, Stern 2005). The sclerotic plaques slow or block neuronal transmission resulting in motor and sensory disturbances and other symptoms. Clinical manifestations include weakness, ataxia, visual disturbances, numbness, paresthesias, heat intolerance, fatigue, depression, pain, and bowel and urinary dysfunction. Symptoms can vary making MS highly unpredictable as well as chronic. The progression of MS depends on several factors including age, intensity of onset, neurological status 5 years post-onset and course of exacerbations and remissions (Goodman & Snyder 2000, Stern 2005).

CLASSIFICATION

In total, 85% of patients present with abrupt onset of symptoms. Classification is based on the clinical course of signs and symptoms. Acute episodes of worsening symptoms (referred to as either relapses or exacerbations) or gradual progression of the disease are hallmarks of the following major classes of MS. Relapsing–remitting MS is characterized by symptoms that develop over a period of a few hours to a few days, followed by recovery and a stable course known as 'remission' between relapses. Approximately 80–85% of patients are initially diagnosed with relapsing–remitting MS. Almost 50% of patients with relapsing–remitting MS eventually develop secondary progressive MS (SP-MS), characterized by gradual neurological deterioration with or without superimposed acute relapses. If there is continual disease progression from onset, with only minor fluctuations, the classification becomes primary progressive MS (PP-MS). PP-MS occurs in approximately 10% of patients, mainly those who are older than

Table 31.1 Classification of MS based on clinical course

Relapsing–remitting	Fluctuating course characterized by sudden onset of new symptoms or reappearance of previous symptoms followed by partial or total remission
Secondary progressive	Absence of remission phases with more rapid progression of symptoms and disability; develops from relapsing–remitting course
Primary progressive	Slow progression of symptoms from onset of disease with no remission of symptoms

40 years at onset. Progressive–relapsing MS, a rare form of the disease, is characterized by gradual neurological deterioration from the onset of symptoms and subsequent superimposed relapses (Goodman & Snyder 2000, Stern 2005). Table 31.1 summarizes each of the major subtypes of MS.

DIAGNOSTIC STUDIES IN THE AGING PATIENT WITH MULTIPLE SCLEROSIS

Magnetic resonance imaging (MRI) with gadolinium is commonly used for the diagnosis of MS (Fig. 31.1). This technique is able to identify white matter lesions and demonstrates the breakdown in the blood–brain barrier that occurs during acute MS activity (when a symptom is present for <6 weeks). However, the physiological process of aging can also produce hyperintense foci in the subcortical region. The older adult with MS presents a challenge in differentiating between new disease activity and a stroke, although changes on MRI resulting from ischemia are typically seen in the vasculature of the brain. Lesions associated with MS extend outwards from the ventricles, brainstem, corpus callosum, cerebellum and spinal cord (Stern 2005).

AGING WITH AND CLINICAL FEATURES OF MULTIPLE SCLEROSIS

The physiological changes that occur during the process of aging present additional challenges for MS patients, caregivers and practitioners. Although many traditional approaches are effective in the management of ailments associated with aging, special thought must be given to addressing such problems in the MS population. One such critical consideration in older adults is their susceptibility to adverse drug side effects because of physiological changes in liver and kidney function. For this reason, pharmacological management of MS symptoms in the older individual can be more challenging. Table 31.2 outlines the various manifestations associated with MS and the issues that require special consideration in the aging MS population (Stern 2005).

One of the hallmarks of MS is fatigue. Individuals with MS frequently have limitations in activities of daily living (ADLs), employment, social relationships, self-care and any activity that requires physical effort. The greatest challenge for clinicians and patients alike is determining what is 'normal' and what is 'pathological' fatigue; pathological fatigue is associated with the disease state. Regardless, for the person with MS, fatigue can limit function 60% of the time (MacAllister & Krupp 2005). Fatigue is considered to be acute if the symptom is new (present for <6 weeks), or chronic if it

has been present for longer than 6 weeks. Fatigue can be intrinsic to MS, i.e. it is made worse by heat; it is also often one of the first symptoms of MS and often precedes a relapse. Its pathophysiology is complex; fatigue has been associated with dysregulation of the immune system and changes in the CNS including neuroendocrine or neurotransmission processes. It can also be considered a secondary complication of MS, for example because of sleep disturbance resulting from nocturnal spasming; incontinence; pain; decreased physical activity and deconditioning; or side effects from medication. Depression, poor sleep and inactivity appear to be interrelated with fatigue (MacAllister & Krupp 2005).

Although depression can be a common mental health issue in the general aging population, this symptom may be related to the neuroanatomical or neurochemical changes associated with MS or to the effects of dealing with a long-term disability. It is one of the most common mood disorders seen with MS and the incidence of depression is three times greater in this population than in the general population. The suicide risk is 7.5 times higher in the MS patient; the suicide risk is not related to the duration or severity of MS but rather to alcohol abuse and living alone (Stern 2005). Other behavioral changes seen in the MS population at any age include emotional lability and euphoria. It is unclear if these other behavioral responses are related to CNS involvement or result from psychological stress because of the limitations and disabilities of MS (Stern 2005).

Another feature closely associated with MS and fatigue is heat intolerance. The symptoms of MS are made worse by heat. Weather, exercise or overexertion can magnify symptoms. The aging MS patient is even more vulnerable to the effects of heat as normal aging decreases sweat gland function (Stern 2005).

The clinical features present in the older adult with MS have far-reaching effects: this patient population is at risk for several other medical conditions. Osteoporosis, increased fall and fracture risk and cardiac disease are serious health concerns for the aging MS patient. The medical conditions and sequelae associated with MS have been aligned into numerous Preferred Practice Patterns (American Physical Therapy Association 2003). Further descriptions of specific Practice Patterns and their use are discussed under Examination below.

Sensory and visual changes, lower extremity weakness, spasticity, cerebellar and corticospinal involvement, heat intolerance and fatigue are often seen in combination in MS; they can be key factors in a debilitating spiral that leads to the medical complications mentioned above. The ability to maintain one's balance requires the integration of multiple sensory and motor systems. Impaired vision, loss of proprioception and vestibular impairment result in a decrease in information regarding postural control in any given environment. Motor control, which stems from the cerebellum, vestibulospinal inputs and corticospinal signals, is also essential in maintaining balance. Spasticity and lower extremity weakness add to the MS patient's imbalance and can also significantly alter the gait cycle. This, in turn, can lead to an increased energy consumption, which can add to fatigue. Limitations in mobility, increased fatigue and depression can lead to a decrease in physical activity, resulting in a lower aerobic capacity. Cardiac disease is more prevalent in the older adult population; this, combined with the decreased activity level and aerobic capacity, means that the older MS patient is at higher risk for cardiopulmonary complications (MacAllister & Krupp 2005, Stern 2005). Of note, swallowing disorders can affect up to 20% of MS patients (Stern 2005). The older adult can also develop deficits such as esophageal reflux and hiatal hernia, which further compound the problem of adequate nutritional intake in the patient with MS.

Sexual disturbance is another feature seen with MS and the general older adult population. Primary sexual dysfunction associated with MS results from CNS lesions that cause diminutions in genital sensation, orgasmic response, erectile function in men and vaginal

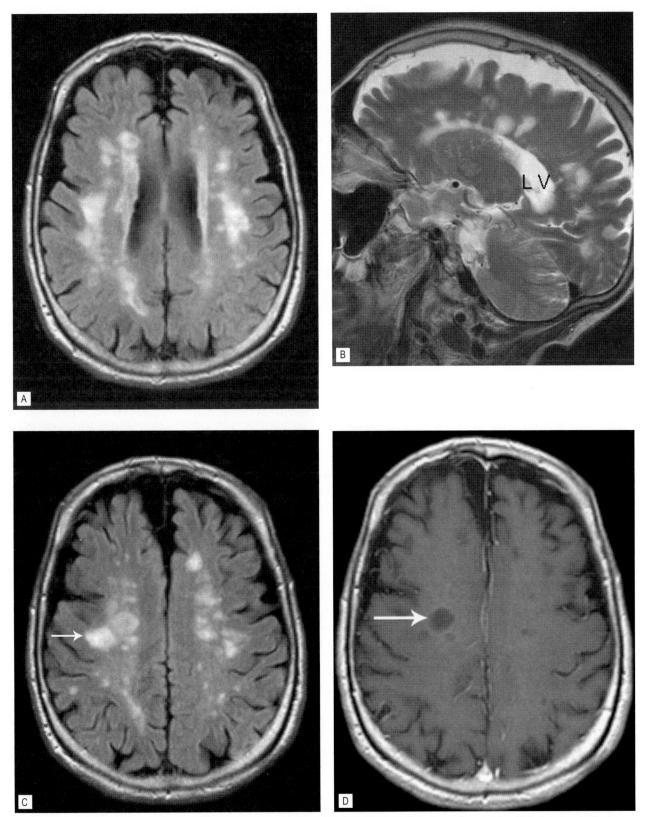

Figure 31.1   MRI images: Axial view (A) and parasagittal view (B) through one of the lateral ventricles (LV) showing typical periventricular T2 hyperintensities in a 70-year-old woman with longstanding MS. Note the typical multiple oval lesions, the so-called Dawson's fingers, many arranged perpendicularly to the ventricles. This is probably best appreciated on the parasagittal view. T2-weighted axial image (C) obtained just superior to the LV, and T1 image at the same level (D) following intravenous contrast. Note that there is no enhancement of any of the lesions. However, on the T1 image, the round lesion is darker than the surrounding white matter (arrow). These are so-called T1 black holes and indicate a more severe white matter injury.

Table 31.2 Clinical manifestations and special considerations in the older adult with MS

Clinical feature	Description	Impact of aging	Treatment considerations
Fatigue	One of the most debilitating symptoms, occurring in over 2/3 of patients. Includes decreased energy; malaise; motor weakness during sustained activities; and difficulty concentrating. Interferes with work, family and social life	Look for secondary causes, e.g. infection; cancer; anemia; hypothyroidism; rheumatological conditions; diseases of the cardiovascular, pulmonary, renal or hepatic systems. Other factors include depression, pain, deconditioning or exposure to heated environment	Medication side effects also contribute: TCAs; benzodiazepines; anticonvulsants; beta blockers; interferons; antispasticity medications. Intervention includes energy conservation and aerobic exercise. Medication: caution with older adults, e.g. use of stimulants, i.e. amantadine, associated with risk of cardiac side effects
Depression	Most common mood disorder; caused by neuroanatomical or neurochemical changes. Incidence 3 × greater than in the general population	Often overlooked because of symptoms of fatigue, decreased activity level and decreased concentration. Depression rating scales have limited utility in the MS population	Use of antidepressants also helpful in pain management. There are depressive side effects from other medications including anxiolytics; beta blockers; methyldopa; clonidine; reserpine; steroids. There is a 7.5 × greater risk for suicide: duration and severity of disease not factors but major depression, living alone and alcohol abuse are
Cognitive dysfunction	Mild cognitive dysfunction; 5–10% have severe condition. Deficits include decreased short-term memory, reasoning, verbal fluency, abstract reasoning and speed of information processing. Intellectual functions intact	In aging, slowing of frontal lobe processes leads to decreased learning rate. Aging MS patient at greater risk for cognitive impairment	Medications may also be a factor, e.g. anticholinergics, antispasmodics, opioids, benzodiazepines, TCAs. Use lists, calendars and journals to assist with memory deficits
Heat intolerance	Frequently associated with increase in severity of symptoms. Excessive heat is caused by weather, overexercising or fever	Elderly vulnerable to hyperthermia because of loss of homeostatic temperature regulation, decreased ANS function, decreased sweat gland function, loss of subcutaneous fat	Outside activities should be performed in early morning; use air conditioning in home and cars; wear light clothes or cooling vests; avoid saunas, hot tubs. Ideal pool temperature 85°F (29.4°C)
Sensory disturbance	Most common initial symptom: affects >50% of patients. Includes paresthesias; numbness; loss of proprioception; neuropathic pain; acute pain because of inflammation; chronic pain from increased muscle tone or musculoskeletal changes	Seen with longer duration of disease, therefore common in older patients. Aging associated with musculoskeletal degeneration; may aggravate symptoms. With aging patient, rule out other etiology of pain, i.e. cervical spondylosis: look for neck and radicular pain; muscle atrophy; decreased deep tendon reflexes	MS patients often under treated for pain. Pain treated with opioid analgesics, NSAIDs, antiseizure medications, antidepressants; antispasticity agents. Intrathecal baclofen pump may be beneficial for intractable pain and spasming. Assess posture and wheelchair seating. Use appropriate assistive devices to decrease strain and overuse of muscles if inefficient gait is observed. Assess skin integrity with sensory loss
Ophthalmological symptoms	Affects 80% of patients. Leads to decreased ADLs and employment. Most common: optic neuritis, internuclear ophthalmoplegia and nystagmus. Symptoms: blurred vision, scotoma, impaired color vision and contrast sensitivity, pain with eye movement	In older population: cataracts, presbyopia, macular degeneration and glaucoma compound visual disturbances. Leads to further isolation and decreased self-care	Environmental adaptations include outlining doorways and stairs. Reduce glare and use magnifiers. Diplopia: eye patching or glasses with prism lenses

(Continued)

Table 31.2 (*Continued*)

Clinical feature	Description	Impact of aging	Treatment considerations
Cerebellar symptoms	Seen in 1/3 of patients. Disabling tremors affect any muscle group. Increases fatigue because of increased energy consumption	Aging also affects balance in general population; cerebellar symptoms may further increase fall risk	No effective medications. Review fall precautions. Home assessment may be helpful to increase safety
Motor loss and spasticity	Present in >60% of patients; results from corticospinal involvement. Lower extremities involved more than upper extremities. Energy requirement increases for activity with spasticity	Weakness associated with aging because of lower motor neuron denervation and atrophy. Rule out secondary causes in aging patient with spasticity: infections, skin breakdown, spinal stenosis with myelopathy	Oral medications for spasticity must be monitored closely. Baclofen: lower initial dose and slower titration decreases risk for sedation and confusion. Benzodiazepines: increased half-life and higher association with agitation and dysequilibrium
Bladder dysfunction	Affects 96% with >10 years' history; detrusor hyperreflexia is most common. Urinary tract dysfunction can lead to bladder or renal stones and frequent UTI	Anatomical and physiological changes because of aging can cause urinary frequency, hesitancy, retention and nocturia. Incontinence can be caused by delirium, atrophic vaginitis, enlarged prostrate, constipation	Elderly sensitive to urological side effects of medications used to treat MS. Take into consideration level of disability; manual dexterity; other medical problems; provide social support for decisions regarding intermittent catheterization vs. indwelling catheter
Bowel disturbance	Constipation most common because of pelvic floor spasticity, decreased gastrocolic reflex, decreased hydration, medication, immobility, weak abdominal muscles	Slowed motility of gastrointestinal tract seen in older adult	Medications (anticholinergics, TCAs, antihypertensives, iron, calcium, opioids) may exacerbate constipation in elderly; regular bowel program may be necessary; rehabilitation to increase mobility may also be beneficial

ADLs, activities of daily living; ANS, autonomic nervous system; NSAIDS, nonsteroidal antiinflammatory drugs; TCA, tricyclic antidepressants; UTI, urinary tract infection.

lubrication in women. Secondary dysfunction is a result of other symptoms of MS, such as bowel and bladder dysfunction. Similar sexual changes are also seen in the general elderly population (Stern 2005).

The effects of aging, a decrease in ambulation and the use of corticosteroids to manage MS are common causes of bone loss and osteoporosis. This decrease in bone density can place the aging patient with MS at risk for falls with a concomitant high risk of bone fractures, especially in the spine and femoral neck (Stern 2005).

QUALITY OF LIFE

Given the clinical features of this disease, the medical needs of the aging MS patient are different from their peers. Although the health-related challenges for individuals with MS are similar to those for others with long-term disabilities, the unpredictability of MS adds to these issues. Several studies have concluded that these issues are present regardless of age, sex or disability. One such issue is a fear of further loss of mobility and independence. Becoming a burden to family and caregivers, physically, financially or psychologically, is another. Nursing home placement is also a significant fear for the aging MS patient. Although these issues are common in others who have a long-term disability, the timing of these problems is unique to MS. Because life expectancy is close to normal, decisions regarding autonomy and

long-term care are made for patients with MS at the age of 55 rather than when they are in their late 70s (Finlayson 2004).

For the effective management of MS throughout the life of the patient, the outcome of any interventions needs to include a quality of life assessment. Three scales are commonly used to quantify quality of life in the individual with MS. The Kurtzke Expanded Disability Status Scale (EDSS) quantifies disability in the MS population (Kurtzke 1983). It evaluates MS according to signs and symptoms observed during a neurological examination. The scale ranges from 0, normal examination, to 10, death (Table 31.3). The Multiple Sclerosis Functional Composite measure consists of a 25-foot walk, nine-hole peg test and paced auditory serial addition test (Fischer et al 1999). The MS Quality of Life Inventory (MSQLI) assesses 10 scales that are generic and MS-specific (DiLorenzo et al 2003). These scales have also been useful in studies on the effects of rehabilitation and exercise.

EXAMINATION

Examination should consist of taking a history, systems review, tests and measures. The physical examination should address cardiopulmonary function, sensory and motor status, posture, balance and coordination, gait and ambulatory status, wheelchair seating and mobility, and endurance. The history/patient interview will help determine and prioritize which tests and measures to carry out. It is

Table 31.3   Kurtzke Expanded Disability Status Scale

0	Normal neurological exam (all grade 0 in FS; mental grade 1 accepted)
1.0	No disability, minimal signs in one FS other than mental
1.5	No disability, more than one grade 1 in FS other than mental
2.0	Minimal disability, one FS grade 2, others 0 or 1
2.5	Minimal disability in two FS with grade 2, others 0 or 1
3.0	Moderate disability in one FS with grade 3, others 0 or 1; or three/four FS with grade 2, others 0 or 1; fully ambulatory
3.5	Fully ambulatory but with moderate disability in one FS with grade 3 and one/two FS grade 2; or two FS grade 3; or five FS grade 2
4.0	Fully ambulatory without aid or rest for at least 500 m, self-sufficient, up and about some 12 h a day despite relatively severe disability of FS grade 4 (others 0 or 1), or combinations of lesser grades beyond limits of preceding step
4.5	Fully ambulatory without aid or rest for at least 300 m, up and about much of day, able to work full day, may have some limits of full activity or require minimal assistance; relatively severe disability consisting of one FS grade 4 (others 0 or 1) or combinations of lesser grades beyond limits of preceding step
5.0	Ambulatory without aid or rest for 200 m; impaired ability to carry out full daily activities; FS of one grade 5 or combination of lesser grades beyond preceding step
5.5	Ambulatory without aid or rest for about 100 m; unable to carry out full daily activities; FS of one grade 5 or combination of lesser grades beyond preceding step
6.0	Intermittent or unilateral constant assistance to walk 100 m with or without rest; more than 2 FS grades 3 + and combinations of lesser grades
6.5	Constant bilateral assistance required to walk 20 m without resting; two FS grade 3 + with combinations of lesser grades
7.0	Unable to walk beyond 5 m even with aid; wheels self in standard wheelchair and transfers independently; up in wheelchair approximately 12 h a day; FS scores are combinations with more than one grade 4+
7.5	Unable to take more than a few steps; may need aid in transfer, cannot be up in chair full day, but wheels self, may require motorized wheelchair, FS as in 7.0
8.0	Restricted to bed or chair, may be up in chair most of day; able to perform self-care functions with effective use of arms; FS as in 7.0
8.5	Restricted to bed much of day; some use of arms; some self-care functions; FS as in 7.0
9.0	Unable to help in bed; can communicate and eat; FS grades mostly 4+
9.5	Totally helpless bed patient; unable to communicate or eat/swallow; almost all FS grade 4+
10	Death due to MS

From Kurtzke JF 1983 Rating neurologic impairment in multiple sclerosis: an expanded disability status scale (EDSS). Neurology 33:1444, with permission.
FS, functional systems.

essential to prioritize what the examination should include and how much can be accomplished in the first session; endurance is limited in the individual with MS and, in addition, the older adult with MS may have endurance that is further compromised because of the physiological changes associated with aging. Obtaining baseline measures of strength, balance, endurance, gait, transfers and community mobility are essential not only for the current episode of care but also for future episodes. Pulmonary function should be assessed, even if it is only a simple measurement such as forced vital capacity. As the course of MS is uniquely unpredictable, it is helpful for the practitioner and patient to have an accurate clinical picture of their status before rehabilitation and to reflect back on it at a later time. This information may be useful in identifying relapses or remissions, quantifying progressive worsening in physical mobility and measuring response to medical interventions. Box 31.1 lists some appropriate tests and measures that are frequently used in the examination of MS patients. As with the examination of any patient, the selection of appropriate tests should reflect the individual's needs. Judicious use of any measurement must bear in mind the physical, emotional and functional components of each patient.

Another comprehensive source for examination measures and intervention strategies is the Guide to Physical Therapist Practice (American Physical Therapy Association 2003). This guide describes physical therapist practice; it defines the role of physical therapists in numerous settings and delineates tests, measures and interventions that are utilized in physical therapist practice. It aligns MS into five Preferred Physical Therapist Practice Patterns and lists an array of current options for the management of patients presenting with the diagnosis of MS. The five practice patterns of MS include 5A, primary prevention/risk reduction for loss of balance and falling; 5E, impaired motor function and sensory integrity associated with progressive disorders of the central nervous system; 6C, impaired ventilation, respiration/gas exchange and aerobic capacity/endurance associated with airway clearance dysfunction; 6E, impaired ventilation and respiration/gas exchange associated with ventilatory pump dysfunction or failure; and 7A, primary prevention/risk reduction for integumentary disorders.

Box 31.1   Standardized tests and measures frequently used in examination of MS patients

Fatigue
- Fatigue Severity Scale

Balance
- Berg Functional Balance Scale
- Tinetti Performance-Oriented Mobility Assessment
- Forward reach
- Dynamic posturography
- Dizziness Handicap Inventory
- ABC Fall Scale

Gait
- Gait Abnormality Rating Scale (GARS)
- Dynamic gait index
- 2-min walk test
- 10-m gait speed
- Sit-to-stand test

Box 31.2   Risk factors for falls in older adults

Intrinsic factors

- Women > men
- ≥80 years
- Incontinence
- Medical conditions
- Medication use
- Low or high physical activity level/exercise[a]
- Sensory: vision, proprioception, vestibular[a]
- Weakness: hips, knees, ankles[a]
- Decreased range of motion[a]
- Balance and gait deficits[a]
- Insight regarding safety, and actual deficits and risk-taking[a]

Extrinsic factors[a]

- Poor lighting
- Clothing too long
- Footwear
- Stairs
- Curbs
- Ramps
- Ice, snow
- Wet surfaces
- Obstacles, clutter

[a]Items that are modifiable factors.

INTERVENTION

Rehabilitation of the older adult with MS should be tailored to the specific needs of the individual. In general, the intervention should be designed to maximize the patient's mobility; educate the patient and caregiver regarding maintenance or improvement of aerobic capacity and endurance without increasing fatigue; and enable the patient to remain independent. All of the patient's impairments should be addressed with the goal of improving function and minimizing disability. In addition, all concurrent medical conditions, which frequently accompany the aging MS patient, need to be considered. As well as the neurological impairments seen with MS, the degenerative musculoskeletal and cardiopulmonary changes also need to be identified and managed during the course of care.

Modifications may need to be made throughout the episode of care. For example, performing balance retraining activities on a compliant foam cushion may be more difficult for the aging patient with severe degenerative joint disease (DJD) in both knees and ankles, and aerobic training activities should be more closely monitored in the elderly patient with MS with a pacemaker. Home exercise programs should be reviewed more carefully, written clearly and possibly enlarged for optimal comprehension and compliance. A review of the home program should occur on a regular basis, ruling out any possible activities that may be worsened by pain or shortness of breath.

As fear of falling and imbalance are significant concerns in the general older adult population, prevention of falls and fall risk modifiers should be included in the rehabilitation of most aging MS patients. Box 31.2 provides a list of modifiable intrinsic and extrinsic factors that can be addressed in physical therapy to reduce fall risk.

Rehabilitation has played a major role in addressing the deficits and improving function in the MS patient population. Exercise is considered the first line of intervention in the treatment of fatigue (MacAllister & Krupp 2005). It not only counteracts deconditioning from inactivity but also has the positive benefits of increasing self-esteem, improving mood, combating social isolation and decreasing the risk of cardiovascular disease (MacAllister & Krupp 2005). Evidence exists that physical therapy can improve function and decrease disability, especially in the MS patient. Recently, there have been numerous studies supporting traditional therapeutic activities and aerobic exercise as a plausible means of increasing endurance, functional activity and even quality of life issues in the older adult with MS. Various physical therapy regimens ranging from sensorimotor adaptation (Rasova et al 2005), individualized programs of therapeutic activities, resistance exercises, balance and gait retraining (Romberg et al 2005) and aerobic exercise on a stationary bike (Romberg et al 2004, Kileff & Ashburn 2005) have had significant positive effects in the MS population at all ages. Outcomes from these studies include increased endurance, ability to walk further, decreased fatigue, decreased depression, decreased disability and improved quality of life (Romberg et al 2004, 2005, Kileff & Ashburn 2005, Rasova et al 2005).

Although there are numerous positive outcomes observed, special consideration should be made when implementing rehabilitation in the older adult with MS. The aging patient with MS may need increased recovery times following exercise. There is also a reduction in training capacity in patients with neuromuscular diseases (Stuerenberg & Kunze 1999). Rigid rules associated with Medicare, i.e. the need for inpatients to receive physical therapy twice daily, may negatively affect the progress of an older adult with MS because overexercising may compound the challenges of fatigue. Exercise prescription should be tailored to each patient carefully; education should include instruction in how to monitor activities and fatigue in an appropriate way. Monitoring fatigue, endurance and aerobic capacity during physical activities and home exercise regimens may help stress the importance of the balance between maintaining physical activity and energy conservation techniques. The Borg Perceived Level of Exertion Scale can assist the patient in assessing their tolerance to exercise (see Chapter 41, Exercise Considerations for Aging Adults).

Gait disturbance is usually caused by weakness, ataxia, sensory loss and spasticity. Achieving independence with mobility can be accomplished with a variety of assistive devices and gait training (Stern 2005). The age of the patient, as well as other demographic and environmental factors and medical conditions, will determine what assistive device is appropriate. Concerns in the aging MS population include energy conservation; seats, baskets and hand brakes may be helpful accessories for a rolling walker. Built-up hand grips are useful for the aging patient with arthritic changes in the hand and wrist. Ankle–foot orthoses will increase knee stability and toe clearance and enable the patient to walk more efficiently. It is necessary to be cautious when selecting the orthosis; a heavy device will increase energy demands during ambulation. For this reason, hip–knee–ankle orthoses are generally avoided (Stern 2005).

PHARMACOLOGICAL MANAGEMENT

Although there is no cure for MS, there are disease-modifying agents. Short-term courses of intravenous corticosteroids are given during exacerbations. Side effects of these drugs include mood changes, hypertension, glucose abnormalities and fluid retention. Long-term or repetitive use is not recommended as this can lead to osteoporosis and cataracts.

With relaxing–remitting MS, two agents are used to decrease the frequency and severity of relapses: interferons and glatiramer acetate (Copaxone). There are three types of interferons: Betaseron, Avonex and Rebif. Side effects for this group include flu-like symptoms, localized reaction at injection site, elevated liver function test and abnormal complete blood counts (CBC). Copaxone mimics myelin protein and its side effects are localized reaction at injection site, chest tightness, flushing and anxiety (Stern 2005).

For those patients with progressive MS, immunosuppressants are used. Because one of the major side effects of these drugs is cardiomyopathy, older patients need to be cautiously monitored (Stern 2005).

Other pharmacological interventions and considerations specific to the manifestations of MS in the older adult population are outlined in Table 31.2.

CONCLUSION

Aging with the chronic, progressive and unpredictable nature of MS is challenging. The clinical consequences of the older adult with MS are far-reaching, affecting literally every aspect of life. It is important to monitor the effects of this disease as well as the medical conditions associated with the aging process, e.g. cancer, stroke, diabetes, arthritis and cardiac disease. Management of the signs and symptoms of MS requires a team effort involving multiple healthcare professionals, the patient and their caregivers, and social supports. Many of the symptoms of MS can be addressed through education on the subjects of energy conservation, provision of appropriate exercise regimens and appropriate compensatory strategies and adaptive equipment. Because fatigue, depression, sleep disturbance and deconditioning are interrelated, an appropriate exercise program is critically important to the rehabilitation of an older adult with MS.

References

American Physical Therapy Association 2003 The Guide to Physical Therapist Practice, 2nd edn. APTA, Alexandria

Cottrell DA, Kremenchutzky M, Rice GP et al 1999 The natural history of multiple sclerosis: a geographically based study. The clinical features and natural history of primary progressive multiple sclerosis. Brain 122(4):625–639

Cruise CM, Lee MHM 2005 Delivery of rehabilitation services to people aging with a disability. Phys Med Rehabil Clin North Am 16:267–284

DiLorenzo T, Halper J, Picone MA 2003 Reliability and validity of multiple sclerosis quality of life inventory in older individuals. Disability Rehabil 25:891–897

Finlayson M 2004 Concerns about the future among older adults with multiple sclerosis. Am J Occup Ther 58:54–63

Fischer JS, Rudick RA, Cutter GR, Reingold SC 1999 The multiple sclerosis functional composite measure (MSFC): an integrated approach to MS clinical outcome assessment. National MS Society Clinical Outcomes Assessment Task Force. Mult Scler 5: 244–250

Goodman CC, Snyder TEK 2000 Differential Diagnosis in Physical Therapy, 3rd edn. WB Saunders, Philadelphia, PA, p 402–403

Kileff J, Ashburn A 2005 A pilot study of the effect of aerobic exercise on people with moderate disability multiple sclerosis. Clin Rehabil 19:165–169

Kurtzke JF 1983 Rating neurologic impairment in multiple sclerosis; and expanded disability status scale (EDSS). Neurology 33:1444–1452

MacAllister WS, Krupp LB 2005 Multiple sclerosis-related fatigue. Phys Med Rehabil Clin North Am 16:483–502

Rasova K, Krasensky J, Havrdova E et al 2005 Is it possible to actively and purposely make use of plasticity and adaptability in the neurorehabilitation treatment of multiple sclerosis patients? A pilot project. Clin Rehabil 19:170–181

Romberg A, Virtanen A, Aunola S et al 2004 Exercise capacity, disability and leisure physical activity of subjects with multiple sclerosis. Mult Scler 10:212–218

Romberg A, Virtanen A, Ruutiainen J 2005 Long-term exercise improves functional impairment but not quality of life in multiple sclerosis. J Neurol 252:839–845

Stern M 2005 Aging with multiple sclerosis. Phys Med Rehabil Clin North Am 16:219–234

Stuerenberg HJ, Kunze K 1999 Age effects on serum amino acids in endurance exercise at the aerobic/anaerobic threshold in patients with neuromuscular diseases. Arch Gerontol Geriatr 28:183–190

Chapter 32

Parkinson's disease

Michael Moran

INTRODUCTION

Parkinson's disease (PD), also known as paralysis agitans, is a progressive neurodegenerative disease that affects approximately 1% of those over the age of 60 years. With the aging of the population, this number is expected to increase. For example, PD currently affects approximately one million people in the US; in coming decades, it is anticipated that this number will triple or quadruple (Pahwa et al 2004). Men and women are equally affected. In Europe, annual incidence estimates range from 5 cases per 100 000 population to 346 cases per 100 000 (von Campenhausen et al 2005).

PD results from a loss of pigmented neurons in the substantia nigra, which leads to a reduction in the production of the neurotransmitter dopamine. The resulting movement disorders are characterized by tremor, rigidity, bradykinesia and postural instability (see Form 32.1 for a sample evaluation). Diagnosis is usually made by observation of signs and symptoms and may be facilitated by positron emission tomography (PET) scans as well as single photon emission computed tomography (SPECT) (Winogrodzka et al 2005). Magnetic resonance imaging (MRI) and computed tomography (CT) can be useful in differentiating PD from other disorders. A clinical presentation that mimics but is different from PD is called Parkinson's syndrome or parkinsonism. Parkinsonism is a frequent cause of functional impairment in the elderly. The diagnosis is based on an evaluation of four signs: resting tremor, akinesia, rigidity and postural abnormalities. Parkinsonism may be caused by PD and can be part of the clinical presentation of other neurodegenerative diseases (Larsen 2005).

SIGNS AND SYMPTOMS

The signs and symptoms of PD vary, depending on the stage of the disease. The early stage may include tremors (often unilateral) and a sense of fatigue. The middle stage usually includes tremors, varying degrees of rigidity and bradykinesia, and postural changes and instability, and the patient may begin to require assistance from caregivers. The final stage of PD includes extensive motor disorders, which result in the patient requiring assistance for movement and the performance of activities of daily living. Cognitive changes (depression, dementia) commonly accompany PD (Poewe 2005).

Tremors are present at rest and usually disappear as a patient attempts to move or during sleep. The term given to the commonly observed repetitive finger movements is 'pill-rolling'. Clinically, it has been observed that PD patients move slowly and with inconsistent acceleration; this bradykinesia is often noticeable when the patient progresses from the early stages of the disease. A complete lack of movement (akinesia) may occur. PD patients can 'freeze' in a certain position (including standing) and then spontaneously begin to move again. Rigidity has been linked to the development of contractures, fixed kyphosis and loss of pelvic mobility. Postural instability most likely reflects central nervous system pathology as well as the musculoskeletal changes mentioned above.

INTERVENTIONS

The management of PD usually combines nonpharmacological and pharmacological treatments. The former should include a multidisciplinary approach involving various therapies (physical, occupational and speech), emphasizing the patient's independence and training of the caregiver. Musculoskeletal changes associated with aging should not be confused with the changes typically seen in PD: a forward-thrust head, increased thoracic kyphosis, posterior pelvic tilt and a slow shuffling gait. Instead, a PD patient should be objectively evaluated using an appropriate device such as the Unified Parkinson's Disease Rating Scale (Table 32.1). The clinical assessment can be video recorded, which allows changes in movement disorders to be more easily tracked.

Nonpharmacological management

Therapeutic intervention should begin as early in the disease state as possible. Avoiding soft-tissue contracture, loss of joint range of motion

Form 32.1 Parkinson's disease evaluation form (circle appropriate score)

Bradykinesia of hands

0   No involvement

1   Detectable slowing of supination/pronation rate evidenced by beginning to have difficulties handling tools, buttoning clothes and with handwriting

2   Moderate slowing of supination/pronation rate, one or both sides, evidenced by moderate impairment of hand function. Handwriting is greatly impaired, micrographia

3   Severe slowing of supination/pronation rate. Unable to write or button clothes. Marked difficulty in handling utensils

Rigidity

0   Undetectable

1   Detectable rigidity in neck and shoulders. Activation phenomenon is present. One or both arms show mild, negative, resting rigidity

2   Moderate rigidity in neck and shoulders. Resting rigidity is positive when patient not on medication

3   Severe rigidity in neck and shoulders. Resting rigidity cannot be reversed by medication

Posture

0   Normal posture. Head flexed forward less than 4 inches (10.2 cm)

1   Beginning poker spine. Head flexed forward up to 5 inches

2   Beginning arm flexion. Head flexed forward up to 6 inches. One or both arms flexed but still below waist

3   Onset of Simian posture. Head flexed forward more than 6 inches. Sharp flexion of hand, beginning interphalangeal extension. Beginning flexion of knees

Upper-extremity swing

0   Swings both arms well

1   One arm decreased in amount of swing

2   One arm fails to swing

3   Both arms fail to swing

Gait

0   Step length is 18–30 inches (45.7–76.2 cm). Turns effortlessly

1   Step length shortened to 12–18 inches. Foot–floor contact abnormalities on one side. Turns around slowly and takes several steps

2   Step length 6–12 inches. Foot–floor contact abnormalities on both sides

3   Onset of shuffling gait. Occasional stuttering gait with feet sticking to floor. Walks on toes. Turns very slowly

Tremor

0   No tremor

1   Less than 1-inch (2.5 cm) amplitude tremor observed in limbs or head at rest or in either hand while walking

2   Maximum tremor envelope fails to exceed 4 inches. Tremor is severe but not constant. Patient still has some control of hands

3   Tremor envelope exceeds 4 inches. Tremor is constant and severe. Writing and feeding are impossible

Face

0   Normal. Full animation. No stare

1   Detectable immobility. Mouth remains closed. Beginning to have features of anxiety or depression

2   Moderate immobility. Emotion shows at markedly increased threshold. Lips parted some of the time. Moderate features of anxiety or depression. Drooling may occur

3   Frozen face. Mouth slightly open. Severe drooling may be present

Speech

0   Clear, loud, resonant, easily understood

1   Beginning of hoarseness with loss of inflection and resonance. Good volume. Still easily understood

2   Moderate hoarseness and weakness. Constant monotone, unvaried pitch, early dysarthria, hesitancy, stuttering, difficult to understand

3   Marked hoarseness and weakness. Very difficult to hear and understand

Self-care

0	No impairment
1	Still provides full self-care but rate of dressing definitely slowed. Able to live alone and still employable
2	Requires help in certain critical areas such as turning in bed, rising from chairs, etc. Very slow in performing most activities but manages by taking time
3	Continuously disabled. Unable to dress, feed self or walk alone

Overall disability (sum of the scores from all categories): 1–9, early stage; 10–18, moderate disability; 19–27, severe or advanced stage

After Turnbull GI 1992 Physical Therapy Management of Parkinson's Disease. Churchill-Livingstone, New York, with permission.

Table 32.1   Unified Parkinson's Disease Rating Scale (Hohn and Yahr Scale)

Stage	Disease state
Stage 0	No signs of disease
Stage 1	Unilateral disease
Stage 2	Bilateral disease, without impairment of balance
Stage 3	Mild to moderate bilateral disease; some postural instability; physically independent
Stage 4	Severe disability; still able to walk or stand unassisted
Stage 5	Wheelchair-bound or bedridden unless aided

From the American Parkinson's Disease Association, with permission.

(ROM), reduction in vital capacity, depression and dependence on others enhances the quality of life of the PD patient. It is important to include caregivers and others who are significant to the patient in goal setting and planning interventions.

Intervention should be goal oriented (restoring or maintaining function is the desired outcome) and individually tailored, based on the stage of disease that the patient is at. Relaxation exercises may be useful to reduce rigidity and there is some support for the idea that strengthening exercises may help to prevent falling (Viliani et al 1999). Stretching and active ROM exercises are vital and the patient should be provided with a home program to facilitate improvement in functional postural alignment. Breathing and endurance exercises can help to maintain vital and aerobic capacities. This is important because PD patients have a high incidence of pulmonary complications such as pneumonia. Balance, transfer and gait activities (including weight shifting) are also recommended.

Balance training should include repetitive training of compensatory steps (Jobges et al 2004) and practice at varied speeds, as well as self-induced and external displacements. Self-induced displacements are necessary to help the patient in tasks such as leaning, reaching and dressing. Displacements of an external origin may be expected if a patient is walking in crowds or attempting to negotiate uneven or unfamiliar terrain. External displacements may be simulated by the use of gradual resistance via rhythmic stabilization.

Transfer training should focus on those activities that can be reasonably expected of the patient. At a minimum, bed mobility and transfers, and chair and commode transfers should be considered. Limitations in active trunk and pelvic rotation may impair a PD patient's mobility in bed. Satin sheets or a bed cradle may reduce resistance to movement from friction. An electric mattress warmer may ease mobility by reducing the need for, and thus the weight of, covers. If the PD patient cannot be taught to perform a transfer independently, accommodations should be considered. Examples include bed rails or a trapeze, a lift chain and a commode with arms.

Specific training may enhance a PD patient's ability to perform some transfers such as sit-to-stand. Recent evidence indicates that strategies designed to facilitate tibialis anterior activation may improve sit-to-stand performance (Bishop et al 2005). However, it is possible that the PD patient may require assistance to perform transfers. Careful instruction and guided practice will help to ensure effective carryover of the learning experience.

Gait training should focus on musculoskeletal limitations that can be quantified. PD patients tend to have limitations in ankle dorsiflexion, knee flexion/extension, stride length, hip extension and hip rotation. Joint mobilization and soft-tissue stretching can be effective in increasing ROM and improving gait. It is important to include trunk mobility (rotation) and upper extremity ROM (large, reciprocal arm swings) in a comprehensive gait-training program for PD patients. Rhythm or music may facilitate movement but the use of assistive devices such as canes and walkers is not always appropriate for PD patients. At times, the use of an assistive device increases a festinating gait or aggravates problems with balance or coordination. Care should be taken to avoid excessive musculoskeletal stress and falls. Conditions such as osteoporosis may predispose a patient to injury.

For PD patients, a primary problem is difficulty in motor planning. Complex tasks such as transferring out of bed and walking to the bathroom have to be broken down into simple components (Bakker et al 2004). It is important for patients and caregivers to remember that verbal and physical cuing (and other forms of assistance) should be oriented toward completion of a number of simple tasks in order to accomplish the overall goals of maintaining function and mobility. Further, it has been noted that stress, fatigue, anxiety or the need to hurry imposed by the caregiver may exacerbate the freezing associated with PD.

When examining and planning interventions for a PD patient, common age-related changes must be considered. For instance, older individuals are more sensitive to glare and benefit from contrasting colors when determining depth. This is especially evident during activities such as gait training on steps. Further, some signs and symptoms of PD have been confused with changes associated with aging. PD patients may present with a reduced or lost sense of smell, handwriting that is difficult or impossible to read and changes in sleep patterns.

Specific nonpharmacological interventions include biofeedback, proprioceptive neuromuscular facilitation, Feldenkrais and the Alexander Technique (Stallibrass 2002). Stretching, active ROM and strengthening exercises should emphasize safety: patients should be placed in a fully supported position initially and progressed to unsupported positions. In addition, spinal mobility must be oriented toward complete full normal rotation, including elongation of trunk musculature. A loss of pelvic motion occurs and can be addressed by means of lateral and anterior/posterior tilts; for instance, the functional task of standing from a seated position can incorporate anterior pelvic tilts. Mobility in bed, such as rolling over, can include

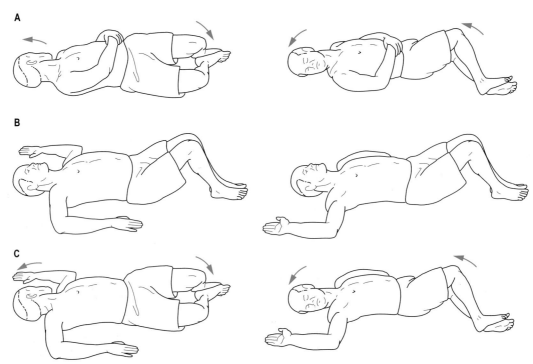

Figure 32.1   A sequence of exercises that can be used in the supine position to increase the range of motion of the neck and trunk. Any combination of motions can be used. (A) Head is slowly rotated side-to-side within the available range of motion while lower extremities are rotated side-to-side in the opposite direction. (B) Upper extremities are positioned in 45 degrees of shoulder abduction with 90 degrees of elbow flexion. One shoulder is externally rotated; the opposite shoulder is internally rotated. From this initial position, the shoulders are slowly rotated back and forth from an internally to an externally rotated position. (C) In an advanced exercise, the head, shoulders and lower extremities are simultaneously rotated from one position to the other.
(From Turnbull GI 1992 Physical Therapy Management of Parkinson's Disease. Churchill-Livingstone, New York, with permission.)

trunk rotation. To improve postural (i.e. balance) responses, a variety of balance activities has been recommended (Hirsch et al 2003). It is important, however, that a variety of tasks are practiced, as skills tend to be task-specific. Examples of some mobility skills are shown in Figures 32.1, 32.2 and 32.3.

The PD patient may experience frustration because of a loss of independence in performing normal activities. This may lead to social withdrawal as symptoms worsen. Social withdrawal can be related to facial involvement – the 'mask' face typical of PD patients, which includes prolonged eyelid closure, slurred speech and drooling. Drooling may be reduced by correcting forward head posture and using speech therapy to address tongue and swallowing dysfunctions. Speech therapy may also assist in improving voice volume and inspiratory muscle strength (Pinto et al 2004). Sucking ice chips for 20–30 min before a meal may help with swallowing and decrease coughing and choking. See Chapter 56 for additional information on dysphagia.

Pharmacological management

Pharmacological management of PD includes dopamine replacement (with Sinemet, a combination of carbidopa and levodopa); dopaminergic drugs that act at the postsynaptic site, such as pergolide (Permax) and bromocriptine (Parlodel); anticholinergic drugs, such as trihexyphenidyl (Artane); and neuroprotective medications (drugs that help prevent further dopaminergic cell death) including selegiline (Eldepryl). A drug that can be used to test for suspected PD is amantadine (Symmetrel), as it is believed to have dopaminergic and anticholinergic properties.

Medications used for PD have a great number of side effects that can hamper rehabilitation. Nausea, vomiting, confusion, lightheadedness, hypotension and dyskinesia are only a few of the clinical signs that may be evident. Some of the clinical problems may be medication-related; Sinemet and Parlodel can cause hallucinations, vivid dreams, leg cramps and daytime drowsiness. In addition, levodopa is associated with the 'on–off' syndrome, in which the PD patient demonstrates periods of time when motor control is intact (on) or not (off). As dosages of levodopa increase, a wearing-off effect may be noted. This is a deterioration of motor performance as the time nears for the next dose of medication. Because of these limitations of levodopa, some physicians delay using it, preferring to start with drugs such as selegiline. Generally, as the disease progresses, finding the right dose of medication becomes difficult and patients may be over- or under medicated (Gladson 2006).

SURGICAL TREATMENT

Surgical treatments are varied as are the reported outcomes (Ansari et al 2002). Specific techniques include basal ganglia stereotactic surgery; thalamotomy, a surgical lesion of the thalamus (which is reported to reduce tremor); chronic thalamic stimulation; and pallidotomy, a

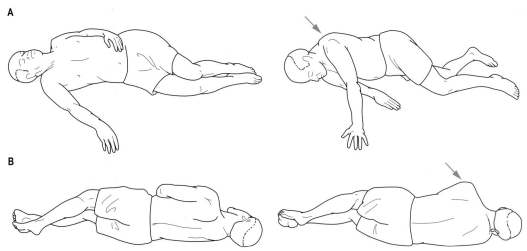

Figure 32.2   In a side-lying position, the thorax is slowly rotated forwards and backwards relative to the pelvis while the upper extremity is protracted and retracted relative to the thorax.
(From Turnbull GI 1992 Physical Therapy Management of Parkinson's Disease. Churchill-Livingstone, New York, with permission.)

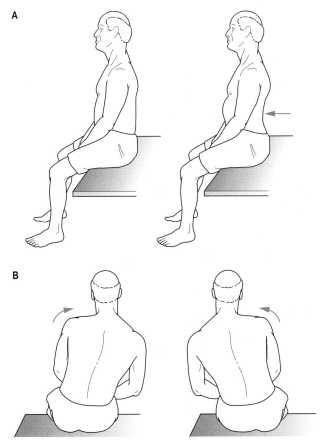

Figure 32.3   Pelvic exercises in the sitting position. (A) The pelvis is anteriorly and posteriorly tilted while the shoulders remain at midline. (B) The pelvis is laterally tilted (by lumbar lateral flexion) while the shoulders remain at midline.
(From Turnbull GI 1992 Physical Therapy Management of Parkinson's Disease. Churchill-Livingstone, New York, with permission.)

surgical lesion of the globus pallidus (which is reported to alleviate bradykinesia more than tremor). Patients apparently demonstrate reduced dyskinesia associated with anti-Parkinson medications following thalamotomy and pallidotomy. Fetal tissue transplant procedures have been carried out in some countries but are banned in others. Techniques for the transplantation of fetal and other cell types are in various stages of research and development. Strategies for using stem cells to benefit patients with PD have been reported in the literature (Olanow 2003, Kim 2004).

COGNITIVE AND SOCIAL ISSUES

Cognitive deficits that have been associated with PD include dementia and depression (mood disorders) (Janvin et al 2005). These deficits are demonstrated by changes in cognitive abilities such as memory, spatial ability, word finding and dealing with new or complex tasks. Cognitive deficits should be considered when planning a treatment program for PD patients, as modifications may be required to accommodate specific patient limitations. Varying the style of interaction and reducing the pace of communication may be helpful. Therapists should use caution when deciding a PD patient is being uncooperative or stubborn, as cognitive deficits may not have been adequately addressed. It is possible that cognitive changes from an earlier injury such as a cerebrovascular accident may already exist. It is important to educate caregivers regarding a patient's cognitive deficits and find strategies to reduce frustration for both.

CONCLUSION

Parkinson's disease is a neurodegenerative disorder that results from a loss of pigmented neurons in the substantia nigra and leads to movement disorders characterized by tremors, rigidity, bradykinesia and postural instability. Therapeutic interventions should begin in the early stages of the disease in order to enhance mobility and quality of life. Pharmacological intervention is a mainstay in the treatment of Parkinson's disease but therapists must be cognizant that the potential side effects of medicines and the on–off syndrome may hamper rehabilitation. Surgical treatment has shown varied results.

References

Ansari SA, Nachanakian A, Biary NM 2002 Current surgical treatment of Parkinson's disease. Saudi Med J 23(11):1319–1323

Bakker M, Munneke M, Keus SHJ, Bloem BR 2004 Postural instability and falls in patients with Parkinson's disease. Ned Tijdschr Fysiother 114(3):63–66

Bishop M, Brunt D, Pathare N, Marjama-Lyons J 2005 Changes in distal muscle timing may contribute to slowness during sit to stand in Parkinson's disease. Clin Biomech 20(1):112–117

Gladson B 2006 Pharmacology for Physical Therapists. Saunders Elsevier, St Louis, MO

Hirsch MA, Toole T, Maitland CG, Rider RA 2003 The effects of balance training and high-intensity resistance training on persons with idiopathic Parkinson's disease. Arch Phys Med Rehabil 84(8):1109–1117

Janvin CC, Aarsland D, Larsen JP 2005 Cognitive predictors of dementia in Parkinson's disease: a community-based, 4-year longitudinal study. J Geriatr Psychiatry Neurol 18(3):149–154

Jobges M, Heuschkel G, Pretzel C et al 2004 Repetitive training of compensatory steps: a therapeutic approach for postural instability in Parkinson's disease. J Neurol Neurosurg Psychiatry 75(12):1682–1687

Kim SU 2004 Human neural stem cells genetically modified for brain repair in neurological disorders. Neuropathology 24(3):159–171

Larsen JP 2005 Diagnosis and treatment of patients with parkinsonism in nursing homes: how to improve quality? Tidsskrift Norske laegeforening 125(12):1669–1671

Olanow CW 2003 Present and future directions in the management of motor complications in patients with advanced PD. Neurology 61(6suppl3):S24–33

Pahwa R, Lyons KE, Koller WC (eds) 2004 Therapy of Parkinson's Disease, 3rd edn. Marcel Dekker, New York

Pinto S, Ozsancak C, Tripoliti E et al 2004 Treatments for dysarthria in Parkinson's disease. Lancet 3(9):547–556

Poewe W 2005 Treatment of dementia with lewy bodies and Parkinson's disease dementia. Movement Disord 20(suppl12):S77–82

Stallibrass C 2002 Randomized controlled trial of the Alexander Technique for idiopathic Parkinson's disease. Clin Rehabil 16(7):695–708

Viliani T, Pasquetti P, Magnolfi S et al 1999 Effects of physical training on straightening-up processes in patients with Parkinson's disease. Disabil Rehabil 21(2):68–73

Von Campenhausen A, Bornschein B, Wick R et al 2005 Prevalence and incidence of Parkinson's disease in Europe. Eur Neuropsychopharmacol 15(4):473–490

Winogrodzka A, Wagenaar RC, Booij J, Wolters EC 2005 Rigidity and bradykinesia reduce interlimb coordination in parkinsonian gait. Arch Phys Med Rehabil 86(2):183–189

Chapter 33

Tremor, chorea and other involuntary movement

Michelle M. Lusardi

INTRODUCTION

Many of the neuromuscular diseases that become more common with advancing age have signs and symptoms that include extraneous or involuntary movement. Some have little impact on functional ability whereas others can significantly compromise an older person's ability to safely or efficiently accomplish functional tasks. In order to select the most appropriate measures of impairment and function, and to develop a plan of care that will enhance safety and function, rehabilitation professionals need to be able to differentiate between the possible causes, characteristics and management of the various involuntary movements and dyskinesias that are encountered when working with older adults. In this section, we define the most common types of dyskinesia, present a scheme for classification of movement dysfunction and review the evidence (such as it is) for examination and functional interventions in individuals who exhibit involuntary movement.

DEFINITION OF TERMS

The word dyskinesia is used when extraneous or unintended motion is routinely observed during postural and/or functional tasks. Tremor is the most commonly occurring form of dyskinesia. Dystonia (fixed abnormal postures) and myoclonus (recurrent hyperactive deep-tendon responses to sudden changes in muscle length) are common in diseases affecting the pyramidal (voluntary) motor systems. Tremors at rest, writhing choreoathetosis and ballism suggest impairment in the extrapyramidal system at the level of the basal ganglia. Tremors that increase in severity with movement often indicate cerebellar dysfunction. Fasciculation, often mistaken for tremor, occurs when there is an adverse drug reaction, or denervation, in which motor units are disconnected from their lower motor neuron.

Tremor

Tremor is an involuntary movement characterized by a rhythmic oscillation around a fixed axis, often congruent with the axis of motion of the affected joint or joints. The frequency (period) and waveform (timing, sequence of muscle activity) of a particular type of tremor is remarkably consistent over time, although the amplitude of the tremor may vary with intraindividual factors (e.g. fatigue, anxiety, stress) or extraindividual factors (e.g. ambient temperature, alcohol or other substance use, environmental conditions or demands) (Bhidayasiri 2005).

Tremor appears to be the result of alternating contraction of striatal muscles on either side of a joint. The underlying central nervous system (CNS) mechanisms of tremor are not clearly understood; there are several interactive factors that may contribute to the motor expression of tremor:

- the oscillating tendencies of the mechanical systems of the joints and muscles;
- short- and long-loop spinal cord and brainstem reflexes;
- closed-loop feedback systems of the higher motor centers, including the cerebellum.

Identifying when a tremor occurs is one strategy for classification: tremor may occur only during movement, only when at rest, when trying to maintain a relatively fixed posture, or under all these conditions. Physiological tremor is a 'normal' phenomenon that is usually so mild that it cannot be easily observed at rest, but becomes more obvious with increasing levels of stress or of fatigue. Most other types of tremor indicate pathology within the CNS (Klein 2005). As in physiological tremor, the amplitude of most types of tremor increases with higher levels of stress, anxiety or fatigue. Most tremors decrease or disappear during periods of sleep.

Fasciculation

Fasciculation (pseudotremor) is a spontaneous, asynchronous contraction of motor units that is often mistaken for tremor (Poolos 2001). On careful observation, fasciculation presents as random twitching rather than the rhythmic oscillating contraction seen in tremor. Fasciculation may be the result of an adverse drug reaction (e.g. excessive caffeine), electrolyte imbalance or sodium deficiency, muscle denervation, nerve root irritation (herniated intervertebral disk or spondylosis) or disease of the anterior horn cell (polio, amyotrophic lateral sclerosis). Fasciculation can sometimes be observed in periods of extreme stress or fatigue, or following excessive strenuous exercise.

Myoclonus

Myoclonus (clonus) is a rhythmic involuntary movement that can resemble tremor (Weiner & Lang 2005). Myoclonus occurs under three circumstances:

1. as the expression of the hyperactive spinal cord-level stretch (deep tendon) reflex related to pathology of the pyramidal system (e.g. stroke, cerebral palsy, multiple sclerosis or spinal cord injury) or, in some instances, occurring in 'normal' individuals who are very anxious, stressed or fatigued;

2. during a partial or generalized seizure as a result of abnormal electrical activity of motor areas of the cerebral cortex;

3. less commonly, as a component of a familial, idiopathic or physiologically induced movement disorder.

Myoclonus associated with hyperactive stretch reflexes can be transient (lasting for several beats) or sustained over a period of time (mimicking tremor). It can be 'triggered' by rapid elongation of affected muscles, as in deep-tendon reflex testing; rapid passive range of motion; or during position change. The peripheral mechanism of myoclonus is the same as that of the stretch reflex: annulospiral 'endings' around intrafusal fibers within the muscle spindle are stimulated by elongation of muscle tissue. Information about change in length is carried to the CNS via 1a afferent neurons in peripheral nerves. These 1a neurons synapse directly with alpha-motor neurons in the anterior horn of the spinal cord or motor cranial nerve nuclei. If stimulated sufficiently, alpha-motor neurons trigger the activation of the motor units of the elongated extrafusal muscle. The resulting contraction elongates the antagonistic muscles on the other side of the joint, triggering the stretch reflex. On reflex testing, individuals with myoclonus are graded as having a 4+ (several beats of clonus) or 5+ (sustained clonus) hyperactive reflex response. Many individuals with myoclonus associated with pyramidal system dysfunction also exhibit a positive Babinski response when the lateral plantar surface of the foot is stimulated (an upward-pointing hallux with fanning of the second to the third toes).

Myoclonus observed during seizure activity may involve a single limb segment (in a partial seizure of the opposite motor cortex) or rhythmic jerking (in a generalized tonic–clonic seizure of the entire cortex). The combination of altered consciousness and myoclonus differentiates the involuntary movement of seizures from tremor. An electroencephalogram (EEG) recorded during either partial or generalized seizure demonstrates abnormal electrical activity of the motor cortex, whereas EEG patterns in those with tremor are likely to be normal.

Hiccups and 'sleep starts' (nocturnal myoclonus) are examples of physiologically triggered myoclonus. Movement-triggered myoclonus has been reported during recovery from severe cerebral hypoxia or ischemia following myocardial infarction or near drowning. Myoclonus may occur as a component of uremic or hepatic encephalopathy. Occasionally, myoclonus may be caused by drug toxicity (e.g. penicillin, tricyclic antidepressant, L-dopa or toxins such as strychnine). Benign essential myoclonus is a relatively rare movement disorder.

Tics

Tics, or mimic spasms, are stereotypical and often complex movements that can resemble myoclonus and tremor as well as the dance-like involuntary movement of chorea (Adams 2001). Tics are often observed as repetitive eye blinking, throat clearing, shoulder shrugging, arm gesturing or skipping while walking. Those who experience tics will describe a sense of increasing muscle tension that can only be relieved when the stereotypical movement occurs. Tics differ from other types of involuntary movement in that they are somewhat under voluntary control and can be suppressed for a length of time. Idiopathic tics often occur for short periods of time, sometimes in childhood, and may be associated with anxiety or other psychological stress factors. Tics associated with Tourette's syndrome may persist over the lifespan and include vocalizations (barking, grunting, echolalia and repetitive swearing) as well as stereotypical facial or extremity movement.

Dystonia

Dystonia is a movement disorder characterized by a sustained positioning or a very slowly changing abnormal synergistic movement (Alarcon et al 2004). It can affect one or more body segments, often observed as tonic abnormal posturing in individuals with longstanding damage to the pyramidal motor system (e.g. 'dinner fork' hand position or severe equinovarus after significant stroke or other acquired brain injury, or spastic cerebral palsy). Dystonic positions are described as 'unnatural'; they cannot be accurately mimicked or recreated volitionally. Individuals with dystonia associated with pyramidal system dysfunction may also exhibit myoclonus and hypertonicity.

Some dystonias are idiopathic and may be familial (e.g. spastic torticollis). Others occur only during one specific motor activity (e.g. writer's cramp or laryngeal dystonia during public speaking). If idiopathic torsion dystonia develops in later life, it most commonly affects axial, facial or upper extremity muscles and may challenge feeding, communication and other activities of daily living. Most idiopathic dystonias are nonprogressive.

Symptomatic dystonias may be associated with damage to the putamen nucleus of the basal ganglia in the forebrain resulting from tumor, ischemia or infarct, or head injury. Dystonia may be one of the signs of progressive degenerative diseases such as supranuclear palsy, Huntington's disease, Wilson's disease or Parkinson's disease. Dystonic postures emerge, along with the reappearance of tonic hindbrain-moderated reflexes, in the end-stages of Alzheimer's disease.

Medications used to manage dystonia and spasticity that impair function include benzatropine mesylate (Cogentin), diazepam (Valium), dantrolene (Dantrium), haloperidol (Haldol), baclofen (Lioresal, Clofen), tizanidine hydrochloride (Zanaflex) and carbamazepine (Tegretol) (Ciccone 2002, Gladson 2005). Severe dystonia may be temporarily treated with injection of botulinum toxin.

Chorea

Chorea is a less common dyskinesia consisting of the random and rapid involuntary contractions of muscle groups, mostly of the extremities or face (Bhidayasiri & Truong 2004). Choreiform movements often occur bilaterally and symmetrically. Proximal and/or distal muscle groups of the extremities may be affected. Typically, muscles of the axial skeleton are not involved and so postural control is not significantly compromised.

Chorea occurs when there is damage to the corpus striatum (basal ganglia), especially the caudate nucleus. Some choreas are hereditary (e.g. Huntington's disease), whereas others are a consequence of another physiological disease or trauma. Choreic movement also occurs with tardive dyskinesia, a complication of the long-term use of certain neuroleptic drugs (e.g. in the management of schizophrenia) or dopamine toxicity (e.g. in the management of Parkinson's disease) (Caligiuri et al 2000).

Although the underlying mechanism of choreiform movement has not been established, several models have been proposed. Surviving neurons in a damaged or degenerating caudate nucleus may become more sensitive to the neurotransmitter dopamine, randomly triggering fragments of motor patterns. Another model suggests that abnormal striatal activity may 'release' long-latency reflexes that would otherwise suppress unwanted movement.

The quality of involuntary choreiform movement is often described as graceful or dance-like. Individuals with chorea learn to blend their involuntary movement with a purposeful movement in an attempt to mask or minimize the unwanted movement (e.g. a choreic movement of the arm over the head might be turned into smoothing of the hair). As with tremor, choreiform movements become more obvious in periods of stress and may disappear during sleep. Pseudochorea has been reported in individuals with impairment of proprioception resulting from multiple sclerosis and other diseases of the posterior columns.

Athetosis

Athetosis is a continuous slow sinuous, and sometimes irregular, writhing movement that occurs when there is unpredictable variation in underlying muscle tone (from hypotonia/low tone to hypertonia/spasticity) (Hallett 2003). Athetosis is mostly observed when it involves muscles of the extremities but it can also involve muscles of the face and postural muscles of the trunk. It is typically bilateral and symmetrical and may be associated with dystonic postures, chorea or spasticity. Individuals with athetosis have difficulty sustaining positions at rest and during volitional movement, which affects the efficacy of postural control when sitting and standing and during transitional functional movement as well as during the skilled movement necessary for activities of daily living.

Athetosis occurs when there has been damage to the corpus striatum (caudate and putamen) in the basal ganglia, most often in children with perinatal ischemia and hypoxia or severe bilirubin toxicity. Athetosis is the basal gangliar form of cerebral palsy and is diagnosed in the first or second year of life. Although the severity of athetosis does not change with maturity, function may become more challenging in aging individuals with athetosis because of typical age-related changes and increased incidence of musculoskeletal and neuromuscular pathologies that are common in later life.

Ballismus

Ballismus (hemiballism) is a rarely occurring movement disorder that is evident as a wild and forceful flinging movement affecting proximal joints of the extremities on one side of the body (Aminoff 2003, Klein 2005). Trunk and facial muscles are usually spared and so bulbar functions (e.g. speaking, swallowing, breathing) are not impaired. The movements of hemiballism are much more stereotypical and disruptive than those seen in chorea. Hemiballism differs from other dyskinesias in that these involuntary motions do not tend to decrease in frequency or amplitude during periods of sleep.

Ballismus is thought to occur when there has been damage or disruption to the subthalamic nuclei in the diencephalon. Alteration of neural output from the subthalamus apparently 'releases' the activity of the globus pallidus nuclei, which unleashes stereotypical synergistic movement of the limb girdle and extremity. It occurs most often as the result of a 'lacunar' stroke of the lenticulostriate branches of the middle cerebral artery, which damages the subthalamus deep in one cerebral hemisphere. Haloperidol (Haldol) is often used to control unwanted and disruptive motion during the acute and early rehabilitation phases of care, and to promote more effective sleeping. Fortunately, hemiballistic movement tends to diminish in both amplitude and frequency in the weeks following a stroke.

Asterixis

Asterixis, an unusual and uncommon dyskinesia, occurs as a brief and recurrent loss of postural tone in antigravity muscles of the extremities and trunk (Aminoff 2003). Asterixis is observed during neurological examination, when the person being assessed exhibits 'flapping' of the hands when asked to hold their arms horizontally with wrists extended against gravity. Asterixis may occur in individuals with hepatic, renal or human immunodeficiency virus (HIV) encephalopathy; pulmonary failure; and malabsorption syndromes. It has also been reported as a consequence of drug toxicity, during anticonvulsant therapies and when there is a lesion interrupting interconnections between the brainstem and thalamus.

Akathisia

Akathisia, often called restless leg syndrome, is a distressing subjective sense of tension and discomfort of the limbs that is often associated with agitation and a need to move around, but that is not always relieved by movement (Weiner & Lang 2005). Those with the clinical diagnosis of akathisia report difficulty sitting or lying still and a powerful urge to move. They may pace or rock in place and often complain of difficulty sleeping. Akathisia can be idiopathic or can be an extrapyramidal side effect of antipsychotic medication. It may be the presenting symptom in someone who is developing tardive dyskinesia.

CLASSIFICATION AND DIFFERENTIAL DIAGNOSIS OF TREMORS

Neurologists and therapists use a variety of subjective and observed characteristics when examining the movement dysfunction of individuals who experience tremor (Hallet 2003, Bhidayasiri 2005). These include when tremors occur, their waveform and amplitude, the body segments affected by the tremor, whether there is a family history, their responsiveness to medications and their association with additional CNS signs and symptoms (Table 33.1).

Because the frequency (period) of most tremors is remarkably stable within and across individuals, one classification strategy focuses on the frequency of the tremor as it typically occurs. This requires electromyographic (EMG) recording or use of a sensitive accelerometer; tremor frequency cannot be reliably assessed by observation alone. Amplitude of tremor is more variable, both within and among individuals (e.g. becoming more pronounced under stressful conditions or with fatigue), and therefore is not a useful indicator of severity of tremor.

A more common way to classify tremor is based on when the tremor is observed. A *resting tremor* occurs in an otherwise relaxed or inactive body part. Resting tremors are commonly observed in individuals with Parkinson's disease (e.g. 'pill-rolling' tremor of the hands) and may also be seen in those with normal pressure hydrocephalus, heavy metal poisoning and neurosyphilis, or as a side effect of the use of neuroleptic medications. A *postural tremor* occurs when a body part (limb or trunk) is maintained in a sustained, often antigravity, position. Postural tremor is frequently a component of essential tremor and may also be observed as senile tremor, Parkinson's

Table 33.1   Comparison of classification strategies for tremor

Type of tremor	Frequency (cps)	Behavior	Mechanism/site of pathology	Response of tremor to medication
Normal physiological	11–13	At rest	Cardioballistic, passive resonance of limb	Increased with sympathetic activity
'Enhanced' physiological	8–12	Postural	Unknown	Increased with epinephrine, isoprenaline, neuroleptics and L-dopa; decreased with alcohol, beta blockers, benzodiazepines
	7–11	Action	Occurs with stress, anxiety, altered metabolic function	
Essential	8–10	Postural, action	Possible interconnections among inferior olivary nucleus, cerebellum and/or red nucleus	Increased with isoprenaline, epinephrine, neuroleptics, L-dopa; decreased with alcohol, beta blockers, primidone, phenobarbitone, benzodiazepines
Muscle fatigue	6	Action	Unknown	No effect
Parkinsonian antagonists	5–7	Postural	Unknown	Decreased with L-dopa, dopamine
	4–5	At rest	Imbalance in long-latency reflex of BG circuit and VL nucleus of the thalamus	Increased with physostigmine, isoprenaline, epinephrine or neuroleptics; decreased with anticholinergics, amantadine, alcohol
Intention	3–5	Action, postural	Cerebellar disease, damage to dentate nucleus, superior cerebellar peduncle or red nucleus	Often increased with alcohol or epinephrine; may be decreased with choline or isoniazid

BG, basal ganglia; VL, ventrolateral.

disease, hereditary motor and sensory neuropathy (Charcot–Marie–Tooth disease) and spastic torticollis. An *action tremor* (kinetic tremor) occurs during volitional movement. In those with essential tremor, the amplitude of an action tremor remains stable throughout the excursion or performance of the movement. Action tremors that worsen (increase in amplitude) during the trajectory of the movement, especially as the movement goal is approached, are referred to as *intention tremors*. Intention tremors are clinically evaluated using 'finger-to-nose' or 'heel-to-shin' movement tasks. Intention tremors are classic signs of cerebellar dysfunction.

Neurologists often evaluate the response to medication as a means of confirming or clarifying the diagnosis of a movement disorder. The amplitude of resting tremors often decreases when anticholinergic medications are administered. The amplitude of essential tremors (whether action or postural) tends to diminish with consumption of alcohol or administration of beta blockers. Cerebellar intention tremors are unresponsive to pharmacological intervention and intensify with alcohol consumption.

Physiological tremor

A fine physiological tremor of 11–13 cycles per second (cps) can be detected in healthy individuals on EMG; this is usually not observable without instrumentation. Because this minimal amplitude physiological tremor is normal in all muscles of the body, it is observed during movement and while holding antigravity positions. Factors that contribute to physiological tremor include the resonant properties of musculoskeletal structures; synchronization of agonist/antagonist motor neuron activity coupled by afferent neurons from the muscle spindle; and the cardioballistic force of the heartbeat. Physiological tremor

affects all muscles of the body simultaneously whereas most pathological tremors tend to affect selected body segments. The amplitude of physiological tremor increases with any mechanism that triggers sympathetic nervous system activity (beta-adrenergic activity and catecholamine release) including stress, anxiety, fright, sleep deprivation, alcohol ingestion, certain classes of cardiac medication, CNS stimulants, exercise and fatigue. The amplitude of physiological tremor increases in hypoglycemia, thyrotoxicosis, alcohol and sedative withdrawal, carbon monoxide exposure and heavy metal poisoning. Toxic levels of certain medications (lithium, bronchodilators, tricyclic antidepressants) may also lead to tremor. Physiological tremor typically becomes more difficult to detect with advancing age.

Essential tremor

Essential tremor can be observed as a postural and/or action tremor, commonly affecting neck and axial muscles, expressed as a nodding rotation of the head or an oscillating flexion/extension movement of the trunk (Sullivan et al 2004). It may be apparent during upper extremity tasks that require holding a fixed proximal position. Involvement of the muscles of the larynx and pharynx may compromise phonation and swallowing. As an action tremor, essential tremor may interfere with the efficiency of fine motor tasks such as writing, grooming or bringing food on utensils toward the mouth. The prevalence of essential tremor is estimated to be between 1% and 7% in those over the age of 40 years. Essential tremor, although considered 'benign' because it is not associated with progressive neuropathology, can significantly interfere with functional activities in older adults. There is often a temporary decrease in symptoms (for approximately 30 min) after ingestion of alcohol. Except when contraindicated by other concurrent conditions [e.g. congestive heart failure, atrioventricular (AV) heart block, asthma, insulin-dependent diabetes], propranolol and other beta-blocker medications are prescribed for long-term management when essential tremor interferes with function. Sedatives, tranquilizers and anticholinergics have little impact on essential tremor. As many as 15% of individuals with Parkinson's disease exhibit an action tremor that is similar to essential tremor; however, this tremor is not responsive to alcohol or beta-blocker medications.

Resting tremor

Tremor at rest that disappears with volitional movement is one of the most common symptoms of Parkinson's disease and may also be seen in other neurological conditions such as normal pressure hydrocephalus, progressive supranuclear palsy and the cumulative encephalopathy in those with repetitive head injury (Jankovic & Eduardo 2002, Krauss & Jankovic 2002). It most often involves oscillating supination/pronation of the forearm or lumbrical flexion/extension of the thumb and fingers (e.g. 'pill-rolling' tremor). Parkinsonian resting tremor has a relatively low period/frequency when compared with other types of tremor. Although the underlying mechanism is unclear, it may be the result of compromised nigral–striatal function. Anticholinergic medications (e.g. trihexyphenidyl/Artane, benzatropine/Cogentin) are more effective in reducing resting tremor than dopamine agonists or L-dopa. Surgical ablation of the contralateral ventral lateral nucleus of the thalamus has been used to reduce the amplitude of severe resting tremor.

Intention tremor

An intention tremor is a tremor that becomes obvious and often exaggerated as the need for precise movement increases (also known as rubral, cerebellar or 'course' tremor) (O'Suilleabhain & Dewey 2004, Weiner & Lang 2005). With intention tremor, there is oscillation of increasing amplitude during voluntary movement, especially as the movement draws to its conclusion. Intention tremor is one of the symptoms of cerebellar dysfunction, especially if there has been damage to the superior cerebellar peduncle because of diffuse axonal injury, multiple sclerosis or infarction/ischemia in the midbrain and upper pons. Because damage to these structures compromises the ongoing 'feedback' necessary for 'error control', intention tremor is most apparent when fine skilled motor tasks are attempted. In addition, intention tremor has been observed in alcohol, barbiturate or sedative intoxication and with high serum levels of some anticonvulsants (e.g. phenytoin/Dilantin and carbamazepine/Tegretol). Intention tremor affects both limb girdle musculature and the more distal joints of the extremities. In very severe cases, there may be observable postural tremor in addition to the classic disruption of goal-oriented volitional movement. Individuals with intention tremor may also exhibit other symptoms of cerebellar dysfunction including nystagmus, hypotonia, dysmetria, movement decomposition and gait ataxia. For reasons not well understood, the amplitude of cerebellar intention tremor often decreases when the eyes are closed.

Neuropathic tremor

Tremor has also been observed in individuals with significant peripheral neuropathy; however, the presentation of neuropathic tremor is much less stereotypical than essential, resting and intention tremors (Adams 2001, Bradley et al 2003). It is not well understood how and why tremor occurs in individuals with neuropathy.

Neuropathic tremor occurs in some, but not all, individuals with longstanding diabetes, end-stage renal disease, chronic alcoholism, hereditary sensory–motor neuropathy (Charcot–Marie–Tooth disease) and infectious neuropathies such as acute Guillain–Barré syndrome. Management of these tremors can be challenging because many of the medications that are successful in controlling extraneous movement are not as effective in the presence of peripheral neuropathy.

Post-traumatic tremor

Individuals of any age who have sustained a mild acquired brain injury may develop an action tremor within 1–4 weeks of the traumatic event, similar to essential tremor (Krauss & Jankovic 2002, O'Suilleabhain & Dewey 2004). However, it is not possible to identify a specific lesion by magnetic resonance imaging (MRI) or computed tomography (CT) scanning. This type of tremor is not particularly responsive to the medications used to control essential tremor. Often, the magnitude of this post-traumatic tremor decreases over time; however, it may remain problematic for some individuals. A delayed-onset post-traumatic tremor, evolving 12–18 months post-injury, has also been reported. Delayed-onset post-traumatic tremor often persists for several years or longer.

Orthostatic tremor

In very rare circumstances, an older adult may experience a tremor only during unsupported standing or during preparation for assuming a standing position. If the tremor is severe, it can interfere with transitional movement (e.g. sit-to-stand) and with postural control (Whitney et al 2003). Orthostatic tremor is usually perceived by the individual as difficulty with stability (unsteadiness) while standing, when not supported by an assistive device or other external support, and is frequently associated with an increased fear of falling. Orthostatic tremor has a higher frequency/faster period (14–18 cps) than most other tremors, although its amplitude tends to be small. Orthostatic tremor does not respond to alcohol or propranolol, the medications used to manage essential tremor, but does respond to clonazepam. Orthostatic tremor can significantly affect quality of life and limit functional ability.

Senile tremor

The term senile tremor is used to describe a mild idiopathic movement disorder that develops in a small percentage of individuals after the seventh decade of life (Louis et al 2000). It is chronic in nature, very slowly progressive, and is diagnosed when there is no familial history of essential tremor. Most commonly, senile tremor occurs as titubation or oscillation of the head and neck or mouth and lips. Senile tremor, although observable and sometimes disconcerting to the individual, has minimal impact on functional ability. Whether this is a distinct movement disorder or a variation of essential tremor is open to debate.

Hysterical tremor

Hysterical tremor, also known as conversion disorder, is a psychiatric condition that appears as involuntary movement, differing in characteristics and consistency from action, intention or resting tremors (Adams 2001, Aminoff 2003). Within an individual, hysterical tremor may 'migrate' from one area of the body to another. Onset is typically abrupt whereas most other types of tremor are insidious. The frequency and amplitude of hysterical tremor are inconsistent and variable over time. In most other types of tremor, the amplitude tends to increase when individuals are given competitive, anxiety-producing cognitive tasks (e.g. beginning at 100 and serially subtracting 7); in hysterical tremor, the amplitude tends to decrease (or completely disappear) when attention is focused elsewhere.

CLASSIFICATION AND DIFFERENTIAL DIAGNOSIS OF DYSKINETIC CONDITIONS

The other types of dyskinetic conditions that are encountered in geriatric rehabilitation are most often associated with a long-term disorder with which the individual has aged; however, some medication-related movement disorders are newly diagnosed.

Huntington's chorea

Huntington's chorea is an autosomal dominant hereditary progressive disorder involving degeneration of the corpus striatum (Bradley et al 2003, Hallett 2003). The gene for Huntington's is located on the short arm of chromosome 4. The first signs and symptoms of the disease appear in midlife as restlessness, emotional lability, neurosis or personality disorders. Over time, cognitive impairment becomes more apparent and choreiform involuntary movement develops, often impairing judgment, locomotion and mobility, speech production and swallowing. As the severity of symptoms increases, functional status deteriorates. Dystonia and rigidity may develop late in the disease process. On CT or MRI, there is marked bilateral degeneration of the caudate nucleus, enlargement of the anterior horn of the lateral ventricles and cerebral atrophy. Treatment of Huntington's disease is symptomatic; choreiform movement can sometimes be managed with dopamine-blocking agents such as haloperidol, respirine or tetrabenzanine. Individuals with Huntington's disease may have to cope with their increasingly debilitating impairments for 10–25 years, until the disease takes their life.

Sydenham's chorea

This type of chorea appears insidiously, usually in childhood, after recovery from rheumatic fever (Janvas & Aminoff 1998). Sydenham's chorea is characterized by a somewhat asymmetrical facial grimacing and a rapid twitching movement of the trunk and proximal extremities on one side of the body. It is often accompanied by emotional lability, pervasive listlessness and hypertonia. There is some suggestion that those with a history of rheumatic fever and Sydenham's chorea in childhood may be more likely to develop other movement disorders later in life.

Wilson's disease

Wilson's disease is an autosomal recessive hereditary disorder of copper metabolism, with a locus on chromosome 13 (Adams 2001, Hallett 2003). If undetected early in life, Wilson's disease can be fatal. Neurological symptoms of poorly managed Wilson's disease include resting or postural tremor, chorea of the extremities, dystonia, pseudobulbar palsy and cognitive dysfunction. The abnormal liver function associated with Wilson's disease eventually leads to chronic cirrhosis. Management with penicillamine, which effectively binds copper, and careful diet can slow progression of the disease. Although initial symptoms typically appear in adolescence and early adulthood, presentation may first occur as late as 60 years of age.

Paroxysmal choreoathetosis

Paroxysmal choreoathetosis (also known as striatal epilepsy) presents as jerking and writhing movements of the limb and trunk when an individual is unexpectedly startled or disturbed (Adams 2001). Paroxysmal choreoathetosis most commonly occurs when there is concurrent CNS pathology, e.g. multiple sclerosis. Individuals with preexisting neurological dysfunction typically bring this condition with them as they move into later life.

Familial choreoathetosis

Familial choreoathetosis is a rare autosomal recessive hereditary movement disorder that is relatively benign (Aminoff 2003). In this condition, the individual experiences intermittent 'attacks' of jerking and writhing choreoathetoid movement that are associated with periods of physical exertion or ingestion of alcohol or caffeine. This is also a lifelong condition that individuals bring with them into later life.

Senile chorea

Senile chorea is a late-appearing movement disorder that evolves in the absence of psychotropic or dopamine therapy, Huntington's chorea, dementia or familial movement disorders (Janvas & Aminoff 1998, Poolos 2001). Also known as oral–facial–lingual dyskinesia, senile tremor primarily affects the muscles of the mouth, tongue and trunk. Although it affects less than 1% of those between the ages of 50 and 59, the prevalence increases to as high as 7% in those over the age of 70. It is important to differentiate the abnormal involuntary movements of senile chorea from the similar facial movements that occur in tardive dyskinesia and the lip and jaw movements commonly observed in older individuals who have lost all of their teeth and are no longer able to wear dentures.

Tourette's syndrome

Tourette's syndrome is an idiopathic movement and behavioral disorder that is characterized by multiple motor and vocal tics (Bradley et al 2003, Hallett 2003). The behavior of those with Tourette's is often described as bizarre and peculiar; many are initially misdiagnosed with a psychiatric illness. Symptoms may occur initially in childhood or adolescence and persist into adulthood and later life. Initial motor tics typically involve the face and eyes, and may eventually include vocalizations (repetitive grunts, barks, throat clearing, cursing, echolalia). Repetitive motor tics of the extremities can resemble chorea. Although the underlying mechanism of the disease is not well understood, it is considered to be a disorder of the basal ganglia that involves excessive levels of the transmitter dopamine. Pharmacological intervention includes dopamine-blocking agents, clonidine, haloperidol or pimozide.

Drug–induced movement disorders

Extrapyramidal dysfunction also occurs as the undesirable side effect of psychotropic drugs and other medications (Caligiuri et al 2000, Lee et al 2005, Morgan & Sethi 2005). Because drug metabolism and excretion mechanisms become less efficient with aging, older adults are more susceptible to drug toxicity and adverse drug reactions; the medications that older adults are prescribed may remain physiologically active for longer periods of time, especially if dosage is not adjusted for age and body composition (Ciccone 2002, Gladson 2005). Classes of medications associated with extrapyramidal side effects are outlined in Table 33.2.

Table 33.2   Medications associated with extrapyramidal side effects

Type of medication	Symptoms	Examples
Psychotropic/neuroleptic	Akathisia, pseudo-Parkinson's chorea, tardive dyskinesia, acute dyskinetic reaction	Phenothiazines (chlorpromazine, triflupromaxine, fluphenazine, perphenazine, trifluoperazine, pericyazine, promazine, mesoridazine); thioxanthenes (thiothizene, chlorprothixene); butyrophenones (droperidol, haloperidol); dibenzapines (loxapine); diphenylbutylpiperidines; indolones (molindone); many sleeping medications
Antidepressants	Chorea, athetosis, akathisia Tremor, myoclonus, pseudo-Parkinson's chorea	Tricyclic antidepressants, mono-oxide inhibitors Lithium carbonate, amoxapine
Stimulants	Postural tremor, chorea	Amphetamines, methadone, methylphenidate, fenfluramine; caffeine, cocaine
CNS depressants/sedatives	Physiological intention tremor, chorea, dystonia	Alcohol; diazepam
Anticonvulsants	Intention tremor, chorea, asterixis	Phenytoin, valproic acid, carbamazepine; phenobarbital, clonazepam
Anti-Parkinson's medications	Akathisia, chorea, dystonia	Amantadine, bromocriptine, L-dopa
Other types of medication	Tremor Chorea, tremor Chorea, dystonia, tremor Tardive dyskinesia Intention tremor, ataxia Chorea	Bronchodilators (theophylline, doxapram); hypoglycemics; corticosteroids Gastrointestinal medications (cimetadine, terfenadine) Antiarrhythmic medications (propranolol, tocainide) Antiemetic medications (prochlorperazine, thiethylperazine, promethazine) Cyclosporin A Estrogen/oral contraceptives

The psychotropic medications most likely to cause iatrogenic extrapyramidal dysfunction include phenothiazines, respirine, benzodiazepines, thioxanthenes and butyrophenones. Tricyclic antidepressants may have similar effects in some individuals. The incidence of drug-induced movement problems in individuals using neuroleptics for long-term management of psychiatric disorders may be as high as 25%. Akathisia is often the initial indicator of iatrogenic extrapyramidal dysfunction, especially in those using medications in the phenothiazine group. Over time, many susceptible individuals develop a condition that mimics Parkinson's disease, including hypokinesia, rigidity, stooped and flexed upright posture, shuffling gait and balance impairment.

An acute dyskinetic reaction occurs within days of initiation of therapy with medications such as phenothiazines, butyrophenones, tricyclic antidepressants, phenytoin, carbamazepine, propranolol and certain calcium-channel blockers. Although this is more common in young adults, it can occur in older adults as well. The relatively sudden onset of choreiform movement of the face, head and neck, or limbs can be frightening but typically resolves as the offending medication is withdrawn.

Tardive dyskinesia is the most severe form of medication-related extrapyramidal movement dysfunction, typically developing 3–12 months into the use of dopamine antagonists (Paulson 2005). Individuals who develop tardive dyskinesia demonstrate involuntary rhythmic choreoathetoid movements of the face, mouth and tongue (e.g. repeated tongue thrusts, lip smacking, sucking, grimacing, blinking). Some may also experience chorea of the extremities and dystonia (e.g. torticollis, occulogyric crisis, opisthotonos). These extrapyramidal signs may develop slowly and progressively worsen until the precipitating medication is reduced in dosage or discontinued; sometimes, symptoms of tardive dyskinesia persist even after the medication is discontinued. If the medication that triggers tardive dyskinesia cannot be discontinued, mild extrapyramidal symptoms can be managed with anti-Parkinson's medication or benzodiazepines. Severe cases of tardive dyskinesia may need to be managed with dopamine-blocking agents, which themselves carry the risk of orthostatic hypotension.

Certain other medications also carry a risk of extrapyramidal side effects. It is not uncommon for individuals taking L-dopa for the long-term management of Parkinson's disease to develop choreic movements of the face, tongue and (less commonly) lower extremities (Elble 2002). The severity of symptoms is dosage related, fluctuating with the levels of circulating L-dopa. Although more frequent administration of smaller doses may reduce the chorea, the disabling bradykinesia and gait disturbance typical of Parkinson's may intensify.

Chorea is an infrequent side effect of anticonvulsant medications such as phenytoin and carbamazepine. If chorea develops, the triggering medication should be withdrawn, even if blood levels are within the therapeutic range. The onset of choreiform movement is one of the many signs of lithium toxicity. Certain CNS stimulants (e.g. amphetamines, methylphenidate) may also induce oral–facial choreiform movement.

REHABILITATION INTERVENTIONS FOR INDIVIDUALS WITH TREMOR AND DYSKINESIA

Although rehabilitation professionals working in geriatric healthcare settings are likely to encounter older individuals who have 'aged' with a concurrent movement disorder (e.g. choreoathetoid cerebral palsy) or have developed dyskinesia associated with a pathology that is more prevalent in later life (e.g. dystonia after stroke, Parkinson's disease), the evidence in the clinical research literature regarding the impact of nonpharmacological and nonsurgical interventions on tremor and other dyskinesias is incomplete. The most compelling evidence is that exercise aimed at preserving or improving cardiovascular fitness, strength and flexibility enhances the functional status of individuals coping with movement disorders by reducing the risk of deconditioning and physical compromise associated with inactivity and a sedentary lifestyle (Bilodeau et al 2000, Reuter 2002, Bilney et al 2003, Robichaud & Corcos 2005, Zesiewicz et al 2005). The use of resting or tone-inhibiting splints and positions may be helpful in slowing secondary musculoskeletal complications (such as severe contracture) in individuals with dystonia. Certainly, functional assessment and training with assistive devices is well warranted to address limitations in mobility, locomotion and activities of daily living in individuals with various types of tremor, dystonia, chorea or athetosis (Guide to Physical Therapist Practice 2003). The evidence regarding the usefulness of cuff weights during functional activities such as feeding (theoretically providing more intense proprioceptive information to the cerebellum) in individuals with intention tremor is conflicting (Meshack & Norman 2002). Periodic reassessment and adjustment of fitness/wellness activities is especially important for those with progressive CNS disorders. In addition, pathologies that result in movement disorders often increase the daily physiological (caloric) demand, while at the same time compromising swallowing, coughing and other bulbar functions. Referral to nutritionists/dieticians and to speech and language pathologists is an important component of the effective interdisciplinary care of individuals with movement dyskinesia.

CONCLUSION

To be most effective in their care of older adults with tremor and other dyskinesias, physical therapists and other rehabilitation professionals must be familiar with the various movement dysfunctions, the etiology and progression of the underlying pathological process and their medical (pharmacological and/or surgical) management. It is especially important to recognize extrapyramidal symptoms of adverse drug reactions and toxicity in older adults. Although rehabilitation interventions may not directly reduce the severity of tremor or other involuntary movement, functional assessment and training have an important role to play and a powerful impact on quality of life as well as in preventing secondary impairments of the musculoskeletal and cardiovascular systems that may occur as a consequence of inactivity.

References

Adams AC 2001 Neurology in Primary Care. FA Davis, Philadelphia, PA

Alarcon F, Zijlmans JC, Duenas G, Cevallos N 2004 Post-stroke movement disorders: report of 56 patients. J Neurol Neurosurg Psychiatry 75(11):1568–1574

Aminoff MJ 2003 Neurology and General Medicine, 3rd edn. Churchill Livingstone, Philadelphia, PA

Bhidayasiri R 2005 Differential diagnosis of common tremor syndromes. Postgrad Med J 81(962):756–762

Bhidayasiri R, Truong DD 2004 Chorea and related disorders. Postgrad Med J 80(947):527–534

Bilney B, Morris ME, Perry A 2003 Effectiveness of physiotherapy, occupational therapy and speech pathology for people with Huntington's disease: a systematic review. Neurorehabil Neural Repair 17(1):12–24

Bilodeau M, Keen DA, Sweeney JP et al 2000 Strength training can improve steadiness in persons with essential tremor. Musc Nerve 23(5):771–778

Bradley WG, Daroff RB, Fenichel G, Jankovic J 2003 Neurology in Clinical Practice, 4th edn. Butterworth Heinemann, Boston, MA

Caligiuri MP, Jeste DV, Lacro JP 2000 Antipsychotic-induced movement disorders in the elderly: epidemiology and treatment recommendations. Drugs Aging 17(5):363–384

Ciccone CD 2002 Pharmacology in Rehabilitation, 3rd edn. FA Davis, Philadelphia, PA

Elble RJ 2002 Tremor and dopamine agonists. Neurology 58(4suppl1):S57–62

Gladson B 2005 Pharmacology for Physical Therapists. WB Saunders, Philadelphia, PA

Guide to Physical Therapist Practice 2003, 2nd edn (revised). American Physical Therapy Association, Alexandria, VA

Hallett M 2003 Movement Disorders: Handbook of Clinical Neurophysiology. Elsevier, Philadelphia, PA

Jankovic JJ, Eduardo T 2002 Parkinson's Disease and Movement Disorders. Lippincott Williams & Wilkins, Philadelphia, PA

Janvas JL, Aminoff MJ 1998 Dystonia and chorea in acquired systemic disorders. J Neurol Neurosurg Psychiatry 65(4):436–445

Klein C 2005 Movement disorders: classification. J Inherit Metab Dis 28(3):425–439

Krauss JK, Jankovic J 2002 Head injury and posttraumatic movement disorders. Neurosurgery 50(5):927–939

Lee PE, Sykora K, Gill SS et al 2005 Antipsychotic medications and drug-induced movement disorders other than parkinsonism: a population-based cohort study in older adults. J Am Geriatr Soc 53(8):1374–1379

Louis ED, Wendt KJ, Ford B 2000 Senile tremor: what is the prevalence and severity of tremor in older adults? Gerontology 46:12–16

Meshack RP, Norman KE 2002 A randomized controlled trial of the effects of weights on amplitude and frequency of postural hand tremor in people with Parkinson's disease. Clin Rehabil 16:481–492

Morgan JC, Sethi KD 2005 Drug-induced tremors. Lancet Neurol 4(12):855–876

O'Suilleabhain P, Dewey RB 2004 Movement disorders after head injury: diagnosis and management. J Head Trauma Rehabil 19(4):305–313

Paulson GW 2005 Historical comments on tardive dyskinesia: a neurologist's perspective. J Clin Psychiatry 66(2):260–264

Poolos NP 2001 Handbook of Differential Diagnosis in Neurology. Butterworth Heinemann, Boston, MA

Reuter I 2002 Exercise training and Parkinson's disease. Physician Sports Med 30(3):43–50

Robichaud JA, Corcos DM 2005 Motor deficits, exercise, and Parkinson's disease. Quest 57:79–101

Sullivan KL, Hauser RA, Zesiewicz TA 2004 Essential tremor: epidemiology, diagnosis, and treatment. Neurologist 10(5):250–258

Weiner WJ, Lang KE 2005 Behavioral Neurology of Movement Disorders. Lippincott Williams & Wilkins, Philadelphia, PA

Whitney SL, Wrisely DM, Musolino MC, Furman JM 2003 Orthostatic tremor: two persons in a balance disorder practice. Neurology Rep 27(2):46–53

Zesiewicz TA, Elble R, Louis ED et al 2005 Practice parameter: therapies for essential tremor. Report of the Quality Standards Subcommittee of the American Academy of Neurology. Neurology 64(12):2008–2020

Chapter **34**

Generalized peripheral neuropathy

Anita S.W. Craig and James K. Richardson

INTRODUCTION

Disorders of the peripheral nerves are common in the elderly and are likely to have a significant impact on the rehabilitation plan. Generalized peripheral polyneuropathies are regularly encountered. It is estimated that 18% of Caucasian Americans and 26% of African–Americans older than 60 have diabetes mellitus; half of these individuals have peripheral neuropathy (PN). Therefore, approximately 10% of Americans over 60 have PN as a result of diabetes and another 10% have PN as a result of other causes, which results in a prevalence of about 20% in the older American population (Richardson & Ashton-Miller 1996). The prevalence of PN in older Americans requiring rehabilitation is undoubtedly much higher. Recognizing a generalized peripheral polyneuropathy and the functional limitations associated with it is important and necessary if a patient is to be successfully rehabilitated. This chapter provides the rehabilitation clinician with knowledge that will allow the recognition and treatment of a functionally significant generalized PN.

RECOGNIZING A GENERALIZED PERIPHERAL NEUROPATHY

PNs can be characterized by the type of nerve fibers affected, whether they affect the nerve axon or myelin and the distribution of affected nerves. The majority of PNs are diffuse and symmetrical in distribution; however, asymmetrical or multifocal neuropathies can be seen in many vasculitic disorders (Craig & Richardson 2003). Neuropathies affecting predominantly small fibers, somatic or autonomic, can be difficult to diagnose as they can present with profound neuropathic pain but have relatively normal physical and electrodiagnostic examinations (Hoitsma et al 2004).

If it is understood that the longer the peripheral nerve, the more greatly it is affected by neuropathic processes, then the signs and symptoms of PN make intuitive sense. Because lower extremities are longer than upper extremities and because sensory nerves are longer than motor nerves (as a result of the former's intraspinal dendritic processes), distal lower extremity sensory function is the first and most severely affected in diffuse PN, followed by distal lower extremity motor function, distal upper extremity sensory function and distal upper extremity motor function. Additionally, nerves that are vulnerable to compressive neuropathies, such as the median and peroneal nerves, may be more susceptible to injury in patients already compromised by PN.

Patients are extremely variable with regard to their insight into PN and so historical features are variable as well. Many patients are acutely aware of their numbness and pain whereas others complain of vague sensory abnormalities such as walking on pillows or simply note that they must be more careful in performing activities requiring balance. When pain or numbness is apparent to the patient, the symptoms are most marked in the forefoot and then lessen proximally. In the upper extremity, symptoms may not occur or may occur in the fingertips only or the hand and distal forearm, depending upon the severity of disease. A typical distribution of nerve dysfunction is demonstrated in Figure 34.1. Motor symptoms are usually not noted but, with severe disease, foot-drop and lessening of hand dexterity may develop. Balance problems that are consistent with PN include difficulty climbing stairs without a railing. Patients often note the insidious onset of the need to touch something while walking, particularly if the floor surface is irregular or the lighting is low. In small-fiber neuropathies, autonomic symptoms may be present including increased or decreased sweating, dry eyes, erectile dysfunction and changes in skin temperature. Clinically significant orthostatic hypotension may be seen in the setting of small-fiber neuropathy associated with diabetes and amyloidosis, which is of particular concern in older populations given the association between postural hypotension and falls.

On examination, there is loss of sensory function in a distal-to-proximal gradient. This is best noted with a 128-Hz tuning fork maximally struck and placed at the base of the great toe, the malleolus and the tibial tuberosity. Accuracy of the test may be improved by first familiarizing the patient with the vibratory stimulus at the clavicle. The examiner should record the number of seconds the patients feels the buzz at each level. The test can also be carried out on the upper extremity by placing the tuning fork at the base of the second finger, the distal radius and the olecranon. In the presence of PN, the number of seconds that the patient feels the vibration increases proximally in the extremities affected. If the patient is able to perceive the

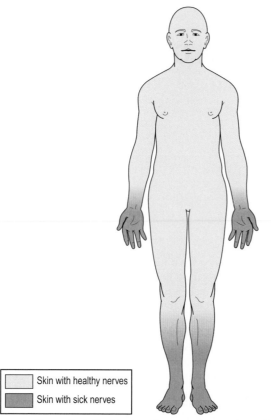

Figure 34.1 The typical distribution of sensory loss and, to a lesser extent, weakness in a patient with mild to moderate peripheral neuropathy.
(From Richardson & Ashton-Miller 1996, with permission from Vendome Group, LLC.)

Table 34.1 Clinical detection of functionally significant peripheral neuropathy

Test or condition	With peripheral neuropathy	Without peripheral neuropathy
Vibratory sense (128-Hz tuning fork)	Obvious gradient	Minimal or no gradient
	Vibration felt at malleolus for <5–10 s	Vibration felt at metatarsophalangeal joint for >10 s
Foot deformities, calluses	Present	Absent
Heel jerk	Absent	Present
Position sense at great toe	<8 of 10 correct responses	≥8 of 10 correct responses
Unipedal stance (three attempts on foot of choice)	≤5 s on each attempt	≥10 s on one of three attempts

From Richardson JK, Ashton-Miller JA 1996 Peripheral nerve dysfunction and falls in the elderly. Postgrad Med 99:169, with permission from Vendome Group, LLC.

maximally struck tuning fork for 10 s or more at the base of the great toe, PN is absent; if a similar patient perceives the same vibration for less than 10 s at the malleolus, PN is likely to be present. Light touch (using a 10-g monofilament) and pinprick sensation can also be used and they produce a similar sensory gradient. In the rare patient with small-fiber neuropathy, pinprick sensation may be diminished whereas vibratory sensation is relatively spared.

Muscle stretch reflexes are also lost in a distal-to-proximal gradient. Loss of Achilles tendon reflexes is almost uniform in PN; patellar tendon and internal hamstring reflexes are progressively less affected. Achilles tendon reflexes can be obtained either by direct percussion of the tendon or by using the plantar strike technique, which may be more reliably obtained in the older population. Proprioception is also affected in functionally significant PN, particularly at the great toe. The inability to correctly identify at least 8–10 small (approximately 1 cm) great toe movements by a noncuing examiner has been correlated with decreased ankle inversion/eversion proprioception (Vanden Bosch et al 1995). Absence of Achilles tendon reflex, with or without facilitation, the inability to perceive at least 8–10 great toe movements and the loss of vibratory sensation within 8 s are predictive of electrodiagnostically confirmed PN in older populations (Richardson 2002).

The intrinsic musculature of the foot is commonly atrophied in PN, which causes changes in foot architecture such that the metatarsophalangeal joints are extended and the interphalangeal joints are flexed ('hammer toes'). Toes move minimally or only in a stiff gross manner. In mild to moderate PN, ankle muscle strength may be more sensitively tested by performing 10–15 resistance maneuvers. In more advanced or severe PN, anterior compartment muscles and, less commonly, posterior calf muscles can atrophy. Usually, by the time these lower extremity changes have occurred, the intrinsic muscles of the hand have begun to weaken and atrophy. Skin lesions or breakdown can be seen in an insensate foot with a predilection for the heel and metatarsal heads. Gross motor function is also affected. Patients may have a positive Romberg's sign in that they are stable when standing with feet together and eyes open but not stable if the eyes are closed, which suggests a deficit in somatosensory input and excessive reliance upon vision for balance. A positive Romberg's sign suggests that the PN is relatively severe; however, many patients with functionally significant PN demonstrate a negative Romberg's sign. A more sensitive test of balance impairment secondary to PN is the assessment of unipedal stance time. If the patient can balance on one foot for 10 s or more (the best of three tries on the foot of choice), functionally significant PN is not likely to be present. If the patient can balance on one foot for only 3–4 s or less, then the PN is functionally significant. It should be noted that the unipedal stance test is not used to identify PN, but rather to determine the extent of loss of balance caused by the PN once it has been identified by the other elements of the clinical examination. In the upper extremity, a patient with functionally significant PN can be identified by the inability to fasten buttons without seeing them (the 'upper extremity Romberg's sign'). Table 34.1 lists the clinical characteristics of a patient with functionally significant PN.

Few other diseases mimic PN. Lumbar stenosis, which is common in older populations, can present in a similar fashion, with gradual-onset numbness and weakness in the distal lower extremities. However, symptoms of lumbar stenosis increase with prolonged standing and walking and improve with sitting or lying down. There is usually some accompanying back pain as well. This contrasts with painful PN, in which the pain is similar at all times or worse at night. On examination, the patient with lumbar stenosis does not usually demonstrate the symmetrical gradient of sensory loss that is found in the PN patient. If there is motor involvement, the patient with lumbar stenosis is likely to have asymmetrical weakness and weakness that commonly involves the gluteal as well as the distal musculature. In

Legend for figure:
☐ Skin with healthy nerves
■ Skin with sick nerves

contrast, the patient with PN has symmetrical weakness that is always most severe distally and improves proximally.

THE FUNCTIONAL RAMIFICATIONS OF NEUROPATHY

PN has a clear impact on the functioning of the older patient in rehabilitation. Two studies have demonstrated that patients with isolated PN are about 20 times more likely to fall than patients without PN (Richardson et al 1992, Richardson & Hurvitz 1995). The subjects in these studies had PN but no other functionally relevant diagnoses and were all community ambulators without assistive devices. PN will undoubtedly have an equal or greater impact on the functioning of rehabilitation patients who have accompanying diagnoses and worse baseline functioning.

Other studies comparing matched older patients with and without PN have demonstrated that PN subjects have impaired ankle proprioception (Vanden Bosch et al 1995) and a decreased ability to maintain a unipedal stance (Richardson et al 1996). The difficulty that PN subjects had with unipedal stance was present regardless of whether the subjects performed the task with preparation time or immediately upon command, with no preparation. This somewhat surprising finding suggests that patients with PN simply cannot do tasks requiring reliable unipedal stance, even if they take their time and are prepared. Therefore, climbing stairs without a support or dressing while standing will always be a challenge, even if done in a calm and leisurely fashion. The other study demonstrated that ankle inversion/eversion proprioceptive thresholds in subjects with PN were about 1.5 degrees but only 0.3 degrees in age- and sex-matched control subjects without PN. The 1.5 degrees of motion at the ankle allows the body's center of mass to travel to the edge of the patient's base of support during unipedal stance without them perceiving the change. As a result, the ability to maintain unipedal stance reliably is impaired.

The inability of the older PN patient to rapidly develop ankle strength contributes to gait dysfunction and the inability to maintain unipedal stance and recover from postural challenges; this is despite clinically normal ankle strength measured by manual muscle testing in patients with mild to moderate PN. In testing of ability to recover from lateral lean, subjects with PN were unable to rapidly develop the torque around the ankle that was necessary to recover (Guitierrez et al 2001). Patients with PN are therefore doubly penalized when their center of gravity is perturbed, as they require a greater excursion to perceive the loss of balance and they lack the ability to quickly generate the muscular torque to compensate, in spite of normal gross strength.

Clinical observation suggests that PN patients rarely fall in optimal environments, i.e. environments that are familiar to the patient and have good lighting and smooth level surfaces. However, irregular surfaces are often a cause of falls; they were found to underlie nearly 80% of the falls in a prospective study of 20 older PN subjects (DeMott et al 2006). Moreover, an increased step-time variability among the older PN subjects in the challenging, but not the standard, environment was associated with falls retrospectively (Richardson et al 2005) and prospectively (Guitierrez et al 2001). Similarly, the difference in gait parameters between patients with PN and those without PN is accentuated in a challenging environment (dim lighting and irregular surface). Specifically, in adapting to the challenging environment, the PN patients demonstrated greater increases in step width–step length ratio and step-time variability, and greater decreases in step length and speed than control subjects. These alterations in gait on an irregular surface have implications for endurance as the altered pattern is less efficient, and for community mobility, where the maintenance of speed on an irregular surface may be critical, for example when crossing a street. In summary, irregular surfaces appear to be a source of falls in older subjects, and gait analysis of PN patients on such surfaces appears to offer improved resolution for the detection of gait abnormalities and a predisposition to fall.

In the older rehabilitation patient, PN is rarely isolated as in the research subjects described above; therefore, PN exacerbates the clinically obvious impairments already present. For example, if a patient with PN has hemiparesis or an above-knee amputation as the primary rehabilitation diagnosis, then the patient's ability to use the 'good' lower extremity is also impaired. If the PN is not recognized, unrealistic expectations or caregiver confusion over difficulty with progression to certain goals develop. Patients with disruption of the other systems that help to maintain balance – the visual and the vestibular systems – have even greater difficulty staying upright if PN is present. Patients with ataxia from cerebellar or vestibular dysfunction and patients with visual or visual–spatial dysfunction have even worse problems when their clinical situation is complicated by PN. The early recognition of PN in such patients allows for the formulation of reasonable goals and an early start to the learning process that enables patients to compensate for PN.

TREATING THE PATIENT WITH PERIPHERAL NEUROPATHY

If PN is identified or suspected clinically, should it be further investigated? The answer depends on the circumstances. Some of the more common causes of PN are shown in Box 34.1. A number of them, for example alcohol abuse, diabetes mellitus, chronic obstructive pulmonary disease (COPD) and critical-care illness, are quite common in the older population. The identification of PN in a patient with any of these disorders, particularly if it has had a gradual onset, does not necessarily mean further investigation is necessary. On the other hand, if PN develops in a patient with no risk factors or it develops in any patient and exhibits a relatively rapid progression, the case deserves further investigation. PN can be the representing manifestation of many treatable systemic diseases. Making that distinction on clinical grounds is challenging; clues to a demyelinating PN are early loss of

---

Box 34.1   Common causes of a generalized peripheral polyneuropathy in older individuals

- Alcohol abuse
- Chronic obstructive pulmonary disease
- Diabetes mellitus
- Monoclonal gammopathy (benign or malignant)
- Neoplasm (especially leukemia, lymphoma)
- Past or long-term use of certain drugs including nitrofurantoin macrocrystals (Macrodantin), phenytoin (Dilantin), lithium, gold compounds, vincristine sulfate (Oncovin, Vincasar PFS), isoniazid, ethambutol HCl (Myambutol), disulfiram (Antabuse)
- Renal disease
- Thyroid disease
- Use of antiarrhythmic drugs [amiodarone HCl (Cordarone)]
- Vitamin B12 deficiency

all reflexes with relative preservation of muscle mass, whereas clues to an axonal PN are maintenance of proximal reflexes and a relatively greater muscle atrophy distally. In general, axonal PN is associated with metabolic disorders or toxins, and demyelinating PN is associated with immune processes that are, at times, related to malignancy. Neuropathies that present with asymmetrical involvement should raise suspicion for autoimmune or vasculitic disorders.

The most important aspect of treatment, in terms of the functional impact of PN, is education. The patient and the patient's family must understand the nature of the disorder – that the patient has lost a special sense in the distal lower (and sometimes upper) extremities. They must further understand that, as a result of this lost special sense, the patient's balance is impaired and compensatory techniques will be necessary to avoid an increased risk of falls.

Visual input must be maximized to compensate for the impaired somatosensory input. Vision should be tested and, if it is impaired, referral to the appropriate health professional is indicated. Equally important, the patient must be taught to use proper lighting. This is particularly significant at night during trips to the bathroom; the temptation to avoid putting on glasses and to leave the lights off so as not to disturb other household members as they sleep must be avoided.

A patient with PN should use proper footwear. The shoes that are best for balance have a wide base of support and thin soles. Thick crepe soles or the heavily cushioned soles of athletic shoes should be avoided. If significant foot deformity exists, custom orthotics, possibly in association with extra-depth shoes to accommodate the foot deformity, should be prescribed. Sometimes, a patient with poor balance finds plastic ankle–foot orthoses that are custom molded to be of benefit; however, care must be taken when fitting them to avoid the initiation of a foot wound. Patients and their families must be educated on the importance of regular skin inspections of insensate areas.

A patient with balance impairment as a result of PN should use support when walking. The use of a cane for stabilization in patients with PN has been studied (Ashton-Miller et al 1996). Subjects were asked to transfer onto an unsteady surface that tilted during mid-transfer and maintain 3 s of unipedal balance (Fig. 34.2). Under such circumstances, the PN subjects failed to maintain their balance without a cane about 50% of the time but succeeded with a cane about 96% of the time. It has been further demonstrated that, to obtain maximal benefit from a cane in preventing a fall, patients must be able to support approximately 25% of their body weight with the cane. The patient should be instructed to place the cane down with each contralateral footstep to assist in preventing falls away from the cane as well as towards it. Patient and family are often reluctant to accept the use of a cane. Acceptance and compliance may be greater if they are told that the cane is a substitute, like glasses or a hearing aid, for a special sense that has been lost and is a way to prevent falls, not a sign of infirmity. The patient also complies better if the cane is used as needed and not all the time. A patient can usually be free of the cane when the lighting is good and the walking surface is firm, flat and familiar. Other interventions can also improve gait parameters and decrease the risk of falls, particularly on irregular surfaces. These include the use of ankle orthoses (AO) with medial and lateral supports and the use of a firm vertical surface for support. All three interventions have been shown to improve step-width variability, which suggests improved medial/lateral stability, and decreased step-width range (Richardson et al 2004). The use of the AO and the vertical wall also improved step-time variability, which has been prospectively associated with falls (Hausdorff et al 2001). Only the use of a cane was associated with decreased walking speed. Advantages of the use of AOs over a cane include the availability of both upper extremities and better walking speed; the disadvantage of an AO is the possibility of skin breakdown.

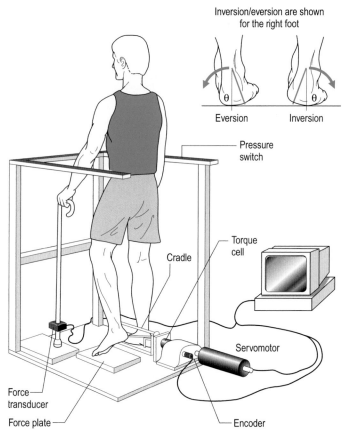

Figure 34.2 The apparatus developed by Dr. J.A. Ashton-Miller to assess the ability of subjects to transfer onto an unstable surface and maintain balance on one foot, with and without vision and/or a cane. This apparatus is also able to help determine ankle inversion/eversion proprioceptive thresholds in subjects with and without PN.

(After Vanden Bosch et al 1995, with permission from WB Saunders.)

There is no evidence that physical training prevents falls in cases of PN; however, a study of a specific exercise program showed that improvements were made in clinical measures of balance (Richardson et al 2001). Subjects with electrodiagnostically confirmed PN were given a series of exercises including bipedal and unipedal toe and heel raises and inversion/eversion exercises; wall slides; unipedal balance exercises; and open chain ankle range-of-motion exercises. In a relatively short period of time, improvements were seen in tandem stance, functional reach and unipedal stance time. Whether these interventions translate to a decreased risk of falls is not proven but, if a patient is interested and motivated, these exercises are simple to teach and well tolerated. Patients with inadequate upper extremity strength should work with grip, shoulder depression and elbow extension so that 25% of their body weight can be supported with a cane if necessary. Strengthening exercises of the hip abductors and abdominal musculature can improve trunk and hip stability and are recommended.

Pain can be a significant problem for a patient with PN, particularly at night. A trial of the topical medication capsaicin is indicated if the patient has the intellectual capacity and manual dexterity to apply it correctly. Although it is cumbersome to use because it must be applied 3–4 times per day and it can make symptoms worse at first, capsaicin has the distinct advantage of causing no systemic side effects, a particularly important point in a debilitated older patient. If the painful area is fairly discrete, a transdermal lidoderm patch can be applied. Other options include a low dosage of one of the tricyclic antidepressants with low anticholinergic effects, for example 10–50 mg of nortryptyline before bed. Other agents include anticonvulsants, such as carbamazepine (Tegretol), phenytoin (Dilantin) and gabapentin (Neurontin); however, the side effects of these drugs limit their use in an older population. Newer medications that have Food and Drug Administration (FDA)-labeled indications for neuropathic pain include duloxetine (Cymbalta) and pregabalin (Lyrica). Transcutaneous electrical nerve stimulation (TENS) can be helpful and, like capsaicin, it has the advantage of producing no systemic side effects.

CONCLUSION

Approximately 20% of older Americans have PN, which is likely to have an impact on rehabilitation. Sensory impairment is usually more prominent than motor impairment and distal lower extremities are affected more than distal upper extremities. These changes usually impair balance control and often lead to falls. Generalized PN usually compounds existing clinical impairments. The patient and the patient's family must be educated about the loss and advised of the potential risk for further injury and how to mitigate risks. The use of assistive devices for mobility, therapeutic exercises for functional activities and medication or TENS for pain is encouraged.

References

Ashton-Miller JA, Yeh MW, Richardson JK et al 1996 A cane lowers the risk of patients with peripheral neuropathy losing their balance: results from a challenging unipedal balance test. Arch Phys Med Rehabil 77:446–452

Craig ASW, Richardson JK 2003 Acquired peripheral neuropathy. Phys Med Rehabil Clin North Am 14:365–386

DeMott TK, Richardson JK, Thies SB, Ashton-Miller JA 2007 Falls and gait characteristics among older persons with peripheral neuropathy. Am J Phys Med 86, in press

Guitierrez EM, Helber MD, Dealva D et al 2001 Mild diabetic neuropathy affects ankle motor function. Clin Biomech 16:522–528

Hausdorff JM, Rios DA, Edelberg HK 2001 Gait variability and fall risk in community-living older adults: a 1-year prospective study. Arch Phys Med Rehabil 82:1050–1056

Hoitsma E, Reulen JPH, de Baets M 2004 Small fiber neuropathy: a common and important clinical disorder. J Neurol Sci 227:119–130

Richardson JK, Ching C, Hurvitz EA 1992 The relationship between electromyographically documented peripheral neuropathy and falls. J Am Geriatr Soc 40:1008–1012

Richardson JK, Hurvitz EA 1995 Peripheral neuropathy: a true risk factor for falls. J Gerontol Ser A Biol Sci Med Sci 50A:211–215

Richardson JK, Ashton-Miller JA 1996 Peripheral nerve dysfunction and falls in the elderly. Postgrad Med 99:161–172

Richardson JK, Ashton-Miller JA, Lee SG et al 1996 Moderate peripheral neuropathy impairs weight transfer and unipedal balance in the elderly. Arch Phys Med Rehabil 77:1152–1156

Richardson JK, Sandman D, Vela S 2001 A focused exercise regimen improves clinical measures of balance in patients with peripheral neuropathy. Arch Phys Med Rehabil 82:205–209

Richardson JK 2002 The clinical identification of peripheral neuropathy among older persons. Arch Phys Med Rehabil 83:1553–1558

Richardson JK, Thies SB, DeMott TK et al 2004 Interventions improve gait regularity in patients with peripheral neuropathy while walking on an irregular surface under low light. J Am Geriatr Soc 52:510–515

Richardson JK, Thies SB, DeMott TK et al 2005 Gait analysis in a challenging environment differentiates between fallers and nonfallers among older patients with peripheral neuropathy. Arch Phys Med Rehabil 86:1539–1544

Vanden Bosch CG, Gilsing M, Lee SG, Richardson JK et al 1995 Effect of peripheral neuropathy on ankle inversion and eversion detection thresholds. Arch Phys Med Rehabil 76:850–856

Chapter 35

Localized peripheral neuropathies

James K. Richardson and Anita S.W. Craig

CHAPTER CONTENTS

INTRODUCTION

Localized peripheral neuropathies are even more common than generalized neuropathies and the two often coincide. Because a diffusely diseased peripheral nervous system is less able to recover from a mechanical insult than a healthy peripheral nervous system, it is a clinical rule that a patient with generalized peripheral neuropathy is at an increased risk for specific discrete neuropathies. In addition, mechanical insults are particularly common in the rehabilitation setting as patients learn alternative strategies for self-care and mobility. Such strategies often involve stressing intact musculoskeletal regions to compensate for regions that are impaired, which increases the risk of nerve trauma in the intact regions. For example, more than 50% of wheelchair athletes have carpal tunnel syndrome (CTS) (Burnham & Steadward 1994). Obviously, early recognition, prevention and, when necessary, treatment of these specific neuropathies are critical for the prevention of further impairment and disability in older patients.

Unfortunately, localized or regional neuropathies are often a particular challenge for the healthcare practitioner (Fuller 2003). The difficulty in diagnosing such problems stems from the fact that even the most articulate patient often has trouble describing the onset, location, quality, and aggravating and alleviating factors of neuropathic pain. Such patients commonly have severe pain but few motor signs to help localize the lesions. Conversely, a patient who has significant weakness because of a peripheral nerve disorder often has few sensory complaints, which can also obscure the diagnosis. However, the proper diagnosis and treatment of these local or regional peripheral neuropathies are often critical to the patient's rehabilitation. Furthermore, some rehabilitative strategies, such as assistive devices and orthotics, are often the cause of peripheral neurological disorders or delayed healing. Finally, peripheral neurological disorders, even when benign, can cause patients and families significant anxiety because they worry that the symptoms represent the progression of a previously existing neurological disease or a new, potentially malignant, entity. Therefore, although it may be challenging at times to obtain, a clear understanding of a patient's peripheral neurological status is of great benefit to the patient and the healthcare practitioner.

In organizing this chapter, the authors considered simply enumerating peripheral neurological disorders by anatomical region. The difficulty with this approach is that a patient does not tell a healthcare practitioner about an 'ulnar mononeuropathy at the elbow' or 'an L5 radiculopathy on the left'. Rather, a patient mentions a numb hand or a foot that drops. Therefore, this chapter will be organized around typical (and nonspecific) symptoms and complaints. The potentially responsible focal neuropathy will be identified for each symptom. The details of clinical presentation and approach to each potentially responsible focal neuropathy will also be discussed.

NUMB HAND

Hand numbness and pain are extremely common complaints. Usually, one of the three nerves that serves the hand distally – the median, radial or ulnar nerves – is at fault. Hand numbness is also a possible presentation of a more proximal process such as a radiculopathy or plexopathy.

Median nerve compression

Although classic median nerve compression at the wrist (CTS) involves the second and third digits (the palmar cutaneous branch to the thenar eminence often branches off proximal to the carpal tunnel), the patient often senses that the 'whole hand is numb'. Examination should focus on sensation in the median distribution (avoiding the thumb). Pinprick sensitivity should be determined by first pricking a noninvolved area and then comparing the sensitivity between sides. Ask, 'If this (the normal side) is 100 percent, how much is this (the affected side)?' It is important not to ask the patient to indicate whether the sensation is sharp or dull because the sharp sensation is often maintained, even in the presence of a clinically significant localized or generalized neuropathy. An additional clue is the presence of Tinel's sign, tingling that radiates from the percussed median nerve at the site of entrapment. The site of entrapment is more distal than is often perceived, approximately 1–2 cm beyond the distal wrist crease. This is the area that should be percussed (Fig. 35.1) (Stewart 1993). Phalen's sign, in which the wrists are held in flexed positions for 30–60 s by pushing the dorsa of the hands together in front of the chest, is often used in examination; however, it is overly sensitive

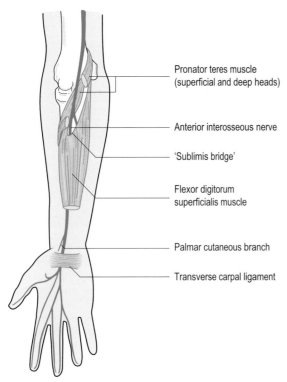

Figure 35.1 The site of compression of the median nerve at the wrist. Note the palmar cutaneous branch taking off proximal to the site of compression.
(From Stewart JD 1993 Focal Peripheral Neuropathies, 2nd edn. Raven Press, New York, p 158, with permission from Lippincott Williams & Wilkins.)

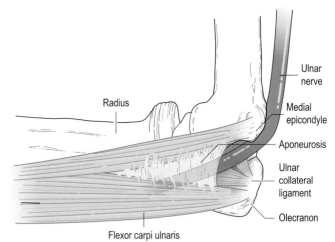

Figure 35.2 The vulnerability of the ulnar nerve to compressive or stretching forces at the elbow is obvious.
(From Kincaid JC 1983 Minimonograph no.31: The Electrodiagnosis of Ulnar Neuropathy at the Elbow. American Association of Electrodiagnostic Medicine, Rochester, MN, with permission.)

because pain of a nature other than that caused by CTS is often elicited. A particularly misleading 'positive' Phalen's test occurs when the hands turn numb because of the stretching of compressed ulnar nerves across the flexed elbows rather than because of median nerve compression at the wrist. Attention should also be paid to the muscles in the hand that are served by the median nerve, those of the thenar eminence. An obvious difference in bulk and strength suggests significant axonal damage to the median nerve and a prolonged, often incomplete, recovery, even with surgical decompression. It is important for the examiner to test the strength of the patient's thumb abductors by opposing them with their own.

Treatment

Treatment requires decreasing the pressure within the carpal tunnel. The pressure in the canal is increased in positions of hyperflexion or hyperextension. Avoidance of wrist extension and gripping is particularly difficult for those who use assistive devices such as walkers and canes. The temporary use of forearm platforms rather than hand grips on assistive devices lessens the pressure on the median nerve without compromising mobility and safety. The use of a splint, which prevents flexion and extension, particularly at night when a patient's tendency is to sleep with the wrist flexed or extended, is recommended. A patient who routinely uses a sliding board is also at risk. Using splints during transfers may allow continued function without repetitively compressing the median nerve. Local steroid injections may offer relief for those who do not respond to conservative measures. Injections have been shown to be superior to surgical decompression at 3 months, with significant clinical improvement in both nocturnal

and diurnal symptoms and functional impairment. Two injections are usually required, administered 2 weeks apart (Ly-Pen et al 2005).

Ulnar nerve compression

The second most common cause of hand numbness is ulnar nerve compression. This occurs most commonly at the elbow. Decreased pinprick response in the ulnar distribution (the fourth and fifth digits), hand-intrinsic muscle wasting and a positive Tinel's sign over the ulnar nerve at the elbow are common findings. When severe, hand-intrinsic wasting leads to a characteristic hand position of hyperextension at the metacarpophalangeal joints and flexion at the interphalangeal joints. The interossei of the hands should be tested against the interossei of the examiner's hands so that a true estimation of strength is possible. This is similar to the testing of the thumb abductors in CTS.

Cause and treatment

The cause of an ulnar neuropathy in an older patient is usually compression at the elbow within the groove between the olecranon and the medial epicondyle, or the stretching of the nerve from a prolonged hyperflexed elbow position (Fig. 35.2) (Kincaid 1983). The latter often occurs while a patient sleeps on one side holding the hand against the neck and chest. Compression commonly occurs in wheelchair users as forearms and elbows rest on wheelchair arms. Men are more likely to develop ulnar mononeuropathies at the elbow (UME) and older age is associated with greater risk, whereas, in women, lower body mass index is a more significant risk factor. This suggests that external compression may be more of a significant factor in the development of UME in women than in men. Treatment is best accomplished by protecting the elbow with an elastic pad, such as those often used by athletes. The pad can be maintained posteriorly during the day to prevent compression and anteriorly during sleep to prevent hyperflexion. If these measures are not successful, ulnar transposition surgery can be performed to remove the nerve from its usual position over a bony prominence. Compression of the ulnar nerve at the wrist is far less common but may occur with direct compression over the wrist and hypothenar eminence. This can be caused by the use of an

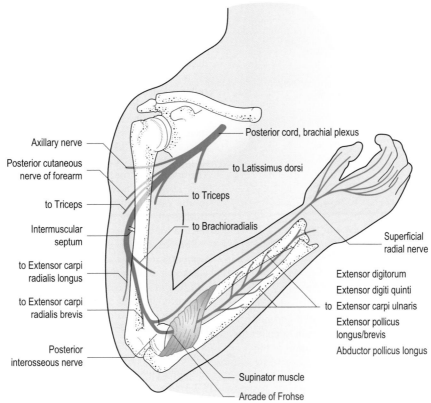

Figure 35.3 The superficial radial nerve in the forearm and the radial nerve as it wraps around the humerus are vulnerable to compressive forces.
(From Lotem M, Fried A, Levy M 1971 Radial palsy following muscular effort: a nerve compression syndrome possibly related to a fibrous arch of the lateral head of the triceps. J Bone Joint Surg Br 53B:500–506, with permission from British Editorial Society of Bone and Joint Surgery.)

assistive device, such as a walker or cane, or with wheelchair propulsion (Richardson et al 2001).

Radial nerve involvement

One of the pitfalls in the treatment of CTS is the development of a radial sensory neuropathy of the distal forearm (Fig. 35.3) (Lotem et al 1971). In this situation, the splint compresses the superficial radial nerve over the distal and radial aspects of the forearm. The only clinical consequence is sensory loss as there is no radial motor function in the hand-intrinsic musculature. The numbness that was initially attributed to CTS persists in the second and third digits of the hand despite the splint. At this point, however, the numbness involves the dorsum of the hand rather than the palmar aspect, but the patient may not recognize or report this subtle change. Decreased pinprick and light-touch sensation in the radial nerve distribution is noted on examination and, usually, a Tinel's sign can be noted with gentle percussion over the superficial radial nerve in the distal forearm. The CTS signs may coexist or may have resolved. Treatment should consist of discontinuing (if the CTS is resolved) or modifying the splint to relieve the compression of the nerve.

The radial nerve can also be affected proximally. This occurs most commonly following a humeral fracture after a fall by an osteoporotic patient but it can also occur after a prolonged compression of the posterolateral humerus (see Fig. 35.3). When the radial nerve is injured proximally, the hand numbness in the radial distribution is accompanied by weakness of the brachioradialis muscle and the

wrist and digit extensors (Fuller 2003). At times, the nerve is not injured acutely at the time of fracture but becomes compressed by bony callus as the fracture heals. This pattern of injury would be most evident to the patient's rehabilitation team. Dynamic orthotics can substitute for some of the extensor functions of the digits until the return of neurological function.

Brachial plexopathy

Another cause of hand numbness that is seen in the older population is an injury to the brachial plexus (see Fig. 35.4). Common causes include trauma, tumors and remote effects from radiation, most commonly to the chest and axilla during treatment for breast or lung cancer. Motor vehicle accidents typically affect the upper trunk; the patient's head is laterally flexed and the shoulders depressed. Such patients experience weakness in the humeral rotators and abductors and the elbow flexors, with numbness involving the lateral aspect of the arm and the first and second digits of the hand more than the fifth. Trauma after surgery usually results from the upper extremity being abducted and externally rotated, which leads to excessive stretching of the lower trunk of the plexus. This results in weakness of the hand-intrinsic musculature and to numbness in the fourth and fifth digits (Fig. 35.4) (Wilbourn 1982).

Tumors – metastatic, recurrent or primary – can cause plexopathy. The two most common tumors to affect the plexus are those of the lung and breast. Classically, these tumors cause shoulder pain and a predominantly lower trunk plexopathy with numbness along the

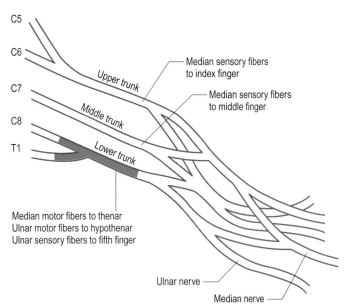

Figure 35.4 The lower trunk of the brachial plexus supplies the hand-intrinsic musculature and supplies sensation to the medial (ulnar) aspect of the forearm and hand; the upper trunk supplies the shoulder musculature and elbow flexors, giving sensation to the lateral aspect of the forearm and hand.
(From Wilbourn A 1982 Case Report no.7: True Neurogenic Thoracic Outlet Syndrome. American Association of Electrodiagnostic Medicine, Rochester, MN, with permission.)

medial aspect of the forearm and hand weakness. Except for Pancoast's syndrome, a carcinoma involving the apex of the lung, it is rare for the brachial plexopathy to be the first manifestation of the tumor. Finally, exposure of the upper chest or shoulder to radiation, for example in lymphoma and breast or lung cancer, can lead to plexopathy. Plexopathy does not occur in every patient who has received radiation therapy, but the likelihood increases with higher doses. Symptoms and signs of plexopathy can occur anywhere from a few months to several years after the completion of radiation therapy. Although it has been suggested that pain and lower trunk involvement are more commonly caused by recurrence of the tumor and upper trunk involvement by radiation effects, it is not possible to distinguish the two based on clinical grounds and a more extensive investigation is indicated.

Regardless of cause, brachial plexopathies that are primarily demyelinating in nature can improve rapidly and leave a fully functional limb. Plexopathies that are associated with significant axon loss typically improve slowly and the patient is usually left with some residual weakness and sensory loss. Atrophy is an important clinical clue to significant axon loss; electrodiagnostic studies can determine much more precisely the degree and distribution of axon loss, thus assisting the rehabilitation clinician with prognosis.

Cervical radiculopathy

Radiculopathy can be a cause of hand numbness in the older patient (Fuller 2003). Although C7 is the most common level affected by acute disk herniations, C5 and C6 are the levels most commonly affected by chronic degenerative changes and are therefore the most commonly affected in the older population.

With a cervical radiculopathy at this level, the patient experiences numbness over the lateral aspect of the forearm and the first and second digits. Weakness occurs predominantly in the humeral rotators and elbow flexors. In a C7 radiculopathy, the third digit feels numb and the elbow extensors and shoulder depressors are weak. With lower cervical radiculopathies (C8 and T1), the fourth and fifth digits are numb and weakness is most prominent in the hand-intrinsic musculature. Atrophy, weakness and decreased reflexes in the proper distribution are clues to the presence of a radiculopathy. In addition, if compression of the nerve roots by simultaneously extending, laterally flexing and rotating the head to the symptomatic side increases upper extremity symptoms and pain (Spurling's sign), radiculopathy is likely. Extension of the neck should be undertaken cautiously in the older patient with vascular or degenerative disease. The addition of axial compression of the head to the above maneuvers, as is often advocated in the Spurling's test, should be avoided in the older patient undergoing rehabilitation. Electrodiagnostic studies should be obtained to assist with specific diagnoses, prognostication and treatment.

Radiculopathies and plexopathies have functional ramifications. Upper plexopathies and high cervical radiculopathies lead to shoulder weakness; this weakness, in turn, predisposes the patient to rotator cuff tendinopathies and impingement. This is particularly true if the extremity is used regularly or is overused, for example during ambulation with a cane or walker. If possible, the extremity should not be used to assist with mobility skills. If this is not possible, the use of a platform rather than a standard cane or walker may be helpful, as these allow the shoulder to bear weight with less internal rotation. C7 radiculopathies cause weakness of shoulder depressors and elbow extensors. As a result, the extremity is much less effective during transfers. It can still assist with ambulation but less effectively; the patient may benefit from a shortening of the cane so that the elbow can lock when the cane is placed on the ground. Lower trunk plexopathies and C8/T1 radiculopathies result in hand and finger weakness. Assistive devices can still be used effectively but compensation for the weakened grip may have to be made. Activities of daily living (ADLs) that require fine motor function become very difficult and adaptive techniques are usually necessary.

Stenosis and myelopathy

It should be noted that the same cervical degenerative processes that cause upper extremity radiculopathies in older patients can cause cervical stenosis and resultant myelopathy (Malcolm 2002); this is particularly true following a fall or motor vehicle accident when the spinal cord is 'shaken' against a narrowed irregular cervical spinal canal. Such patients have weak atrophied upper extremities and minimally atrophied, often spastic, lower extremities; these changes are sometimes associated with bowel or bladder dysfunction. Muscle stretch reflexes give the best clinical clues. Depressed reflexes in the upper extremities associated with hyperactive reflexes and extensor plantar (Babinski) responses in the lower extremities suggest a cervical myelopathy. If this syndrome is suspected, then appropriate imaging studies and neurosurgical consultation are indicated.

FOOT-DROP

Foot-drop, or dorsiflexor weakness, is a common observation or complaint in the older population. Both upper motor neuron dysfunction leading to equinovarus posturing and lower motor neuron dysfunction can cause functionally significant foot-drop. This section focuses on the latter. The common areas of peripheral nerve compression that lead to foot-drop are demonstrated in Figure 35.5 (Stewart 1993).

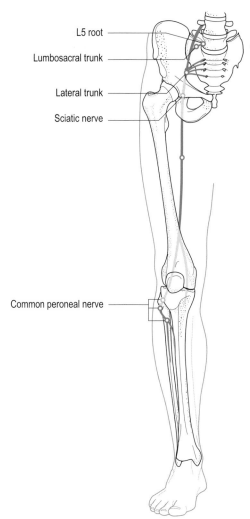

L5 root

Lumbosacral trunk

Lateral trunk

Sciatic nerve

Common peroneal nerve

Figure 35.5   The common sites of compression or trauma that lead to foot-drop.
(From Stewart JD 1993 Focal Peripheral Neuropathies, 2nd edn. Raven Press, New York, p 355, with permission from Lippincott Williams & Wilkins.)

Common peroneal neuropathy

Probably the most frequent cause of foot-drop is a common peroneal neuropathy at the fibular head. Older patients in rehabilitation have many risk factors for such a lesion. Common peroneal neuropathy typically occurs in patients with prolonged hospitalization, weight loss, knee replacement surgery, plaster casts and fractures of the fibular head or neck (Fuller 2003). Weakness occurs in the ankle dorsiflexors and evertors. Numbness and decreased sensation are present along the anterolateral calf and dorsum of the foot. At times, Tinel's sign can be found over the peroneal nerve just inferior and posterior to the fibular head. Significant wasting of the musculature of the anterior and lateral compartments suggests significant axon loss and a prolonged or incomplete recovery. Electrodiagnostic studies can further clarify both diagnosis and prognosis. Treatment should protect the peroneal nerve from further mechanical trauma. Weight gain and careful positioning in bed to prevent knee hyperflexion and pressure over the area are helpful. As the patient becomes ambulatory, it is imperative that the ankle–foot orthosis prescribed to compensate for the foot-drop does not prolong it by putting pressure on the peroneal nerve adjacent to the fibular head.

Deep peroneal neuropathy

Less commonly, foot-drop can be caused by a deep peroneal neuropathy. The common peroneal nerve divides into the superficial and deep branches just distal to the fibular head. The deep branch provides innervation of the anterior compartment muscles, which are the ankle dorsiflexors and toe extensors, plus sensation to a small space between the dorsal aspects of the first and second toes. Lesions to the deep peroneal nerve are commonly caused by anterior compartment syndromes that result from high pressure within the anterior compartment caused by tissue trauma, tibial fracture or hemorrhage. Compartment syndromes are usually handled surgically in the acute care setting. The deep peroneal nerve is not influenced by external compression forces or positioning and so little can be done in the rehabilitation setting to influence the course of recovery, either positively or negatively. It is important to follow the guidelines mentioned above for the common peroneal nerve so that a lesion more proximal to the peroneal nerve does not develop.

L5 radiculopathy

Another cause of foot-drop is a low lumbar (usually L5) radiculopathy (Fuller 2003). This can develop as the result of an acute disk herniation, which is uncommon in older populations, or more gradually as the result of degenerative changes. Such patients usually have a long history of low back pain with or without leg pain. It should be kept in mind that tumor can be a cause of back pain and radiculopathy, especially in patients over 50. Clinical clues that suggest a malignant cause of back pain and radiculopathy include an age greater than 50, insidious onset, pain for more than 1 month and a history of any kind of cancer. Worsening pain at night is almost universal in patients with a malignant cause of back pain, but it also occurs commonly in benign causes of back pain. As a result, the absence of night pain is reassuring and suggests that the source of pain is not malignant, but the presence of night pain is less diagnostically helpful.

L5 radiculopathy can be differentiated clinically from a lesion at the fibular head by a variety of clinical findings. A patient with an L5 radiculopathy usually has the following: weakness in the hip abductors and knee flexors; loss of an internal hamstring reflex on the affected side; a positive straight-leg raising sign (straight-leg raising causes pain or dysesthesia in the anterolateral calf and dorsum of the foot); and absence of Tinel's sign at the fibular head. If the cause of the radiculopathy is not known, appropriate imaging studies should be performed. If the cause is benign, electrodiagnostic studies can provide prognostic information. As the patient begins to ambulate, it is important to use an orthosis to accommodate the foot-drop and also to support the weakened gluteal musculature by using a cane in the opposite hand. This helps to avoid a trochanteric bursitis on the affected side and difficulty during the swing phase of gait on the contralateral side.

Sciatic neuropathy

Despite the fact that the sciatic nerve contains fibers that give rise to both the tibial and peroneal nerves, a sciatic neuropathy can cause foot-drop. The reason for this is that the peroneal division of the sciatic nerve lies in a more lateral and superficial position as it travels through the buttock and proximal posterior thigh and is thus more vulnerable to external forces. Although in such instances, foot-drop, or dorsiflexion weakness, is the predominant finding, close examination usually suggests that there is some degree of tibial division involvement as demonstrated by a decreased ankle muscle stretch reflex or plantar flexor weakness or both. In addition, sensation commonly decreases in both the peroneal and tibial distributions (Fuller 2003). Risk factors for sciatic neuropathies in older patients include hip surgery, repeated intramuscular injections in the hip, cachexia, malpositioning (hips flexed for too long, lying supine on an operating-room table) and a history of trauma to the hip or pelvis. Avoiding pressure over the posterior thigh and buttock, such as that caused by sitting on a ledge, and avoiding a prolonged time either supine or with hips flexed are important to allow healing. Ankle–foot orthotics are important functionally but must be carefully fitted to prevent the development of a more distal peroneal neuropathy at the fibular head or a foot wound.

Lumbosacral plexopathy

Several disorders that are common among older patients can affect the lumbosacral plexus which, in turn, can cause foot-drop. These include radiation exposure, proximal diabetic neuropathy and retroperitoneal disorders such as hematomas, aortic aneurysms, malignancies and abscesses. Radiation plexopathy does not occur in the lumbar region as frequently as it does in the cervical region. When it does occur, symptoms develop a few months to several years after the radiation therapy and are associated with relatively painless weakness. Proximal diabetic neuropathy typically causes symptoms in the thigh and hip although more distal involvement is possible and will be discussed in a later section (see under Diabetic neuropathy). Retroperitoneal hematomas can occur in any anticoagulated patient; the resultant neurological compromise is usually related to hemorrhage into the psoas muscle. Usually, the thigh muscles are more affected than the distal muscles. Postural lightheadedness or weakness is often associated with retroperitoneal hemorrhages as large amounts of blood can be lost from the intravascular space into such lesions.

Several tumors that are common among older populations occur in the retroperitoneal area and lead to plexopathy. These include lymphoma and carcinomas of the prostate, bladder, kidney, cervix and colon. In 15% of cases, the initial manifestation of retroperitoneal tumors is lumbosacral plexopathy. Sensory and motor symptoms develop, as does pain.

All of these diagnoses have serious ramifications. If foot-drop develops and there are also proximal signs or symptoms suggestive of a plexopathy (weakness of the knee extensors, hip flexors and abductors and numbness proximal to the knee), proper diagnostic studies should be carried out as soon as possible. This typically involves investigation of the area with magnetic resonance imaging (MRI) or computed tomography (CT) and electrodiagnostic studies.

THIG NUMBNESS OR WEAKNESS

Thigh numbness or weakness is a common problem in the older patient involved in rehabilitation. If there is no numbness and the complaints are bilateral, a muscular cause such as disuse or a metabolic myopathy is the likely underlying cause. This section focuses on patients who have associated numbness or unilateral symptoms.

Meralgia paresthetica

One of the most benign and common causes of thigh numbness is entrapment of the lateral femoral cutaneous nerve, often referred to as meralgia paresthetica (Fuller 2003). This nerve is purely sensory and often gets entrapped between an external force and the inguinal ligament or anterior superior iliac spin, as shown in Figure 35.6 (Smorto & Basmajian 1979). The nerve then travels distally, supplying the anterior and lateral thigh. Entrapment can occur because of belts or restraints and commonly occurs because of thoracolumbosacral orthoses (TLSOs). Anxiety often develops in patients with TLSOs when meralgia paresthetica develops, as well as in their families and healthcare

providers, as there is a natural concern that spinal instability is developing along with progressive neurological compromise. Patients can be reassured if the numbness is just over the anterior and lateral aspects of the thigh, and the knee muscle stretch reflex and quadriceps muscle bulk are maintained. Further confirmatory evidence is sometimes available if Tinel's sign is found when the skin just medial and inferior to the anterior superior iliac spine is percussed. If the diagnosis is clear, no further studies are needed; although electrodiagnostic evaluation can rule out other diagnoses, it is surprisingly ineffective in confirming the presence of meralgia paresthetica and is generally not indicated.

The natural history of meralgia paresthetica is spontaneous resolution. If present, tightness of the rectus femoris and iliotibial band muscle tendon complexes should be corrected and this correction can help to hasten improvement. Avoiding compression medial to the anterior superior iliac spine will prevent the prolongation of the syndrome. If symptoms become severe or longlasting, injection with local anesthetics and corticosteroids may be helpful; surgical treatment is also efficacious.

Upper lumbar radiculopathy

Thigh numbness and weakness resulting from an upper lumbar radiculopathy are more common among older than younger patients. One of the reasons is that as patients age, the L4/L5 and L5/S1 disks degenerate, decreasing movement at these interspaces. As motion and stress increase in the upper lumbar segments, disk displacement, injury and degenerative changes become more likely. An upper level (L2, L3 or L4) radiculopathy may result. The patient experiences unilateral knee weakness and numbness of the anterior and medial thigh. On examination, there is evidence of muscle wasting, which can be subtle and is best found by looking for side-to-side differences in vastus medialis oblique mass or measuring circumferences 10 cm above the superior pole of the patellae. Other findings include decreased sensation over the anterior and medial thigh and a reverse straight-leg raising sign. This occurs when the patient experiences dysesthetic pain into the anterior thigh while lying prone and having the thigh passively extended by the examiner at the same time as maintaining knee flexion at about 90 degrees. The side-lying position can be used as well if care is taken that lumbosacral motion is not substituted for true hip extension. Imaging studies are indicated in older patients to rule out malignant causes of radiculopathy. If the patient does not improve, electrodiagnostic studies are indicated to provide information concerning the location and severity of the lesion.

Retroperitoneal and femoral neuropathy

Thigh numbness and weakness can result from any of the retroperitoneal processes described in the section on foot-drop. As is true for foot-drop, a careful examination usually demonstrates abnormalities of reflex, sensation or strength in the gluteals or leg muscles and in the thigh, which leads the examiner to suspect a plexopathy. In anticoagulated patients, however, an isolated femoral neuropathy can develop because of a hematoma in the iliacus muscle. (The close relationship between the iliopsoas musculature and the femoral nerve can be seen in Fig. 35.6.) The patient keeps the lower extremity flexed at the hip and bruising may be seen in the proximal thigh. Loss of patellar reflex and knee extension strength on the affected side are usually present; sensory loss may be less remarkable and occurs over the anterior or lateral thigh and medial knee and leg.

Diabetic neuropathy

Proximal diabetic neuropathy (also known by other terms including diabetic amyotrophy, diabetic polyradiculopathy, diabetic radiculoplexopathy) is included in this section as the major clinical manifestation

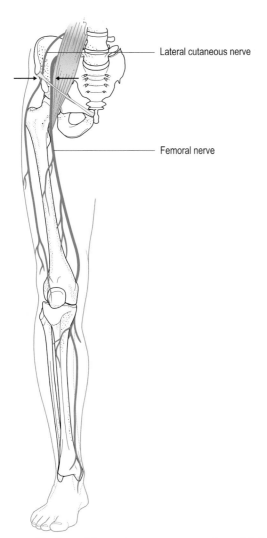

Lateral cutaneous nerve

Femoral nerve

Figure 35.6 The lateral femoral cutaneous nerve is at risk for compression medial to the anterior iliac spine, whereas the femoral nerve is vulnerable to compression by hematoma and other retroperitoneal processes.
(Redrawn from Smorto MP, Basmajian JV 1979 Clinical Electroneurography: An Introduction to Conduction Testing, 2nd edn. Williams & Wilkins, Baltimore, MD, p 59, with permission from Lippincott Williams & Wilkins.)

often involves the thigh. However, it should be recognized that proximal diabetic neuropathy may involve multiple roots or multiple lesions at the level of the lumbosacral plexus. Commonly, the patient experiences the abrupt or subacute onset of pain in the hip and thigh. Lower extremity weakness soon develops and has a predilection for the anterior thigh musculature. The pain usually diminishes as the weakness develops, and the weakness is often accompanied by dramatic weight loss. Often, the pain and weight loss lead to a search for neoplasm. Most patients have evidence of a generalized polyneuropathy at the onset of the proximal diabetic neuropathy. Similarly, most patients are known to have diabetes when proximal diabetic neuropathy develops but it can be the presenting manifestation of diabetes (Polydefkis et al 2003). Symptoms are usually bilateral but often so asymmetric that the less affected side is not functionally impaired.

Although there is no clear way to influence the recovery of the nerves from the presumed metabolic or vascular insult associated with proximal diabetic neuropathy, it makes good clinical sense to maximize the patient's neuromuscular anabolism by optimizing glycemic control and instituting a graded therapeutic exercise regimen. Joint protection with orthotics, particularly to stabilize the knee, is often indicated. Careful education of patient and family to prevent falls is critical, as the majority of these patients have peripheral neuropathy as well as marked proximal weakness. Pain control can be difficult. Tricyclic antidepressants (preferably with low anticholinergic side effects), anticonvulsants, capsaicin and transcutaneous electrical nerve stimulation (TENS) units may be helpful. Pain lessens after the first few weeks or months and strength returns slowly over a period of 6–18 months. A full recovery occurs in slightly less than 50% of patients, but most have sufficient recovery to develop functional mobility skills. When the patient walks again it is important to avoid superimposed compression neuropathies as described above; the median, ulnar and peroneal nerves are at particular risk.

CONCLUSION

Localized peripheral neuropathies are common complaints; they manifest as numbness, weakness and radicular pain. The common causes of these clinical problems have been discussed for upper and lower extremities. Accurate diagnosis is crucial for prognosis and effective treatment, which is aimed at reducing compression or entrapment; educating the patient and family; teaching the proper use of protective equipment, orthotics or assistive devices; preventing further injury; controlling pain; and restoring function.

References

Burnham RS, Steadward R 1994 Upper extremity peripheral nerve entrapments among wheelchair athletes: prevalence, location and risk factors. Arch Phys Med Rehabil 75(5): 519–524

Fuller G 2003 Focal peripheral neuropathies. J Neurol Neurosurg Psychiatry 74(suppl2):ii20–ii24

Kincaid JC 1983 Minimonograph no.31: The Electrodiagnosis of Ulnar Neuropathy at the Elbow. American Association of Electrodiagnostic Medicine, Rochester, MN

Lotem M, Fried A, Levy M 1971 Radial palsy following muscular effort: a nerve compression syndrome possibly related to a fibrous arch of the lateral head of the triceps. J Bone Joint Surg Br 53B:500–506

Ly-Pen D, Andreu JL, de Blas G et al 2005 Surgical decompression versus local steroid injection in carpal tunnel syndrome. Arthritis Rheumatol 52(2):612–619

Malcolm G 2002 Surgical disorders of the cervical spine: presentation and management of common disorders. J Neurol Neurosurg Psychiatry 73:34–41

Polydefkis M, Griffin JW, McArthur J et al 2003 JAMA 290:1371–1376

Richardson JK, Green DF, Jamieson SC et al 2001 Gender, body mass, and age as risk factors for ulnar mononeuropathy at the elbow. Musc Nerve 24:551–554

Smorto MP, Basmajian JV 1979 Clinical Electroneurography: An Introduction to Conduction Testing, 2nd edn. Williams & Wilkins, Baltimore, MD, p 59

Stewart JD 1993 Focal Peripheral Neuropathies, 2nd edn. Raven Press, New York

Wilbourn A 1982 Case Report no.7: True Neurogenic Thoracic Outlet Syndrome. American Association of Electrodiagnostic Medicine, Rochester, MN

UNIT **4**

Neoplasms

UNIT CONTENTS

Neoplasms of the brain

Stephen A. Gudas

INCIDENCE

Primary tumors of the central nervous system have an annual incidence rate of between 4.8 and 20 per 100 000 population; on average, this results in 18 500 new cases and 12 760 deaths annually in the US (Jemal et al 2005). Between 2000 and 2002, the rates were similar in Canada and Israel for men, and for both genders in New Zealand, Spain and the UK. Deaths in women were less frequent in Canada (4.4%), Israel (3.4%) and Japan (1.1%) (Cancer Mondial 2006).

The actual age incidence is bimodal, with an early peak in infancy and childhood and another more sustained peak in the fifth to eighth decades. In adults, primary brain cancer is the 13th most frequent of all cancers. Because brain tumors affect the organ of intellect, humanity and function, they evoke powerful emotional and psychosocial sentiments. Contemporary neurooncology stresses some of the more hopeful clinical features of these tumors. Approximately 50% of patients with primary brain tumors are now successfully treated, many with an excellent long-term prognosis (Thapar & Laws 1995). Older patients may be treated suboptimally, as comorbidity and age discrimination may influence the treatment choices (Basso et al 2003, Brandes & Monfardini 2003).

Some very unique therapeutic considerations govern the diagnosis and management of tumors in the central nervous system, where the distinction between benign and malignant histology is not an absolute concept. A benign tumor of the brain will be just as lethal if it recurs and is surgically ineradicable as one that is similarly located but frankly malignant in histology. The brain lacks a defined lymphatic drainage system; this, in conjunction with the fact that brain neoplasms rarely, if ever, metastasize outside the central nervous system, gives these tumors special significance (Thapar & Laws 1995). Tumors can be locally progressive and invasive, compressing structures from their own substance. Cerebral edema, especially in metastatic lesions, complicates the clinical picture and may be responsible, in part, for the symptomatology that is observed.

The exact pathophysiology and etiological features of most brain tumors remain obscure, despite the fact that, in small discrete groups of subpatients, a genetic predilection to brain tumor development has been identified. There is an increased incidence in patients with neurofibromatosis; familiar clustering has been observed (Blatt et al 1986, Brandes & Monfardini 2003). Other syndromes carrying an increased incidence of brain tumor development are uncommon, which means that the vast majority of brain tumors arise, or appear to arise, spontaneously. However, the fact that as many as 7% of patients with primary brain tumors have a blood relative with a history of brain tumor is intriguing and demands further study (Thapar & Laws 1995). Although there is currently scant evidence supporting a viral etiology of brain tumors, the concept cannot be completely ignored, considering the relationship between cerebral lymphomas and the Epstein–Barr virus (O'Neil & Illig 1989).

Results of studies implicating environmental carcinogens in brain tumor etiology and development have been conflicting. There are some questionable positive statistical associations between brain tumor occurrence and working in the rubber, petrochemical and farming industries. Much work remains to be done regarding the etiology and pathogenesis of brain tumors. This chapter will concentrate on primary and secondary tumors of the brain. Tumors of the spinal cord and pituitary gland are excluded; they are much less common than primary or secondary brain tumors, although they are just as important clinically for those elderly individuals who develop them.

CLINICAL RELEVANCE

Brain tumors are classified on the basis of both cellular origin and histological grade. Tumor location, independent of tumor pathology, may be a critical factor governing therapy and prognosis (Taphoom et al 2005). Although neurons themselves have an extreme tissue density in the central nervous system, they have no reproductive capabilities and, therefore, are rarely the cause of tumors. Glial cells, on the other hand, have tremendous replicative ability and are the most common cell of origin of central nervous system tumors and account for more than half of all primary brain tumors. Tumors may also arise from the meninges, choroid plexus, blood vessels and primitive embryonal cells. Primary lymphomas of the brain, once uncommon and accounting for only 1–2% of brain tumors, have seen an appreciable rise in incidence in the last two decades, partly because they tend to occur in patients with acquired immunodeficiency syndrome (AIDS), transplant recipients and those who are immunocompromised.

The astrocytomas, graded from I to IV depending on their differentiation and degree of malignancy, are the most common tumors seen by healthcare practitioners. The glioblastoma multiforme is a grade IV astrocytoma, characterized by cellular atypia, high mitotic activity, florid endothelial proliferation and necrosis. These tumors are the classical type that can kill a patient in less than 6 months. They most often occur in patients between 45 and 65 years of age, which is somewhat later than lower grade gliomas (Thapar & Laws 1995). Oligodendrogliomas comprise 30% of brain tumors and are characterized by a somewhat earlier age of occurrence, slow growth, calcification and indolent course; however, they are still seen in the elderly population. Meningiomas make up approximately 20% of brain tumors, have a 3:1 female–male ratio, occur more commonly in elderly individuals and carry a good prognosis with surgical removal. Regardless of tumor type, tumor recurrence after surgical removal is common and the tumors typically recur with a higher grade pathology, rendering difficult treatment decisions.

The brain has a surprisingly good tolerance for the compressive and infiltrative effects of an expanding cranial lesion but, in time, all tumors produce symptoms via several mechanisms: increased intracranial pressure, compression or destruction of brain tissue or cranial nerves and local electrochemical instability, which results in seizures (Thapar & Laws 1995). Headache occurs in 30% of patients at diagnosis, and 70% will have headache during the course of the disease. Papilledema, increased intraoptic pressure, occurs in 50–70% of patients and is often detected early. Seizures are the presenting symptom in about one-third of patients and will occur in 50–70% of patients during the disease course.

Tumors in subcortical areas tend to be less epileptogenic. Altered mental status occurs in about 15–20% of cases; this is more commonly caused by tumors of the frontal lobe. Focal neurological signs are characterized by gradual and progressive loss of neurological function – this is especially important when the frontoparietal lobe is involved; hemiparesis and loss of sensation are of interest to rehabilitation clinicians. Tumors of the temporal lobe often cause seizure activity whereas tumors of the occipital lobe, uncommon in comparison to other brain areas, cause homonymous hemianopsia. Tumors of the cerebellum cause headaches, vertigo, ataxia, akinesia, and nausea and vomiting, all symptoms that can profoundly affect function. Many tumors cause considerable brain edema and this increased swelling may result in false localizing signs.

Computed axial tomography (CAT) scans and magnetic resonance imaging (MRI) have revolutionized the diagnosis of brain tumors. The former will detect 90% or more of tumors whereas the latter provides much greater anatomical detail and resolution in multiple planes, and is particularly useful in visualizing the skull base, brainstem and posterior cranial fossa. Cerebral angiography is rarely indicated, perhaps only when excessive vascularity is anticipated in surgery; however, outlining the blood supply of a brain tumor preoperatively can be of help to the surgeon in the planning approach and technique, especially in areas affording limited accessibility.

Metastatic complications of cancer are an escalating clinical problem, with brain metastases occurring in 20% of patients with cancer. Lung and breast tumors are the most common primary tumors, followed by renal cell carcinoma and melanoma (Patchel 1991). Although usually occurring late in the clinical course of a malignancy, brain metastases are being seen earlier in some cancers, particularly lung carcinoma, where it is not uncommon to present with brain metastases as the first symptom of cancer. Tumors are more common in the frontal and parietal lobes because of the extensive vascular territory of the middle cerebral artery. Multiple metastatic lesions, many of them subclinical, are present in over one-half of cases. Solitary brain lesions may present a diagnostic problem in the face of an unknown primary tumor; histological confirmation may be necessary. Unlike primary brain tumors, the evolution of symptoms in brain metastases is rapid, often measured in days to weeks. This may be partially a result of cerebral edema, which is disproportionate when compared with edema caused by primary brain tumors. The symptoms caused by brain metastases are, in other ways, similar to those caused by a primary lesion.

THERAPEUTIC INTERVENTION

The treatment of malignant brain tumors is guided by the principle that it is worthwhile to prolong the lifespan of patients, as most of this remaining time is qualitatively good. Serious functional loss tends to occur late in the course of brain tumors. For virtually all types of brain tumor, surgical resection is the most important form of initial therapy. Surgery establishes the tissue diagnosis, quickly relieves intracranial pressure and the mass effect, and achieves the oncological cytoreduction that will facilitate later adjuvant or first-line chemotherapy (Basso et al 2003). Collectively, many advances in neurosurgical techniques, including lasers, intraoperative ultrasound and computer-based stereotaxic resection procedures, have afforded new dimensions to neurosurgical approaches and strategies. Even if not curative, tumor resection is a reasonable goal provided that a neurological deficit is not imposed. Corticosteroids are a mainstay because they relieve cerebral edema, believed to be responsible for much of the symptomatology that is observed. Corticosteroids can sometimes produce dramatic improvements in clinical function and neurological status. The clinician treating a patient on prolonged corticosteroids should be aware of the increased risk of osteoporotic fracture.

Radiation therapy is a proven effective method of treatment for most brain tumors. The elderly may exhibit a poor clinical course and lower tolerance to radiation therapy; therefore, prospective randomized studies should be performed to define the best option for efficacy in light of the toxicity and effect on quality of life (Chinot 2003, Tanaka et al 2005). Older and younger individuals do not differ significantly in their response to radiation therapy; therefore, age alone should not be a consideration in decision making. At the very least, a short-term survival advantage is obtained from radiation therapy and so it is often used in conjunction with surgery in tumor treatment. Effects of radiation therapy can be divided into acute and chronic; the acute brain syndromes seen as a result of edema and irritation of the brain microvasculature are self-limiting and respond well to steroid administration. Long-term chronic effects are fortunately uncommon and they include brain necrosis, endocrine disturbances and neurooncogenesis. The newer techniques of interstitial brachytherapy and stereotaxic radiotherapy employ different radiation physics compared with conventional external beam radiation; they are designed to deliver a highly concentrated, discrete and well-controlled dose of radiation directly to the tumor, sparing uninvolved brain tissue in the process. As the availability of these procedures has increased, so have the favorable clinical results that are reported.

Although chemotherapy has not made major breakthroughs in brain tumor treatment, some brain tumors in children have responded well. Chemotherapy can provide modest increases in survival for some patients but the gains may be overshadowed by other variables, such as age, performance status and neurological deficit. Immunotherapy has some clinical appeal, as brain tumors cause a marked reduction in immunocompetence. The potential use of biological response modifiers is being explored.

REHABILITATION

In terms of rehabilitation, clinical problems frequently arise that are amenable to therapeutic intervention. Any patient with a hemiparesis or other motor syndrome secondary to the tumor or its treatment will respond to therapeutic strategies structured to return and enhance motor function. All neurophysiological approaches are appropriate and may be tried sequentially or concomitantly. The efficacy of many of the standard exercise and facilitative approaches is empirical, and the choice of treatment is sometimes by trial and error. Postural and balance control exercises may be necessary, even in the absence of frank hemiparesis. For balance and coordination problems, location of the tumor may be a factor; rehabilitation may be more efficacious with cerebellopontine angle tumors than with posterior fossa tumors (Karakaya et al 2000). Pain management and proper breathing exercises are useful in many patients. Because so many patients exhibit symptoms attributable to brain edema, relief of this complication with corticosteroids will assist the healthcare practitioner in bringing improved clinical function to the patient.

Wheelchair prescription and management, evaluation for assistive devices and teaching skills used in activities of daily living (ADLs) and related activities are tantamount to a good functional outcome. The various therapeutic disciplines should combine their efforts in a team approach, each field contributing its own expertise. Nutrition intake should be monitored to prevent malnourishment, dehydration or excessive weight gain. To this end, patients should be evaluated for dysphagia, as dehydration and aspiration pneumonia can result from swallowing difficulties (Wesling et al 2003). Nursing must attend to skin, bowel and bladder integrity, as well as infection control. Social interaction with other patients may be crucial to success. Family involvement and teaching are also integral; psychosocial support and intervention are very helpful, especially when the family is confronted with an individual who has altered mental status and severe motor/sensory deficit. Formal rehabilitation in an inpatient rehabilitation center setting is sometimes indicated, and the rehabilitation professional should be available to assist in this transition when it occurs. Patients may make functional gains during and after inpatient rehabilitation, but the gain in quality of life may not be significant until 1 month or more post-discharge (Huang et al 2001). Also, quality of life may not correlate well with functional outcome in rehabilitation.

In summary, the treatment of primary and metastatic tumors of the central nervous system offers unique and challenging clinical opportunities for the healthcare practitioner. Because the clinical course may be prolonged and sometimes indolent, the rehabilitation staff should be on hand to provide the services necessary to bring patients to their highest level of function. Newer and more exciting treatment techniques, particularly in the delivery of radiation therapy, will result in increased survival in selected patients and longer periods when the healthcare professional will be needed to respond to the clinical syndromes and rehabilitative problems that ensue.

References

Basso V, Monfardini S, Brandes AA 2003 Recommendations for the management of malignant gliomas in the elderly. Expert Rev Anticancer Ther 3(5):643–654

Blatt J, Jaffe R, Deutsch M, Adkins JC 1986 Neurofibromatosis and childhood cancers. Cancer 57:1225–1228

Brandes AA, Monfardini S 2003 The treatment of elderly patients with high grade gliomas. Semin Oncol 30(6suppl19):58–62

Cancer Mondial 2006 International Agency for Research for Cancer, World Health Organization. Available: http://www-dep.iarc.fr/. Accessed 14 Feb 2006

Chinot OL 2003 Should radiotherapy be standard therapy for brain tumors in the elderly? Considerations. Semin Oncol 30(6suppl19):68–71

Huang ME, Warlella JE, Kreutzer JS 2001 Functional outcomes and quality of life in patients with brain tumors: a preliminary report. Arch Phys Med Rehabil 82(11):1540–1546

Jemal A, Murray T, Ward E et al 2005 Cancer statistics 2005. Cancer J Clin 55(1):10–30

Karakaya M, Kose N, Otman S, Ozgen T 2000 Investigation and comparison of the effects of rehabilitation on balance and coordination problems in patients with posterior fossa and cerebellopontine angle tumors. J Neurosurg Sci 44(4):220–225

O'Neil BP, Illig JJ 1989 Primary central nervous system lymphoma. Mayo Clin Proc 64:1005–1009

Patchel RA 1991 Brain metastases. Neurol Clin 9:817–823

Tanaka M, Ino Y, Nagawaka K et al 2005 High dose conformal radiotherapy for supratentorial malignant glioma; an historical comparison. Lancet Oncol 6(12):953–960

Taphoom MJ, Stopp R, Coens C et al 2005 Health-related quality of life in patients with glioblastoma: a randomized controlled clinical trial. Lancet Oncol 6(12):937–944

Thapar K, Laws E 1995 Tumors of the Central Nervous System. In: Murphy GP, Lawrence W, Lenmhard RE (eds) American Cancer Society Textbook of Clinical Oncology, 2nd edn. American Cancer Society, Atlanta, GA, p 378–411

Wesling M, Brady S, Jensen M et al 2003 Dysphagia outcomes in patients with brain tumors undergoing inpatient rehabilitation. Dysphagia 18(3):203–210

Chapter **37**

Neoplasms of the breast

Stephen A. Gudas

INCIDENCE

Breast carcinoma remains one of the most challenging diseases for healthcare practitioners and their patients. The disease's extensive metastatic capability, combined with intriguing responses to treatment, make breast cancer a compelling enigma for all involved in oncology. Until just a few years ago, breast cancer was the number one cause of cancer death in women in the US, and is now surpassed only by cancer of the lung. Similarly, breast cancer is one of the leading causes of cancer-related deaths in many other countries (see Box 37.1. It is estimated that 40 870 people will die of breast cancer in the US in 2006 (Jemal et al 2005). Breast cancer death rates had been stable for over 50 years but have just recently begun to decrease. During this time, there has been a 15% increase in breast cancer incidence among women aged 55 years or older and a concomitant decrease among women younger than 55 (Harris et al 1992). Individuals with breast cancer are now living for considerably longer periods of time, and survivorship has increased appreciably. Screening for breast cancer in the elderly is also important (Walter & Covinski 2001). The recognition that breast cancer is a treatable disease has set the stage for numerous clinical trials utilizing various forms of treatment; however, there are sometimes barriers to participation in clinical trials for older patients with breast carcinoma (Trimble et al 1994, Kemeny et al 2000). These barriers can range from comorbidities in the patient to investigator bias.

The median survival of patients with metastatic breast cancer is longer than 5 years, a considerable improvement from just a decade or so ago (Henderson 1995, Francheschi & LaVecchia 2001). As many as 10% of those who have metastatic disease will live for more than a decade. During this long interval, symptoms arise which may lead to functional disability. Thus, many geriatric patients with breast cancer will have problems related to both the disease process and its treatment.

Breast cancer in the geriatric patient does not differ greatly from that in younger individuals (Balducci & Yates 2000, Diab et al 2000). It is common for clinicians to encounter patients with longstanding

---

Box 37.1 The leading causes of cancer deaths in the US in 2005

Men

1. Lung carcinoma
2. Prostate carcinoma
3. Colon and rectal carcinoma

Women

1. Lung carcinoma
2. Breast carcinoma
3. Colon and rectal carcinoma

Other leading causes of cancer death include carcinoma of the pancreas, stomach and esophagus in men, and carcinoma of the ovaries, pancreas and stomach in women.

From Jemal et al 2005.

---

indolent disease. Considering treatment, women aged 70 or more who are enrolled in clinical trials are similar to their younger counterparts with regard to response rates, time interval to disease progression, survival and effects of chemotherapy (Christman et al 1992, Dees et al 2001). Many elderly patients with breast cancer suffer from intercurrent diseases that not only significantly reduce their life expectancy but also increase their operative risk. However, despite a high percentage of deaths from concomitant diseases, long-term survival of the elderly breast cancer patient is possible and comparable to the general population with breast cancer.

CLINICAL RELEVANCE

The clinical relevance of breast cancer to the rehabilitation professional is engendered across the disease process: from detection to primary treatment, through a long period of metastatic disease, should it occur, and culminating in terminal patient care. Many forms of breast cancer are now treated with simple lumpectomy, segmental mastectomy or axillary node dissection. These procedures have not replaced the modified radical mastectomy, which is still necessary in many patients (Fisher et al 2002). In a modified radical procedure, the breast and the axillary lymphatics are removed but the pectoralis major and minor are preserved. The patient is often discharged from hospital with surgical drains still in place, to be removed at the first clinical visit the following week. Although aggressive manipulation of the shoulder may not be indicated during the first few days, a temporary loss of abduction and forward flexion may be commonly observed.

The percentage of elderly patients undergoing immediate or delayed reconstruction is less than the percentage of younger individuals; however, more elderly patients are opting for breast reconstruction when it is feasible (Francheschi & LaVecchia 2001). Age alone should not be a factor in decision-making; the functional abilities and overall health of the elderly patient should take more importance. More extensive disease, such as a neglected or aggressive tumor that becomes attached to the chest wall or muscles, will naturally require a more extensive surgical approach to result in a definitive cure.

The functional disabilities seen following mastectomy or breast-conserving procedures are usually temporary and respond favorably to physical therapy intervention. Elderly patients who do not gain their full range of motion within 6–8 weeks following surgery are not likely to do so (Lauridsen et al 2005). The reasons for this observation are not entirely clear; a sedentary patient combined with an overly cautious therapist may be contributory factors. The window of opportunity to avoid functional decreases in range and function is not a large one, and an aggressive approach to these patients during the second month following surgery is warranted in otherwise healthy elderly individuals (Nay et al 1999).

Edema of the ipsilateral arm occurs in a significant percentage of cases. The incidence of this complication has declined considerably over the last few decades, largely because of early detection, improved radiation therapy and more limited surgical techniques and, most importantly, early and comprehensive management to effect control. In some cases, edema is severe and neglected, resulting in a grossly enlarged upper extremity with resultant loss of range and function. This is usually preventable with active rehabilitation interventions. Complex lymphedema therapy, which involves bandaging, exercises and specialized massage, can be of immense benefit to patients with lymphedema (Mosely et al 2005).

Few cancers can match carcinoma of the breast in terms of metastatic patterns; the disease spreads both lymphatically and hematogenously and the latter process can actually occur well before the primary cancer is detected and initial treatment begun. The skeleton is the most common site of bloodborne spread. Lesions favor the axial skeleton because of Batson's vertebral plexus of veins; the pelvis, spine, ribs, upper femora, upper humeri and scapulae are most frequently involved. Lesions are most often lytic, but blastic-predominating and mixed patterns may occur. Large lytic lesions in the long bones carry the greatest risk of pathological fracture. The proximal femur is the area of most concern. In bony metastatic disease, pain usually heralds positive radiographs. Occasionally, however, pain may be severe in the absence of both radiographic evidence of the disease and scan positivity.

Differential diagnosis is extremely important. A patient who has no specific cause of pain, especially back or pelvic pain; a history of cancer; is awakened at night; gets no relief with rest; and is not responding/presenting like the typical back or shoulder pain patient should receive further workup. If radiography is negative, a bone scan or MRI may be integral in detecting metastatic bone disease.

Occasionally, axillary metastases and local recurrence in the chest wall produce troubling edema and complex wound care problems. More common are metastases to other organs, following or concomitant to bone metastases. The liver, pleura, lungs, central nervous system and intra-abdominal area can all be involved, with each area producing its particular array of symptoms. Liver metastases cause fatigue, early coffee or strong food intolerance, anorexia, metabolic disturbances and weakness – all rehabilitative problems. Pleural effusions are painful, debilitating and require frequent thoracentesis. Chest tubes may be in place, which limit mobility and function. Lung metastases are of several types. Parenchymal rounded lesions eventually coalesce but do not affect pulmonary function or cause symptoms until a critical amount of lung tissue is compromised. On the other hand, lymphangitic metastases, where the tumor is within the lymphatics of the lung, cause an early and distressing pulmonary syndrome of cough, dyspnea and intense sputum production. Metastases to the brain cause symptoms and signs that are comparable to primary brain tumors. Older individuals may not be diagnosed as readily because of concomitant illnesses and comorbidity.

Metastatic breast carcinoma, the second leading cause of epidural spinal cord compression after lung cancer, is a medical emergency. Sudden or subacute onset of sensory disturbances and motor weakness of the lower extremities in a metastatic breast cancer patient with known spinal disease warrants prompt attention. The pattern and degree of weakness may fluctuate and often the neurological condition improves with treatment, which is less likely in traumatic spinal injury. This presents a dynamic and sometimes frequently changing clinical picture to the healthcare practitioner. Metastases of any type will debilitate the patient. Pain may be one of the major limiting factors in any rehabilitative effort and, therefore, adequate pain control is tantamount to successful rehabilitative intervention. Older patients undergoing chemotherapy will need to be monitored for neutropenic infections, anemia and management of mucositis (Carrera et al 2005).

It is clear that breast cancer is a complex disease process, resulting in a multiplicity of rehabilitation issues that are important for the clinician. Because patients are living longer with treatable metastatic disease, these issues will continue to pose unique and challenging problems to the clinicians who diagnose and treat them.

THERAPEUTIC INTERVENTION

The therapeutic treatment of and rehabilitative intervention in the elderly patient with breast cancer is comprehensive and ongoing throughout the disease process. Preoperative physical therapy screening in a sound clinical practice is important, as the information imparted can do much to allay fears and establish a good clinical rapport with the patient. In an elderly patient, the common existence of premorbid functional loss of range of motion in the shoulder on the operated side underscores the value of preoperative intervention when possible. If a preoperative visit is not carried out, a physical therapy visit on the day after surgery is desirable. After a modified radical mastectomy or a lumpectomy with axillary node dissection, glenohumeral flexion and abduction should be limited to 90 degrees until the surgical drains have been removed (Chen & Chen 1999). It is also necessary to proceed gently with other shoulder movements, such as extension and external rotation. Because the hospital stay of all patients having this procedure is short, early and consistent intervention assures optimal functional and physical return. The actual timing of exercise after surgery has been studied by several authors and results suggest that the incidence of seroma formation is not increased by waiting several days after breast surgery before beginning exercises (Schultz et al 1997, Nay et al 1999, Shamley et al 2005).

A scoliotic curvature is common in elderly women and should be a consideration when treating the elderly post-mastectomy patient. This curve may be present before surgery; when the curve results from surgery and the weight imbalance that follows, positioning, trunk range of motion and strengthening exercises, and chest wall and breathing exercises may offset any problems.

Various exercises are utilized to regain shoulder range and function; no single program has proved to be superior to another in terms of functional results. Most regimens call for a gradual stretch of the pectoralis major muscle; pulley exercises and wall climbing are often used (Box et al 2002, Morimoto et al 2003). External rotation emphasis, slowly bringing the clasped hands behind the head, is another standard approach. Recall that many geriatric patients may already have a functional loss in external rotation before surgery. Early monitoring for lymphedema is essential. The fitting of elastic compression garments has become a large part of the care of these individuals. The success of sequential pneumatic intermittent compression devices to decrease or control lymphedema is variable, even among younger patients. More important, perhaps, has been the acceptance of complex lymphedema therapy into mainstream postoperative care. The program is multidimensional and includes manual lymph drainage techniques followed by specific exercise, meticulous skin care and wrapping with elastic material of specific pressure. Complex lymphedema therapy has gained favor in clinical practice as an approach to lymphedema management, and certified lymphedema therapists should be consulted when swelling is an issue (Hwang et al 1999). Lymphedema prevention through patient and family education is perhaps more integral to control.

Older breast cancer patients tend to have more bony and soft tissue disease than their younger counterparts and sometimes an indolent clinical course may be seen where bony metastases predominate (Ratner 1980). However, even in older women with extensive bony disease, the lesions may be largely asymptomatic. Pain is made worse by activity, particularly weight-bearing. If a patient experiences a pathological fracture and is treated surgically or has the procedure performed prophylactically, aggressive rehabilitative therapy is warranted when the patient can tolerate it. Internal fixation of the femur facilitates nursing care, potentiates ambulatory ability and makes transportation of the patient easier. Ease of transportation is important in facilitating limb positioning during radiation therapy treatment. Early mobilization with cautious weight-bearing needs to be instituted and graduated exercises need to be performed for a maximum functional outcome to be expected. Strength and range of motion can be restored and the complications of a bedridden patient can be avoided.

Orthotic devices to relieve weight-bearing may be tried but extensive bracing should be avoided in the moribund patient, unless used for pain control. Thoracolumbar stabilization with an orthotic device may be required if the spine is heavily involved with tumor and has become unstable. Patients with liver metastases have poor exercise tolerance and this must be respected, while weighing up the difficulties that accompany the immobile patient. Pleural effusions and lung metastases will respond to chest physical therapy techniques when pulmonary symptoms require intervention. Epidural spinal cord compression is approached assertively, with all rehabilitation techniques pertinent to traumatic spinal cord injury being applicable. The changing weakness patterns, as well as the fairly frequent and sometimes dramatic motor return that is seen, merit intense rehabilitative efforts. Lastly, the importance of supportive and palliative care for terminally ill geriatric breast cancer patients is integral to total patient care and is most appreciated by those patients who need it.

Breast cancer rehabilitation in the elderly patient begins with diagnosis, continues through the early postsurgical phase and is both reactive and active. As metastases spread and cause specific symptoms and disabilities, rehabilitation plays a major role in preventing immobility. Palliative and comfort care round out the intervention and, with patients living for an appreciably longer time, the period of rehabilitative care may span decades. Breast cancer in the elderly is a treatable disease and rehabilitation is an integral part of this treatment.

References

Balducci L, Yates J 2000 General guidelines for the management of older patients with cancer. Oncology 14:221–227

Box RC, Reul-Hirshe HM, Bullock-Saxton JE, Furnival CM 2002 Shoulder movement after cancer surgery: results of a randomized controlled study of postoperative physiotherapy. Breast Cancer Res Treat 75(1):35–50

Cancer Mondial 2006 International Agency for Research for Cancer, World Health Organization. Available: http://www-dep.iarc.fr/. Accessed 14 Feb 2006

Carrera I, Balducci L, Extermann M 2005 Cancer in the older person. Cancer Treat Rev 31(5):380–402

Chen SC, Chen MF 1999 Timing of shoulder exercise after modified radical mastectomy – a prospective study. Changgeng Yi Xue Zu Zhi 22(1):37–43

Christman K, Muss HB, Case LD et al 1992 Chemotherapy of metastatic breast cancer in the elderly. The Piedmont Oncology Association experience. J Am Med Assoc 268:57–62

Dees EC, OReilly S, Goodman SN et al 2001 A prospective pharmacologic evaluation of adjuvant chemotherapy in women with breast cancer. Cancer Invest 18:521–529

Diab SG, Elled RN, Clark GM 2000 Tumor characteristics and clinical outcome in elderly women with breast cancer. J Natl Cancer Inst 92:550–556

Fisher B, Bryant J, Dignam J et al 2002 Tamoxifen, radiation therapy or both for prevention of ipsilateral breast tumor recurrence after lumpectomy in women with invasive breast cancer one centimeter or less in size. J Clin Oncol 20:4141–4149

Francheschi S, LaVecchia C 2001 Cancer epidemiology in the elderly. Crit Rev Oncol Hematol 39(3):219–226

Harris JR, Lippman ME, Veronesi U 1992 Breast cancer. N Engl J Med 327:319–324

Henderson IC 1995 Breast cancer. In: Murphy GP, Lawrence WL, Lenmhard RE (eds) American Cancer Society Textbook on Clinical Oncology, 2nd edn. American Cancer Society, Atlanta, GA p 198–220

Hwang JH, Kwon JY, Lee KW et al 1999 Changes in lymphatic function after complex physical therapy for lymphedema. Lymphology 32:15–21

Jemal A, Murray T, Ward E et al 2005 Cancer statistics 2005. Cancer J Clin 55(1):10–30

Kemeny M, Muss HB, Kornblith AB et al 2000 Barriers to participation of older women with breast cancer in clinical trials. Proc Soc Clin Oncol 19:602a

Lauridsen MC, Christiansen P, Hessor I 2005 The effect of physiotherapy on shoulder function in patients surgically treated for breast cancer: a randomized study. Acta Oncologica 44(5):423–424

Morimoto T, Tamura A, Ichihaia T et al 2003 Evaluation of a new rehabilitation program for postoperative patients with breast cancer. Nurs Health Sci 5(4):275–282

Moseley AL, Piller NB, Carati CJ 2005 The effect of gentle arm exercise and deep breathing on secondary arm lymphedema. Lymphology 38(3):136–145

Nay M, Lee TS, Kay SW et al 1999 Early rehabilitation program in postmastectomy patients; a prospective clinical trial. Yonsei Med J 40(1):1–8

Ratner LH 1980 Management of cancer in the elderly. Mount Sinai J Med 47:224–231

Schultz I, Bauholm M, Rondal S 1997 Delayed shoulder exercise in reducing seroma frequency after modified radical mastectomy: a prospective randomized study. Ann Surg Oncol 4(4):293–297

Shamley DR, Barker K, Simonite V et al 2005 Delayed vs. immediate exercise following surgery for breast cancer: a systematic review. Breast Cancer Res Treat 90(3):262–271

Trimble EL, Carter CL, Cain D et al 1994 Representation of older patients in cancer treatment trials. Cancer 74:2208–2214

Walter LC, Covinski KE 2001 Cancer screening in elderly persons. A framework for individualized decision-making. J Am Med Assoc 285:2750–2756

Chapter 38

Gastric and colon neoplasms

Stephen A. Gudas

INCIDENCE

Gastric cancer

Until 1940, gastric carcinoma had the highest mortality rate of all cancers. Despite the fact that the treatment and overall survival rate for gastric cancer patients in the US has not changed appreciably in the past 50 years, the number of stomach cancer deaths has decreased considerably during this same period (Correa 1988). In other areas of the world, stomach cancer is the most common form of cancer. In 1995, the age-standardized rate for stomach cancer deaths in Mexico in men over the age of 60 was 66.7 per 100 000. In 1994, similar data from Venezuela showed a rate of 116.1 per 100 000 for men and 70.3 per 100 000 for women. In the UK, the respective figures are 65.1 and 31.8 per 100 000 (Cancer Mondial 2006).

Ongoing studies are attempting to delineate the purported dietary factors that are believed to play a major role in the geographical differences in the incidence of stomach cancer. The role of *Helicobacter pylori* remains to be fully elucidated and described (Hunt 2004). In 2005, there will be an estimated 21 860 new cases of stomach cancer in the US and approximately 11 550 deaths (Jemal et al 2005). Stomach cancer is now the third most common gastrointestinal neoplasm, after colorectal cancer and pancreatic cancer. There is a slight male preponderance and the incidence is greater in older men, peaking between 50 and 70 years of age (Lawerence & Zfass 1995).

Atrophic gastritis seems to be more common in countries that have a high incidence of gastric cancer, an association only partly explained by the natural progression of a dysplasia or inflammatory process to frank cancer. Similarly, there is a slight increase in the risk of gastric cancer in individuals who have undergone a partial gastric resection for peptic ulcer disease. The stimulus for this pathological chain of events has not been clearly defined. Although nitrosamines can produce carcinoma of the stomach in animal experiments, the synthesis of these compounds is blocked by normal stomach acid; however, this may explain the increased incidence of gastric carcinoma in individuals with pernicious anemia and the accompanying achlorhydria.

Colon cancer

In the US, colon cancer is the third leading cause of cancer death for both men and women, with approximately 104 950 new cases per year and 56 290 deaths (Jemal et al 2005). This is surpassed only by lung cancer and breast cancer in women and lung cancer and prostate cancer in men. The average age at diagnosis is between 60 and 70 years (Bader 1986). In patients with both gastric cancer and colon cancer, two-thirds of cases occur in individuals over the age of 65 (Enzinger & Mayer 2004). The average survival rate for colorectal cancer is about 50%, and that figure has increased only slightly over the last three decades (Stelle 1995). There has been a trend to finding more proximal bowel tumors in both younger and elderly populations. This may be partly because of the increased access to the proximal bowel with the use of current colonoscopy procedures (Au et al 2003).

There are several known predisposing conditions for colon cancer, the most common of which are ulcerative colitis and familial polyposis. In ulcerative colitis, length of disease is as important a factor as severity of symptoms in the progression of the disease to malignant transformation. If there is a strong predisposition to the development of colon cancer, a partial colectomy with preservation of sphincter function is possible and has been a rather remarkable clinical advance in recent years for the prevention of colon cancer. All patients with familial polyposis will eventually have malignant degeneration of one or more polyps. Despite the benefit of prophylactic colectomy for selected patients, the majority of colon cancer patients are termed 'sporadic'. However, in the future, with major breakthroughs in the molecular biology of colon adenocarcinoma, medical genetics may be able to define a population of additional individuals with premalignant colon phenotypes to which model systems of genetics and screening can be applied, allowing polyps that are believed to presage colon cancer to be found and treated at an earlier stage.

CLINICAL RELEVANCE

Gastric cancer

Gastric cancer most often arises from the distal portions of the lesser curvature of the stomach. However, there seems to be an increasing trend towards a more proximal origin. In the US, by the time that gastric cancer has been diagnosed and the patient comes to surgery, the tumor has already penetrated the muscular layers of the gastric wall and can frequently be seen on the outer serosal surface of the stomach (Donati & Nano 2003, Dicken et al 2005). The tumor frequently involves anatomical structures that are in close proximity to the stomach, with involvement of the pancreas and the transverse mesocolon being most frequent. In addition, gastric cancer spreads via the peritoneal surface of the abdominal cavity, making survival less certain if ascites or peritoneal tumor implants are present. In almost two-thirds of patients, gastric cancer will already have spread to the abdominal lymphatics when the patient is surgically explored; sentinel lymph nodes are usually involved and are therefore sampled (Donati & Nano 2003). The gastric area is richly supplied lymphatically and this, along with an intricate mixture of vessels and nervous tissue, results in the rapid spread of the tumor and surgery that is risky and fraught with difficulty. Once regional lymphatics on the greater and lesser curvatures are involved, spread to the lymphatics along the hepatic and splenic vessels occurs and survival is much less certain.

Hematogenous dissemination of gastric cancer occurs late in the course of the disease; dissemination is most often to the liver via the portal vein but other distant sites may be involved. Spread may be asymptomatic; 25% of patients at autopsy show lung metastases, but they are not usually detected clinically prior to death. This is because of both the silent nature of parenchyma metastases until they are well advanced and the fact that other pressing issues and symptomatology may supersede pursuing pulmonary metastases in the later stages of gastric cancer.

Clinically, gastric carcinoma presents most often with vague epigastric discomfort, postprandial pain or early satiety in eating. Because these somewhat nonspecific symptoms may be attributed to simple gastritis or dietary indiscretion, the elderly especially may delay seeking medical attention. Anemia, weakness and weight loss may all occur, alerting the patient to a more serious source of the discomfort. The physical examination of the elderly patient with gastric cancer may often be unrevealing, except when advanced disease is present (Sial & Catalano 2001). A palpable tumor in the upper abdomen is not a common presentation but, when it does occur, it is usually a poor prognostic sign. A thorough workup is indicated in any elderly individual who exhibits persistent symptomatology. This is needed to evaluate the patient's risk and optimize surgical, chemotherapeutic and palliative outcomes (Sial & Catalano 2001). An upper gastrointestinal endoscopy accompanied by biopsy of the suspected lesion will provide the diagnosis in over 95% of cases. Endoscopic ultrasound evaluation is a relatively new technique that shows some promise in that it enables the clinician to visualize all the walls of the stomach (Dicken et al 2005).

Colon cancer

Colon cancer spreads through the bowel wall, and the tumor node metastases (TNM) classification system has begun to replace the Duke's ABC terminology (related to size and depth of bowel invasion). In classic colon or rectal carcinoma, spread occurs sequentially from the bowel to pericolonic nodes or the rectal mesentery and its nodes, to more regional nodes and eventually to venous channels. Because of the portal venous system, metastases most often occur in the liver, and much has been written concerning the various techniques and approaches to treat metastatic hepatic disease. The lungs and bone may also be involved, usually late in the course of the illness. Interestingly, direct extension of a rectal or low colonic tumor into the sacral area and eventual involvement of the lumbosacral plexus sometimes occurs, causing varying syndromes of plexopathy or nerve compression. Tumor compression neuropathies are usually a late event in the progression of colon cancer. In addition to the carcinoembryonic antigen (CEA) that is commonly followed in these patients, there are other potential tumor markers in the marrow that may be determinants of metastatic proclivity to certain distant sites.

Following selected patients for detection and observation of metastatic expression is good clinical practice in the geriatric population.

Diagnosis of colon cancer is difficult despite the more widespread use of the digital exam and sigmoidoscopy, and the use of complete colonoscopy for high-risk patients. Circumferential or 'apple-core' lesions of the lower colon are usually the cause of changes in bowel habits, where almost complete obstruction may lead to a paradoxical diarrhea. More proximal lesions may cause weakness because of anemia from slow blood loss. Melena, blood in the stool, is a frequent and sometimes presenting sign of colon cancer. Frank obstruction is most common in the left colon, where the pain may be colicky. In rectal cancer, the pain may be gnawing and constant, the melena is bright red and tenesmus may occur. Liver metastases may compromise hepatic function, causing the patient to become weak and moribund. Other sites of metastases produce symptomatology that is specific to their location and occasionally function.

THERAPEUTIC INTERVENTION

Gastric cancer

In gastric carcinoma, surgery is the only effective method of treatment where cure is the goal, and this approach is utilized for palliation as well. Survival rates remain low except in those with early carcinoma, which is not frequently diagnosed. The mortality rate from surgery is the same for fit elderly patients and younger patients (Kemeny 2004). All patients are carefully screened and newer noninvasive diagnostic imaging has done much to assist in selectively identifying curable patients as opposed to those who require a palliative procedure. Unfortunately, only 40% of patients can be considered potentially curable. Distal, proximal or total gastrectomy may be performed, with various methods and pouches used to restore or assure continuity of the alimentary tract. Resection of adjacent organs may be required, making cure less likely. Careful abdominal exploration at the time of surgery is necessary to not only avoid unnecessary radical procedures but also confirm the histological diagnosis. For the 60% of patients who are not curable but potentially operable, some type of palliative resection is usually done to relieve symptoms and prolong survival.

Because the common reason for palliation is anatomical unresectability, radiation therapy is often employed where surgery has failed. Postsurgical external beam radiation therapy may be used to relieve obstruction or control bleeding. Although some surgeons are trying intraoperative radiation therapy, trials are pending or in progress and the results are inconclusive. Many chemotherapeutic trials of various preparations have taken place over the years, with most regimes including 5-fluororacil (Enzinger & Mayer 2004).

The gastric cancer patient usually needs rehabilitation postsurgery, including assistance in mobilization and ambulation to avoid complications and to get the alimentary tract functioning again. Barring serious complications, older patients should be mobilized out of bed gently but definitely on the first postoperative day. Mild exercise programs are also helpful in restoring muscle strength and functional mobility.

After recovery from gastrectomy, long-term sequelae are more important than short-term ones. The former includes the 'dumping syndrome', where gastric transit is greatly accelerated; this can result, for example, from the loss of pyloric function controlling food entry into the duodenum. This can usually be controlled by diet and the more frequent employment of gastric reservoirs during surgery. Anemia and accompanying weakness may occur if there is impairment of iron absorption or loss of intrinsic factor when large portions of the stomach are removed (Lawerence & Zfass 1995). Metastatic disease is typically confined to the abdomen but distant hematogenous metastases may be seen late in the disease process. Treatment is organ specific, depending on the site of metastatic disease.

Colon cancer

Colon cancer is also primarily treated surgically, with the creation of a temporary or permanent colostomy if the distal colon or rectum is resected (Gingold 1981). More proximal tumors may allow end-to-end colonic anastamosis, a less radical and less dysfunctional procedure. During the surgical procedure, the entire lesion is removed, analysis of the depth of invasion through the colonic wall is performed and lymphatic drainage is analyzed (Sobrero & Guglielmi 2004). Intraoperative ultrasonography allows observation of the adjacent and noncontiguous abdominal organs. When utilizing less extensive procedures for low rectal cancer, where a low anterior resection is common, a major limiting factor is the lack of adequate preoperative staging techniques. The inability to define microscopic lymphatic spread contributes to the failure rate of surgical intervention. Sphincter preservation approaches, especially desirable in the elderly, should not result in sacrifice of curative surgical principles. Elderly surgical patients seem to tolerate the surgery reasonably well and chronological age alone is not a deterrent to surgery (Sobrero & Guglielmi 2004).

The creation of a temporary or permanent colostomy or ileostomy engenders loss of voluntary control of bowel function. Ostomy rehabilitation has become a specialty in its own right, and enterostomal therapists and wound care specialists are called upon to manage postcolostomy care and instruction. The diversification of collecting devices, skin adhesives and related appliances has been remarkable over the last few decades. A regular elimination schedule, skin protection and odor control are a few of the many issues addressed in the postoperative care of these patients. Like gastric cancer patients, the postoperative colon cancer patient needs gentle but persuasive out-of-bed mobilization and exercises as required. Healthcare practitioners must also keep in mind the special problems of the elderly patient. Liver metastases are common and the healthcare worker involved with these patients should be alert to the decreased exercise tolerance, generalized weakness and cachexia that can occur. Even patients with widespread metastases from colon cancer can benefit from a therapeutic program that emphasizes exercise, ambulation and pain control.

There have been many clinical trials of radiation therapy and chemotherapy in the treatment of colon cancer. Most recently, it has been shown that concurrent or subsequent radiation therapy and chemotherapy affords a survival advantage and more trials are under way (Wasil & Lichtman 2005). An interdisciplinary team approach is the best method for supporting and rehabilitating the patient. It is of interest that less than 10% of gastric and colon cancer cases are unresectable at surgery and approximately 50% of patients will be alive and free of disease 5 years after treatment. These results are encouraging and continue to improve.

References

Au HJ, Mulder KE, Fields AL 2003 Systematic review of management of colorectal cancer in elderly patients. Clin Colorectal Cancer 3930:172–173

Bader JF 1986 Colorectal cancer in patients older than 75 years of age. Dis Colon Rectum 29:728–734

Cancer Mondial 2006 International Agency for Cancer Research. Available: http://www-dep.iarc.fr/. Accessed 14 Feb 2006

Correa PA 1988 A human model of gastric carcinogenesis. Cancer Res 48:3519–3554

Dicken BJ, Bigam DL, Cass C et al 2005 Gastric adenocarcinoma: review and considerations for future directions. Ann Surg 241(1):27–39

Donati D, Nano M 2003 The role of lymphadenectomy in gastric cancer in elderly patients. Minerva Chir 58:281–289

Enzinger PC, Mayer RJ 2004 Gastrointestinal cancer in older patients. Semin Oncol 31(2):206–219

Gingold BS 1981 Local treatment for carcinoma of the rectum in the elderly. J Am Geriatr Soc 29:10–16

Hunt RH 2004 Will eradication of Helicobacter pylori infection influence the risk of gastric cancer? Am J Med 117(suppl15A):865–915

Jemal A, Murray T, Ward E et al 2005 Cancer statistics 2005. Cancer J Clin 55(1):10–30

Kemeny NM 2004 Surgery in older patients. Semin Oncol 31(20):175–184

Lawerence W, Zfass A 1995 Gastric neoplasms. In: Murphy GP, Lawerence WL, Lenmhard RE (eds) American Cancer Society Textbook on Clinical Oncology, 2nd edn. American Cancer Society, Atlanta, GA, p 281–293

Sial SH, Catalano MF 2001 Gastrointestinal tract cancer in the elderly. Clin North Am 30(2):565–590

Sobrero A, Guglielmi A 2004 Current controversies in the adjuvant therapy of colon cancer. Ann Oncol 15(suppl14):39–41

Stelle G 1995 Colorectal cancer. In: Murphy GP, Lawerence WL, Lenmhard RE (eds) American Cancer Society Textbook on Clinical Oncology, 2nd edn. American Cancer Society, Atlanta, GA, p 236–251

Wasil T, Lichtman SM 2005 Treatment of elderly cancer patients with chemotherapy. Cancer Invest 23(60):537–547

Chapter **39**

Neoplasms of the skin

Stephen A. Gudas

INCIDENCE AND CLINICAL RELEVANCE

Skin cancer is one of the most common forms of cancer in humans (Betchel et al 1980). In the US, it accounts for almost one-quarter of all cancers diagnosed (Miller 1991) and kills an estimated 10 000 individuals annually (Jemal et al 2005). In total, 53% of skin cancer-related deaths occur in those over the age of 65 (Syrigos et al 2005). The worldwide variation in the number of cases of melanoma (one type of skin cancer) and the subsequent deaths per year for both sexes is presented in Table 39.1 (Globocan 2006).

Skin cancer tends to be a disease of the middle-aged and elderly (Stevenson & Ahmed 2005), and age alone should not be an obstruction to seeking optimal treatment. The most common forms of skin cancer are basal cell carcinoma (BCC), squamous cell carcinoma (SCC) and malignant melanoma. Other rarer types occur and the skin can also be the site of metastatic tumors. In this chapter, each of the three most common types of skin cancer will be discussed, with emphasis on incidence, clinical relevance and therapeutic intervention.

When working with patients, all practitioners, especially physical therapists and nurses, should be ever vigilant for any skin changes that may warrant further evaluation. Careful inspection of the skin of any body part under examination should be part of a complete physical therapy evaluation. Figure 39.1 depicts the differences between common skin moles and skin cancers.

BCC, the most common of the skin cancers, occurs primarily on sun-exposed skin surfaces (those areas of skin exposed to ultraviolet light). Although historically this disease affected more men than women, there is currently only a slight male preponderance. It is commonly a disease of older individuals; however, it is becoming more common in younger people, with some cases being diagnosed in only the third decade of life. Increased sun exposure, as culturally defined, and depletion of the protective ozone layer in the atmosphere, believed to be a result of increased air pollution, are both believed to play a role in the etiology of this disease. Those who work outdoors or who participate in extensive outdoor recreation are at most risk; cumulative exposure to ultraviolet light over time is the strong unifying factor. Ionizing radiation can also be implicated as causative; the resultant BCC occurs after a long latency period and is usually in the area of previous

Table 39.1 Worldwide variation in the number of cases of skin melanoma and subsequent deaths

	Cases		Deaths	
	Men	Women	Men	Women
World	79 043	81 134	21 952	18 829
North America	32 338	25 123	5258	3131
North Africa	446	361	269	232
South America	3575	3968	1334	1033
Eastern Asia	2114	1745	1056	971
Northern Europe	5576	6932	1571	1361
Australia/ New Zealand	5683	4511	832	483

From the Globocan 2002 database. Available: http://www-dep.iarc.fr/ GLOBOCAN_frame.htm.

irradiation. The immune system may play an, as yet, undefined role but this is less well appreciated compared with SCC.

BCCs are locally destructive but rarely, if ever, metastasize (Freidman et al 1995). Metastases usually occur in long-standing head and neck BCCs. The tumor follows the path of least resistance and so muscle, cartilage and bone are invaded late in the course of the illness. The primary lesion may vary in size and appearance but is most often of the nodular-ulcerative variety. The margin of the lesion typically demonstrates a pearly, raised or rolled border, with reactive telangiectasis and central necrosis. A superficial multicentric variant can occur, more commonly on the trunk and extremities than the head and neck, the latter being the most frequent sites of BCC.

SCC of the skin is a tumor of the keratinizing cells of the epidermis and its behavior is like SCC arising elsewhere in the body. It is the second most common skin cancer and the risk of occurrence increases dramatically with age (McNaughton et al 2005). For SCC, the mean age at diagnosis is 68.1 and 72.7 years for men and women, respectively, with very few cases occurring before the age of 40. The factors that initiate or promote the development of SCC are the same as those for BCC; both are sun-exposure related and light-skinned poorly tanning individuals are at most risk. Other predisposing factors are exposure to ionizing radiation and chemical carcinogens, both usually incurred in the workplace. The list of chemical carcinogens is extensive and is growing.

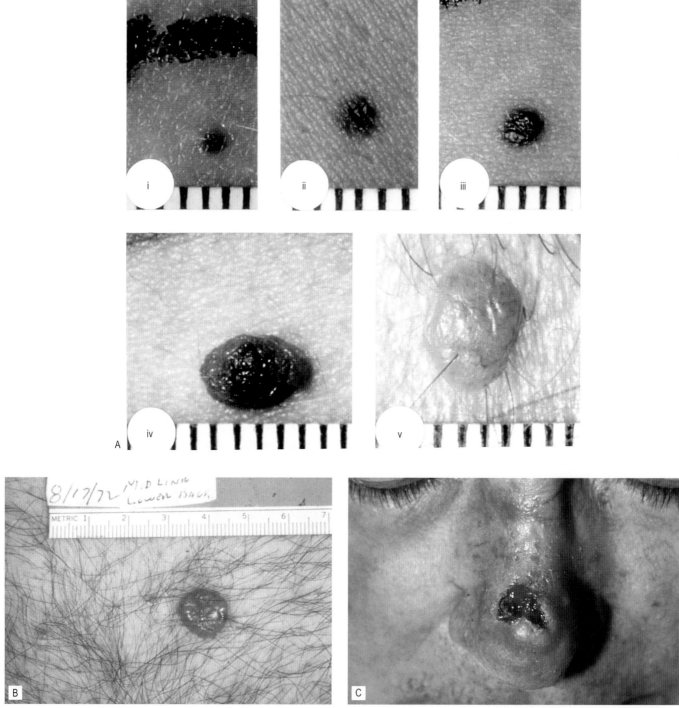

Figure 39.1 The differences between common skin moles and skin cancers. (A) Natural history of commonly acquired nevi (National Cancer Institute). Ordinary moles begin as uniformly tan or brown macules, 1–2 mm in diameter (i), expand to a larger macule (ii), progress to a pigmented papule that may be minimally (iii) or obviously (iv) elevated above the surface of the skin, and terminate as a pink or flesh-colored papule (v). These lesions are junctional (i, ii), compound (iii, iv) and dermal (v) nevi respectively. Note their smooth borders and clear demarcation from the surrounding skin. (B) Basal cell carcinoma. Small, reddish/brownish papule, often with telangiectatic blood vessels. May appear translucent and, when it is, is described as being 'pearly' in color. May have a central depression with rolled borders. (C) Squamous cell carcinoma (National Cancer Institute). Tends to arise from premalignant lesions and actinic keratoses; surface is usually scaly and often ulcerates (as shown here).

Unlike BCC, SCC has a propensity to metastasize to regional lymph nodes and distant sites. The metastatic potential of SCC is determined by tumor size, location, extent of cellular differentiation, whether mucocutaneous or purely cutaneous and a host of other factors. SCC tumors may present in a variety of ways, from a non-healing ulcer to a plaque-like lesion that is raised and erythematous. SCC typically lacks the pearly raised border and telangiectasia of BCC.

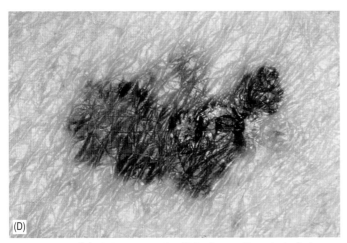

Figure 39.1 (D) Melanoma: color (Skin Cancer Foundation). A melanoma with coloring of different shades of brown, black or tan. Part of the ABCDs for the detection of melanoma.

Malignant melanoma develops from the malignant transformation of the melanocyte, a cell of neural-crest origin that produces melanin pigment (Testori et al 2004). It is surprising that the disease is not more common, considering that most individuals have numerous pigmented moles or other lesions. Melanoma accounts for about 3% of all cancers and is increasing in incidence, mainly as a result of increased sun exposure (Swetter et al 2004). In the last few years, the survival rate has increased from 60% to 84%; this is not only because of newer and more intense methods of detection but also because of improved treatments. Melanoma may appear as a change in an existing mole, with rapid growth, bleeding or a change in color (Vrist et al 1995). However, the lesion can also arise de novo; the increased incidence in the last few years has caused some public concern for all pigmented nevi.

Four patterns of melanoma are seen: superficial spreading melanoma, nodular melanoma, lentigo melanoma and acral lentigo melanoma. The last two varieties occur almost exclusively in the elderly and carry a better prognosis because they tend to stay in situ longer (Stevenson & Ahmed 2005). The nodular type has the worst prognosis because of the great depth of invasion, which may be unapparent at quick visual inspection. Pathological staging of melanoma is based on the microscopic assessment of thickness and level of invasion, the latter expressed as Clarke's level I–IV.

Melanoma does not kill by local extension of disease, but rather by distant metastases. No other human tumor approaches the metastatic potential and virulence of an aggressive melanoma (Testori et al 2004). Virtually any organ in the body can be invaded but the regional lymph nodes are often involved first. Distant sites that can be invaded are the brain, lung and bone. Prognostic factors are multiple and variable, and depend on the stage of the disease at diagnosis. Tumor thickness is the most important and dominant variable; other factors include site, sex, age of the patient, ulceration, number of nodes involved and length of disease. Older patients may not seek treatment and diagnosis early compared with younger individuals with pigmented tumors (Testori et al 2004). Melanomas can metastasize years after the primary lesion has been successfully treated, a fact not often appreciated among healthcare workers.

THERAPEUTIC INTERVENTION

BCC and SCC are treated primarily by either surgery or radiotherapy. Curettage and electrodessication are commonly used for small tumors, with total surgical excision saved for larger lesions. The Mohs micrographic technique, a method employed for SCC and BCC, allows maximum conservation of normal tissues. Wide surgical margins are necessary; the fact that BCC and SCC can spread deeply into the tissue must be respected and recognized in surgical treatment procedures. Alternative removal methods include lasers, cryosurgery and radiation therapy, the last being a paradoxical method of treatment as it can also induce the development of cancer. Radiation therapy is best used for small lesions or in patients who cannot or will not tolerate a surgical procedure.

Both SCC and BCC can be treated with these methods but the propensity for SCC to metastasize must be considered. All therapies are designed to result in total tumor removal, the primary goal in treating these cancers. Recurrence rates are high in certain areas and in certain histological variants; this may call for more extensive surgery or an alternate technique. Many older individuals can be freed from tumors with the techniques described above. Follow-up visits are essential to promptly diagnose recurrent or new primary tumors. A person who has had at least one BCC or SCC is at a higher risk of developing a second tumor; careful vigilance and frequent skin checks are necessary.

Malignant melanoma demands some special consideration regarding treatment, as regional lymph node involvement may be high and subclinical, and the relatively strong metastatic potential of these tumors must be taken into account in treatment planning. A therapeutic node dissection is employed in stage III (large and/or deep primary lesion) patients, whether or not the nodes are clinically involved. Specific guidelines have been established for the accepted surgical margin, depending on thickness and size of the primary lesion. Patients undergoing a prophylactic or definitive groin dissection for a melanoma of the lower extremity are prone to lymphedema, and complex lymphedema evaluation and therapy are indicated. Most patients are fitted with a compression garment. Patients with enlarged regional nodes have a greater than 85% chance of having hematogenous dissemination of their cancer, and the survival rate at 10 years is less than 10%. This does not mean that palliative surgery for stage IV patients cannot be used, as it is commonly practiced to remove surgically accessible lesions and may palliate the patient significantly.

The response rates of metastatic melanoma to chemotherapy are encouraging, and many trials are being conducted to determine optimal drugs and dose scheduling. Immunotherapy and gene therapy have been studied in melanoma more than in other tumors, with varying degrees of patient response and success. All of the approaches are really experimental but can provide palliation and relief of distressing symptoms. Unfortunately, cures are few once the disease has metastasized to distant areas. This drives and underscores the importance of the intense research that is carried out in melanoma.

BCC and SCC are treated with chemotherapy and other methods when the disease is extensive or unresectable, or when there are local or distant metastases. Healthcare practitioners can do much to assist the patient in treatment planning and decision-making. It is of note that, because of the common location of tumors on the head and neck and exposed areas, and the sometimes cosmetically disfiguring surgery that is required for their removal, psychosocial intervention is important to total patient care. Noncomplicated surgical removal does not usually require rehabilitation intervention, except where function is compromised or the surgery is extensive. Caution should be utilized when applying manual stretching techniques, massage, heat or electrical stimulation to areas of previous surgery or when using exercise techniques. The surgical site should be examined carefully.

Like lung cancer, skin cancer is largely preventable. Healthcare practitioners should assist in efforts to educate the public in limiting sun exposure and reducing their exposure to chemical carcinogens that can cause skin tumors.

References

Betchel MA, Cullen JP, Owen LG 1980 Etiological agents in the development of skin cancer. Clin Plastic Surg 7:265–270

Friedman RJ, Rigel DS, Nossa R, Durf R 1995 Basal cell and squamous cell carcinoma of the skin. In: Murphy GP, Lawrence WL, Lenmhard E (eds) American Cancer Society Textbook on Clinical Oncology, 2nd edn. American Cancer Society, Atanta, GA, p 330–342

Globocan 2002 Melanomas, of the Skin in Males and Females. Available: http://www-dep.iarc.fr/GLOBOCAN_frame.htm. Accessed 23 March 2006

Jemal A, Murray T, Ward E et al 2005 Cancer Statistics 2005. Cancer J Clin 55(1):10–30

McNaughton SA, Marks GC, Green AC 2005 Role of dietary factors in the development of basal cell carcinoma and squamous cell carcinoma of the skin. Cancer Epidemiol Biomarkers Prev 14(7):1596–1607

Miller SJ 1991 Biology of basal cell carcinoma. J Am Acad Dermatol 24:1–8

Stevenson D, Ahmed J 2005 Lentigo melanoma: prognosis and treatment options. Am J Clin Dermatol 6(3):151–164

Swetter SM, Geller AC, Kirkwood JM 2004 Melanoma in the older person. Oncology 18(9):1187–1196

Syrigos KN, Tzannov I, Katirtzoglov N et al 2005 Skin cancer in the elderly. In Vivo 19(3):643–652

Testori A, Stanganelli I, DellaGrazia L et al 2004 Diagnosis of melanoma in the elderly and surgical implications. Surg Oncol 13(40):211–221

Vrist MM, Miller DM, Maddox WA 1995 Malignant melanoma. In: Murphy GP, Lawrence WL, Lenmhard RE (eds) American Cancer Society Textbook on Clinical Oncology, 2nd edn. American Cancer Society, p 304–311

Chapter 40

Neoplasms of the prostate

Stephen A. Gudas

INCIDENCE

Prostate cancer is the most common male cancer in the US, accounting for approximately 32% of all newly diagnosed cancers in men (Jemal et al 2005). It is also the second leading cause of cancer deaths in men in the US, accounting for 13% of all male cancer deaths (Koys & Bubley 2001, Calabrese 2004). In 2005, it is estimated that there were 232 000 new cases of prostate cancer diagnosed in the US, with 30 000 deaths (Jemal et al 2005). The rates of prostate cancer vary between different populations (Table 40.1), and there are factors that may lead to familial clustering of cases (Gronberg 2003). The median age of onset is 70 years, making it a distinct geriatric problem; the incidence increases for each decade after the age of 50. It is a curious fact that the incidence of histological prostate cancer at autopsy increases with advancing age, from 5–14% for individuals in their 50s to 40–80% for those in their 90s (Kassahian & Graham 1995). This is rather constant across cultures and countries, although the incidence of frank prostatic cancer is low in Japan, for example. With the aging of the population, it is expected that the incidence of prostate cancer will rise.

Although the exact etiology of prostate cancer is unknown, there appears to be a hormonal relationship as many tumors respond to orchidectomy, implying that testosterone augments cancer growth in men. The precise factors that serve to facilitate or enhance the gradual, if not multistep, transition of a benign epithelial cell to adenocarcinoma are unknown. Cancer of the prostate has been found to occur at a disproportionately higher rate in certain industrial workers – those who work with cadmium, tire and rubber, and sheet metal (Carter 1989). The exact reason for this increased incidence is unknown. Familial factors may play a role but this has not been fully elucidated.

CLINICAL RELEVANCE

Almost 60% of prostate cancer patients will have clinically localized cancer at diagnosis, making cure a real possibility. Frequently,

Table 40.1 Worldwide variation in rates of prostate cancer deaths[a]

Country	Crude rate per 100 000 population
Australia/New Zealand	27.6
Canada	25.8
Caribbean	25.7
China	0.9
Ecuador	13.6
Egypt	2.1
Iraq	1.5
Northern Europe	35.9
South African Republic	10.8
South America	13.1
United Kingdom	33.5
United States	22.8
World	7.1

From the Globocan 2002 database. Available: http://www-dep.iarc.fr/GLOBOCAN_frame.htm.
[a]Estimates for 2002 based on data from 2–5 years previously.

resectable tumors are asymptomatic or patients have a few symptoms of urinary tract obstruction, such as difficulty in initiating and/or stopping micturition. In the absence of infection, marked bladder symptoms should warrant a search for prostate cancer. If the clinical presentation is advanced, there will be symptoms of bladder outlet obstruction and anuria, uremia, anemia and anorexia will ensue. Patients are very ill at this juncture and most will have sought medical attention.

The digital rectal exam still finds most primary prostate cancerous tumors. Approximately 50% of palpable nodules in the prostate are proven to be carcinoma. The prostate-specific antigen (PSA) is a prostate marker that is useful in the early detection of prostate cancer (Catalona et al 1991, Stenman et al 2005). PSA levels are determined after a nodule is palpated on digital examination. If the level of PSA is above 10 ng/ml, there is a 66% chance that a subsequent biopsy will be

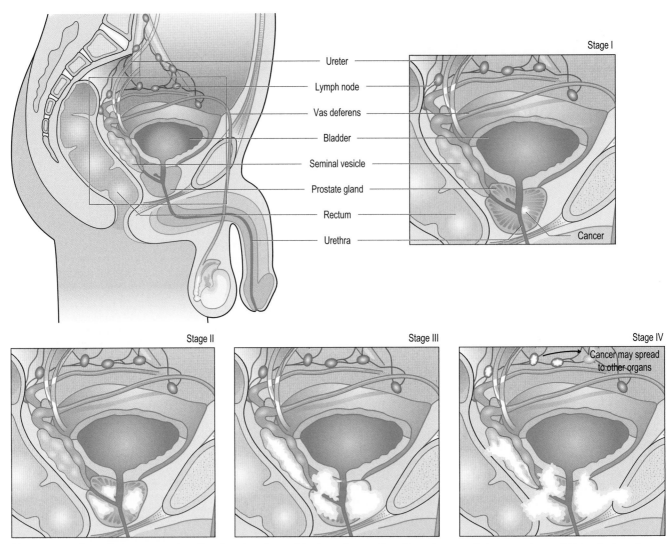

Figure 40.1   Prostate cancer staging. Drawing showing a side view of normal male anatomy and close-up views of stage I, stage II, stage III and stage IV cancer. As prostate cancer progresses from stage I to stage IV, the cancer cells grow within the prostate, through the outer layer of the prostate into nearby tissue and then to lymph nodes or other parts of the body.
(From the National Cancer Institute, with permission.) Author: Terese Winslow (artist).

positive. The use of PSA levels as a screening tool for the general geriatric male population is still under investigation. However, a baseline PSA should be taken in men after the age of 50 and repeated at intervals. Because the early detection of prostate cancer is only now becoming a reality, it will be some time before the effect of the PSA tool on the natural history of the disease and survival in patients can be fully evaluated. Continued investigation will be necessary to determine the true value of both screening and clinical staging procedures (see Fig. 40.1 for a representation of staging for prostate cancer). Prostatic acid phosphatase (PAP) is used to detect metastatic disease, as elevated levels signify spread to at least the lymph nodes (Syrigos et al 2005).

Prostate carcinoma, like breast and lung cancer, spreads both lymphatically and hematogenously, with the regional lymphatics involved in over 60% of cases at diagnosis. Most patients who die of prostate cancer have relatively successful local tumor control. Metastatic disease develops in the vast majority of fatal cases and, as in breast cancer, the favored site is the bone. Similarly to tumors of the chest or chest wall, Batson's vertebral plexus of veins allows easy access to the axial skeleton. In total, 70% of patients develop bony metastases, most commonly in the sacrum, pelvis, lumbar spine and femur (Winell & Roth 2005). The osseous metastases may cause considerable pain and disability, making management of these patients a challenging clinical problem. For reasons that are not entirely clear, the metastases are usually blastic rather than osteolytic, and occasionally mixed patterns are seen. For this reason, pathological fracture through metastatic lesions is seen much less frequently in prostate carcinoma than in metastatic breast cancer. Bony pain, however, may be severe and out of proportion to the extent of bone involvement or the number of bones involved.

Spinal involvement may lead to epidural spinal cord compression (Benjamin 2002). As in breast and lung cancer, this complication has increased markedly, partly because of the fact that patients are living longer with spinal disease, long enough to develop the complication. Epidural spinal cord compression is treated in the same way as compression arising from other primary tumors; full spinal cord rehabilitation efforts are employed as tolerated by the patient. Surgery plus radiation therapy was found to be better than radiation alone in allowing patients to remain ambulatory and continent.

Other distant organs may be involved, usually late in the disease course, with the lungs, liver and pleura the most common sites (Hall et al 2005). Occasionally, prostate cancer can spread beyond the regional pelvic lymph nodes to other lymphatics, such as lumbar, para-aortic and even mediastinal and chest nodes. Large tumors here can also compress organs in close contiguity, causing symptoms that are referable to that organ. Patients with widespread metastatic disease from prostate cancer are quite debilitated and appear older than their stated age.

THERAPEUTIC CONSIDERATIONS

Although, at present, there is no cure for patients with extensive bone or visceral metastases, surgery, radiation therapy, hormonal therapy and chemotherapy have all been used to combat this disease with varying degrees of success. A radical prostatectomy through the retropubic route is the surgical method of choice; this involves resection of the prostate gland, seminal vesicles and a section of the bladder neck. At the time of this procedure, pelvic lymph nodes are removed and sampled for tumor involvement. Although pelvic lymphadenectomy is not therapeutically curative when spread is present, it offers palliation and allows for precise staging, as these nodes are the first sites of metastatic disease in the majority of cases. A laparoscopic approach to the pelvic node dissection can be employed in patients with suspected node involvement but for whom radical prostatectomy is not an option. A nerve-sparing procedure is employed, in which the capsular and periprostatic nerves are spared, and offers a greater chance for preserving potency in many patients. In the past, impotence as an operative sequelae was an almost certainty in radical prostatectomy. Even in older individuals, preservation of sexual function can be an important issue that needs to be addressed so that appropriate psychosocial intervention can be begun, if desired.

Highly focused modern radiotherapeutic techniques enable a large dose of radiation (60–70 Gy) to be delivered to the patient with relatively little morbidity. Pelvic lymph nodes can also be irradiated. However, the major role of radiation therapy is still to control bone pain from metastases, at which it is extremely effective. Patients can also undergo a surgical or chemical orchidectomy with good local or systemic control of disease for 2–3 years (Pienta & Smith 2005). A wide variety of chemotherapeutic agents have been employed and it is currently accepted that chemotherapy increases survival in patients with hormone-refractory prostate carcinoma. Current regimens employ docetaxel, mixantrone and zolendromic acid. No

schedule of drugs is uniformly efficacious and research in this area continues. Cancer cells exist in complex humeral microenvironments that afford multiple therapeutic targets. Bisphosphonates, which inhibit osteoclast action, have been shown to be effective in hormone-refractory prostate cancer (Pienta & Smith 2005).

It appears that both radiation therapy and surgery are equally effective, especially in early disease. For large tumors, with expected spread beyond the prostate gland, biological recurrence is seen in 90% of patients at the end of 3 years. On occasion, the clinical course of prostate cancer is indolent and carries a slow decline in function and mobility. There will be comorbidities in the elderly and extensive bony lesions notoriously lead to general debilitation.

In terms of rehabilitation, it is important to remember that patients with prostate cancer, even the elderly, will generally survive for more than 1–2 years and that therapeutic intervention, designed to maximize function and mobility, are standard in patient management. For patients who undergo surgical treatment, it is important to begin gentle exercises and assume the erect bipedal posture as soon as possible because postoperative pain encourages hip/trunk flexion, which may develop into contractures. Severe spinal involvement may lead to restricted motion and a bedfast condition, and even turning and positioning may require assistance. Most patients are elderly and, as mentioned previously, they will have concomitant diseases that themselves influence function. Light range-of-motion exercises and ambulation with appropriate assistive devices, usually a walker, can both be used and should be encouraged in all patients. Examples of appropriate exercises are active shoulder abduction and flexion, scapular mobilization, and active hip flexion and knee flexion from supine. Although bony lesions are usually osteoblastic, lytic lesions may occur and fractures are treated accordingly. Orthotic devices to stabilize the spine in extensive disease tend not to be tolerated well in the elderly and weight and pressure of a brace may actually aggravate symptoms and bone pain in some patients. Degenerative joint disease of the spine may complicate the clinical picture. Transcutaneous electrical nerve stimulation (TENS) can be used on occasion for pain control, lessening the amount of narcotics needed for effective analgesia.

In summary, in the US, prostate carcinoma ranks as number one for incidence and number two for cancer deaths in men. With the possibility of diagnosing the illness in its early stages, when it is confined to the prostate itself and therefore curable by surgery/radiation, many more survivors of prostate cancer will be found among the elderly. Prostate cancer is an example of a cancer that demonstrates both an increase in survival rates and the length of survival time. Healthcare practitioners will need to respond with appropriate interventions and treatments to assure that this trend continues.

References

Benjamin R 2002 Neurologic complications of prostate cancer. Am Fam Physician 65(9):1834–1840

Calabrese DA 2004 Prostate cancer in older men. Urol Nurs 24(4):258–264

Carter BS 1989 Epidemiologic evidence regarding predisposing factors to prostate cancer. Prostate 16:187–194

Catalona WJ, Smith DS, Ratliff TL et al 1991 Measurement of prostate-specific antigen in serum as a screening test for prostate cancer. N Engl J Med 324:1156–1160

Gronberg H 2003 Prostate cancer epidemiology. Lancet 361(9360):859–864

Hall WH, Jani AB, Ryu JK et al 2005 The impact of age and comorbidity on surgical outcomes and treatment patterns in prostate cancer. Prostate Cancer Prostatic Dis 8(1):22–30

Jemal A, Murray T, Ward E et al 2005 Cancer statistics 2005. Cancer J Clin 55(1):10–30

Kassahian VS, Graham SD 1995 Urologic and male genital cancer. In: Murphy GP, Lawrence WL, Lenmhard KE (eds) American Cancer Society Textbook of Clinical Oncology, 2nd edn. American Cancer Society, p 311–330

Koys J, Bubley GJ 2001 Prostate cancer in the older man. Oncology 15:1113–1119

Pienta J, Smith DC 2005 Advances in prostate cancer chemotherapy: a new era begins. Cancer J Clin 55(5):300–318

Stenman UH, Abrahamson PA, Ari G 2005 Prognostic value of serum markers for prostate cancer. Scand Urol Nephrol Suppl 216:64–81

Syrigos KN, Karapanagiotov E, Harrington KJ 2005 Prostate cancer in the elderly. Anticancer Res 25(6c):4527–4533

Winell J, Roth AJ 2005 Psychiatric assessment and symptom management in elderly cancer patients. Oncology 19(11):1479–1490

UNIT **5**

Cardiopulmonary disease

UNIT CONTENTS

Chapter 41

Exercise considerations for aging adults

Pamela Reynolds

INTRODUCTION

All exercise requires the coordinated function of both the heart and lungs, as well as the peripheral and pulmonary circulations, to transport nutrients and exchange the oxygen required to support muscular contraction and movement. Age-related cardiovascular and pulmonary changes have been described earlier (see Chapters 6 and 7). This chapter primarily presents an overview of endurance or aerobic exercise considerations for normal age-related changes. Other chapters discuss appropriate exercise interventions for specific cardiovascular and pulmonary pathologies (see Chapters 44–47) as well as additional information related to muscle strengthening (see Chapter 16).

The availability of oxygen and the body's ability to utilize it during physical activity is a key performance factor of therapeutic exercise and related interventions. The Fick equation, $V_{O_2} = CO \times a{-}v_{O_2}$, concisely represents this concept, where V_{O_2} represents the volume of oxygen/min/unit of body weight that is utilized during a specific activity; CO is cardiac output; and $a{-}v_{O_2}$ is arteriovenous difference. $V_{O_2(max)}$ is the maximum amount of oxygen that the body can obtain and utilize for any physical activity. This can also be described as a person's physical fitness level or functional capacity. The amount of oxygen that the body can obtain and effectively utilize is dependent on two factors: (i) the delivery of oxygen-rich blood to metabolically active tissues, especially muscles; and (ii) the ability of these tissues to extract and utilize the delivered oxygen. The delivery factor or central component is dependent on CO, which is a product of heart rate (HR) and stroke volume (SV). The peripheral component is represented by the arteriovenous difference ($a{-}v_{O_2}$), or the difference between the oxygen content of the arterial blood entering the metabolically active tissue and the amount of oxygen left in the venous blood that is returned to the heart. Cardiopulmonary dysfunctions are usually a result of impairments in the delivery system (McArdle et al 2000).

EXERCISE CONSIDERATIONS

When developing an exercise program or prescription, it is important to consider the following:

- medical screening or clearance;
- informed consent;
- baseline functional capacity;
- consideration of the mode, intensity, frequency and duration;
- gradual progression;
- safety;
- motivation;
- regular reevaluation.

Screening and informed consent

Aging has some immutable factors that increase a person's risk for exercise. Many disorders do not demonstrate significant clinical signs during regular daily activities but they may become evident during exercise. The American College of Sports Medicine (ACSM 2000, 2006) defines individuals at moderate risk of having coronary artery disease as men aged 45 or over and women aged 55 or over, or those who meet the threshold for two or more of the risk factors shown in Box 41.1. Thus, by virtue of age alone, all elderly individuals fall

---

Box 41.1 Risk factors for coronary artery disease

1. Family history: myocardial infarction or sudden death in first-degree relative (male before the age of 55 and female before the age of 65)
2. Current cigarette smoking
3. Hypertension: $\geq 140/90$ mmHg
4. Dyslipidemia: total serum cholesterol >200 mg/dL; or LDL >130 mg/dL and HDL <40 mg/dL
5. Impaired glucose fasting or diabetes mellitus: fasting blood glucose ≥ 100 mg/dL on at least two separate occasions
6. Obesity: body mass index > 30 kg/m^2
7. Sedentary lifestyle/physical inactivity: sedentary jobs involving sitting for a large part of the day and no regular exercise

From ACSM 2000, 2006, with permission from Lippincott Williams & Wilkins.

within this category. High-risk individuals are defined as anyone having one or more of the signs and symptoms listed in Box 41.2 or known cardiovascular, pulmonary, or metabolic disease.

Medical examination and exercise testing are recommended for both categories of individuals before beginning vigorous exercise training. Vigorous exercise is defined as activities requiring more than six metabolic equivalents (METs) of functional capacity. For the elderly in the moderate-risk category only, who plan to engage in moderate exercise training, medical screening is not necessary. Moderate exercise training entails activities requiring three to six METs. However, although training at this level may be designated as screening 'not necessary', it should not be deemed inappropriate. Examination and evaluation should always guide a clinician's decisions in this area (ACSM 2000, 2006). It is also important to identify the medications that a patient is taking. Regular use of cardiovascular drugs, tranquilizers, diuretics and sedatives can affect the physiological response to exercise.

Patient/clients who are receiving skilled therapeutic rehabilitation services regularly sign informed consent forms before treatment. Informed consent is an important ethical and legal consideration, particularly for health promotion services that may not be covered by insurances. The participant should know the purposes and risks associated with an exercise program and testing.

Baseline functional capacity

Establishing a baseline functional capacity is essential for those who intend to participate in an exercise program. As the individual progresses through the exercise program, comparison of the initial exercise test with subsequent tests will provide feedback regarding the individual's success in the program. Such assessments have been shown to play a significant role in decreasing attrition rates in exercise programs.

The selection of a graded exercise test should take into consideration the purpose of the test, desired outcome and the individual being tested. A graded exercise test protocol must effectively challenge the patient/client but not be too aggressive. Figure 41.1 gives the metabolic costs of selected treadmill tests (ACSM 2000, 2006). Tests can be categorized into single-stage and multi-stage tests. An example of a single-stage exercise test is the 6- or 12-min walk test (Steffen et al 2002). Multi-stage exercise tests include treadmills, cycle ergometers and step tests. The Naughton–Balke, modified Balke (Table 41.1) and modified Bruce treadmill protocols are recommended for deconditioned individuals or patients with cardiovascular or respiratory disease (ACSM 1991). Heart rate, blood pressure, respiratory rate and possible electrocardiogram (ECG) responses should be recorded minimally at rest, immediately upon completion of testing and until the person regains their pretest or resting measures. It is also highly recommended that vital signs be monitored throughout the stages of the test.

Box 41.2 Symptoms or signs suggestive of cardiopulmonary disease

1. Pain, discomfort (or other angina equivalent) in chest, neck, jaw, arm or other areas that may be ischemic in nature
2. Shortness of breath at rest or with mild exertion
3. Dizziness or syncope
4. Orthopnea or paroxysmal nocturnal dyspnea
5. Ankle edema
6. Palpitations of tachycardia
7. Intermittent claudication
8. Known heart murmur
9. Unusual fatigue or shortness of breath with usual activities

From ACSM 2000, 2006, with permission from Lippincott Williams & Wilkins.

METS	1.6	2	3	4	5	6	7	8	9	10	11	12	13	14	15	16
Balke Speed				3.4 miles/h												
Balke % grade			2	4	6	8	10	12	14	16	18	20	22	24	26	
Balke Speed			3.0 miles/h													
Balke % grade			0	2.5	5	7.5	10	112.5	15	17.5	20	22.5				
Naughton Speed	1.0	2.0 miles/h														
Naughton % grade	0	0	3.5	7	10.5	14	17.5									
METS	1.6	2	3	4	5	6	7	8	9	10	11	12	13	14	15	16
O$_2$, mL/kg/min	5.6	7	14		21			28		35		42		49		56
Clinical status	Symptomatic patients															
	Diseased, recovered															
	Sedentary healthy															
	Physically active subjects															
Functional class	IV	III		II		I normal										

Figure 41.1 Metabolic cost of selected treadmill test protocols. One metabolic equivalent (MET) signifies resting energy expenditure, equivalent to approximately 3.5 mL of oxygen uptake/kg of body weight/min. Unlabeled numbers refer to treadmill speed (top) and percentage grade (bottom).
(From Wenger NK, Hellerstein HK 1992 Rehabilitation of the Coronary Patient, 3rd edn. Churchill-Livingstone, New York, p 150, with permission.)

Considerations for exercise prescription

In 1995, the Centers for Disease Control (CDC) and the ACSM recommended that 'every US adult should accumulate 30 minutes or more of moderate-intensity physical activity on most, preferably all, days of the week' (Pate et al 1995). In 1996, the Surgeon General's Report, *Physical Activity and Health* (US Dept of Health and Human Services 1996), advised that: 'Significant benefits can be obtained by including a moderate amount of physical activity (e.g. 30 minutes of brisk walking or raking leaves, 15 minutes of running or 45 minutes of playing volleyball) on most, if not all, days of the week. . . . Additional health benefits can be gained through greater amounts of physical activity.'

The components of an exercise prescription include mode(s) or the type of exercise, intensity, duration, frequency and progression of physical activity. 'These five components apply when developing exercise prescriptions for people of all ages and fitness levels, regardless of the individual health status' (ACSM 2006).

Mode of exercise

Activities can be classified into two groups: continuous or sustained activities and discontinuous or intermittent exercise. Any activity that requires work from large muscle masses for a prolonged period of time will elicit an exercise training response from the cardiovascular and pulmonary system. Discontinuous or intermittent exercise activities are often required for those with low functional capacities or any condition that limits performance, such as chronic obstructive lung disease, intermittent claudication, moderate cardiovascular disease and orthopedic limitations. Examples of a continuous and intermittent walking protocol are illustrated by the Senior's Walking Exercise Program in Tables 41.2 and 41.3 (Reynolds 1991).

Intensity

Prescribing the appropriate exercise intensity is the most difficult challenge in designing an exercise program. The two most common methods for prescribing and monitoring exercise intensity are HR and rating of perceived exertion (RPE). Because there is a linear relationship between HR and percent functional capacity (VO_2), HR is used to set an exercise intensity range. Exercise intensities of 60–80% are generally recommended for the younger population. However, in the elderly, an exercise intensity of 40% of the HR reserve has demonstrated aerobic and functional training adaptations (Pate et al 1995, ACSM 2000, 2006).

One of the oldest and easiest methods of computing intensity is to use the percent of maximum HR (zero to age-predicted maximum). Age-predicted maximum HR is calculated by subtracting the person's age from 220, with a potential adjustment of ±10–15 beats per minute (b.p.m.). However, this is a very conservative method that is especially inaccurate at lower intensity target ranges. Therefore, the Karvonen method is recommended for setting exercise intensity

Table 41.1 Naughton–Balke and modified treadmill protocols

	Speed (mph)	% Grade	Time (min)	METs
Naughton–Balke treadmill protocol	3 (constant)	2.5	2	4.3
		5	2	5.4
		7.5	2	6.4
		10	2	7.4
		12.5	2	8.4
		15	2	9.5
		17.5	2	10.5
		20	2	11.6
		22.5	2	12.6
Modified Balke treadmill protocol	2	0	3	2.5
	2	3.5	3	3.5
	2	7	3	4.5
	2	10.5	3	5.4
	2	14	3	6.4
	2	17.5	3	7.4
	3	12.5	3	8.5
	3	15	3	9.5

From ACSM 1991, with permission from Lea & Febiger.

Table 41.2 Seniors' Walking Exercise Program protocol: continuous walking protocol[a]

	Time (min)	Frequency (times/week)
Walk	45–50	3
Walk	34–38	4
Walk	27–30	5
Walk	23–25	6
Walk	17–19	8 (or twice a day, 4 times a week)

From Reynolds (1991), with permission from Wolters Kluwer.
[a]1. At the start of the walking program, do not allow the client to walk for longer than the time indicated on the exercise test. 2. To increase the client's motivation and sense of control, the client should choose how often (frequency) they will exercise per week. 3. The client should determine how long they would like to walk and set that as the time goal. 4. Expect to progress at a rate of 2–5 min/week until the time goal has been achieved.

Table 41.3 Seniors' Walking Exercise Program protocol: intermittent walking protocol[a]

Stage	Exercise (min)	Rest (min)	Total exercise (min)
1	2	1	6
2	3	1	9
3	4	1	12
4	5	1	15
5	6	1	18
6	7	1	21

From Reynolds (1991), with permission from Wolters Kluwer.
[a]Repeat each walk/rest cycle three times. Do not progress to the next stage until three cycles can comfortably be completed within set exercise tolerance parameters. Recommended frequency, 5–7 times per week.

range; this uses the HR reserve, which is the difference between resting HR and maximum HR. If the results from a graded exercise test are available, then the maximum HR achieved in this test is utilized as the maximum HR. If not, the age-predicted maximum HR formula is used (ACSM 2000, 2006). The calculation of the target HR range for exercise intensity ranging from 40–60% in an individual of 70 years with a resting HR of 60 b.p.m. is illustrated in Box 41.3.

Individuals with cardiovascular disease are frequently taking medications, such as digoxin or beta blockers, which blunt the HR response to exercise. Measures such as Borg's RPE can also be used to prescribe intensity (see Table 41.4). RPE is a widely used measure, which quantifies the subjective sensation of physical exertion. It correlates closely with several measurable variables such as peak VO_2 and percent HR reserve. It can be used to prescribe intensity, especially

Box 41.3   Calculating target heart rate range with the Karvonen method

Maximal heart rate	220	
Subtract age	−70	
Equals	150	
Subtract resting heart rate	−60	
Equals heart rate reserve	90	90
Multiply by % intensity	×40	×60
Equals	36	54
Add back resting heart rate	+60	+60
Target heart rate range for 40–60%	96 b.p.m. to 114 b.p.m.	

Table 41.4   Borg's original and revised rating of perceived exertion (RPE)

Original category RPE scale		Revised category–ratio scale	
Value	Description	Value	Description
6		0	Nothing at all
7	Very, very light	0.5	Very, very weak
8		1	Very weak
9	Very light	2	Weak
10		3	Moderate
11	Fairly light	4	Somewhat strong
12		5	Strong
13	Somewhat hard	6	
14		7	Very strong
15	Hard	8	
16		9	
17	Very hard	10	Very, very strong
18		•	Maximal
19	Very, very hard		
20			

From Borg GA (1982). Scales © American College of Sports Medicine, with permission from Lippincott Williams & Wilkins.

when a person is taking a medication that alters the cardiopulmonary response to exercise. The original category RPE scale is numbered from 6–20. Although the numbering system may appear unusual, it correlates HR with a specific number. For instance, the number '11', described as 'fairly light' exertion, generally corresponds to a HR of 110. An RPE of 11–16 associates closely with exercise intensities of 50–75%. Numerous studies have demonstrated reproducible results among a wide variety of individuals using this scale. The newer category–ratio scale, numbered from 0–10, was designed with the perception that exercise intensity appears to increase as a power function rather than a linear progression. It allows for more fine tuning for subjective responses to small increases in objective exercise intensity. Whichever method is used, it is critical that all individuals are educated in its application to ensure that ratings are reliable and valid.

Duration

Duration is inversely proportional to intensity. A conditioning response is the result of the interaction of intensity and duration of exercise. The lower the intensity, the longer the duration needs to be. The ACSM (2000) recommends 20–60 min of continuous or intermittent (10-min bouts) aerobic activity, accumulated throughout the day.

Frequency

Frequency refers to the number of exercise sessions per week that are included in the exercise prescription. It depends on a person's initial functional capacity. The ACSM (2000) recommends an exercise frequency of 3–5 times per week for individuals who have a higher functional capacity and can tolerate a greater exercise intensity. The frequency of exercise for those with a low functional capacity should be more frequent, even daily. Multiple brief daily sessions are advised for patient/clients with an aerobic capacity of less than three METs.

Progression of physical activity

The rate of exercise progression depends on several factors including the individual's functional capacity, medical status, age, activity preference and individual goals. Increases in the patient/client's exercise intensity or duration are made as the person adapts to training within the constraints of avoiding musculoskeletal injury or debilitating fatigue. The ACSM offers an example of exercise progression using intermittent exercise for individuals with a functional capacity of less than and greater than four METS (Table 41.5) (ACSM 2006).

Parameters for progression that have guided this author for over 10 years involve monitoring the patient/client's HR, blood pressure and respiratory rate/rhythm/pattern during exercise and through recovery, in conjunction with related signs and symptoms such as pain, sweating and fatigue. Progression in the exercise program is advised when the individual recovers their near-resting HR and blood pressure within 5 min, and respiratory rate and effort within 10 min. Although the latter measure may seem long, it is especially necessary for patients with respiratory pathologies. Resting or baseline respiratory effort for patient/clients with respiratory pathologies is often 1+ on the dyspnea scale (see Table 41.6). Any exercise program will increase their dyspnea level, which should never be allowed to go above 3+. Because the respiratory system is already compromised, return to baseline will take longer.

Exercise participants should be strongly encouraged and taught to monitor their HR, blood pressure and respiratory effort and share the information with their therapist. Minimally, an individual should know how to monitor their pulse and breathing. They should also be aware of the signs of exercise intolerance. Guidelines to ending an exercise session are listed in Box 41.4. Maintaining an activity log, such as the one in Form 41.1, provides useful feedback to both the participant and health professional.

Progress is recognized as an increase in the individual's $V_{O_{2(max)}}$ or an increase in the MET level of activity. Increased distance, speed, repetition and weights all indicate improved exercise or workload tolerance. This improved response can be verified when retesting the patient using the same pretest protocol. An individual having a positive training response will achieve the established workloads at a lower HR and systolic blood pressure. There have been some observations that the older adult with cardiac disease may experience a greater relative improvement in response to an exercise program than their younger counterparts. A possible explanation is that, because exercise has not been part of their regular physical activity for several years, there is a greater percentage of improvement from their baseline (Williams 1996).

Box 41.4   Guidelines for termination of an exercise session

These signs and symptoms are general indicators of exercise intolerance:

1. Severe breathlessness: only able to speak in two to three word sentences
2. Drop in heart rate of >10 b.p.m. with an increased or continuous steady workload
3. Drop in systolic blood pressure of >20 mmHg while exercising
4. Light-headedness, dizziness, pallor, cyanosis, confusion, ataxia
5. Loss of muscle control or fatigue
6. Onset of angina, tightness or severe pain in chest, arms or legs
7. Nausea or vomiting
8. Excessive rise in blood pressure: systolic blood pressure ≥220 mmHg or diastolic blood pressure ≥110 mmHg
9. Excessively large rise in heart rate of >50 b.p.m. with low-level activity
10. Severe leg claudication: 8/10 on a 10/10 pain scale
11. ECG abnormalities: ST-segment changes and multifocal premature ventricular contractions >30% of complexes
12. Failure of any monitoring equipment

Table 41.5   Example of exercise progression using intermittent exercise

	Week	% FC	Total minutes at % FC	Minutes of exercise	Minutes of rest	Repetitions
Functional capacity (FC) > 4 METs	1	50–60	15–20	3–5	3–5	3–4
	2	50–60	15–20	7–10	2–3	3
	3	60–70	20–30	10–15	Optional	2
	4	60–70	30–40	15–20	Optional	2
Functional capacity (FC) ≤ 4 METs	1	40–50	10–15	3–5	3–5	3–4
	2	40–50	12–20	5–7	3–5	3
	3	50–60	15–25	7–10	3–5	3
	4	50–60	20–30	10–15	2–3	2
	5	60–70	25–40	12–20	2	2
	6	Continue with two repetitions of continuous exercise with one rest period, or progress to a single continuous bout				

From ACSM Guidelines for Exercise Testing and Prescription.

Table 41.6   Assessing dyspnea

Dyspnea scale[a]	Interpretation[b]
1 Light, barely noticeable	0 Breathing normally 1+ Noticeable only to individual but not observer
2 Moderate, bothersome	2+ Use of accessory muscles noted by observer
3 Moderately severe, very uncomfortable	3+ Only able to speak in two to three words between breaths
4 Most severe or intense dyspnea ever experienced	4+ Unable to speak and must stop activity

[a]From ACSM (2006).
[b]From Reynolds (2000); referred to by colleagues as author's 'Talk Test'.

COMPONENTS OF AN EXERCISE SESSION

When the exercise prescription has been established, it should be integrated into a comprehensive physical conditioning program. The training program has three primary components: warm-up, stimulus or endurance phase, and cool-down. Sometimes, recreational activities are added between the stimulus and cool-down phase. The beginning warm-up phase usually lasts for 5–10 min. The purpose is to facilitate the transition from rest to exercise. It reduces susceptibility to musculoskeletal problems, which is especially important in the elderly. Activities may include flexibility or stretching exercises and low-intensity exercise that will be progressed to a higher intensity in the stimulus phase.

The activities in the stimulus phase vary according to the individual goals of treatment and may include flexibility, resistance and/or endurance (cardiovascular and pulmonary) training. This phase can last for 20–60 min. When both endurance and resistive training are part of an exercise program, they are usually done on alternate days of the week and not on the same day.

Cool-down is an important component of a safe program for both healthy individuals and patient/clients with disease. It decreases exercise-induced circulatory changes, including returning HR and blood pressure to baseline. It also facilitates the dissipation of body heat produced by exercise and attenuates venous return, reducing the potential for post-exercise dizziness and hypotension. This phase lasts for 5–10 min and usually includes exercise with diminishing intensity and stretching (ACSM 2006).

In summary, Williams (1996) offers a well-rounded exercise training program for older adults with cardiac disease (Box 41.5). His recommendations incorporate all of the considerations that have been discussed in this section.

Form 41.1 Prototype activity log to be used by patients with cardiovascular disease in order to record specific exercise considerations before and after exercising

Activity Log

Name _____

Date _____

Time of day _____

Heart rate before exercise _____

Heart rate after exercise _____

Heart rate 5 min after exercise _____

Blood pressure before exercise _____

Blood pressure after exercise _____

Blood pressure 5 min after exercise _____

Exercise activity and minutes of activity _____

Pain (Y = yes; N = no). If yes, where? _____

Fatigue, tiredness _____

Weakness _____

Sweating (amount?) _____

Shortness of breath? How long? _____

Rating of perceived exertion after exercise (RPE) _____

Other comments _____

Box 41.5   General recommendations when initiating an exercise training program for elderly patients with cardiac disease

- *Warm-up*: 5–10 min of stretching and light activity involving the large muscle groups before each session
- *Intensity*: 50–80% of peak oxygen uptake attained at the most recent exercise test, corresponding to 60–85% of the peak heart rate at same test
- *Frequency*: participation 3–5 days/week
- *Duration*: 20–40 min of aerobic exercise broken up into shorter periods, allowing for 1- to 2-min rest intervals when appropriate
- *Mode*: upper and lower extremity exercise using treadmill walking, leg ergometry and arm ergometry
- *Cool-down*: 5–10 min of activity similar to warm-up
- *Flexibility*: 10–15 min of static stretching 'of the muscles of each major body section', including head and neck, shoulders, chest, trunk, hips, legs, knees and ankles
- *Resistive training*: 12–15 repetitions of a modest work load (25% of body weight for larger muscle groups, such as the quadriceps femoris muscle, and 10% of body weight for smaller muscle groups, such as the triceps muscles), 4–8 stations, 2–3 sessions/week; always performed after the regular exercise session to provide for adequate warming of various muscle groups and to reduce likelihood of injury

From Williams (1996), with permission from American Physical Therapy Association.

CONCLUSION

Motivating and maintaining exercise participation is difficult to achieve. Research has demonstrated a greater than 50% dropout rate from most supervised exercise programs after 6 months (US Dept of Health and Human Services 2000). Exercise approaches that highlight organization and safety but focus more on the individual personal goals have better program compliance. This approach also assumes that the participant's commitment to exercise is a personal one and an opportunity for self-expression (Prochaska & DiClemente 1982). The goal is to encourage safe progression of exercise activity to an unsupervised environment based on education and enjoyment.

References

American College of Sports Medicine (ACSM) 1991 ACSM's Guidelines for Exercise Testing and Prescription, 6th edn. Lea & Febiger, Philadelphia, PA

American College of Sports Medicine (ACSM) 2000 ACSM's Guidelines for Exercise Testing and Prescription, 6th edn. Lippincott Williams & Wilkins, Philadelphia, PA

American College of Sports Medicine (ACSM) 2006 ACSM's Guidelines for Exercise Testing and Prescription, 7th edn. Lippincott Williams & Wilkins, Philadelphia, PA

Borg GA 1982 Psychophysical basis of perceived exertion. Med Sci Sports Exerc 14(5):377–381

McArdle WD, Katch FI, Katch VL 2000 Essentials of Exercise Physiology, 2nd edn. Lippincott Williams & Wilkins, Philadelphia, PA

Pate RR, Pratt M, Blair SN et al 1995 Physical activity and public health: a recommendation from the Centers for Disease Control and Prevention and the American College of Sports Medicine. JAMA 273:402–407

Prochaska J, DiClemente C 1982 Transtheoretical therapy, toward a more integrative model for change. Psych Theory Res Pract 19:276–288

Reynolds P 1991 Seniors Walking Exercise Program. Focus Geriatr Care Rehabil 4(8)

Reynolds P 2000 Cardiopulmonary Considerations for Evaluation and Management of the Older Adult (Monograph). American Physical Therapy Association, newsletter

Steffen TM, Hacker TA, Mollinger L 2002 Age- and gender-related test performance in community-dwelling elderly people: six-minute walk test, Berg balance scale, timed up and go test, and gait speed. Phys Ther 82:128–137

US Department of Health and Human Services 1996 Physical Activity and Health: A Report of the Surgeon General, Washington DC

US Department of Health and Human Services 2000 Healthy People 2010: Understanding and Improving Health, Washington DC

Williams MA 1996 Cardiovascular risk-factor reduction in the elderly patients with cardiac disease. Phys Ther 76:469–480

Chapter **42**

Clinical development and progression of heart disease

Timothy L. Kauffman, Pamela Reynolds and Joanne Dalgleish

INTRODUCTION

Heart disease can begin early in the young adult with the formation of atherosclerotic plaques on the walls of the coronary arteries. These plaques lead to a decreased flow of blood through the coronary arteries resulting in less oxygen-rich blood perfusing the heart muscle; At this point in time, the individual is diagnosed as having coronary artery disease (CAD). When the heart muscle is not perfused with enough blood to meet its demand for oxygen, the result is myocardial ischemia, which presents as angina. As CAD becomes worse, angina symptoms become more frequent and intense, which ultimately leads to an acute myocardial infarction (AMI).

Heart disease is the single leading cause of death in the world and is likely to increase (Anderson & Smith 2005). Worldwide, ischemic heart disease is estimated to cause 12.6% of all deaths annually (7.2 million deaths) (WHO 2005). In the US, heart disease accounts for 28.5% of all deaths (Anderson & Smith 2005). Unfortunately, this is no longer the exclusive problem of established market economies. The projected increases in deaths from ischemic heart disease in the Western economies between 1990 and 2020 are 32% for females and 45% for males. In India, the same projected increases are 115% and 127% respectively; in Latin America, they are 144% and 148% respectively; in Asian and Pacific Islanders, 143% and 148% respectively; and in sub-Saharan Africa, 125% and 141% respectively. The worst increases are projected for the Middle East; 148% for females and 174% for males (Milan Declaration 2004).

Arteriosclerosis is the most common cause of CAD. It generally refers to the thickening and hardening of the arterial walls, specifically in the cardiac vessels. The underlying pathology in aortic aneurysms and arterial disease of the vessels in the lower limbs and brain is also arteriosclerosis (Hillegas & Sadowsky 2001).

The normal aging process affects the arterial walls in a slow but continuous fashion. The most common feature is symmetrical thickening of the innermost wall (intima), which manifests as increased smooth muscle and connective tissue. The lipid content in the arterial wall, which is an accumulation of phospholipids and cholesterol, also increases with age. These normal age-related intimal changes are diffuse, whereas atherosclerotic disease causes focal raised lesions in addition to the aging process. The normal changes that occur with aging result in a gradually increasing rigidity of the vessel walls. Larger arteries can become dilated, elongated and tortuous, which lead to the development of aneurysms, especially in areas of bifurcation, at vessel curvatures and at points with little external support (see Chapter 9 for further information about age-related changes in blood vessels).

ATHEROSCLEROSIS

Atherosclerosis is a patchy, nodular form of arteriosclerosis. The lesions are distributed irregularly, with the aorta usually becoming involved early and often being the area most severely affected. Patchy changes also occur in the cerebral vessels, especially in the carotid, basilar and vertebral arteries. The proximal portion of the internal carotid artery is a commonly affected site, with a concentration of lesions located near the bifurcation. Peripherally, lesions are more common in the legs than the arms, with the majority of atherosclerotic plaques found in the larger proximal vessels such as the femoral and iliac arteries. Atherosclerosis of the coronary arteries is also commonly widespread. The most usual site of plaques is within the main part of each vessel, just after it arises from the proximal ascending aorta (Blessey & Irwin 1996). However, lesions can be distributed through the branch vessels as well. The degree of lumen narrowing is variable; however, after the plaque reaches 40% or more of the internal elastic lamina, luminal stenosis may occur (Orford & Selwyn 2005). The saphenous vein and internal mammary artery are common vessels for coronary artery bypass grafts (CABGs); the same process of atherosclerosis can subsequently develop in these vessels, making CABG necessary again.

Angiographic visualization of deformity to a vessel lumen is still the best evidence of silent atherosclerosis. Doppler probes to measure blood flow, in conjunction with ultrasound, are excellent techniques for determining the location of atherosclerotic plaques and narrowing of lumens in carotid and femoral vessels but not for coronary or other, more deeply set, blood vessels.

The development of atherosclerosis has recently been linked to inflammation, and research has therefore focused on the role of infections in the development of CAD (Singh & Deedwania 2005).

Inflammation and infection, such as with *Chlamydia pneumoniae,* generate proinflammatory cytokines that promote increases in adhesion molecules and procoagulants. C-reactive protein (CRP), an inflammatory marker, has been shown to be a good prognosticator for CAD.

When multiple risk factors are present, the possibility of atherosclerosis escalates. Traditionally, the most significant risk factors in the causation and acceleration of atherosclerotic disease are generally hypercholesterolemia, hypertension and cigarette smoking. Other factors that play an important role include age, gender and genetics. Some influence is also exerted by body habitus (obesity), diet, hyperglycemia and diabetes mellitus, sedentary lifestyle, stress and personality type (Mosca et al 2004, Orford & Selwyn 2005). However, more recent studies indicate that male gender is no longer considered to be a differentiating risk factor, for example the percentage of deaths in the US from heart disease in 2002 was 28.4% for males and 28.6% for females (Anderson & Smith 2005).

The clinical outcomes of atherosclerosis can be improved by removing or reversing a single risk factor or group of risk factors. In particular, alteration of diet, reduction of blood cholesterol levels, treatment of hypertension and cessation of smoking are the major targets to prevent the progression of atherosclerotic disease. Physical activity has been shown to reduce the negative effects of some of these factors. Exercise allows an individual to attain or maintain a higher metabolic rate, which allows better caloric intake tolerance – one can enjoy a few more calories without gaining weight. Reduction of blood cholesterol and blood pressure along with successive reductions or elimination of reliance on blood pressure lowering medications are other benefits of exercise (Thompson et al 2003). The general rehabilitation exercise considerations presented in Chapter 41 are all applicable to individuals with atherosclerosis. (Further evidence is available in DeTurk & Cahalin 2004 and Hillegas & Sadowsky 2001).

MYOCARDIAL ISCHEMIA

Myocardial ischemia results from a deficient blood supply to the heart muscle because of either obstruction or constriction of the coronary vessels. Underlying this deficiency is an imbalance between the oxygen supply and demand of the myocardial muscle cells. The majority of diseased coronary arteries have fixed obstructions in the form of atherosclerotic lesions that lead to anginal symptoms. However, the ischemia can also be caused by spasms of the coronary artery walls, also known as Prinzmetal's angina. Both are equally capable of reducing the supply of blood and therefore of oxygen to the myocardial muscle cells.

Ischemia produces major changes in two of the important functions of a myocardial cell: electrical activity and contractility. Alteration in electrical activity generates many of the electrocardiogram (ECG) arrhythmias. Impairment of myocardial contractility affects the function of the left ventricle and results in a reduced ejection fraction (the amount of blood pumped out with each heartbeat) and decreased cardiac output, which further compromises the blood supply to the coronary arteries.

Angina pectoris

The term 'angina pectoris' describes paroxysmal or spasmodic chest pain that is usually caused by myocardial cell anoxia and is typically precipitated by exertion or excitement. It is estimated that 6.3 million Americans experience angina (Alaeddini et al 2006). Stable angina is characterized by episodic chest pain that usually lasts for 5–15 min, is provoked by exertion or stress and is relieved by rest or sublingual nitroglycerin. The pain almost always has a retrosternal component

and commonly radiates into the neck, jaw and shoulders and down the left or the left and right arms. Radiation to the back is also possible. Additional symptoms, such as lightheadedness, palpitations, diaphoresis, dyspnea, fatigue, nausea or vomiting, may accompany the pain. Females and elderly individuals are more likely to present with atypical symptoms (Tan et al 2005). The specific ECG changes seen with ischemia are usually indicated by ST-segment depression of more than 1 mm, which occurs in about 50% of cases during an acute attack (Alaeddini et al 2006).

Unstable angina represents a clinical state between stable angina and acute myocardial infarction (AMI). It is also referred to as crescendo or preinfarction angina. The clinical definition of unstable angina includes any of the following subgroups: (i) exertional angina of recent onset, usually within the past 4–8 weeks (which means that all newly diagnosed angina is essentially unstable); (ii) angina of worsening character, either with increasing severity of pain, increasing duration of pain, increasing frequency of pain or increasing requirement for nitroglycerin; and (iii) angina at rest. Also included within this group of unstable anginas is postinfarction angina, which, as its name suggests, occurs after an AMI. It is important to remember that it can occur within days or weeks of an acute infarction or even months to years later (occurring after an angina-free period dating from the AMI). Those who experience angina after successful coronary artery bypass surgery are yet another group of individuals who are considered unstable. Once again, the onset of pain may occur several months or years after surgery.

Unstable angina is thought to be caused by a progression in the severity and extent of coronary atherosclerosis, coronary artery spasm or bleeding into non-occlusive plaques in the coronary artery. It eventually results in complete occlusion of the artery. Studies have shown that those with unstable angina have a 40% incidence of acute infarction and a 1% incidence of death within a 3-month period. With intensive education, treatment and avoidance of coronary risk factors, the risk of infarction drops to 8% and early death to 3%. Therefore, it is vital to recognize, hospitalize and treat patients with unstable angina.

Another form of angina is variant or Prinzmetal's angina. It occurs primarily at rest and often without any precipitants, although exposure to cold air has been known to precipitate it. Unlike the other types of angina, the exercise capacity in those with variant angina is preserved. There is also a tendency for the pain to occur at about the same time each day. Arrhythmia or conduction disturbances may accompany episodes of variant angina. Considering that up to one-third of variant angina sufferers have no atherosclerotic disease of the coronary vessels, the current theory of pathogenesis is that variant angina is caused by the spasm of one or more of the coronary arteries. Spasm is not isolated to variant angina; it also seen in individuals with typical angina and AMI. Unlike other forms of angina, history alone is not adequate to diagnose variant angina. Also, unlike other forms of angina, an episode of variant angina actually causes ST-segment elevation on an ECG.

Rehabilitation considerations for the person with angina

Differentiating angina pain from non-angina and musculoskeletal pain is challenging. The person experiencing the angina initially denies it and passes it off as a musculoskeletal pain. It is commonly described as pressure, squeezing or tightness in the substernal area. However, there are other individuals whose angina presents in atypical areas such as the jaw, neck, epigastric area or back. Table 42.1 presents some guidelines for differential diagnosis (Irwin & Blessey 1996).

Angina can be quantified for evaluation purposes in two ways. First, the rate pressure product (RPP), also called the double product,

Table 42.1   Differentiation of nonanginal discomforts from angina

Stable angina	Nonanginal discomfort (chest wall pain)
Relieved by nitroglycerin (30 s to 1 mm)	Nitroglycerin generally has no effect
Comes on at the same heart rate and blood pressure and is relieved by rest (lasts only a few minutes)	Occurs any time, lasts hours
Not palpable	Muscle soreness, joint soreness, evoked by palpation or deep breaths
Associated with feelings of doom, cold sweats, shortness of breath	Minimal additional symptoms
Often seen with ST-segment depression	No ST-segment depression

From Irwin & Blessey (1996), with permission from Mosby.

Table 42.2   Angina levels: an individual's subjective response to discomfort

Level 1	First perception of discomfort or pain in the chest area; does not require one to stop physical activity
Level 2	Discomfort that increases in intensity, extends in distribution, or both, but is tolerable; patient slows activity in an attempt to decrease angina level
Level 3	Severe chest pain that increases to intolerable levels; patient must stop activity, take nitroglycerin, or both
Level 4	The most severe pain imaginable (infarction-like pain)

From Temes WC 1994 Cardiac rehabilitation. In: Hillegass E, Sadowsky HS (eds) Essentials of Cardiopulmonary Physical Therapy. WB Saunders, Philadelphia, PA, p 643, with permission.

is closely correlated with the myocardial oxygen requirement. It is calculated by multiplying the heart rate by the systolic blood pressure. When these measures are calculated at the onset of angina symptoms or ECG instability (ST-segment depression > 1 mm), it is referred to as the angina threshold. A person with stable angina usually develops symptoms at a consistent level of the RPP. Exercise training programs can therefore be designed to keep the person from reaching the anginal threshold by closely monitoring heart and systolic blood pressure. Second, the subjective experience of the intensity of angina can be graded on a scale such as the one developed at Ranchos Los Amigos Medical Center (Table 42.2) (Temes 1994).

An individual known to have angina should always carry nitroglycerin medication with them. When angina symptoms begin, one tablet of nitroglycerin should be taken every 5 min. If the angina pain is not relieved after three tablets or 15 min, emergency care should be sought immediately.

ACUTE MYOCARDIAL INFARCTION

The vast majority of people with AMI have CAD but there is no universal agreement about exactly what precipitates the acute event. Current concepts concerning the immediate cause of AMI include the interaction of multiple trigger factors: progression of the atherosclerotic process to the point of complete occlusion; hemorrhage at the site of an existing, narrowing coronary artery embolism; coronary artery spasm; and thrombosis at the site of an atherosclerotic plaque. Previous approaches to the treatment of AMI, such as resting the cardiovascular system while monitoring and treating only the complications, if they develop, is being replaced by interventions that are aimed at reversing the precipitating causes of the infarction (Circulation 2005).

Like ischemia, infarction produces changes in the electrical depolarization and contractility of myocardial cells. These functions are important and derangement in one or both of them can cause the common complications of AMI. During the first few hours after the onset of pain, there are areas of infarction interspersed with or surrounded by areas of ischemia; therefore, in the early phases, infarction is not a completed process. These ischemic areas can be saved by the early application of medical and surgical therapy. The overall amount of infarcted myocardium remains one of the most critical factors in determining the prognosis, especially future morbidity and mortality.

Arrhythmias such as tachycardias, ventricular ectopy, bradycardias and atrioventricular blocks are commonly seen in AMI and are the major manifestations of the disruption of the electrical depolarization of the myocardial cells and the specialized conducting system. The major result of impaired contractility is the failure of the left ventricular pump. Heart failure usually develops if 25% of the left ventricular myocardium is damaged. Cardiogenic shock is also common and involves more than a 40% impairment of left ventricular function (Circulation 2005). If the papillary muscles of the mitral valve are involved, acute mitral valve regurgitation may develop and cause acute pulmonary edema and hypotension. Rupture of the myocardial wall or ventricular septum, resulting from autolysis in the infarcted area, can also occur and cause cardiac tamponade or an acutely acquired ventricular septal defect. Both of these conditions can present as sudden death after AMI.

Clinical aspects of AMI

The classic symptom of AMI is retrosternal chest pain, which is usually the same as angina pain but lasts for more than 15–30 min. Individual variation in the site and radiation of the pain, and also in the nature and severity of the pain, is very common. Associated features such as dyspnea, diaphoresis, palpitations, nausea and vomiting are common accompaniments but not all are present all of the time. The degree of heart muscle damage and extent of infarction is usually independent of the presence of associated features or the severity of the pain. A long duration of pain often indicates more damage. AMIs in elderly patients, as opposed to those in younger individuals, are likely to present with no pain or with a noncardiac type of pain or altered mental status (Garas & Zafari 2006). Longitudinal studies indicate that up to 25% of myocardial infarctions are not recognized clinically but are diagnosed later in routine ECGs performed for unrelated conditions. In addition, individuals with diabetes are more susceptible to silent (painless) myocardial infarction.

The physical examination can be quite normal. Mild to moderate increases in pulse rate are common despite the fact that inferior infarcts are usually associated with bradycardia. The pain and the activation of the sympathetic nervous system can cause elevation of blood pressure. However, if left ventricle function is impaired by the pain, hypotension is more likely. Abnormal S3 and S4 heart sounds can usually be auscultated. New systolic murmurs may cause great concern as they can indicate that there is muscle damage affecting the cardiac valves or causing regurgitation or that rupture of the septum has occurred.

AMIs may involve the full or partial thickness of the myocardial wall. Full-thickness infarctions are referred to as transmural; partial wall thickness infarctions are subendocardial or nontransmural. In the clinical setting, they are referred to respectively as Q-wave and non-Q-wave infarctions, depending on the presence or absence of pathological Q waves on the ECG. Mortality and complications depend on the extent of myocardial damage rather than on the presence of Q waves; however, Q-wave AMIs do tend to be larger and produce more myocardial necrotic tissue. On the whole, non-Q-wave infarctions result in lower in-hospital mortality but also in a far greater number of complications, especially recurrent infarction and postinfarct angina.

Diagnostic tests

Electrocardiography is an important diagnostic test for an AMI. However, only 50% of AMIs show diagnostic changes on the initial ECG. The classical AMI produces a progression of ECG changes that include ST-segment elevation, T-wave inversion and development of significant Q waves. Both the pain and the ECG changes resolve with relief of the ischemia and infarction. Localization of the AMI is important for prognosis, as the type and incidence of complications vary with the site and size of infarction.

Damage to cardiac muscle cells results in the release of enzymes into the bloodstream. Both the American College of Cardiology and the American Heart Association state that troponin levels show the best specificity and sensitivity for the diagnosis and prognosis of AMI. Serum levels increase within 3–12 h of the onset of chest pain, reach peak levels in 24–48 h and decrease to baseline in 5–14 days (Garas & Zafari 2006). Previously, the diagnostic standard was to monitor increases of creatinine phosphokinase–myocardial band (CK–MB), which occur within 3–12 h after chest pain starts, peak within 24 h and decrease to baseline in 2–3 days. However, the sensitivity and specificity are not as high as for troponin levels. Serial blood testing for cardiac enzyme levels in the setting of suspected AMI is now routine and is especially useful when ECG changes are nonspecific or absent. CK–MB may also be elevated after cardiac surgery and cardiopulmonary resuscitation (Garas & Zafari 2006).

Echocardiography is a form of ultrasound that is used to identify abnormalities in wall motion of regional cardiac muscles and also to observe the function of the cardiac valves. Its primary use is in the detection of complications of AMI that may need surgical intervention, such as rupture of the myocardial wall or valve damage. It is also used after AMIs to determine the extent of impairment to cardiac function.

Radionuclide scans are also used to detect both ischemia and infarction. Two radionuclides, thallium-201, which is taken up by normal myocardial cells, and technetium-99 (also labeled sestamibi), which is deposited in infarcted myocardial tissue, are commonly used to determine the amount of cardiac tissue involved in AMIs.

Complications of AMI

Lethal arrhythmias are most common during the prehospital phase of an AMI. The site of infarction does not usually influence the incidence of arrhythmias but it does play an important role in the type of arrhythmias that occur. For example, sinus tachycardia is more common with anterior AMIs, whereas sinus bradycardia frequently accompanies inferior AMIs. Atrial fibrillation usually occurs within the first 48 h after an AMI and is often associated with heart failure.

Nearly all patients with acute AMIs have premature ventricular contractions (PVCs), and their significance in heralding more serious arrhythmias is still an issue for debate. Ventricular tachycardia always requires intervention and, in a hemodynamically unstable patient, immediate cardioversion is essential (Garas & Zafari 2006). Ventricular fibrillation can occur early in the development of an AMI. It is nearly always successfully managed with defibrillation, if this equipment is available.

AMIs can also damage the conducting system, which leads to complete or third-degree heart block. The risk of developing complete heart block is dependent on the site of infarction and the presence of preexisting conduction disturbances, such as first- or second-degree conduction disturbances, in conjunction with bundle-branch or fascicular blocks (Garas & Zafari 2006).

AMIs nearly always produce an impairment in left ventricle pumping ability. The greater the area of damage, the more likely it is that symptoms will be clinically apparent. Clinical findings, ranging from no cardiac failure to mild failure and worsening pulmonary edema to cardiogenic shock, correlate with an increasing likelihood of mortality, for example there is a 5% mortality risk in cases with no cardiac failure and an 80% risk with cardiogenic shock.

Cardiac wall rupture at the site of infarction occurs more often in those with persisting postinfarction hypertension, in the elderly and in those having a first AMI. The mortality rate from cardiac wall rupture is about 95%, with 50% of the cases occurring in the first 5 days after AMI and 90% in the first 14 days postinfarction. Immediate surgical intervention and repair are essential for survival. The risk of both venous thrombosis and pulmonary embolism is higher after an AMI because of the prolonged bedrest required. Atrial fibrillation, obesity and old age also contribute to this risk.

The return to physical activity

Early mobilization of individuals after an AMI, using a symptom-limited rehabilitation approach, is very important in the postinfarction period. In the acute setting, the physician determines the upper limits of exercise while considering the deconditioning effects of bedrest and lack of exercise. For individuals who are asymptomatic and do not show signs of ischemia, tolerance of exercise is more important than exercising at a specific heart-rate intensity. Box 41.4 presents guidelines for termination of an exercise session and these should be followed. Also, the American College of Sports Medicine offers general criteria for exercising starting initially in the in-patient setting and can be followed after hospital discharge. Their guidelines suggest that the rate of perceived exertion from the board scale (from 6–20) should be less than 13. This ranges in a description fashion from very, very light to fairly light. The value of 13 is described as "somewhat hard." For the post-MI, the heart rate should remain less than 120 beats per minute or the resting heart rate should not elevate more than 20 beats per minute (the arbitrary upper limit). The intensity post-surgery should be resting heart rate +30 beats per minute (arbitrary upper limit). The intensity of exercise post-myocardial infarction may be to tolerance if asymptomatic.

Again, according to the American College of Sports Medicine, the duration of exercise can be intermittent with bouts lasting 3–5 minutes. Rest periods may be taken at the patient's discretion lasting 1–2 minutes and should be shorter than the exercise bout of duration. The total duration may be up to 20 minutes.

The frequency of exercise with early mobilization should be 3–4 times per day (days 1–3) and in later mobilization, two times a day beginning on day 4. The exercise bout can be progressed initially with increasing the duration of 10–15 minutes of exercise and then increase intensity (American College of Sports Medicine 2000).

CONCLUSION

Atherosclerosis leads to the development of CAD and ischemic heart disease. Angina is a symptom of myocardial ischemia. Angina pectoris is a retrosternal symptom, and other complaints of pain to the neck, jaw, shoulders and upper extremities result from myocardial anoxia, usually precipitated by exertion or excitement. Angina is commonly denied and dismissed as a musculoskeletal complaint. Appropriate therapeutic exercise training programs must be designed to prevent the patient from reaching the anginal threshold. If anginal pain is not relieved within 15 min, emergency care should be sought because of the likelihood of having suffered an AMI. Progressively increasing myocardial ischemia will ultimately lead to an AMI or the need for coronary artery bypass surgery. Much like angina, the classic symptom of AMI is retrosternal pain; however, in AMI, the pain lasts for more than 15–30 min without relief from rest or sublingual nitroglycerin. It is crucial to seek medical attention early because of the possibility of reversing the ischemia and preventing further infarction. AMIs can cause conduction problems that result in arrhythmias and ventricular fibrillation and, possibly, left ventricular failure. It is important to resume physical activity with caution.

Acknowledgment

The authors would like to acknowledge the suggestions of Roddy P. Canosa, DO, FACC.

References

Alaeddini J, Alimohammadi B, Shirani J 2006 Angina pectoris online. Available: http://www.emedicine.com/med/topic133.htm. Accessed March 7 2006

American College of Sports Medicine (ACSM) 2000 Guidelines for Exercise Testing and Prescription. Williams & Wilkins, Baltimore, MD

Anderson RN, Smith BL 2005 Deaths: leading causes for 2002. Natl Vital Stat Rep 53(17):1–89

Blessey AL, Irwin S 1996 Atherosclerosis: overview of the basic mechanism of atherogenesis, pathophysiology, and natural history. In: Irwin S, Tecklin JS (eds) Cardiopulmonary Physical Therapy, 3rd edn. Mosby-Year Book, St Louis, MO

Circulation 2005 Part 8: stabilization of the patient with acute coronary syndromes, 112:IV89–IV110. Available: http://www.circulationaha.org. Accessed March 7 2006

DeTurk WE, Cahalin LP 2004 Cardiovascular and Pulmonary Physical Therapy. McGraw-Hill Medical Publishing Division, New York

Garas S, Zafari AM 2006 Myocardial infarction. Available: http://www.emedicine.com/med/topic1567.htm. Accessed March 7 2006

Hillegas EA, Sadowsky HS 2001 Essentials of Cardiopulmonary Physical Therapy, 2nd edn. WB Saunders, Philadelphia, PA

Irwin S, Blessey AL 1996 Patient evaluation. In: Irwin S, Tecklin JS (eds) Cardiopulmonary Physical Therapy, 3rd edn. Mosby-Year Book, St Louis, MO

Milan Declaration 2004 Positioning technology to serve global heart health. Available: http://www.internationalhearthealth.org/Publications/milan_declaration.pdf. Accessed March 7 2006

Mosca L, Appel L, Benjamin E et al 2004 Evidence-based guidelines for cardiovascular disease prevention in women. Arterioscler Thromb Vasc Biol 24: 29–50

Orford J, Selwyn A 2005 Atherosclerosis. Available: http://www.emedicine.com med/topic182.htm. Accessed March 7 2006

Singh V, Deedwania P 2005 Coronary artery atherosclerosis. Available: http://www.emedicine.com/med/topic446.htm. Accessed March 7 2006

Temes WC 1994 Cardiac rehabilitation. In: Hillegass E, Sadowsky HS (eds) Essentials of Cardiopulmonary Physical Therapy. WB Saunders, Philadelphia, PA

Tan W, Moliterno D, Filby S 2005 Unstable angina online. Available: http://www.emedicine.com/med/topic2606.htm. Accessed March 7 2006

Thompson P, Buchner D, Piña I et al 2003 Exercise and physical activity in the prevention and treatment of atherosclerotic cardiovascular disease. Arterioscler Thromb Vasc Biol 23: 42–49

World Health Organization (WHO) 2005 What is the deadliest disease in the world? Available: http:// www.who.int/features/qa/18/en/. Accessed December 8 2005

Chapter 43

Cardiac arrhythmias and conduction disturbances

Pamela Reynolds

Cardiac rhythm originates from and is controlled by specific areas within the heart itself. These areas are called intrinsic pacemakers and are responsible for the propagation of electrical impulses that generally travel from the right atrium to the apex of the heart, and activate both atria and ventricles in the process. Although these impulses can pass from cardiac muscle cell to adjacent cardiac muscle cell, there is a preferential tract that they follow along specialized conducting tissue situated within the myocardium that minimizes conduction time. This pathway is detailed in Fig. 43.1.

The primary intrinsic pacemaker is the sinoatrial (SA) node, situated at the junction of the superior vena cava and the right atrium. Electrical impulses travel from the SA node through the atria to the atrioventricular (AV) node, which sits on the right side of the interatrial septum. The rate of SA node discharge is controlled by the autonomic nervous system. Sympathetic stimulation increases the firing rate whereas parasympathetic activity (vagal stimulation) lowers the rate (Weiderhold 1988, Hillegass 2001, Mammen et al 2004).

Beginning at age 60, there is a pronounced decrease in the number of pacemaker cells in the SA node. By the age of 75, less than 10% of the cells found in the young adult remain. Similar changes occur in the AV node and bundle of His but to a lesser extent (Kantelip et al 1986).

The depolarization of the atria corresponds to the P wave on the electrocardiogram (ECG). The impulse conduction is slowed as it traverses the AV node, allowing time for atrial contraction to be completed before ventricular contraction. This slowing or delay corresponds to the P–R interval on the ECG. After passing through the AV node, the impulse passes into the bundle of His, down the interventricular septum and then divides into the right and left bundle branches that supply impulses to the right and left ventricles respectively. The ventricular depolarization corresponds to the QRS complex on the ECG. The ST segment and T wave on the ECG are produced by ventricular repolarization. Specifically, the ST segment

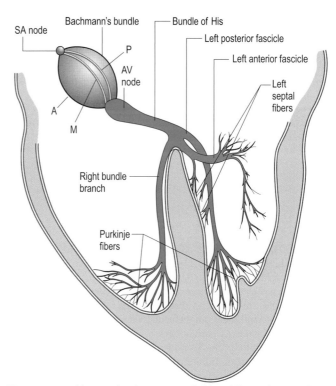

Figure 43.1 The conduction system. A, M and P are the anterior, medial and posterior interatrial tracts.
(From Goldman MJ 1979 Principles of Clinical Electrocardiography, 10th edn. Lange Medical Books, Los Altos, CA, with permission.)

is the absolute refractory period in which no depolarization of the ventricles can occur. T-wave repolarization is also known as the relative refractory period. During this time, the ventricles can be stimulated to contract but the heart is still electrically unstable, and depolarization in this period can progress to ventricular tachycardia (Weiderhold 1988).

Each wave, segment and interval has certain normal characteristics, which are identified in Figure 43.2. Variances are usually indicative of different heart impairments. For instance, changes in the ST segment and T wave classically demonstrate some type of myocardial ischemia. Depression of the ST segment by more than 0.1 mm is generally indicative of ischemia and may also produce symptoms of angina. T-wave inversion is usually a sign of ischemia and/or an evolving

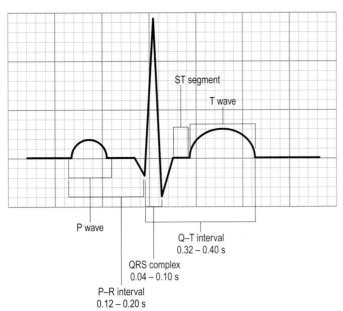

Figure 43.2 Graphic of ECG with all wave segments identified. Normal P–R interval measures between 0.12 s and 0.20 s. The normal duration for the QRS interval is between 0.04 s and 0.10 s. Normal R–R intervals are regular and equally distanced; if irregular, the distance between the shortest and longest is <0.12 s. Normal values for the Q–T interval depend on the heart rate. A normal ST segment is elevated or depressed by <1 mm. (From Hillegass E 1994 Electrocardiography. In: Hillegass E, Sadowsky HS (eds) Essentials of Cardiopulmonary Physical Therapy. WB Saunders, Philadelphia, PA, with permission.)

(Labels in figure: ST segment; T wave; P wave; Q–T interval 0.32 – 0.40 s; QRS complex 0.04 – 0.10 s; P–R interval 0.12 – 0.20 s)

myocardial infarction. Other abnormalities are discussed in the following text.

Many areas of the heart can depolarize spontaneously and rhythmically. The rate of ventricular contraction will be controlled by the area with the highest frequency of discharge. The SA node normally has the highest rate and therefore the ventricles will follow the rate set by the SA node. The normal cardiac cycle is termed normal sinus rhythm because it originates in the SA node and is conducted along the normal electrical pathway of the heart. Disturbances to cardiac rhythm and conduction are classified in several ways, for example (i) heart rate; (ii) site of origin for the delay or block; (iii) whether rhythm is regular or irregular; (iv) mechanism of the arrhythmia; and (v) the ratio of atrial to ventricular depolarization (P waves–QRS complexes).

BASIC RHYTHM DISTURBANCES AND IMPLICATIONS

Abnormal cardiac rhythms can arise in the atrial muscle, the junctional region between the atria and ventricles or in the ventricular muscle. These arrhythmias may be slow and sustained (bradycardias), occur as early single beats (extrasystoles or ectopic beats) or be sustained and fast (tachycardias). Rhythm disturbances may decrease cardiac output and potentially lead to orthostatic hypotension and possibly heart failure. If the ventricular rate is too fast, the volume of blood pumped with each contraction decreases. When the heart beats too slowly, the contractions are not adequate to supply the body's demands. In the normal adult, heart rates between 40 and 160 beats per minute (b.p.m.) are usually well tolerated as physiological

adaptations are able to maintain an adequate cardiac output and blood pressure. However, problems can arise in those with significant vascular disease if the heart rate drops below 50 b.p.m. or goes above 120 b.p.m. These alterations to rate can cause tissue ischemia, with the heart being especially susceptible.

Different areas of the heart are able to initiate the depolarization sequence if the SA node fails or, if conduction is blocked, another area will fire a depolarizing impulse and keep the heart beating. These secondary sites have lower depolarization frequencies than the SA node to avoid competition between pacing sites. As the heart is controlled by whichever site is discharging most frequently, the SA node with a rate of about 70 b.p.m. is the primary site of impulse initiation. If the SA node fails, control will be assumed by a focus either in the atrial muscle or around the AV node (junctional region). Both of these have spontaneous depolarization frequencies of 40–60 b.p.m. If these fail, or conduction through the bundle of His is blocked, a ventricular focus will take over, with a rate of about 30–40 b.p.m. (Weiderhold 1988, Mammen et al 2004). Therefore, the major mechanisms that cause bradyarrhythmias are either depression of SA node activity or blocks within the conducting system. In either situation, a supplementary pacemaker takes over to control the heart rate. If these supplementary pacemaker cells are located above the bifurcation of the bundle of His, the rate will be adequate enough to maintain cardiac output. Any bradyarrhythmia that causes hemodynamic compromise of the heart muscle requires urgent medical intervention.

Junctional impulses can arise from the AV node or above the bifurcation of the bundle of His. The impulse then spreads retrogradely or backwards through the atria and antegradely towards the ventricles. Depending on the site of origin and the conduction velocity of the impulse, and the refractory periods of the atria and ventricles, activation of the atria may occur before, during or after depolarization of the ventricle.

Any part of the heart can depolarize earlier than it should and, if it initiates a heartbeat, this is called an extrasystole or ectopic beat. Atrial ectopic beats cause abnormally shaped P waves on the ECG, whereas junctional ectopic beats may have no P wave or a P wave immediately before or after the QRS complex, depending on the site of the ectopic focus within the junctional region. The QRS complexes for atrial and junctional ectopic beats have the same configuration as in normal SA rhythm. Ectopic beats arising in the ventricles do not travel down the normal bundle branches. Therefore, they evoke abnormally shaped QRS complexes, frequently referred to as wide and bizarre, which are easily recognized on an ECG tracing.

Tachycardia refers to a clinical state in which the heart rate is over 100 b.p.m. Regardless of whether an ectopic focus is within the atria, the junctional (AV nodal) region or the ventricles, it can fire rapidly and repeatedly causing a sustained tachycardia. Bradycardia refers to a heart rate that is less than 60 b.p.m. Urgent treatment is needed if there is hemodynamic compromise of the cardiac muscle or rhythms develop that have the potential to become life-threatening (Weiderhold 1988, Hillegass 2001).

The following discussion of the common types of rhythm disturbance will be categorized according to the anatomical site of the disturbance: supraventricular (atrial), junctional or ventricular. Each will then be divided into the type of arrhythmia: slow, fast or ectopic. Conduction blocks are discussed separately as a cause of bradycardia.

ATRIAL ARRHYTHMIAS

SA arrhythmia

In SA arrhythmia, the vagal nerves and changes in respiration can alter the rate of SA node discharge. The ECG is normal except for the

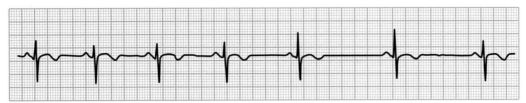

Figure 43.3   Sinus arrhythmia consisting of normal P–QRS–T configuration with increasing and decreasing intervals between complexes.
(From Thys D, Kaplan J 1987 The ECG in Anesthesia and Critical Care. Churchill Livingstone, New York, with permission.)

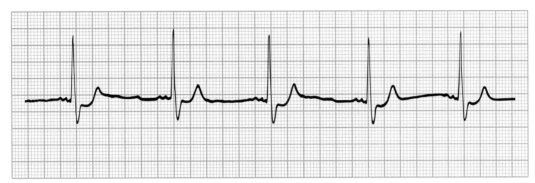

Figure 43.4   ECG tracing illustrating sinus bradycardia with a rate of approximately 50 beats per minute.
(From Weiderhold R 1988 Electrocardiography: The Monitoring Lead. WB Saunders, Philadelphia, PA, p 189, with permission.)

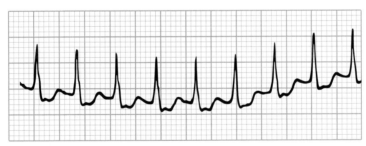

Figure 43.5   Atrial tachycardia.
(From Cohen M, Michel TH 1988 Cardiopulmonary Symptoms in Physical Therapy Practice. Churchill Livingstone, New York, p 146, with permission.)

variable lengths of the R–R intervals (Fig. 43.3). Variations are common, especially with changes in the rate of respiration. This rhythm is very prevalent in young people and tends to decline with aging. No treatment is required (Weiderhold 1988, Hillegass 2001, Mammen et al 2004).

SA bradycardia

SA bradycardia is a regular SA rhythm but with a SA node rate below 60 b.p.m. (Fig. 43.4). The ECG has normal P waves and P–R intervals and a 1:1 conduction ratio between the atria and ventricles, but an atrial rate of less than 60 b.p.m. It represents a suppression of the SA node discharge rate, usually in response to normal physiology in athletes, during sleep and with stimulation of the vagus nerve. It may be drug related, especially narcotics, beta blockers and calcium-channel blockers. Pathologies that may produce a bradycardia rhythm include acute myocardial infarction, increased intracranial pressure, hypersensitivity of the carotid sinus and hypothyroidism.

If evidence of hemodynamic compromise is present, then treatment is needed. Drug treatment can be useful in the short term; however, in those with symptomatic recurrent or persistent bradycardia, internal cardiac pacing is indicated (Weiderhold 1988, Hillegass 2001, Mammen et al 2004).

SA tachycardia

SA tachycardia is an acceleration of the SA node impulse discharge rate (Fig. 43.5). The ECG has normal P waves and P–R intervals and a 1:1 conduction ratio between the atria and ventricles. The atrial rate is increased to between 100 and 160 b.p.m. The tachycardia may result from a normal physiological response, as seen in infants and children with exertion and emotions, especially anxiety. It may be drug related, for example from the use of atropine, epinephrine (adrenaline), alcohol, nicotine and caffeine. It may also reflect a pathological process such as fever, hypoxia, anemia, hypovolemia or pulmonary embolism. In many of these conditions, the increased rate is

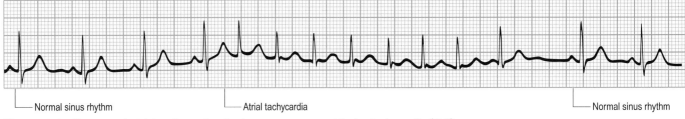

Normal sinus rhythm   Atrial tachycardia   Normal sinus rhythm

Figure 43.6   Paroxysmal atrial tachycardia, also known as supraventricular tachycardia (SVT).
(From Phillips RE, Feeney MK 1990 The Cardiac Rhythms, 3rd edn. WB Saunders, Philadelphia, PA, p 154, with permission.)

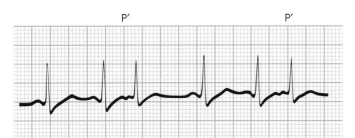

Figure 43.7   Premature atrial contractions. P' indicates premature atrial contraction on ectopic beat.
(From Summerall CP III 1991 Lessons in EKG Interpretation, 2nd edn. Churchill Livingstone, New York, p 139, with permission.)

the result of the heart increasing cardiac output in an attempt to meet the increased circulatory demands. Treatment of the underlying condition is indicated, especially in those with preexisting cardiac disease, as increased cardiac output may further exacerbate any heart problems (Weiderhold 1988, Hillegass 2001, Mammen et al 2004, Larry & Schaal 2006).

Supraventricular tachycardia

Supraventricular arrhythmias include any rhythm in which the depolarizing impulse occurs above the level of the AV node. These rhythms all have a normal QRS complex following depolarization. Supraventricular tachycardia (SVT, also known as paroxysmal atrial tachycardia) is a regular rapid rhythm that arises from any site above the bifurcation of the bundle of His (Fig. 43.6). Sensations of palpitations and light-headedness are common with SVT. In those with coronary heart disease, angina pain and dyspnea may occur because of the rapid heart rate. SVT also commonly occurs in those with poor left ventricular function, heart failure and pulmonary edema. Treatment includes discontinuation of any causative drugs, use of a variety of antiarrhythmic medications to control rate and the use of vagal maneuvers (such as carotid sinus massage, Valsalva and immersion in cold water) to slow the atrial rate. The physician may also perform a synchronized cardiac conversion, especially with an unstable patient with hypotension, pulmonary edema or severe chest pain (Weiderhold 1988, Hillegass 2001, Mammen et al 2004, Larry & Schaal 2006).

Premature atrial contractions

Premature atrial contractions (PACs) originate from ectopic pacemakers located anywhere in the atrium other than the SA node (Fig. 43.7).

The ECG shows ectopic P waves that appear sooner than the next expected SA beat. The ectopic P wave has a different shape and/or direction to a normal P wave. The ectopic P wave will not be conducted if it reaches the AV node during the absolute refractory period but it will be conducted with delay (longer P–R interval) during the relative refractory period. PACs that are conducted through the AV node, bundle of His and the bundle branches will have typical QRS complexes. PACs may appear at any age and are often seen in the absence of heart disease. It is generally believed that stress, fatigue, alcohol, tobacco and caffeine may precipitate PACs, although nothing has been proven yet. Frequent PACs are seen in chronic lung disease, ischemic heart disease and digitalis toxicity. Treatment involves cessation of precipitating causes and management of underlying disorders. If the PACs produce symptoms or sustained tachycardias, drug therapy should be implemented, with the aim of suppressing the PACs (Weiderhold 1988, Hillegass 2001, Mammen et al 2004, Larry & Schaal 2006).

Atrial fibrillation

Atrial fibrillation occurs when there are multiple areas of the atrial myocardium continuously discharging and contracting (Fig. 43.8). Depolarization and contraction are so disorganized and irregular that the atria quiver rather than contract uniformly. The atrial rate is usually above 400 b.p.m., whereas the ventricular rate is slower because it is limited by the AV node refractory time. The ECG shows fibrillatory atrial activity instead of P waves and an irregular ventricular response (Weiderhold 1988, Hillegass 2001, Mammen et al 2004, Larry & Schaal 2006).

There are primarily two problems with atrial fibrillation. First, the atria do not depolarize and, consequently, there is no contraction of the atria. Contraction of the atria can add up to 30% to the ventricular volume, therefore, without it, cardiac output can decrease by up to 30%. Cardiac output is usually not affected in individuals who have a ventricular response of less than 100 b.p.m.; however, in an individual with a resting heart rate of more than 100 b.p.m. or who exercises, signs of hemodynamic compromise may quickly be demonstrated. Second, there is a danger of blood coagulating in the fibrillating atria; a mural thrombus may form and subsequently lead to an embolus. In total, 30% of all patients with atrial fibrillation develop emboli (Hillegass 2001).

Atrial fibrillation can occur either as a paroxysmal burst or a sustained rhythm. Rheumatic heart disease, hypertension and ischemic heart disease are conditions in which atrial fibrillation commonly occurs. Treatment depends on the overall condition of the patient. Drugs can be used in the more stable patient. Response is best in those in which the atrial fibrillation is treated shortly after onset. In individuals who become hemodynamically compromised, cardiac conversion or a pacemaker are other treatment choices (Weiderhold 1988, Hillegass 2001, Mammen et al 2004).

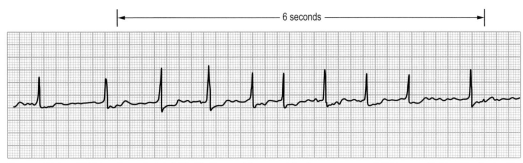

Figure 43.8   ECG tracing of atrial fibrillation, with a ventricular response of 80 b.p.m. Notice the lack of P waves and the irregular rhythm.
(From Hillegass E 1994 Electrocardiography. In: Hillegass E, Sadowsky HS (eds) Essentials of Cardiopulmonary Physical Therapy. WB Saunders, Philadelphia, PA, p 377, with permission.)

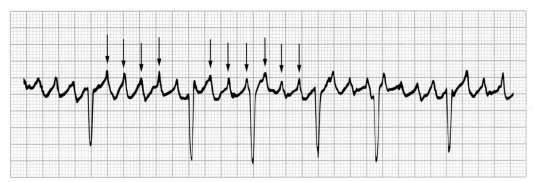

Figure 43.9   ECG tracing of atrial flutter waves (arrows) with a variable block.
(From Weiderhold R 1989 Electrocardiography: The Monitoring Lead. WB Saunders, Philadelphia, PA, p 218, with permission.)

Atrial flutter

The exact mechanism involved in the development of atrial flutter is unknown but the problem seems to involve a small area of the atrium only (Fig. 43.9). The ECG characteristics include a regular atrial rate of 250–350 b.p.m. and sawtooth-shaped flutter waves in place of P waves. Atrial flutter rarely occurs in the absence of preexisting heart disease. Incidence is highest in those with ischemic heart disease or acute myocardial infarction but it can also be a complication of congestive cardiomyopathies, myocarditis, pulmonary embolus, blunt chest trauma and dioxin toxicity. Atrial flutter can occur as a transient arrhythmia between SA rhythm and atrial fibrillation. Treatment consists of cardiac conversion or medical therapy depending on the clinical status of the patient (Weiderhold 1988, Hillegass 2001, Mammen et al 2004, Larry & Schaal 2006).

Tachycardia–bradycardia syndrome (sick sinus syndrome)

Sick sinus syndrome occurs when there are problems with both impulse generation and conduction, at or above the AV node region. Clinically, a variety of arrhythmias may be seen; fortunately, most are transient. The main arrhythmias include atrial fibrillation, junctional tachycardia, SVT and atrial flutter. Intermittent SA bradycardia, prolonged SA arrest and SA node block with AV node conduction abnormalities are the most common bradycardias. Symptoms reflect the presence of a fast or slow heart rate. Symptomatic bradycardia

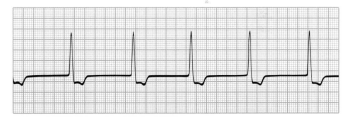

Figure 43.10   Junctional rate with sinus node arrest.
(From Cohen M, Michel TH 1988 Cardiopulmonary Symptoms in Physical Therapy Practice. Churchill Livingstone, New York, p 151, with permission.)

usually requires a permanent pacemaker (Weiderhold 1988, Hillegass 2001, Mammen et al 2004).

Junctional rhythm

Under normal circumstances, the SA node discharges at a faster rate than the AV node, so the pacemaker at the AV junction is overridden. If the SA node discharge is slow or fails to reach the AV node, a junctional escape beat (Fig. 43.10) may occur, usually at a rate of 40–60 b.p.m. Generally, these escape beats do not conduct back into the atria, so a QRS complex without a P wave is seen on the ECG. Whenever there is a long enough pause before an impulse reaches the AV node, the junctional pacemaker can elicit a junctional beat. Sustained junctional escape rhythms may be seen with congestive heart failure, dioxin toxicity or myocarditis.

Junctional tachycardia

An enhanced junctional impulse may override the SA node and produce either an accelerated junctional rhythm (rate 60–100 b.p.m.) or a junctional tachycardia with rates greater than 100 b.p.m. Accelerated junctional rhythm or junctional tachycardia can occur with inferior myocardial infarction or dioxin toxicity. If the enhanced rhythm is sustained and produces symptoms of hemodynamic compromise or ischemia, therapy for the underlying cause is required. Acute therapy to increase the SA rate may also be needed. At higher rates, it is difficult to differentiate SVT from junctional tachycardia because, if the P wave is present, it is lost in the QRS complex and not visualized (Weiderhold 1988, Hillegass 2001, Mammen et al 2004).

VENTRICULAR ARRHYTHMIAS

Premature ventricular contractions

Premature ventricular contractions (PVCs) are impulses that arise from single or multiple areas within the ventricles. The ECG shows a premature, widened and often bizarre QRS complex with no preceding P wave (Fig. 43.11). The ST segment and T wave of the PVC are opposite in direction to the major QRS deflection. Most PVCs do not affect the SA node discharge and it will therefore trigger the next impulse after the refractory period. If conducted to the atria, a PVC will cause a retrograde (inverted) P wave. PVCs are common, even in those without heart disease. They occur frequently in individuals with ischemic heart disease and are universally found in those with acute myocardial infarction. This highlights the underlying electrical instability of the heart and the added risk of developing ventricular tachycardia. Other common causes of PVCs include congestive heart failure, hypoxia, dioxin toxicity and hypokalemia. Treatment of PVCs is important in those with acute myocardial ischemia or infarction where maintenance of cardiac output is critical. The treatment of chronic ectopy depends on balancing the underlying heart disease, the origin of the ectopy and the presence of symptoms against the risks of side effects from antiarrhythmic drugs (Weiderhold 1988, Hillegass 2001, Mammen et al 2004, Larry & Schaal 2006).

Ventricular tachycardia

Ventricular tachycardia is the occurrence of three or more beats from a ventricular ectopic pacemaker at a rate of more than 100 b.p.m. (Hillegass 2001). The ECG findings are wide QRS complexes because of aberrant conduction, heart rates greater than 100 b.p.m. (usually 150–200), a regular rhythm and a constant QRS axis. Ventricular tachycardia can occur in a nonsustained manner, usually as short bursts of a few seconds that then spontaneously terminate (Fig. 43.12), or in a sustained fashion with longer episodes and symptoms of hemo-dynamic instability. The latter requires immediate

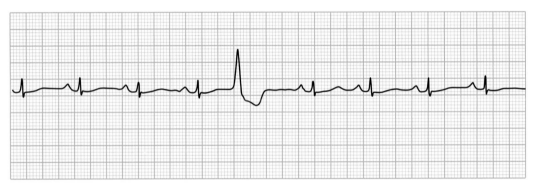

Figure 43.11   ECG tracing of an isolated premature ventricular complex. Note that there is no P wave preceding the QRS complex.
(From Weiderhold R 1989 Electrocardiography: The Monitoring Lead. WB Saunders, Philadelphia, PA, p 82, with permission.)

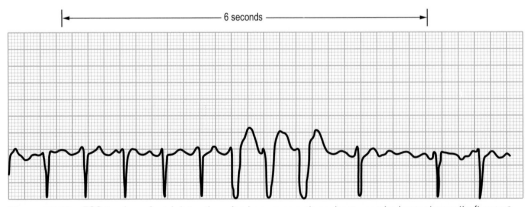

Figure 43.12   ECG tracing of a triplet, otherwise known as a three-beat ventricular tachycardia (beats 6, 7 and 8).
(From Hillegass E 1994 Electrocardiography. In: Hillegass E, Sadowsky HS (eds) Essentials of Cardiopulmonary Physical Therapy. WB Saunders, Philadelphia, PA, p 387, with permission.)

treatment. A danger with sustained ventricular tachycardia is that is can deteriorate into ventricular fibrillation. Ventricular tachycardia is rare in individuals without underlying heart disease. Ischemic heart disease and acute myocardial infarction are the most common causes of ventricular tachycardia. Unstable patients are treated with cardiac conversion, whereas more stable patients receive intravenous antiarrhythmic drugs (Weiderhold 1988, Hillegass 2001, Mammen et al 2004).

Ventricular fibrillation

Ventricular fibrillation is the totally disorganized depolarization and contraction of the ventricular myocardium so that no effective ventricular or cardiac output occurs. The ECG shows a fine to coarse zigzag pattern with no detectable P waves or QRS complexes (Fig. 43.13). There is no blood pressure or pulse detectable in ventricular fibrillation. In an awake and responsive person, an ECG pattern of ventricular fibrillation is usually a result of loose lead artifact or electrical interference. Ventricular fibrillation is the most common complication of severe ischemic heart disease, with or without acute myocardial infarction. It can occur suddenly without preceding hemodynamic deterioration or after a period of left ventricular failure and/or circulatory shock. Other etiologic factors include dioxin toxicity, blunt chest injury, hypothermia, severe electrolyte abnormalities and myocardial irritation from intracardiac catheter or pacemaker wires. Treatment is immediate defibrillation; several attempts may be necessary. Antiarrhythmic medications are used as adjuncts to cardiac conversion (Weiderhold 1988, Hillegass 2001, Mammen et al 2004).

CONDUCTION DISTURBANCES

SA node block

In normal sinus rhythm, the SA node discharge traverses the atria and paces the heart. SA node block can occur when the impulses are either delayed or have their propagation blocked. The block can be divided into first-, second- and third-degree types. First-degree block results from a delay in impulse conduction out of the SA node to the atria. With second-degree block, some impulses get through whereas others do not. Third-degree block is when the SA node discharge is completely blocked, meaning that no P waves originate from the SA node. SA node block can result from myocardial disease, especially acute inferior myocardial infarction. Drug toxicity and myocarditis can also cause this type of block. Treatment is dependent on the underlying cause, the associated arrhythmias and whether hemodynamic compromise is present. Specific drugs can increase SA node discharge and aid conduction. Recurrent or persistent bradycardia, especially if symptomatic, may require an artificial cardiac pacemaker (Weiderhold 1988, Hillegass 2001, Mammen et al 2004).

First-degree atrioventricular (AV) block

First-degree heart block is characterized by a delay in AV conduction. In other words, after the SA node discharges, it takes longer for the impulse to reach the AV node. Although each impulse is conducted to the ventricles, the rate is slower than normal, leading to prolongation of the P–R interval by more then 0.20 s [or more than five small boxes on the ECG tracing (Fig. 43.14)]. It is occasionally

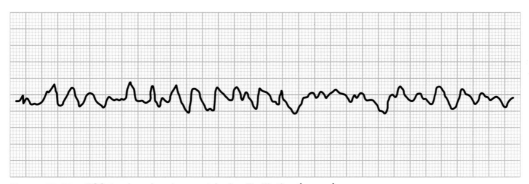

Figure 43.13   ECG tracing showing ventricular fibrillation (coarse).
(From Hillegass E 2001 Electrocardiography. In: Hillegass E, Sadowsky HS (eds) Essentials of Cardiopulmonary Physical Therapy. WB Saunders, Philadelphia, PA, p 410, with permission.)

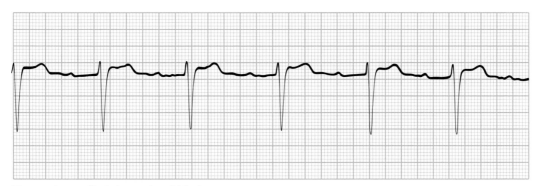

Figure 43.14   First-degree heart block.
(From Weiderhold R 1988 Electrocardiography: The Monitoring Lead. WB Saunders, Philadelphia, PA, p 87, with permission.)

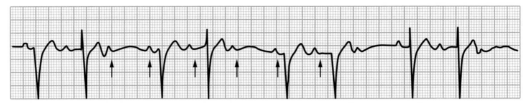

Figure 43.15   ECG tracing showing type I second-degree heart block (Wenckebach's). The arrows identify the P waves. Notice the progressive lengthening of the P–R interval until finally a P wave exists without a QRS complex.

(From Phillips RE, Feeney MK 1990 The Cardiac Rhythms, 3rd edn. WB Saunders, Philadelphia, PA, p 255.)

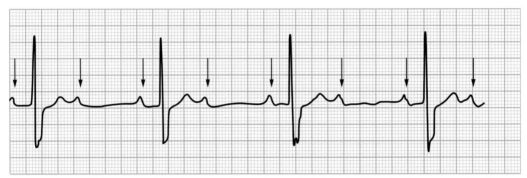

Figure 43.16   ECG tracing of type II second-degree heart block (Mobitz II) with a heart rate of 37 b.p.m. Note the two P waves for every QRS complex.

(From Hillegass E 1994 Electrocardiography. In: Hillegass E, Sadowsky HS (eds) Essentials of Cardiopulmonary Physical Therapy. WB Saunders, Philadelphia, PA, p 383, with permission.)

found in normal hearts but is more commonly seen with acute myocardial infarction, drug toxicity and myocarditis. Generally, nerve conduction velocity is known to slow with the aging process; first-degree heart block may be a functional result of this decrease. Generally, first-degree heart block is relatively benign. No treatment is required unless more serious conduction disturbances are also present (Weiderhold 1988, Hillegass 2001, Mammen et al 2004).

Second-degree AV block

Second-degree AV blocks are subdivided into Mobitz I (or Wenckebach) and Mobitz II blocks. The Wenckebach phenomenon describes the progressive lengthening of the P–R interval, a dropped beat and repetition of the cycle (Fig. 43.15). There is progressive prolongation of AV conduction and the P–R interval until an atrial impulse is completely blocked by a refractory AV node. After the dropped beat, which is seen as a P wave not followed by a QRS complex, the AV conduction returns to normal and the cycle repeats itself with either the same (fixed) or a different (variable) conduction ratio. This block is usually transient and can be associated with an acute inferior myocardial infarction, dioxin toxicity, myocarditis or cardiac surgery. Specific treatment is not required unless the ventricular rate is slow enough to reduce cardiac output and produce signs of hemodynamic compromise. Drugs can be used to increase the rate but, if unsuccessful, a ventricular pacemaker is needed (Weiderhold 1988, Hillegass 2001, Mammen et al 2004).

In the Mobitz type II form of second-degree block, one or more beats may not be conducted at a single time and the P–R interval

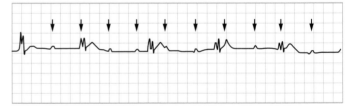

Figure 43.17   Electrocardiogram tracing showing third-degree heart block, also known as complete heart block. Notice how the P waves have their own regular rhythm (arrows) without interrupting the rhythm of the QRS complex. There is no communication between atrial firing and ventricular firing.

(From Hillegass E 1994 ECG. In: Hillegass E, Sadowsky HS (eds) Essentials of Cardiopulmonary Physical Therapy. WB Saunders, Philadelphia, PA, p 405, with permission.)

remains constant before and after the nonconducted atrial beats. There are more P waves than QRS complexes (Fig. 43.16). This type of block frequently occurs with bundle-branch (or fascicular) problems and the QRS complexes are consequently widened. Type II block means that there is structural damage to the conducting system, which is usually permanent and may proceed suddenly to complete heart block, especially in the setting of acute myocardial infarction. Emergency treatment is required if the ventricular rate is slow enough to produce symptoms of hemodynamic compromise. In most

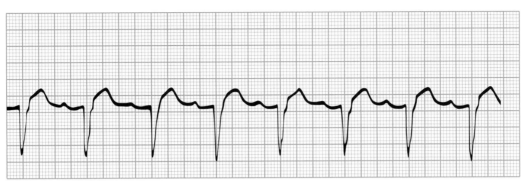

Figure 43.18   Bundle branch block demonstrating a wide QRS complex with a normal sinus rhythm. (From Cohen M, Michel TH 1988 Cardiopulmonary Symptoms in Physical Therapy Practice. Churchill Livingstone, New York, p. 157.)

cases, especially those that occur in conjunction with acute myocardial infarction, insertion of permanent cardiac pacemakers is usually indicated (Weiderhold 1988, Hillegass 2001, Mammen et al 2004).

Third-degree (complete) AV block

In third-degree AV block, none of the impulses initiated above the ventricles is through the normal AV conduction system. The ventricles are paced by ectopic impulses generated somewhere in the ventricles and at a slower rate than the atrial rate, which continues to originate from the SA node (Fig. 43.17) (Hillegass 2001). If the block occurs at the level of the AV node, a junctional pacemaker (rate 40–60 b.p.m.) takes over. The resultant QRS complexes are narrow, as the rhythm originates before the bifurcation of the bundle of His. When the block occurs below the AV node, a ventricular rhythm at a rate of less than 40 b.p.m. drives the ventricles. This is usually inadequate to maintain cardiac output. The QRS complexes are wider than normal. Blocks of the SA and AV nodes develop frequently in patients with acute myocardial infarction. Although most are transient, they may persist for several days. Blocks that originate below the bifurcation of the bundle of His indicate structural damage to the distal conducting system and are seen with extensive acute anterior myocardial infarction. External pacing or drugs may be used in the short term to accelerate the ventricular escape rhythm until insertion of a pacemaker can be completed (Weiderhold 1988, Hillegass 2001, Mammen et al 2004).

Bundle-branch blocks (fascicular blocks)

Bundle-branch or fascicular blocks can include one, two or all three fascicles. As illustrated in Fig. 43.1, the bundle of His bifurcates into the right bundle branch and left bundle branch, which almost immediately divides into the left anterior and posterior branches. The block occurs when one of the three major conduction pathways below the AV node and bundle of His has an obstruction to the passage of the depolarization impulse. It can be recognized by a widening of the QRS complex and an interval length of more than 0.11 seconds (Fig. 43.18). Conduction blocks in the fascicles can be caused by a wide variety of conditions such as ischemia, cardiomyopathies, valvular heart problems (especially aortic), myocarditis, cardiac surgery and degenerative processes that affect the conduction tissue (Weiderhold 1988, Hillegass 2001, Mammen et al 2004, Larry & Schaal 2006).

REHABILITATION CONSIDERATIONS FOR INDIVIDUALS WITH CARDIAC ARRHYTHMIAS AND CONDUCTION DISTURBANCES

The underlying reason for an irregular heart rate cannot be determined by palpation of a pulse. As discussed in the previous sections, some irregularities in rate can be relatively benign, whereas others can lead to potentially lethal arrhythmias. It is imperative that the etiology of the underlying arrhythmia be identified and understood to enable the development of an appropriate treatment plan, either through a prudent chart review or by contacting the physician. It is irresponsible to treat all individuals with cardiovascular disease with the same cardiac precautions. Exercise progression should be response and symptom guided (Weiderhold 1988, Hillegass 2001, Mammen et al 2004, Larry & Schaal 2006).

Atrial arrhythmias without conduction disturbances are generally less serious than ventricular arrhythmias. Any individual with an arrhythmia that leads to hemodynamic compromise and decreased cardiac output should be monitored closely for signs of exercise intolerance. Irwin and Blessey (1996) have ranked atrial arrhythmias from least to most serious as follows: (i) premature atrial contraction and premature junctional beats; (ii) atrial fibrillation; (iii) supraventricular tachycardia; and (iv) atrial flutter, which is considered a block. They rank ventricular arrhythmias from least to most serious as follows: (i) unifocal PVCs; (ii) multifocal PVCs; (iii) coupled PVCs (R-on T PVCs); (iv) ventricular tachycardia; and (v) ventricular fibrillation.

CONCLUSION

The most common cardiac arrhythmias and conduction disturbances have been described. Some of these abnormalities are more serious than others. Differentiating between the less serious and the potentially life-threatening arrhythmias cannot be completely assured by taking a pulse and auscultating heart sounds. A thorough cardiac evaluation is therefore essential. Before beginning an exercise program for a patient with known cardiac pathology, it is important that the therapist understands the implications of the patient/client's cardiac arrhythmias so that they are treated neither too aggressively nor undertreated.

References

Hillegass E 2001 Electrocardiography. In: Hillegass E, Sadowsky HS (eds) Essentials of Cardiopulmonary Physical Therapy, 2nd edn. WB Saunders, Philadelphia, PA, p 380–420

Irwin S, Blessey RL 1996 Patient evaluation. In: Irwin S, Tecklin JS (eds) Cardiopulmonary Physical Therapy, 3rd edn. Mosby-Yearbook, St Louis, MO, p 106–141

Kantelip JP, Sage ES, Duchene-Marullaz P 1986 Findings on ambulatory electrocardiography monitoring in subjects older than 80 years. Am J Cardiol 57:398–401

Larry JA, Schaal SF 2006 Dysrhythmias and selected conduction defects. In: ACSM's Resource Manual for Guidelines for Exercise Testing and Prescription, 5th edn. Lippincott Williams & Wilkins, Philadelphia, PA, p 289–302

Mammen BA, Irwin S, Tecklin JS 2004 Common cardiac and pulmonary clinical measures. In: Irwin S, Tecklin JS (eds) Cardiopulmonary Physical Therapy: A Guide to Practice, 4th edn. Mosby-Yearbook, St Louis, MO, p 177–244

Weiderhold R 1988 Electrocardiography: The Monitoring Lead. WB Saunders, Philadelphia, PA

Chapter 44

Heart failure and valvular heart disease

Chris L. Wells

INTRODUCTION

Despite the increase in diagnostic procedures and medical management, heart disease continues to be one of the most common causes of morbidity and mortality in the US. With the rise in life expectancy, increases in hypertension, obesity, diabetes mellitus and sedentary lifestyles are contributing to the incidence of coronary artery disease. This chapter will briefly discuss heart failure and valvular disease.

HEART FAILURE

Heart failure is defined as the inability of the heart to pump blood at a sufficient rate to meet the metabolic demands of the body. Heart failure can be the result of many different diseases; therefore, it is important to complete a thorough evaluation of the patient with heart failure to identify the underlying pathology and any factors that exacerbate the heart failure. The heart may compensate for years before the patient reaches a level of dysfunction that leads to the clinical presentation of heart failure. In many cases, it is an acute event that places additional stress, beyond the heart's ability to circulate a sufficient blood flow, leading to clinical heart failure. Exacerbation of other chronic diseases, such as renal insufficiency, pulmonary embolism or infection, cardiac arrhythmias and uncontrolled hypertension, and poor dietary consumption, can precipitate the insidious onset of clinical signs and symptoms associated with heart failure.

Coronary artery disease leading to myocardial impairment is one of the most common causes of heart failure (LaBresh et al 2004, Tenenbaum & Fisman 2004); however, there are many other diseases, such as valvular lesions, viral infections, myocardial dysfunction and pulmonary disease, that can also lead to the development of heart failure. Along with the diagnosis, it is important to identify factors that exacerbate heart failure or lead to an uncompensated state, such as excessive fluid consumption, arrhythmias, systematic infection and kidney failure. Understanding the pathology and contributing factors can aid in the delivery of prompt and appropriate medical intervention.

Congestive heart failure (CHF) is a clinical syndrome that occurs when cardiac pump function is inadequate to meet the circulatory demands of the body. One of the consequences of pump dysfunction is fluid retention; fluid leaves the vascular system and is stored in various parts of the body, hence the term 'congestive heart failure'. When the left ventricular pump function is impaired, it is unable to sufficiently pump blood forward, leading to a rise in vascular pressure. This leads to excess fluid being stored in the pulmonary interstitium to decrease the workload of the left ventricle. Left ventricular dysfunction is commonly associated with an increase in stress to the right ventricle. Right ventricular myocardial dysfunction leads to an increased blood volume in the venous system and liver. The engorgement of the venous system can lead to fluid retention in the lower extremities and abdomen (referred to as ascites).

Heart failure can be categorized in many ways. Myocardial pump dysfunction can be described as an acute or a chronic state. Heart failure can be classified as predominately left heart failure or right heart failure, or as biventricular failure. It can also be classified as systolic failure, where the myocardial contraction is ineffective in circulating blood forward into the pulmonary and systemic circulations, or diastolic dysfunction, where the ventricles do not relax to allow for sufficient filling.

Causes of ventricular failure

To understand the mechanism of heart failure, it is important to understand the basic cardiac cycle. Blood flows from the venous system and the pulmonary capillary beds into the right and left atria respectively. Once there is a sufficient volume and, therefore, enough pressure in the atria, the atrioventricular, tricuspid and mitral valves will open to allow filling of the ventricles. When the atria contract, another 15–20% of the blood volume is delivered into the ventricles and the atrioventricular valves close. The right and left ventricles then begin to contract, generating enough force to open the semilunar, pulmonic and aortic valves and eject blood into the pulmonary circulation for gas exchange and into the systemic circulation to meet the metabolic demands of the body's cells.

The most common cause of right ventricular failure (RVF) is left ventricular pump dysfunction. Failure to pump blood forward into the aorta leads to a backflow of blood and an increase in pressure within the left atrium and pulmonary system. The right ventricle is not anatomically designed to pump under elevated pressure, which leads to failure. Right heart failure may result from pulmonary hypertension caused by pulmonary diseases such as emphysema and from pulmonary embolism, mitral or tricuspid valve disease, restrictive or hypertrophic cardiomyopathies and viral or idiopathic myocarditis.

Left ventricular failure (LVF) results in lower systemic cardiac output. It can be caused by the long-term adverse effects of hypertension, aortic or mitral valve disease and coronary artery disease. Coronary artery disease can cause pump dysfunction because of the long-term subtle effects of myocardial ischemia or because of an acute ischemic event, such as an abrupt rupture of an atherosclerotic plaque, which leads to a myocardial infarction. Less frequently, LVF may also occur because of a systemic condition such as septic shock. During this critical medical state, the left ventricle attempts to increase cardiac output to meet the high oxygen demand of the body. The stress from this physiological imbalance may lead to the left ventricle being unable to meet the body's needs, resulting in LVF.

Contributing factors

There are several factors that can lead to the heart no longer being able to circulate a sufficient blood flow to meet the metabolic demands of the body. These factors can either increase the body's needs or further decrease cardiac output. Cardiac arrhythmias such as atrial fibrillation can decrease cardiac output in the presence of myocardial pump dysfunction. In atrial fibrillation, which is one of the most common arrhythmias associated with heart failure, the atria do not contract as a unit and therefore the ventricles do not deliver the last 15–20% of blood volume, causing the loss of the 'atrial kick'. In the presence of pump dysfunction, the loss of filling means that there is not a sufficient stretch of the ventricular myocardium, which leads to further output loss. The compensatory mechanism for the loss of the atrial kick is an increase in heart rate, which further impairs filling, increases oxygen demand and decreases output. Tachycardiac rhythms can increase the oxygen demands of the myocardium and decrease output by shortening the filling time. Bradycardiac rhythms allow for sufficient filling but may not be sufficient to maintain output. Finally, arrhythmias generated from the ventricles can directly lead to insufficient filling and contraction.

Acute myocardial ischemia or infarction is another factor that can further impair the contractile properties of the heart and directly impair output. The improper utilization of medications can also precipitate heart failure. The discontinuation of medications such as diuretics and beta blockers, which are commonly used to manage blood pressure and volume status, can lead to the development of CHF. Improper prescription/administration and monitoring of the therapeutic levels of medications like antiarrhythmics and calcium-channel blockers can also contribute to heart failure.

Poor dietary choices including increased sodium intake or the consumption of large amounts of fluids have also been linked to the onset of CHF. In addition, stress brought on by emotional disturbances, extreme temperatures (see Chapter 10 for a description of thermoregulation) or overexerting oneself beyond the ability of the heart to meet demands can lead to an increase in pump dysfunction. The body's response to this pump dysfunction is to increase the output of the sympathetic nervous system, which is already in an elevated state. This elevated state is associated with the increase in heart rate, which leads to further oxygen demand. In the presence of pump dysfunction, the impaired myocardium is unable to further increase stroke volume. This results in the heart being unable to meet the body's demand and leads to cardiac decompensation and heart failure. Please refer to Chapter 41 for guidelines on starting and stopping exercise training in patients with heart disease.

In cases of anemia, the heart tries to compensate by increasing cardiac output to meet oxygen demands. When there is myocardial pump dysfunction, the heart may not be able to sustain this increased stress. Anemia and the increased workload may lead to further ischemia and precipitate heart failure. Anemia is a common comorbidity in the elderly and is a probable factor to manage during the postoperative period. The therapist must consider the increase in oxygen demand during functional mobility training in an individual with both anemia and heart disease. It is therefore important to monitor vital signs closely.

Individuals with heart failure, atrial fibrillation and sedentary lifestyles are at an increased risk of developing a deep vein thrombus, particularly of the lower extremities. The development of a deep vein thrombus can increase the risk of the individual suffering an embolic stroke or a pulmonary embolism. If the pulmonary embolism is clinically significant, it can result in increased pulmonary arterial pressure or pulmonary hypertension. This rise in pulmonary arterial pressure will further compromise heart function by straining the right ventricle. Individuals with heart failure are also more susceptible to pulmonary infections because of a decrease in activity level. Pulmonary vascular congestion can place additional demands on a failing cardiopulmonary system.

Clinical manifestations

The most common symptoms associated with heart failure are dyspnea, fatigue and exercise intolerance. Dyspnea and tachypnea can be related to many factors including pulmonary vascular congestion and the increased work of breathing, a decrease in cardiac output to meet peripheral tissue demand, disuse atrophy, alterations in skeletal muscles and renal dysfunction. The patient will report a progressive shortness of breath with exertion, to dyspnea at rest, as pump dysfunction progresses. Box 44.1 describes the signs and symptoms associated with right and left heart failure; however, it is important to note that it is uncommon to see isolated unilateral heart failure.

Fatigue and exercise intolerance associated with heart failure are still currently under investigation to better understand this complex clinical disorder. Exercise intolerance is defined as 'the reduced ability to perform activities that involve dynamic movement of large muscles because of symptoms of dyspnea or fatigue' (Pina et al 2003). The failing heart has a limited ability to increase cardiac output on demand. A rise in stroke volume and heart rate is blunted, leading to a depressed cardiac output and response that is insufficient to meet the rise in metabolic demand. Heart rate response is also reduced with age, which also contributes to the limited cardiac response in the elderly.

In heart failure, there are several factors that limit exercise tolerance which are linked to peripheral abnormalities. There is a reduction in blood flow to skeletal muscles because of the increase in vasoconstriction, elevation of the renin–angiotensin system and the impaired endothelial mechanism regulating peripheral blood flow. There is also a decrease in blood distribution to active muscles when compared with healthy individuals. The skeletal fiber makeup in patients with heart failure is also altered; there is a reduction in type I fibers and an increase in type II fibers, which reduces the aerobic capacity of the individual. Finally, in response to the skeletal metabolic acidosis that occurs in the early phase of exercise, there is a further increase in vasoconstriction that amplifies exercise intolerance (Pina et al 2003).

The therapist needs to keep in mind that there is a poor link between the resting ejection fraction, which is the percentage of blood flow ejected upon contraction, and exercise tolerance. Exercise tolerance, and therefore rehabilitation potential, appears to be more related to the heart's ability to respond to the increase in metabolic demand by increasing stroke volume and heart rate (Fransciosa et al 1981, Pina et al 2003).

Box 44.1   Common signs and symptoms of right and left heart failure

Right heart failure

- Peripheral edema
- Pitting edema
- Ascites
- Jugular vein distension
- Hepatojugular reflux
- S3 heart sound
- Abdominal discomfort/anorexia

Left heart failure

- Orthopnea
- Paroxysmal nocturnal dyspnea
- Exercise intolerance with fatigue and weakness
- Pulmonary rales
- Dyspnea on exertion
- Dry cough in supine
- Unexplained mental status changes

Therapeutic intervention

The number of cases of CHF continues to rise as life expectancy increases and there are medical and surgical advances in managing heart disease. The first line of intervention is in the prevention of heart disease by reducing the associated risk factors, such as smoking, hypertension and diabetes. The American Heart Association recommends that everyone participate in at least 30 min daily of moderately intense activity, eat sensibly and maintain a proper body weight. Medical management includes the proper treatment of hypertension, dyslipidemia, hypercholesterolemia and diabetes. Diuretics can be used to lower blood volume along with beta blockers and angiotensin-converting enzyme (ACE) inhibitors to treat hypertension. When pump dysfunction becomes significant, inotropic medications like dubutamine can be used to improve contractility; antiarrhythmics are also helpful in the management of heart failure. The use of pacemakers and implantable cardiac defibrillators are options that have shown success in the management of serious arrhythmias. Surgical management is appropriate to correct valvular dysfunction, and coronary artery bypass grafting can be carried out to restore myocardial perfusion. In the US, clinical trials are being conducted to examine the use of implantable mechanical assistive devices, such as the Heartmate and Novacor, as destination therapy in older patients with LVF.

Exercise has become a key component in the medical management of heart failure. Many studies have documented the improvements in aerobic capacity and muscle performance with exercise in subjects with heart failure (Shephard & Franklin 2001, Pina et al 2003, Levinger et al 2005, Senden et al 2005). There are improvements in the peripheral abnormalities for patients who participate in a routine exercise program. Improvements in the strength and endurance of respiratory muscles has also been documented and is associated with a decreased level of dyspnea with exertion. Finally, there is an improvement in the quality of life (Shephard & Franklin 2001, Stevenson et al 2004, van den Berg-Emons et al 2004).

VALVULAR DISEASE

The heart has four valves, which function to keep blood flowing in a unidirectional manner with myocardial contraction. The opening and closing of the valves operates on the principles of volume/pressure. As blood returns to the heart via the venous system, the atria fill while all of the valves are closed. Once there is a sufficient volume within the atria, the increased pressure opens the atrioventricular (tricuspid and mitral) valves. The tricuspid valve separates the right atrium and right

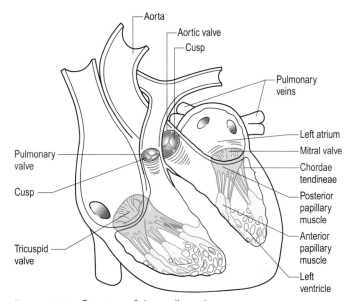

Figure 44.1   Structure of the cardiac valves.
(From Myers R 1995 Saunders Manual of Physical Therapy Practice. WB Saunders, Philadelphia, PA, p 196, with permission from Elsevier.)

ventricle, and the mitral valve is located between the left atrium and left ventricle. The atria contract, fill the ventricles and the valves then close. The ventricles contract to generate a pressure that is sufficient enough to overcome the pressure within the pulmonary trunk and aorta. At that time, the semilunar valves (pulmonic and aortic) open to eject blood from the right and left ventricles respectively.

The atrioventricular valves have several components that can be damaged, resulting in various clinical signs and symptoms. The annulus is composed of fibrous rings that provide a secure attachment for the leaflets, or cusps. The space at the edge of the annulus where the leaflets insert is referred to as the commisure. The leaflets are made of a strong fibrous material and function as doors that allow unidirectional blood flow in the presence of a pressure gradient. The margins of the leaflets are thin and are stabilized by the chordae tendineae cordis, strong fibrous cords that originate from the papillary muscle and insert into the leaflet margins. When myocardial contraction occurs, the papillary muscle contracts as well, making the chordae tendineae cordis taut. It is this relationship that prevents the leaflets from inverting and causing a backwards flow of blood through the heart (see Fig. 44.1).

The semilunar valves are similar in function but are structurally different from the atrioventricular valves. There are three cusps per valve; they have a concave–convex shape, with the convexity facing the ventricles. After the ventricles begin to relax, there is a tendency for the blood to flow backwards toward the ventricles. The concavities of the cusps fill with blood and the pressure from this blood secures the approximation of the cusps. The pulmonic valve is a more delicate structure than the aortic valve, which must be rugged to function under the high pressure that exists.

Valvular dysfunction is commonly categorized by the alteration in blood flow across the valve, valvular stenosis or regurgitation. A stenotic valve describes the narrowing of the opening of the valve. This condition interferes with the flow of blood through the valve and places an increased oxygen demand on the myocardium. Over time, a stenotic valve will cause hypertrophy and dilatation of the chambers. Regurgitation, which is also referred to as a valvular insufficiency, is defined as backflow of blood across the valve, leading to an enlargement of the cardiac chamber before the dysfunctional valve. In either situation, the end result is an increase in oxygen demand, myocardial ischemia and eventually heart failure. The two dysfunctions are not mutually exclusive of one another; a valve can be categorized as stenotic and insufficient.

Causes of valvular disease

Valvular dysfunction has many causes depending upon the valve in question and the age of the individual. Today, one of the primary causes of valvular dysfunction is hereditary factors related to congenital valve deformity, compounded by the increasing lifespan (Anonymous 2005a). Rheumatic heart disease (RHD) is another common cause of valvular disease, despite the decreased incidence of rheumatic fever in the US. Mitral stenosis and aortic regurgitation are commonly associated with RHD (Anonymous 2005a). RHD is a complication of group A streptococcal infection and rheumatic fever, which causes acute carditis. This infection typically occurs in childhood to adolescence, but the valvular dysfunction may not be apparent until later in life. An individual who experiences recurrent streptococcal infections (e.g. strep throat) should seek medical attention for proper treatment to minimize the risk of developing rheumatic fever and consequentially RHD (Anonymous 2005a). There is also an increased incidence of valvular disease with aging, particularly aortic stenosis and mitral regurgitation (Anonymous 2005a, 2005b). Other causes of valvular dysfunction include infectious endocarditis, trauma, dilated cardiomyopathy, myocardial infarction, pulmonary hypertension and heart failure.

Many individuals with valvular dysfunction will be asymptomatic until myocardial function is significantly impaired such that cardiac output is no longer maintained at an appropriate level because of the development of arrhythmias. It is important to understand normal cardiopulmonary physiology in order to understand the adverse effects of valvular disease. This understanding leads to a comprehension of the typical clinical presentation and guides the effective and efficient assessment of the patient. The therapist should be particularly familiar with aortic and mitral stenosis and regurgitation.

Aortic stenosis is a clinically significant valvular dysfunction because of the impact on left ventricular function. The narrowing of the aortic valve leads to increased pressure across the valve and an increase in the oxygen demand of the left ventricle. This leads to increased coronary vascular resistance and, consequently, to a decrease in myocardial perfusion. This may lead to myocardial infarction and ventricular arrhythmias. During exercise, the left ventricle may not be able to increase stroke volume in the presence of decreased systemic vascular resistance. This can result in a drop in

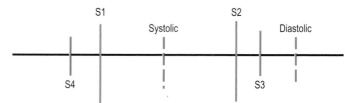

Figure 44.2 This graph represents the normal and common abnormal heart sounds that can be heard across one cardiac cycle. S1 represents the closure of the atrioventricular valves; S2 represents the closure of the semilunar valves; S3 is referred to as a ventricular gallop; and S4 is referred to as an atrial gallop. Systolic murmur can be associated with stenosis of one of the semilunar valves or insufficiency of one of the atrioventricular valves. Diastolic murmur can be associated with stenosis of one of the atrioventricular valves or insufficiency of one of the semilunar valves.

systolic pressure, ventricular arrhythmias and syncope. Over time, the heart attempts to compensate for the aortic stenosis with left ventricular hypertrophy. The left atria dilate, which leads to the onset of atrial fibrillation and eventually to CHF. Aortic stenosis is typically underestimated and patients usually present for medical care because of heart failure, angina, a presyncopal or syncopal episode, or progressive shortness of breath.

Although RHD is the underlying etiology of aortic regurgitation, the valve may become insufficient from infectious endocarditis, aortic root aneurysm or dissection. Regurgitation, the backflow of blood into the left ventricle, results in hypertrophy with dilatation, an increase in myocardial oxygen demand, possible ischemia and heart failure.

Mitral stenosis is primarily the result of RHD. In the elderly, RHD only causes mild to moderate dysfunction and the progression of the dysfunction is related to fibrotic or calcification of the valve related to aging (Anonymous 2005a, 2005b). The narrowing of the mitral valve causes an enlargement of the left atrium and increasing pulmonary vascular pressure. The development of pulmonary hypertension strains the right ventricle and eventually leads to right heart failure. Just as in aortic stenosis, the dilation of the atria and development of atrial fibrillation increases the risk of thromboembolic events and either pulmonary embolism or cerebral vascular accident (i.e. brain attack).

Mitral regurgitation is most commonly associated with myocardial infarction with papillary muscle impairment or rupture. As with mitral stenosis, regurgitation leads to left atrial enlargement, pulmonary hypertension and right heart failure, as well as eccentric left ventricle hypertrophy as the heart attempts to maintain cardiac output.

Clinical manifestations

The signs and symptoms of valvular dysfunction vary according to which valve is malfunctioning and the severity of the malfunction. The ultimate key is the degree to which the malfunction affects cardiac output. Valvular disease can be clinically detected by the alteration in normal heart sounds and the presence of abnormal heart sounds (Fig. 44.2). Exercise intolerance increases as the heart's compensatory mechanisms fail to maintain an efficient cardiac output to meet the metabolic demand of the body. The increase in volume and pressure within the left atrium either from stenosis or regurgitation causes an increase in pulmonary vascular resistance and eventually leads to the signs and symptoms of right heart failure. Patients may present with progressive dyspnea, orthopnea and paroxysmal nocturnal dyspnea and rales upon auscultation. In the case of acute valvular dysfunction, the patient may rapidly develop pulmonary edema and respiratory failure, requiring mechanical ventilation of the patient. Aortic stenosis is commonly associated with angina, a pre-syncopal episode or syncope, arrhythmias and signs of CHF, as described previously.

Stenosis and regurgitation of tricuspid or pulmonic valves are less common but both may contribute to right atrial enlargement, atrial fib-rillation and the development of right heart failure with pitting periph-eral edema and jugular vein distension. Tricuspid and pulmonic valvular impairment also affects the filling of the left ventricle.

Therapeutic interventions

Often, medical intervention is initiated when the patient presents with the adverse consequences from the valvular dysfunction. Medical treatment will focus on the management of angina, CHF, cause of dyspnea, arrhythmias and syncopal episodes. Patients will com-monly be prescribed beta blockers, calcium-channel blockers and/or diuretics to manage hypertension. Antiarrhythmic medications, such as digoxin or amiodarone, may be used to control atrial and ventricu-lar arrhythmias. An implantable pacemaker and/or automatic implantable cardiac defibrillator may be necessary to control arrhyth-mias that are life-threatening or impair ventricular function.

There are several invasive procedures that can be considered to correct the valvular dysfunction. Percutaneous balloon valvulo-plasty is a nonsurgical approach for stenosis. A catheter is positioned across the lumen of the valve and inflated to decrease the stenosis. For mitral stenosis, another nonsurgical option is a percutaneous mitral commissurotomy, in which the leaflet of the valve is cut via a catheter. In both of these options, there is a risk of restenosis and complica-tions of valvular regurgitation.

When medical management has reached its maximal benefit or when ventricular function is impaired or myocardial ischemia needs to be resolved, surgical intervention is the therapy of choice (Yacoub & Cohn 2004). Depending on the valve involved, the patient's anatomy and the surgeon's training, a mediastinal or anterior thoracotomy may be the surgical approach.

There are many factors that must be considered when the surgeon and patient are determining if the valve should be repaired or replaced. Some of these factors may include the age of the patient, the risk associated with the use of anticoagulation, the risk of infections and the extent of the anatomical disorder of the valve. If the valve needs to be replaced, it must be decided whether the replacement should be a mechanical or biological valve. Age, past medical history and lifestyle all contribute to the decision regarding the type of valve replacement that is used (Vahanian & Palacios 2004, Yacoub & Cohn 2004).

Surgery to repair an impaired valve is becoming more refined and applied more frequently. A repair may involve one or more proce-dures to restore the function of the native valve. An annuloplasty involves the implantation of an artificial ring to help support the fail-ing annular ring, which is needed to support the leaflets and permit proper closure of the valve. For a faulty and fused leaflet, a commis-surotomy or partial resection can be completed to increase valve lumen diameter. The surgeon can shorten, reposition or implant an artificial chordae tendineae to correct regurgitation.

Exercise is contraindicated in a patient with severe aortic or mitral valve disease (particularly aortic stenosis) who is symptomatic at rest. It is important that the therapist works closely with a cardiolo-gist to develop hemodynamic parameters as guidelines to monitor the patient during the rehabilitation process. For these patients, the role of rehabilitation is to focus on interval functional exercises, energy conservation and job simplification to minimize functional limitation, disability and aid the patient achieve end-of-life goals.

CONCLUSION

In 2004, it was reported that there were over 800 000 new cases of acute coronary syndrome, over 700 000 new cases of stroke and over 500 000 new cases of CHF (Sousa et al 2005). These data clearly illus-trate the clinical relevance of proper examination, prevention and effective intervention in reducing the number of cardiac incidences as well as minimizing functional limitations and disability. It is impor-tant to identify the precipitating causes of heart failure; early detec-tion of valvular dysfunction and prompt medical intervention can preserve heart function. It is important that the therapist is an active member of the patient's healthcare team to ensure that screening for hypertension, education to reduce other cardiac risk factors and appro-priate medical referrals are sought. The therapist is therefore a vital member of the healthcare team, providing services across the spec-trum of preventive and rehabilitative medicine to optimize the patient's quality of life in the community.

References

Anonymous 2005a Heart valve diseases. US National Library of Medicine. Available: http://www.nlm.nih.gov/medlineplus/heartvalvediseases.html. Accessed December 12 2005

Anonymous 2005b Valvular disease. Merck. Available: http://www.merck.com/mrkshared/mmg/sec11/ch89/ch89a.jsp. Accessed December 12 2005

van den Berg-Emons R, Balk A, Bussmann H, Stam H 2004 Does aerobic training lead to a more active lifestyle and improved quality of life in patients with congestive heart failure. Eur J Heart Fail 6(6):95–100

Fransciosa J, Park M, Levine T 1981 Lack of correlation between exercise capacity and indexes of resting left ventricular performance in heart failure. Am J Cardiol 47:33–39

LaBresh K, Ellrodt A, Gliklich R et al 2004 Get with the guidelines for cardiovascular secondary prevention: pilot results. Arch Intern Med 164:203–209

Levinger I, Bronks R, Cody D et al 2005 Resistance training for chronic heart failure patients on beta blocker medications. Int J Cardiol 102(3):493–499

Pina I, Apstein C, Balady G 2003 Exercise and heart failure. A statement from the American Heart Association Committee on exercise, rehabilitation and prevention. Circulation 107:1210–1225

Senden P, Sabelis L, Zonderland M et al 2005 The effect of physical training on workload, upper leg muscle function and muscle areas in patients with chronic heart failure. Int J Cardiol 100(2):293–300

Shephard RJ, Franklin B 2001 Changes in the quality of life: a major goal of cardiac rehabilitation. J Cardiopulm Rehabil 21(4):189–200

Sousa J, Costa M, Tuzcum M et al 2005 New frontiers in interventional cardiology. Circulation 111:671–681

Stevenson W, Chaitman B, Ellenbegen K et al 2004 Clinical assessment and management of patients with implantable cardioverter devices presenting to nonelectrophysiologist. Circulation 110:3866–3869

Tenenbaum A, Fisman E 2004 Impaired glucose metabolism in patients with heart failure. Pathophysiology and possible treatment strategies. Am J Cardiovasc Drugs 4(5):269–280

Vahanian A, Palacios I 2004 Percutaneous approaches to valvular disease. Circulation 109:1572–1579

Valvular Heart Disease 2005 Valvular heart disease. Available: www.gilmanheartvalve.org. Accessed December 12 2005

Yacoub M, Cohn L 2004 Novel approaches to cardiac valve repair from structure to function: part II. Circulation 109:1064–1072

Chapter 45

Cardiac pacemakers and defibrillators

Chris L. Wells

INTRODUCTION

The heart has specialized cells called conduction cells that generate an electrical impulse and cause myocardial contraction. As well as the conduction system, the myocardium also possesses electrical properties that facilitate cardiac function. The myocardium has automaticity and excitability; this allows an electrical impulse to be self-generated, altering the resting potential of the myocardial cells. The heart readily conducts the impulse if the threshold is reached, which leads to myocardial contraction. Finally, in the all-or-none principle, which is specific to cardiac muscle, if an electrical impulse is sufficient, complete depolarization and full contraction of the myocardium occurs.

In the presence of a cardiac disease or disorder, and through the natural process of aging, there is an increased incidence of dysfunction of the conduction system. This dysfunction may be benign and not disrupt general heart function or it can have life-threatening consequences. The source of the conduction dysfunction, its rate and occurrence or frequency determines the clinical significance. The bottom line for the clinician is how the arrhythmias affect myocardial perfusion and what happens to cardiac output. In the presence of ischemic heart disease, a fast conducting rhythm, such as supraventricular tachycardia (SVT), rapid ventricular rate or atrial fibrillation, will decrease the diastolic filling time, which leads to a decline in myocardium perfusion and further ischemia, resulting in a vicious cycle. The same tachycardiac arrhythmias can lead to a decrease in cardiac output because of the decrease in filling time. In the presence of myocardial or pump dysfunction, the ventricles rely on volume to improve the contractile force, which is known as the Frank–Starling law. However, with the decrease in the filling time there is a decrease in the volume entering the ventricles and a loss of myocardial stretch, which results in a decrease in contractility. Bradycardiac rhythms allow sufficient time for ventricular filling but the rate may be too slow to maintain the cardiac output needed to meet the metabolic demands of the body. The loss of cardiac output is associated with the following common clinical signs and symptoms: lightheadedness, dizziness, visual disturbances, altered mentation, syncope and increased risk of falls.

Cardiac arrhythmias may be temporary or permanent, depending on the etiology. Transient arrhythmias may be caused by significant alterations in electrolytes. This may result from gastrointestinal distress because of nausea, vomiting and diarrhea, or from the use of medications, such as diuretics and potassium supplements. Transient arrhythmias may also be caused by myocardial hypersensitivity resulting from heart catheterization, open heart procedures, myocardial infarct or trauma. More permanent arrhythmias may be caused by ischemic disease that directly impairs the cells of the conduction system. This may lead to various conduction arrhythmias, such as heart blocks, atrial or ventricular bradycardia or tachycardia. Heart failure is commonly associated with atrial fibrillation and ventricular ectopy. Aging may also lead to a significant loss of conduction cells, which results in sick sinus syndrome.

PACEMAKERS

Approximately 300 000 people in the US undergo pacemaker implantation annually for the management of arrhythmias (Gregoratos 2005). The prevalence per year of pacemaker implantation varies across Europe, with 200 cases per million people in Eastern Europe and over 400 cases per million in western Europe (Vardas and Ovsyscher 2002). Permanent pacemakers have been shown to improve the quality of life, oxygen consumption, exercise tolerance and survival of patients with life-threatening arrhythmias and decrease their need for hospitalization (Abraham et al 2002). The pacemaker is able to sense or detect the intrinsic electrical activity of the heart and deliver an electrical impulse in the absence of intrinsic activity. The pacemaker causes the action potential that leads to depolarization and contraction of the myocardium, which allows the ejection of blood from the heart into the systemic and pulmonary circulations.

There are specific indications for utilization of a pacemaker including sinus node dysfunction and ineffective communication between atrial and ventricular conduction pathways. Sinus node dysfunctions are commonly associated with bradycardia, periods of lack of conduction and brady–tachy syndrome in which the heart rate varies from very slow to very fast (Woodruff & Prudente 2005). Pacemakers may also be used to control atrial arrhythmias such as atrial fibrillation, and atrioventricular blocks, which are impairments in the transmission of the atrial electrical impulse to the ventricles. The presence of a block of the ventricular bundle branches may also be an indication for a pacemaker (Woodruff & Prudente 2005).

Temporary and permanent pacemakers

Pacemakers can be classified as temporary or permanent. In the case of an acute dysfunction of the conduction system, a temporary pacer may be used to stabilize the patient's rhythm and hemodynamics. It is common practice for the surgeon to place pacer wires on the epicardial surface of the heart (atrial, ventricle or both) during an open-heart procedure because a patient can often have transient arrhythmias after heart surgery; these can result from the myocardium becoming irritable from the trauma of surgery, imbalances of electrolytes, disruption of the acid–base balance and alterations of blood gases. The wires are passed transthoracically and secured to the anterior chest wall. In an urgent situation, the heart can be temporarily paced via transcutaneous electrode pads. Finally, a temporary pacemaker can be initiated using a transvenous approach, typically through the jugular or subclavian vein.

If it is determined that the disturbance of the patient's conduction system is irreversible and interferes with heart function, a permanent pacemaker will be implanted with the patient's consent. The pacemaker will be individually programmed to meet the conduction needs so that efficient cardiac function can be maintained.

Details of pacemaker function

The pacemaker comprises two components. The first component is the pulse generator that contains the electronic program and the energy system that generates the electrical stimuli. It is implanted underneath the skin in the right or left pectodeltoid area or subpectoral in patients that are very thin, to prevent erosion of the skin. The second component of the pacemaker is the lead or wire that senses the activity of the native conduction system and delivers the impulse to the myocardium. The leads for permanent pacemakers are typically attached to the endocardium of the right atrium and right and/or left ventricle via the transvenous approach. Leads can be placed using an epicardial approach at the time of an open-heart procedure.

The program within the pacemaker generator can sense the intrinsic activity of the conduction system and delay the release of an electrical impulse. In the absence of intrinsic activity, the generator can deliver an electrical impulse that causes the depolarization of the myocardium. There are three general modes for pacing the heart. In a fixed-rate or asynchronous mode, the pacemaker paces the heart at a constant rate, regardless of intrinsic electrical activity or physiological need. This mode does not respond to the metabolic needs of the body and the patient reaches an exercise plateau quickly. Because of this limitation, a fixed mode is not commonly used at present. The second mode is referred to as the demand or inhibited mode. In this mode, when the pacemaker senses the intrinsic activity it inhibits the generator from releasing its electrical stimuli. In the absence of intrinsic activity, the pacemaker generates a pulse. The third mode is the triggered or synchronous mode that paces when the conduction system fails to pace; this mode also paces in unison with the conduction system when it senses intrinsic activity.

The pacemaker can be referred to by the number of chambers that it interacts with and is dependent upon the underlying pathology. Single-chamber pacemakers sense and stimulate the atria or ventricles on the basis of the intrinsic activity. In dual pacing, the delivery of an electrical impulse to the ventricles is timed with the depolarization of the atria in order to maintain the proper relationship between the atria and ventricles; this is referred to as atrioventricular synchrony (Woodruff & Prudente 2005).

Pacemaker universal reference system

There is a universal reference system that is used to describe the function of the pacemaker. This is very important and enables any clinician

Table 45.1 Generic codes for pacemakers

Position	Codes
I (pacing chamber)	O, A, V, D (A + V)
II (sensing chamber)	O, A, V, D (A + V)
III (response to sensing)	O, I, T, D (T + I)
IV (programmability)	O, R, S, M, C
V (multisite pacing)	O, A, V, D (A + D)

A, atrium; C, communicating; D, dual; I, inhibited; M, multi; O, none; R, rare; S, simple; T, triggered; V, ventricle.

who is working with the patient to have a basic understanding of the pacemaker. The details of the generic pacemaker code are shown in Table 45.1. The first letter of the code represents the chambers in which the pacemaker will pace. The second position of the code tells the clinician where the pacemaker senses conduction system activity. The third letter of the code represents how the pacer will respond to the activity that it senses. The fourth and fifth positions of this coding system are less frequently used. The forth code refers to the programming. With the rate program® feature, the pacer can sense an increase in physiological demand, such as occurs during exercise. This is achieved by either sensing changes in thoracic impedance or movement because of increased respiratory rate or sensing changes in blood gases. When the pacemaker senses the increase in metabolic needs, it paces at a faster rate. The fifth code position refers to the chamber in which the pacemaker can 'tachypace' the heart in an attempt to control atrial and/or ventricular tachycardias.

Two of the more common types of pacemaker are the VVI and the DDDR. A VVI pacer is one that will pace the ventricle (V), sense conduction activity within the ventricle (V) and, if intrinsic activity is detected, inhibit the release of an electrical stimulus (I). A DDDR pacemaker is a device that paces and senses activity within both the atria and ventricles, and that can pace or hold pacing depending on the activity of the conduction system within the atria and ventricles. It can internally increase the pacing rate when the metabolic demand is higher (Zaidan et al 2005).

More recently, pacemakers are being implanted for the management of heart failure. About 30% of patients with a diagnosis of heart failure suffer from bundle-branch blocks that result in the delay of intraventricular conduction. In this therapy, referred to as cardiac resynchronization therapy (CRT), atrial and ventricular conduction are synchronized and both ventricles are paced (Vesty et al 2004). Clinically, CRT is also referred to as biventricular pacing or 'Bi-V' pacing. The positive effects of Bi-V pacing include an improvement in intraventricular depolarization, contractility and cardiac output, which results from improvements in the wall motion of the ventricles, particularly the intraventricular septum. It also decreases mitral regurgitation and the restrictive pattern of the heart (Vesty et al 2004). Several studies have documented improvements in the quality of life, exercise tolerance and ejection fraction, a decrease of 40% in the death rate and decreased hospitalization rates (Abraham et al 2002, Young et al 2003, Cannon & Prystowsky 2004). Some investigators have reported ventricular remodeling with the use of Bi-V pacing in patients with heart failure (Vesty et al 2004).

There are several complications related to the utilization of pacemakers that the clinician should be aware of when caring for a patient. During the implant procedure, the patient may experience a pneumothorax, hemothorax or cardiac tamponade. It is possible for the leads to be displaced, which leads to pacemaker dysfunction;

malplacement of the lead may also stimulate the diaphragm or cause other cardiac arrhythmias. The patient may also develop a hematoma, infection or skin erosion at the site of the pacemaker generator (Woodruff & Prudente 2005).

Pacemaker dysfunction can be classified according to three categories. 'Inappropriate sensing' means that the pacemaker is either undersensing or oversensing. In undersensing, the pacemaker does not detect the intrinsic activity of the conduction system, which leads to improper pacing. When a pacemaker is oversensing, it does not appropriately detect the lack of conduction activity and inhibits the pacemaker from actually firing an impulse. This is clinically more critical as the patients will be more symptomatic because of the loss of conduction, contraction and cardiac output. 'Loss of capture' means that the pacemaker does not generate a strong enough impulse to cause myocardial depolarization. This may be caused by battery failure, lead dysfunction, an increase in the capture threshold because of fibrosis and necrosis at the lead site, or the use of certain medications. Finally, 'failure to fire' means that the pacemaker fails to release an impulse when it should. This can be caused by a failure of the lead, battery failure or oversensing (Woodruff & Prudente 2005).

Therapeutic intervention

There is little established data on rehabilitation in individuals with pacemakers. The following section includes the author's recommendations, which are based upon years of experience and unpublished protocols at the University of Maryland Medical System.

Specific care must be taken when the therapist is treating a patient with a temporary pacemaker. The clinician should understand the reason for the use of the pacemaker and how reliant the patient is on the pacemaker. Before mobilizing the patient, the clinician needs to ensure that the connections of the pacer leads are secure and that the wires and temporary pacemaker are handled with care. It is crucial that the clinician monitors the patient's vital signs and responses to any activity. It is helpful for the therapist to document if there is an increase or decrease in pacing reliance based upon the activity and the intensity of the activity.

When the patient no longer needs temporary pacing, either because there is medical stability of the cardiac rhythm or because there has been a placement of a permanent pacemaker, it is important that the patient is monitored after the removal of the temporary transthoracic epicardial leads. There is a risk of epicardial bleeding when the leads are removed, which is done at the bedside before the patient is discharged from hospital. The clinician should monitor the patient for signs of tamponade or pericardial inflammation. The signs and symptoms of cardiac tamponade include tachycardia, a decrease in systemic arterial blood pressure, diminished heart sounds, dyspnea, orthopnea and jugular venous distension. The adverse effects of inflammation include pain, hypotension, diminished heart sounds and tachycardia.

The protocol for rehabilitation after the placement of a permanent pacemaker varies from facility to facility. Typically, the involved upper extremity is immobilized for the first 24h to decrease pain, protect against bleeding or the development of a hematoma at the site of the generator implant, and to decrease the risk of lead displacement. It is safe for the patient to ambulate even if he or she needs to use an assistive device. If a hematoma does not develop, range-of-motion (ROM), strengthening and functional training can be resumed within the tolerance of the individual. If a hematoma does develop, the patient may experience neurological symptoms because of compression of the brachial plexus. The upper extremity may be immobilized until there are signs that the bleeding has stopped and the hematoma is stable. Some physicians will instruct the patient to avoid resistive

overhead activities for 2 weeks after implantation, but active ROM and activities of daily living are safe to resume. It is important that treatment guidelines be established between the rehabilitation service and the electrophysiology department to maximize the patient's recovery.

Before working with a patient who has a permanent pacemaker, the therapist should know which mode of pacing has been programmed into the device because the mode affects a patient's cardiovascular tolerance to exercise. Exercise tolerance is dependent on the underlying disease, the type of pacemaker and the degree to which the patient is dependent on the pacer to maintain cardiac output. Patients with fixed-rate pacemakers are unable to elevate their heart rate to accommodate higher demand, so the therapist must recognize this limitation and adjust the treatment plan accordingly. A pacemaker set on dual mode, for example the DDDR pacemaker, allows the patient's heart rate to vary according to demand. Such a patient would not be expected to have an exercise limitation because of the existing conduction abnormality. Exercise tolerance is also dependent on the patient's level of fitness. It is also important to evaluate the cardiovascular response to exercise to ensure that the patient is tolerating the exercise and that the pacer is working appropriately. Finally, the clinician should talk to the patient to make sure that the pacemaker is appropriately inspected for proper function and to assess battery life.

There are special concerns that the physical therapist must consider when working with a patient who has a pacemaker. Modalities such as transcutaneous electrical nerve stimulation (TENS), shortwave and microwave diathermy, neuromuscular stimulators and ultrasound should not be used in the region of the pacemaker (Woodruff & Prudente 2005). Superficial heat and cold should be safe to use once the surgical incision has healed, but the tissue directly over the generator should be insulated for protection. If there are any questions regarding the use of a modality or specific rehabilitation technique, the cardiologist should be consulted. The therapist should also be aware that the muscular activity of pectorals, abdominals and the diaphragm can lead to artifacts, which can result in inappropriate sensing (oversensing) and underpacing. Therefore, it is important for the therapist to continue to monitor the patient's vitals, symptoms and heart rate regularity when new exercises are introduced or the intensity is increased. If the patient complains of lightheadedness or presents with syncope, low blood pressure and decreased tolerance to activity, the patient should be referred to the cardiologist to assess the function of the pacemaker.

DEFIBRILLATORS

When a patient has a history of presyncope, syncope, cardiac arrest or heart disease, with documented significant ventricular arrhythmia, an automatic implantable cardiac defibrillator (AICD) may be the intervention of choice. Approximately 100 000 AICDs are implanted annually (Stevenson et al 2004). In Europe, it is more difficult to determine the actual rate of utilization of AICDs but it is estimated to be about 453 cases per million people in the UK and 93.3 cases per million in Italy per year (Plummer et al 2005, Proclemer et al 2005). This device delivers a strong enough electrical impulse to depolarize the entire myocardium, in the hope that the sinus node will resume control as the primary pacemaker. The use of AICDs decreased the mortality rate by 40% over 1 year and 30% over 3 years for patients with a low ejection fraction (Cannon & Prystowsky 2004).

In many incidences, a generator can be implanted that has the capacity of a pacemaker and an AICD in one unit. The generic codes for AICDs are shown in Table 45.2. In patients with brady-tachy arrhythmias, the pacemaker/AICD can be programmed to pace at a

Table 45.2 Generic codes for AICDs

Position	Codes
I (shock chamber)	O, A, V, D (A + V)
II (antitachycardia pacing chamber)	O, A, V, D (A + V)
III (tachycardia detection)	E, H
IV (antibradycardia pacing chamber)	O, A, V, D (A + V)

A, atrium; D, dual; E, electrogram; H, hemodynamic; O, none; V, ventricle.

minimal rate when the rate becomes to slow. When the rate becomes too fast, the pacemaker will attempt to overpace the heart to recapture the rhythm and then slow the rate down again. This is referred to as 'tachypacing'. If this program does not work, the AICD may deliver a low level shock (5–10 J) in an attempt to convert the rhythm to a more stable rate. If this is unsuccessful or the generator interprets the rhythm as ventricular tachycardia or fibrillation, the AICD will fire a more significant shock (30–50 J) to convert this life-threatening rhythm to a more stable rhythm (Cannon & Prystowsky 2004). The use of a pacemaker/AICD has been shown to improve survival, exercise tolerance and quality of life and decrease hospitalization for patients with heart failure (Schron & Domanski 2003).

The AICD is also comprised of a generator and leads. The generator is inserted in the left or right pectodeltoid area. The older models were larger and were inserted in the submuscular or subcutaneous left upper quadrant of the abdomen. The endocardial lead is placed in the right ventricular apex via a transvenous approach (Stevenson et al 2004). When there is also a pacemaking program, leads are placed in the right atria and possibly the left ventricle for pacing function.

Most AICDs function in the following manner. The AICD monitors the heart rate and rhythm for abnormalities. It is programmed to detect a preset rate and, if that rate is exceeded, the device is activated. There is a delay in the response of the defibrillator to provide a chance for the abnormal rhythm to convert back to a normal rhythm. If the arrhythmia continues beyond the delay, the generator charges, takes a second look at the rhythm and delivers an electrical shock if the abnormality is still present. The goal is to depolarize the myocardium and return the patient's heart to a more stable rhythm.

Therapeutic intervention

It is important that a therapist is aware when working with a patient who has an AICD. In the acute phase, the immobilization of the upper extremity and restoration of arm function follows the same guidelines as described above for pacemakers. If the AICD generator is implanted in the abdominal wall, the patient should be instructed in proper body mechanics to protect the incision. It is also helpful to teach the patient splinting so that pain caused by movement and coughing can be decreased.

The patient and therapist should know the rate at which the generator becomes activated as well as the length of time of the delay. One of the goals of therapy is to determine what are safe activities and proper resistance or workloads for exercise, so that a high enough heart rate is achieved to provide benefit from the exercise but not high enough to activate the AICD. The therapist can provide the cardiac electrophysiologist with vital information in setting the heart rate boundary.

The therapist should recognize that there are psychological effects in almost 90% of patients with AICDs. These patients suffer from depression and anxiety, and will self-limit and therefore decrease their quality of life because they are fearful of the firing of the AICD. There is an elevated fear of death and a change in body image, which may interfere with intimate relationships. There is also a loss of control and increase in self-doubt and helplessness (Schermann & Keung 2005). Providing education about exercise, self-monitoring and the function of the AICD is important. It is also important that the clinician make sure that the patient is undergoing routine check-ups to ensure that the AICD is working appropriately to prevent false firing and sense appropriately and that the battery is active.

If the patient's heart rate rises above the preset rate, the patient should sit down and be instructed to cough or perform a Valsalva maneuver. These maneuvers may cause vagal stimulation, which may result in a decrease in heart rate and prevent a shock. The therapist should monitor the patient's vital signs and notify the cardiologist if the defibrillator delivers a shock. The clinician may feel the shock if in contact with the patient at the time of defibrillation but it will not be harmful. Complications involved in the use of an AICD are similar to the complications discussed above for pacemakers.

CONCLUSION

Disturbance or dysfunction of normal heart conduction can result in decreased cardiac output, which leads to symptoms of lightheadedness, altered vision or mentation and syncope and balance/fall dysfunction. Temporary and permanent conduction problems may be treated by inserting a pacemaker or, in cases of life-threatening arrhythmias, an AICD. These devices can improve the patient's safety and tolerance to exercise and participation in work and recreational activities and can therefore improve quality of life. In such circumstances, the therapist must be aware of certain treatment concerns and must know the set mode of pacing before exercising a patient. Vital signs should be monitored during exercise to determine the patient's tolerance. To prevent harm, the clinician should know the relative and absolute contraindications of various modalities in a patient who has a pacemaker and/or AICD implanted.

References

Abraham W, Fisher W, Smith A et al 2002 Cardiac resynchronization in chronic heart failure. N Engl J Med 346(24):1845–1853

Cannon D, Prystowsky E 2004 Evolution of implantable cardiovertor defibrillators. J Cardiovasc Electrophysiol 15(3):375–385

Gregoratos G 2005 Indications and recommendations for pacemaker therapy. Am Fam Physician 71(8):1563–1570

Plummer CJ, Irving RJ, McComb JM 2005 The incidence of implanted cardiac defibrillators in patients admitted to all coronary care units in a single district. Eurospace 7(3):266–272

Proclemer A, Ghidina M, Cicuttini G et al 2001 The Italian implanted cardiac defibrillator registry: a survey of the national activity during the years of 2001 and 2003. Ital Heart J 6(3):272–280

Schermann M, Keung E 2005 The year in clinical electrophysiology. J Am Coll Cardiol 4(5):790–795

Schron E, Domanski M 2003 Implantable devices benefit patients with cardiovascular disease. J Cardiovasc Nurs 18(5):337–342

Stevenson W, Chaitman B, Ellenbegen K et al 2004 Clinical assessment and management of patients with implantable cardioverter devices presenting to nonelectrophysiologist. Circulation 110:3866–3869

Vardas P, Ovsyscher E 2002 Geographic differences of pacemaker implant rates in Europe. J Cardiovasc Electrophysiol 13(suppl1):S23–S26

Vesty J, Rasmusson K, Hall J et al 2004 Cardiac resynchronization therapy and automatic implantable cardiac defibrillators in the treatment of heart failure. J Am Acad Nurse Pract 16(10):441–450

Woodruff J, Prudente L 2005 Update on implantable pacemakers. J Cardiovasc Nurs 20(4):261–268

Young J, Abraham W, Smith A et al 2003 Combined cardiac resynchronization and implantable cardioversion defibrillation in advance congestive heart failure: the MIRACLE ICD Trial. J Am Med Assoc 289(20):2685–2694

Zaidan J, Atlee J, Belott P et al 2005 Practice advisory for perioperative management of patients with cardiac rhythm management devices: pacemakers and implantable cardioverter defibrillators. Anesthesiology 103(1):186–198

Chapter 46

Invasive cardiac procedures

Chris L. Wells

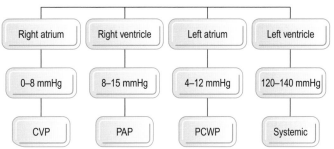

Figure 46.1   This illustration defines the clinical name of the pressures within each of the chambers of the heart and their average values. CVP, central venous pressure; PAP, pulmonary arterial pressure; PCWP, pulmonary capillary wedge pressure.

INTRODUCTION

Invasive procedures for the treatment of cardiac pathologies, such as catheterization, angioplasty and bypass surgery, have become commonplace over the past 30 years. Over 1.3 million invasive cardiac procedures are completed annually (Arjomand et al 2003, Maziarz & Keutlar 2004) and there have been many advances in the surgical management of cardiac disease. The age and number of comorbidities of elderly patients have increased the complexity of the procedures performed; unfortunately, however, these factors have also continued to affect the outcomes. This chapter will briefly discuss the various invasive procedures for the management of heart disease, particularly coronary artery disease.

CATHETERIZATION

Cardiac catheterization has become a standard procedure in the diagnosis of heart disorders and disease and in the assessment of cardiac function (see Fig. 46.1 for a description of the clinical name of the pressures within each of the chambers of the heart and their average values). A right heart catheterization (RHC) can be used to assess the volume and pressures within the cardiopulmonary system and is completed by placing a catheter within the right side of the heart, typically via the internal jugular, femoral or brachial veins. This catheter can measure how much blood is returning to the heart, referred to as preload, by recording the pressure within the right atrium, which is called central venous pressure. The physician can measure the function of the right ventricle and pulmonary vascular system by measuring the volume and pressure within the right ventricle. The catheter can be passed into the pulmonary trunk and used to indirectly measure the preload of the left side of the heart, which is referred to as the pulmonary capillary wedge pressure. This procedure can also be used to estimate blood gases, cardiac output and function of the tricuspid and pulmonic valves and to detect septal defects. Finally, RHC can be used to diagnose pulmonary hypertensive diseases, assess extent and location of embolism, take a tissue biopsy and evaluate the responsiveness to medications used to improve heart function and decrease pulmonary hypertension (Guillinta et al 2004).

A left heart catheterization (LHC) is commonly used to diagnose coronary atherosclerosis; this helps to determine the state of perfusion of the myocardium. The catheter is passed into the arterial system through the femoral or brachial arteries. At the time of the coronary arteriography, a ventriculography can be completed for assessment of left ventricular function including description of wall motion and function of the mitral and aortic valves and measurement of the ejection fraction, blood gases and the blood volume of the left ventricle and cardiac output. Heart catheterization can also be used to assess the health of the extracardiac major blood vessels of the body (DiMario & Sirtaria 2005).

Therapeutic intervention

Activity restrictions will vary depending on whether a patient has a RHC or a LHC. If the patient undergoes only a RHC, once the catheter is removed from the vein, pressure is applied to the site for 2–5 min to ensure that bleeding has stopped. The patient is then allowed out of bed and can resume activities as tolerated and as medically indicated. After undergoing a LHC, direct pressure is applied for 5–20 min or until the bleeding has stopped after which a pressure dressing is applied and the limb immobilized. The physician may insert a vascular plug or a suture to seal the puncture site of the artery but the patient will typically need to be on bedrest. If the femoral artery is the site for catheterization, the patient will be on bedrest for 4–6 h. If the brachial artery is the site for the LHC, the patient may be allowed out of bed in 2–4 h but the extremity will need to be elevated and immobilized for 4–6 h. When the patient and the extremity are permitted to be mobilized, it is important for the clinician to inspect the arterial site for bleeding or the development of a hematoma before and after the therapeutic intervention. If bleeding persists or a hematoma has developed, it is critical to notify the physician in order to control the bleeding and assess the artery for the development of an aneurysm. There is also the risk of renal dysfunction because of the dye that is used during the arteriography.

ANGIOPLASTY

There are several procedures that may be performed in the cardiac catheterization laboratory when a diagnosis of coronary atherosclerosis has been confirmed. A discrete noncalcified lesion that is in the proximal artery is the best lesion for a percutaneous transluminal coronary angioplasty (PTCA) procedure. Angioplasty should be considered for one- or two-vessel disease except when there is significant disease involving the left main artery (Michaels & Chatterjee 2002). Heart function and comorbidities, such as diabetes mellitus and acute myocardial infarction (MI), should also be taken into account when the specific invasive procedure is selected because they may decrease the favorable outcome of a PTCA (Arjomand et al 2003).

By performing a PTCA, it may be possible for the cardiologist to open the occluded artery and restore blood flow. A guide wire and catheter are inserted using the same procedure as in LHC. The guide wire is advanced through the atherosclerotic lesion and a dilatation catheter balloon is inserted over the guide wire. The balloon is then inflated, with the goal of redistributing the atherosclerotic plaque. The result is an enlargement of both the lumen and the overall diameter of the vessel. The balloon is then deflated and an angiography repeated to assess the effectiveness of the PTCA. The patient is typically administered heparin or bivalirudin to decrease the risk of thrombus formation and nitroglycerin may be administered into the coronary artery to prevent vasospasm. The PTCA can be repeated if necessary or be performed on other involved arteries.

The catheter sheath is typically not removed immediately and the patient is taken to the recovery room for monitoring to ensure hemodynamic stability and resolution of ischemia and anginal symptoms. It is recommended that the sheath be removed within 5 h to reduce the risk of complications such as bleeding. This decreases the length of stay and, in addition, it has been shown that patients who have a sheath in place for more than 7 h have an increased mortality rate (Galli & Palatrik 2005).

Although PTCA is a minimally invasive procedure and is associated with an approximate acute success rate of 90%, it is associated with several complications. Venous thrombosis and embolization may occur, causing a cerebrovascular accident (CVA) or occlusion of another coronary vessel and creating further ischemia or infarction. During the procedure, there is a risk of perforating or dissecting the coronary artery, which could lead to tamponade or MI. Tamponade or artery dissection requires emergency surgical intervention to stop bleeding and preserve myocardial function. The catheter can also cause life-threatening arrhythmia, and bleeding, infection and the development of a pseudoaneurysm may occur at the entrance site of the catheter, usually the femoral artery. PTCA is associated with a complication rate of 4.1%; in total, 29% of these complications are caused by arterial dissection. The restenosis rate is 4% and, of patients who suffer from restenosis, the arterial closure leads to MI in up to 50% of cases. About 30% of patients will require surgical intervention. Finally, there is a 5% mortality rate for patients who suffer from PTCA complications (Arjomand et al 2003).

Despite the advances in medical technology, there is a 30% chance of restenosis within the first year after a PTCA. Restenosis within the first 6 months post-PTCA is associated with cell proliferation, macrophage infiltration, platelet agitation and neovascularization (Hedman et al 2003) that leads to narrowing or occlusion of the coronary artery. After 6 months, it is believed that restenosis is caused by further progression of the coronary artery disease.

STENTS

The use of an endovascular stent in PTCA has been associated with a decreased rate of restenosis compared with the use of a PTCA alone. The benefit of stents is that a larger lumen can be achieved and there is a decrease in elastic recoil of the artery (Arjomand et al 2003). These stents may also be placed after a PTCA when there is an acute restenosis. In the US, over a million stents are used annually but there still is a 15–20% restenosis rate (Radke et al 2003), which has the same cellular mechanism as described above. The stent is guided into place across the atherosclerotic plaque over the guide wire. Once in position, the stent either self-expands or a balloon is inflated to disrupt the lesion and dilate the coronary artery to restore myocardial perfusion.

Further advances in stent technology have been made to address the complication of restenosis. Stents vary in size, length, thickness and drug coating over the stent. A stent can be coated with heparin or another drug that actively interrupts the development of restenosis. Thus, drug-coated or drug-eluding stents can be covered with such drugs as sirolimus or rapamycin. Sirolimus actually decreases endothelial function and affects platelet physiology (Lemos et al 2003) and rapamycin inhibits cell proliferation (Arjomand et al 2003). At the time of the catheterization, a glycoprotein IIb/IIIa inhibitor, such as abciximab, eptifibatide or tirofiban, may be injected before stent placement to decrease thrombosis formation (Arjomand et al 2003). Along with a drug-eluding stent, the patient is typically placed on anticoagulant medication for at least 6 months to decrease risk of thrombosis formation.

When stenosis occurs, there are several options to treat the ischemic state. Another stent can be placed within the present stent to reopen the lumen; this is known as 'stent-in-stent therapy'. Also, a PTCA, atherectomy, or laser or radiation therapy can be selected to reopen the lumen (Radke et al 2003).

ATHERECTOMY

There are four general types of atherectomy procedure that can be used to debulk or remove a thrombosis or atherosclerotic plaque and restore coronary blood flow. Atherectomy can be used independently or in conjunction with PTCA or stent deployment. The primary function of the atherectomy is to mechanically remove the plaque. A directional atherectomy (side-cutting) is best used when the lesion is located at a bifurcation or is eccentric and complicated. The rotational atherectomy uses a circular abrasive method and an atherosclerotic extraction device with cutting blades at the end of the endovascular instrument to debulk the artery. Laser has been successfully used to vaporize tissue in the case of 'in-stent' stenosis. Finally, a cutting balloon angioplasty, which is an atherotomy as opposed to an atherectomy, excises the lesion and dilates the artery by using a balloon catheter with a microsurgical blade (Arjomand et al 2003).

As well as the complications mentioned for PTCA, atherectomy can also cause microembolic activity that can result in arterial occlusion of distal smaller arteries. This can lead to focal ischemia and infarction.

LASERS

The atherosclerotic lesion can be managed by an ablative laser atherectomy procedure. Direct ablation by laser is indicated for a lesion in a saphenous vein graft, in aorta–coronary artery ostial stenosis, for a fibrotic or calcified lesion, for a lesion that affects a diffuse area or in stent restenosis. Based upon the cellular makeup of the plaque, the correct wavelength can vaporize the lesion. The most common complication of this application of lasers is perforation of the vessel (Arjomand et al 2003).

Lasers are also being used to conduct the Maze procedure for the treatment of atrial fibrillation and transmyocardial revascularization. These procedures will be briefly discussed later in this chapter (see under 'Maze procedure').

RADIATION

Intracoronary radiation, also known as brachytherapy, is being utilized to manage restenosis of treated coronary artery disease. The use of isotopes inhibits smooth muscle proliferation, delays the healing process and prevents the remodeling of the treated arteries. When brachytherapy is used in stent restenosis, there is a reduction of further restenosis by 50% (Arjomand et al 2003).

Therapeutic intervention

The therapeutic intervention during the acute phase after a catheterization procedure is similar to that described above for a LHC. Because the patient has been diagnosed with coronary artery disease and there is the risk of restenosis, it is important that the clinician educates the patient in the importance of compliance with routine medical check-ups and the use of medications and that the patient is able to recognize the signs and symptoms related to MI. In the long term, it is important that the patient begins to minimize his or her cardiac risk factors, such as cessation of smoking, management of hypertension and diabetes and proper diet and weight management, and participate in a regular exercise program.

CORONARY ARTERY BYPASS SURGERY

In the presence of multivessel coronary disease, complex diffuse lesions, left main arterial disease, multivessel disease with left ventricular dysfunction and in patients with diabetes, coronary artery bypass graft (CABG) surgery is the invasive procedure of choice (Ghali et al 2000, Grip et al 2004). The purpose of performing CABG surgery is to restore perfusion to viable myocardium by diverting blood around the atherosclerotic plaque to perfuse the myocardium distal to the occlusion.

Typically, the surgical approach is a median sternotomy but, more recently, CABG procedures are being carried out using an anterior thoracotomy approach. The approach that is used depends on the involved arteries, heart function, stability of the conduction system, the need for cardiopulmonary bypass support and the surgeon's training.

The vascular tissue that is harvested for the bypass procedure can be either arterial or venous in nature. Traditionally, the saphenous vein has been used to bypass the lesion by making an anastomosis of the vein to the aortic root and to a point distal to the lesion or stenosis. The vein is sutured in the reverse direction to prevent the valves within the veins from obstructing blood flow. Other sources of grafts or conduits continue to be investigated because the saphenous vein graft (SVG) has a modest rate of stenosis. In total, 15% of SVGs will become occluded within the first year because of hyperplasia and accelerated atherosclerosis and 50% are occluded within 10 years (Verma et al 2004).

The left, right or both internal thoracic (mammary) arteries (IMA) are common grafts for bypassing the left anterior descending artery. The left mammary artery, which has a 90% patency rate 10 years after the surgical procedure (Verma et al 2004), is most commonly used because the use of the right mammary artery or both IMA is associated with sternal wound complications (Knot et al 2004). Other arteries of the torso, such as the right gastroepiploic and inferior epigastric arteries, have been used as conduits but are not commonly used because of the difficulty in harvesting the arteries, which are small and fragile and associated with wound complications (Verma et al 2004).

The radial artery is another viable graft option if there is sufficient perfusion to the hand and forearm. In total, 88% of radial artery conduits are still patent 10 years after surgery. The radial artery is susceptible to vasospasm and lower patency when it is used to bypass the left circumflex or right coronary artery. It is also less viable for women (Knot et al 2004, Verma et al 2004).

Traditionally, when undergoing this procedure, the patient was placed on a cardiopulmonary bypass (CPB) to stop the heart and allow the CABG surgery to be completed. The CPB circulates blood to allow for full cardiopulmonary support while the heart is not beating and the grafts are sutured in place. This is a necessary procedure based upon the size and location of the coronary arteries, hemodynamic stability and left ventricular function. Unfortunately, there are adverse effects associated with CPB, particularly in the geriatric population. These adverse effects are related to the inflammatory response by cellular and humeral mediators that can lead to myocardial, renal and neurological dysfunction and coagulopathies, and small embolic activity that may impair cerebral function. These complications can also lead to respiratory failure and multisystem organ failure (Verma et al 2004).

It is believed that there is a decrease in mortality and a decrease in the incidence of stroke and central nervous system dysfunction when the CABG surgery is completed off CPB. However, it has not been determined how this will affect the long-term outcome for patients (Verma et al 2004).

Certain risks are involved when a patient is undergoing a CABG. The surgery may be complicated by MI, arrhythmia, incisional and sternal infections, failure to wean from mechanical ventilation, bleeding, stroke or acute renal failure. The procedure also carries a 1–3% mortality rate, which can be higher in patients with postoperative complications or in patients with coexisting disease like diabetes, declining left ventricular function and untreated heart failure.

Minimally invasive direct coronary artery bypass

Depending upon the blood vessels that are occluded, the stability of the patient and the function of the heart, the surgeon may opt to perform the bypass through a small anterior thoracotomy, referred to as minimally invasive direct coronary artery bypass (MIDCAB). The goal of a thoracotomy approach is to decrease the surgical trauma caused by a median sternotomy, improving recovery and reducing the length of the hospital stay. The MIDCAB is performed through a small anterior thoracotomy incision in the left fourth or fifth intercostal space. Typically, the left IMA is the conduit of choice to bypass the left anterior descending artery. The inferior epigastric artery or the saphenous vein can also be used as a conduit, but this is rare.

There are two major advantages to this surgical procedure: the patient does not have to be placed on CPB during surgery and a median sternotomy is avoided. MIDCAB is also referred to as a keyhole procedure. It is usually selected over the traditional CABG in cases of isolated left anterior descending (LAD) arterial disease, with or without additional vessel stenosis that can be managed with PTCA. When the patient undergoes a MIDCAB and PTCA, it is commonly referred to as a hybrid procedure. Patients who are at high risk for developing complications from CPB or median sternotomy are candidates for a MIDCAB.

Therapeutic intervention

Immediate postoperative precautions should be followed but the clinician should be aware that the postoperative precautions may vary from facility to facility. There is little published research to guide the clinician in the appropriate care of patients in the acute postoperative period; consequently, the information provided in this section is the clinical advice from this author. Commonly, the incisions are covered with only a dry dressing in the immediate postoperative phase and in the presence of a draining wound. If the saphenous vein is harvested, the involved lower extremity will typically be Ace-wrapped for 24–48 h to control edema.

In terms of shoulder range of motion (ROM), when a median sternotomy is the surgical approach, activity is performed within the tolerance of the patient, particularly flexion and abduction to 90 degrees and external rotation with abduction from 0 to 60 degrees. If the patient has a long history of diabetes associated with poor healing or is cognitively impaired or unable to report pain upon movement, ROM should be limited to 90 degrees of flexion only and external rotation performed only at 0 degrees of abduction.

Acute care rehabilitation includes restoring functional mobility, increasing ambulation tolerance and preparing for discharge. Strengthening and functional mobility exercises are also performed within the patient's tolerance and using proper body mechanics to protect the sternum and incision. Female patients who wear a 'C-cup' or larger size of bra should wear a bra that does not have an underwire, to decrease the tension of the incision.

For a patient who has undergone a median sternotomy and been classified as uncomplicated, functional mobility should begin as soon as the patient is alert and hemodynamically stable. Out-of-bed activities may begin as early as 3–6 h in the postoperative period. The supine-to-sit transfer should begin with the patient placing a pillow across the chest and rolling to a sidelying position. If the patient rolls to right sidelying, the right arm should splint the sternum while the left upper extremity assists in the roll, keeping the left humerus anterior to the midaxillary line. From the sidelying position, the right upper extremity continues to splint the sternum while the left upper extremity is positioned across the torso onto the bed to push the body upward into a sitting position.

For getting into and out of a chair, the patient should be instructed on weight-shifting on to an elbow; this will unweight the contralateral pelvis and enable the pelvis to be moved forwards or backwards. Moving from 'sit' to 'stand', the hands can be placed on the knees or on the arm rest but the work should be performed through the lower extremities. It is safe to allow the patient to use an assistive device if necessary; in the case of a wheelchair, the patient should instructed not to position the hands any further back than the top of the wheel. Patients are typically instructed to comply with sternal precautions for appropriately 10 weeks.

Patients who have undergone a thoracotomy procedure do not have to follow strict upper extremity precautions. ROM can be completed according to tolerance. Splinting across the surgical site helps to decrease pain and improves the patient's willingness to cough, participate in deep breathing exercises and initiate mobility training. There are no restrictions for transfers; if necessary, the clinician should assist the patient in transfer modifications to decrease the incisional pain.

At the University of Maryland Medical Center, patients are classified into low, moderate and high risk for sternal complications. Patient are classified as moderate risk for sternal complications if they have a significant history of poorly controlled diabetes, a history of type I diabetes of greater than 10 years, a history of systemic corticosteroid use, moderate truncal obesity or if the surgeon used a bilateral IMA graft. Other moderate-risk patients are those with comorbidities that require partial or weight-bearing as tolerated for the upper extremities in order to permit mobility. These patients may be placed in a device that approximates the upper rib cage, such as a sheet wrapped around the thorax or a 'heart-hugger' device, to increase the stability of the sternum. Once the sternum is stabilized, functional mobility can be instructed as described above. The clinician should routinely inspect the incision for healing and assess the patient for sternal stability. Figure 46.2 describes mobility training in patients using moderate sternal precautions.

Patients who are classified as high risk have a known history of wound complications, nonunion fractures and impaired mental status. These patients are instructed to splint the sternum and rib cage with both upper extremities and avoid the use of upper extremities during transfers. Family training to assist with functional mobility is very important for these patients. ROM exercises are limited to shoulder flexion to 70 degrees and external rotation is completed only at 0 degrees abduction. If the patient is unable to comply with precautions and follow commands, ROM exercises are delayed for 10–21 days to simplify the patient's education. If mental status improves, ROM and functional mobility can be advanced to promote functional independence. Patients classified as having a moderate to high risk of sternal complications are instructed to follow precautions for at least 12 weeks and sternal healing should be confirmed by radiography.

Rehabilitation during the acute phase of recovery should also address pulmonary care and include education about cardiac risk factors (e.g. cessation of smoking), the proper use of medications and the need for a sensible diet. Instruction in the use of the incentive spirometer, splinting and coughing techniques, and early ambulation should be emphasized to reduce the risk of atelectasis or pneumonia. It is recommended that patients ambulate at least three times a day with a goal of ambulating for at least 10 min in each session. Postoperative education should also include a home exercise program that includes increasing walking tolerance to 30 min a day for 5 days a week over the next 6 weeks of recovery. The patient and family should be instructed on which signs and symptoms to monitor so that any postoperative complications can be identified. The patient should avoid lifting more than 10 lbs (5 kg) and should not drive until the surgeon or clinician discontinues the sternal precaution. The patient should sit in the back seat of a vehicle with a pillow across the chest underneath the seat belt; the patient should not sit in the front seat of a vehicle if it is possible that an airbag may be activated. The goal for discharge is to achieve medical stability, restore functional mobility and complete all the education necessary within 3–5 days of surgery.

The focus of rehabilitation in the subacute phase is to restore the patient's ability to perform the activities of daily living and low-level aerobic exercise. Upper extremity ROM is progressed to within normal limits. Walking and cycling are the most common modes of exercise. The aerobic program usually begins with timed intervals based upon the patient's tolerance, with the goal of achieving 15–20 min of exercise daily. Referral to outpatient cardiac rehabilitation to begin phase II can occur as early as 2–3 weeks postoperatively; this typically ranges from 24 to 36 visits during which electrocardiogram and vital sign responses to exercise are monitored. The goal of this phase of rehabilitation is to raise the patient's tolerance to the point where 40 min of aerobic exercise can be completed. Once the surgeon has confirmed that the sternum is healed, the patient can begin weightlifting using light to moderate weights. Questions regarding a return to work and recreational activities are entertained at this time. If the patient is returning to a job that requires physical labor, the clinician should design a work-hardening program to enable the patient to successfully re-enter the workforce and decrease the risk of work-related injuries.

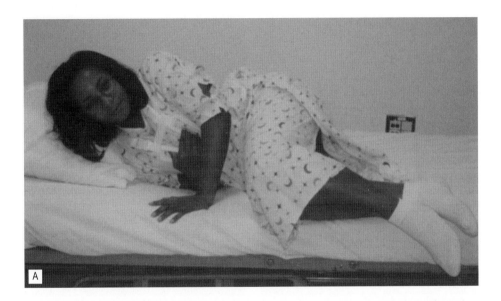

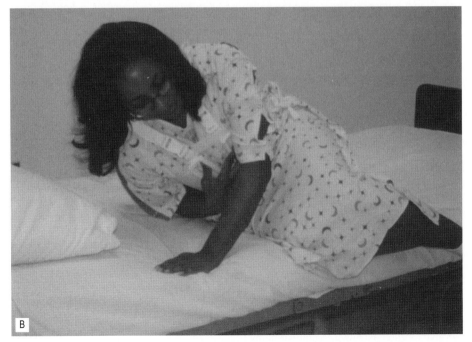

Figure 46.2   (A and B) These photographs illustrate how the patient is instructed to progress out of bed using a heart hugger. Please note that the patient is using the right upper extremity to splint the chest wall and that the elbow is held tightly against the rib cage to prevent the patient from abducting the arm.

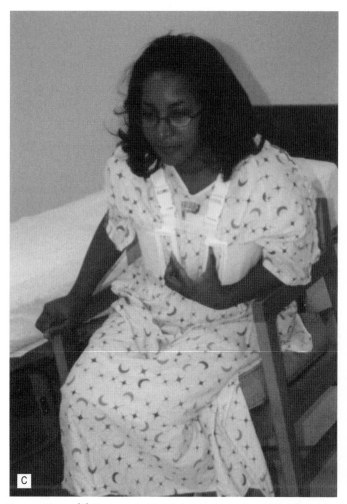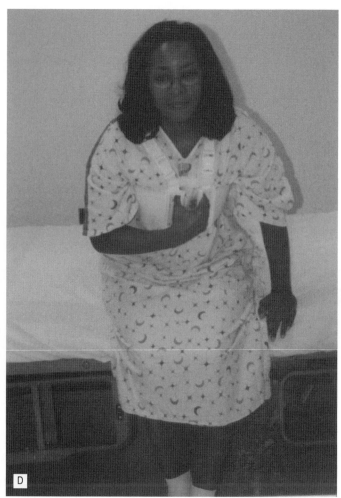

Figure 46.2   (C) During scooting it is important to remind the patient to keep the upper extremities in front of the trunk. (D) The upper extremity (–ies) can be used to move from 'sit' to 'stand' but the patient should visually check to make sure that their hand(s) is properly placed in front of the trunk before pushing.

VALVULAR PROCEDURES

In the case of moderate to severe valvular disease, the valve can be dilated, repaired or replaced. In balloon valvuloplasty, a procedure that is carried out via catheterization for a noncalcified stenotic valve, the balloon catheter is placed across the valve. The balloon is then inflated to dilate the lumen and thus decrease the pressure across the valve. This procedure may be complicated by hypotension, myocardial wall perforation, tamponade, arrhythmia, an embolic event, rupture of the chordae tendineae cordis or papillary muscle, MI and valvular regurgitation. A valvotomy is a palliative procedure performed in a younger patient with an uncomplicated noncalcified stenotic lesion. This open procedure allows the surgeon to see the valve and to resect an atrial thrombus, a common finding. The surgeon can correct the fusion of the leaflets or chordae tendineae cordis and split the papillary muscles to improve the function of the valve. An annuloplasty involves the repair of the annulus, particularly necessary in cases of regurgitation. The annulus can be reduced in size to correct the insufficiency or a stent can be put in place to stabilize valve function. Finally, a commissurotomy involves the surgical splitting of the commissure to correct a stenotic valve (Vahanian & Palacios 2004, Yacoub & Cohn 2004).

In the case of a complicated calcified lesion, a symptomatic patient with moderate to severe disease or the failure to repair a defect, the diseased valve can be replaced by either a mechanical or a biological valve. The mechanical valve, composed of metal or synthetic materials, is a ball or disk mechanism that responds to pressure changes. The most common valve is a St Jude valve. It is highly durable and is the valve of choice for the younger patient. The disadvantage of the mechanical valve is that it makes an audible sound and requires anticoagulation drugs to be taken for life because of the risk of thromboembolic complications. Biological valves can be obtained from animal or human tissue. A heterograft is composed of porcine or bovine tissue. Human valves are harvested from cadavers, but the availability is low. The advantage of a biological valve is that it preserves the normal function of the valve and is fairly nonthrombogenic; however, it is of limited durability and has a tendency to have a smaller orifice, which creates a stenotic state. The selection of the type of valve depends on the age of the patient and the risk of anticoagulation (Vahanian & Palacios 2004, Yacoub & Cohn 2004). The reader is referred to Chapter 44 on Heart Failure and Valvular Heart Disease for further information on the management of valvular disease.

Therapeutic intervention

The rehabilitation of the patient who has undergone valvular repair or replacement is similar to that of patients who have undergone myocardial revascularization (see the discussion above on immediate post-CABG rehabilitation). Patients who are placed on anticoagulation therapy should be educated to be cautious when participating in contact recreational sports and vigorous weight-lifting activities. They should also be educated on the importance of follow-up medical checks to monitor anticoagulation levels and the signs and symptoms of bleeding.

MAZE PROCEDURE

One of the complications of heart disease is the development of atrial fibrillation. This is an irregular conduction rhythm that interferes with proper filling of the ventricles and increases the risk of thrombus formation within the atrium, which increases the risk of stroke.

Although atrial fibrillation is considered to be very unpredictable with regard to heart rate, the pattern of depolarization is more predictable than once thought. With this in mind, it is possible to disrupt the pathway of depolarization within the atria, with emphasis on the left atrium, to ablate the arrhythmia. The Maze procedure involves making surgical incisions or lesions with a laser in a precise pattern to create alleys that only allow one way for atrial depolarization to occur (Cox 2004).

The Maze procedure can be performed alone through an anterior thoracotomy or, more commonly, in conjunction with another open heart procedure. With the most recent Maze procedure, the Maze III, the surgeon also excises the appendage of the left atrium and concentrates the laser around the pulmonary veins (Gillinov & McCarthy 2004).

In the acute phase of recovery, it is not uncommon for the patient's heart to revert back into atrial fibrillation because the myocardial tissue is irritated and inflamed. It is important for the clinician to monitor and be able to recognize the signs and symptoms of atrial fibrillation. Typically, for the first three months after the procedure, the patient will be placed on antiarrhythmic medication to decrease the risk of developing atrial fibrillation. In total, 38% of patients will develop atrial fibrillation in the acute and subacute phase of recovery (Palazzo 2000). The patient should undergo cardioversion and have their medication adjusted to prevent recurrence of the arrhythmia.

TRANSMYOCARDIAL REVASCULARIZATION

A patient who suffers from disabling angina that is nonresponsive to medical therapy but who is not a candidate for the bypass procedure because of diffuse distal coronary disease may be a candidate for transmyocardial revascularization (TMR). Since the acceptance of enhanced external counterpulsation therapy, fewer isolated TMR procedures are being performed. In today's practice, the surgeon is more likely to perform a TMR in conjunction with a CABG or valvular procedure (Yang et al 2004). The TMR procedure involves the use of a laser and the approach can be percutaneous, thoracoscopical or, most commonly, a left anterolateral thoracotomy in the fifth or sixth intercostal space. When the left ventricle is fully distended with blood and depolarization has begun, a laser is fired through the myocardium. The laser makes a 1-mm channel through the wall of the left ventricle and the laser beam is absorbed by the blood in the chamber. Several channels are made through the myocardium. Direct pressure is applied to the epicardial surface to stop bleeding into the pericardial sac. A suture may also have to be placed at the entrance of the laser to control bleeding (Horvath 2004, Yang et al 2004).

The exact mechanism that enables TMR to improve myocardial perfusion is still unknown. One theory states that perfusion is improved because blood is allowed to pass directly into the myocardium from within the chamber. The use of the laser may also stimulate the formation of collateral circulation, which further improves perfusion. The procedure may also decrease angina because of the denervation of the myocardium at the channel sites (Horvath 2004).

Therapeutic intervention

The rehabilitation process is similar to that recommended for the patient who has undergone a medial sternotomy, but with a few differences. With the incision being made in the intercostal space, no sternal precautions need be taken. Upper extremity ROM, strengthening and functional mobility can progress within incisional tolerance. The rehabilitation progress may be slower for the patient who has undergone a TMR secondary to coronary artery disease with impaired overall myocardial perfusion. In this patient population, it is important to educate on the signs and symptoms of myocardial ischemia and focus training on functional strengthening and functional activities, for example walking, to promote independence. Education regarding work simplification and energy conservation may also be a key component of the rehabilitation process.

VENTRICULAR RECONSTRUCTION

When the ventricle becomes dilated as a consequence of ischemic heart disease or develops an aneurysm as a result of a large transmural myocardial infarction, the ventricle is unable to generate a sufficient contraction to maintain cardiac output and the patient develops heart failure. The surgeon may consider a procedure to reconstruct the ventricle and improve the efficiency of muscle contraction. The aneurysm can be resected, known as aneurysectomy, which may also improve anginal symptoms and decrease ventricular arrhythmia. A section of the ventricular wall can be excised and a polyester mesh wrapped around the ventricle to act as a girdle; this provides flexibility to the ventricle to allow for filling and strengthened ejection. This is known as the Acorn Corcap procedure and is currently under clinical trial. Surgeons have also used a portion of the latissimus dorsi to wrap around the ventricles, known as dynamic cardiomyopathy; however, this procedure is associated with a high mortality rate. Also under investigation is the myosplint procedure. In this procedure, epicardial pads are secured to the ventricular wall and transventricular wires pass through the wall to connect them. This increases wall tension and results in a restructuring of the shape of the ventricles and therefore an improvement in their function (Lee et al 2004). These procedures are primarily used for left ventricular pump dysfunction and failure but may be used in patients with severe right ventricular failure.

VENTRICULAR ASSIST DEVICES

Until recently, the use of ventricular assist devices (VADs) was reserved for younger patients who were suffering end-stage heart failure and waiting for heart transplantation. The VAD was implanted as a bridge to transplant in patients whose condition was refractory to medical care. More recently, in the US, clinical trials have begun to explore the use of VADs in older patients who are not candidates for heart transplantation. The goal of these trials is to support the function of the failing left ventricle so that the patient can regain functional independence and improve their quality of life. The investigators in these clinical trials are also hoping that the use of VADs will decrease the number of

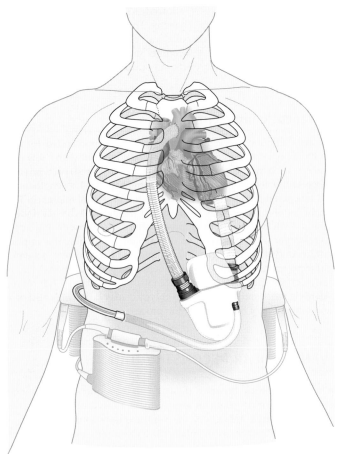

Figure 46.3 The Novacor is a ventricular assist device (VAD) that supports the left ventricle. The position of the VAD within the body and its interface with the cardiovascular system is shown, along with the actual pump, its cannulas that allow for filling and emptying of the pump and the drive line that connects the pump to the computer, controller and power source.
(From WorldHeart Inc., Oakland, CA. Available: www.worldheart.com., with permission.)

hospital admissions and the cost of healthcare for patients with end-stage heart failure.

Currently, three clinical trials are exploring the use of left VADs (LVADS) as surgical management for end-stage heart disease. The permanent use of VADs is referred to as destination therapy. The RELIANT trial is studying the performance and outcome of the Novacor VAD compared with the HeartMate I (see Fig. 46.3). The other clinical trials are investigating the use of the HeartMate II and

the DeBakey VAD. Physical therapy plays a critical role in preparing these patients to return home and restore an active role within their families and communities.

The mechanics of how these LVADs support left ventricular function vary among each of the devices but are based upon using the normal physiology of circulating blood to support the metabolic demand of the body. The surgeon places an inflow cannula in the apex of the left ventricle that drains blood into the pump. The pump then returns a sufficient amount of blood to support the body's needs into the aorta through an outflow cannula. With the Novacor and HeartMate, the pumps fills with blood before it ejects the blood into the systemic circulation, modeling the function of the left ventricle. The HeartMate II and DeBakey devices actually constantly circulate blood from the left ventricle to the aorta; consequently, there is frequently a loss of peripheral pulses. With all these devices, the pump is implanted within the body and has a drive line that exits the body, typically at the right abdominal wall, to connect to a 'controller' or computer that runs the pump and a power source.

These studies are still recruiting patients and collecting data, so the potential role of VADs for destination therapy is still unanswered at this time. The primary complications of these devices are stroke and infections.

Therapeutic intervention

The general rehabilitation of patients who have undergone a VAD implantation is very similar to that of patients who have undergone a CABG procedure. The most important thing that clinicians need to do in preparing to work with these patients is to complete any training and demonstrate competency, as defined by the facility and the device's manufacturers, to ensure that they understand how the device functions, what the various alarms mean and what the appropriate sequence of actions should be when an alarm goes off. The clinician needs to remember that the VAD is supporting left ventricular function and so cardiac output should be stable; this should allow the patient to participate in an aggressive rehabilitation program to restore function, improve activity tolerance, permit a possible return to work and improve quality of life.

CONCLUSION

In the evaluation and treatment of cardiac pathology, various invasive techniques exist. Some are only minimally invasive, whereas others require extensive surgical techniques. Care providers must be aware of the specific invasive techniques used and their associated precautions. Immediate postoperative wound care is a concern for all of these techniques. In most cases, rehabilitation should commence within 24 h of surgery. The goal of care is to return the patient to as normal a lifestyle as possible within weeks to months and within the limits of individual cardiac and coexisting pathologies.

References

Arjomand H, Turi Z, McCormick D, Goldberg S 2003 Percutaneous coronary intervention: historical perspectives, current status, and future directions. Am Heart J 146:787–796

Cox J 2004 Cardiac surgery for arrhythmias. J Cardiovasc Electrophysiol 15(2):250–262

DiMario C, Sirtaria N 2005 coronary angiography in the angioplasty era: projections with a meaning. Heart 91:968–976

Galli A, Palatrik A 2005 What is the proper activated clotting time (ACT) at which to remove a femoral sheath after PCI: what are the best 'protocols' for sheath removal? Crit Care Nurse 25(2):88–95

Ghali W, Quan H, Norris C et al 2000 Prognostic significance of diabetes as a predictor of survival after cardiac catheterization. Am J Med 109:543–548

Gillinov A, McCarthy P 2004 Surgical treatment of atrial fibrillation. Cardiol Clinic 22:147–157

Grip L, Albertsson P, Schiersten F 2004 Survival benefits of CABG and PCI: facts and speculations. Scand Cardiovasc J 38(1):36

Guillinta P, Peterson K, Ben-Yehunda D 2004 Cardiac catheterization techniques in pulmonary hypertension. Cardiol Clinics 22:401–415

Hedman M, Hartikainen J, Syvanne M et al 2003 Safety and feasibility of catheter-based local intracoronary vascular endothelial growth factor gene transfer in the prevention of postangioplasty and instent restenosis in the treatment of chronic myocardial ischemia: phase II results of the Kuopio Angiogenesis trial (KAT). Circulation 107:2677–2683

Horvath K 2004 Mechanisms and results of transmyocardial laser revascularization. Cardiology 101:37–47

Knot U, Friedmand D, Patterson G et al 2004 Radial artery bypass grafts have an increased occurrence of angiographyically severe stenosis and occlusion compared to left internal mammary artery and saphenous vein grafts. Circulation 109:2086–2091

Lee R, Hoercher K, McCarthy P 2004 Ventricular reconstruction surgery for congestive heart failure. Cardiology 101:61–71

Lemos P, Lee C, Degertelem M et al 2003 Early outcome after Sirolimus-eluding stent: implantation of patients with acute cardiac syndrome. J Am Coll Cardiol 41(11):2093–2099

Maziarz D, Keutlar T 2004 Cost considerations in selecting coronary artery revascularization therapy in the elderly. Am J Cardiovasc Drug. 4(4):219–225

Michaels A, Chatterjee K 2002 Angioplasty versus bypass surgery for coronary artery disease. Circulation 106:e187–190

Palazzo T 2000 Frequently asked questions about the Maze procedure. June 21, 2000. Available: http//www.members.aol.com/mazern,mazefaq.htm. Accessed December 12 2005

Radke P, Kaiser A, Frost C, Sigwart U 2003 Outcome after treatment of coronary in stent restenosis. Eur Heart J 24:266–273

Vahanian A, Palacios I 2004 Percutaneous approaches to valvular disease. Circulation 109:1572–1579

Verma S, Fedate P, Szmitko R, Badicuala M 2004 Off-pump coronary artery bypass surgery: fundamentals for clinical cardiologists. Circulation 109:1206–1211

Yacoub M, Cohn L 2004 Novel approaches to cardiac valve repair from structure to function: part II. Circulation 109:1064–1072

Yang E, Barsness G, Gerth B et al 2004 Current and future treatment strategies for refractory angina. Mayo Clinic Proc 79(10):1284–1292

Chapter 47

Pulmonary diseases

Chris L. Wells

INTRODUCTION

Lung disease can be classified based on its clinical characteristics. It is common to classify pulmonary diseases as obstructive, restrictive (also known as pulmonary fibrosis) or vascular.

Chronic obstructive pulmonary disease (COPD) is a generic term to describe many lung pathologies that result in the trapping or retention of air upon exhalation. Emphysema and chronic bronchitis are two common obstructive diseases that affect people in the sixth decade of life. Asthma and cystic fibrosis are also considered to be obstructive lung diseases; they are typically diagnosed early in life, although asthma can develop across the lifespan.

Pulmonary fibrosis refers to diseases that cause a scarring of the lung tissue, for example interstitial pulmonary fibrosis and occupational lung diseases such as silicosis, farmer's or coal worker's pneumoconiosis and sarcoidosis. The result of the scarring causes a restriction or reduction of the lung's compliance, which is the ability of the lung to expand upon inspiration.

When a lung disease results in the destruction of the massive pulmonary vascular bed, pulmonary hypertension develops within the pulmonary system. Pulmonary hypertension in the elderly can be the result of a long-standing progressive obstructive or restrictive lung disease, stenosis of the mitral valve, which causes a chronic rise in pressure in the pulmonary vascular bed, or a pulmonary embolism.

In a complete classification of lung pathology, there are three more categories of lung disease that are recognized by clinicians: infectious diseases such as pneumonia and tuberculosis, pulmonary oncology and diseases of the pleural lining. This chapter will briefly discuss obstructive, restrictive and infectious diseases, their clinical presentation and therapeutic interventions.

CHRONIC OBSTRUCTIVE PULMONARY DISEASE

Emphysema and chronic bronchitis

Emphysema is defined as irreversible anatomical enlargement of the airspaces that are distal to the terminal bronchioles (Fig. 47.1). There is destruction of the acini, which are the functional units of the lung where gas exchange occurs in individuals without fibrosis. Emphysema can be classified based on the location of the anatomical disruption. Centrilobular emphysema is the type of emphysema most commonly associated with smoking and involves the enlargement and destruction of the first- and second-order respiratory bronchioles with the alveoli remaining intact. It most commonly affects the upper lobes and results in a mismatch between ventilation and perfusion. Panacinar emphysema is found in the elderly and in patient's who have a genetic form of emphysema called α1-antitrypsin deficiency. This form of emphysema affects all of the respiratory bronchioles in a uniform pattern. Paraseptal emphysema involves the peripheral secondary lobules and is not typically associated with progressive end-stage disease but with an increased risk and incidence of pneumothorax. Finally, paracicatrical emphysema is characterized by irregular enlargements of the acini with fibrosis, usually adjacent to a previous pulmonary lesion (Hogg 2004).

Emphysema is the second most common of the obstructive diseases, with only asthma having a higher incidence. There is a definite increase in the incidence of emphysema in the fifth decade and a continued increase into the seventh decade. Because the lungs have a vast amount of surface area to allow for sufficient gas exchange, many individuals will be asymptomatic in the early stages of the disease unless the activity level is at a high intensity; under such conditions, emphysema may contribute to the fatigue and shortness of breath caused by deconditioning and the aging process (Higenbottam 2005). The level of disability or functional limitation is dependent on the extent of lung destruction, not the type of emphysema.

Chronic bronchitis is a clinical diagnosis that presents as a persistent productive cough that produces sputum for more than 3 months per year for at least two consecutive years in the absence of another definable medical cause for the sputum production such as pneumonia. The disease is associated with hyperplastic glands and an increase in goblet cells of the epithelial lining. There is a marked decrease in the ratio of goblet cells to ciliated cells, leading to hypersecretion of mucus, which overwhelms the mucociliary clearance (Fig. 47.2). The end result is the overproduction and retention of sputum, which causes airway obstruction, inflammation of the respiratory bronchioles, narrowing or occlusion of the small airways from mucus plugs and

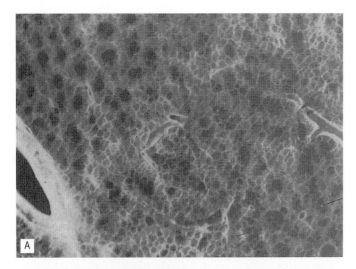

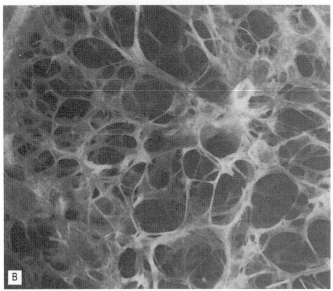

Figure 47.1 Comparison of normal lung tissue (A) with the pathological changes observed in lung tissue damaged by emphysema (B).
(From Heard B 1969 Pathology of Chronic Bronchitis and Emphysema. Churchill Livingstone, London.)

hypertrophy of the smooth muscle, resulting in an increased risk of pulmonary infections.

Contributing factors

Several contributing factors have been linked to emphysema and chronic bronchitis, the most common of which is cigarette smoking. Smoking increases the aggregation of neutrophils and alveolar macrophages, which begin the immune response to rid the body of foreign materials. One theory suggests that emphysema is the result of an imbalance between the protective antiprotease enzymes that protect the delicate structures of the lungs and the protease enzymes that lyse or break down tissue. This imbalance leads to the loss of the elastic recoil of the lung architecture. The small airways depend upon the adjacent elastic tissue of the parenchyma to recoil and assist with expiration and to provide airway stability to allow for effective inspiration. Another theory currently under examination is the role that

smoking plays in the observed elevated rate of apoptosis or cell death of the alveolar cells, followed by the failure to repair the structures to a functional state. There is also an increase in platelet and neutrophil aggregation, which destroys the small capillary bed. This leads to a decrease in the gas exchange function of the lungs and pulmonary hypertension (White et al 2003, Higenbottam 2005).

Exposure to air pollutants and occupational factors is also associated with an increased incidence of emphysema and chronic bronchitis. There is an increased incidence in the development and progression of COPD as the number of respiratory infections increase. The increased frequency and dose exposure to systemic steroids, for example prednisone, has also been linked to the progression of COPD. Finally, genetic factors that have been linked with a predisposition to emphysema and chronic bronchitis.

Clinical manifestation

Emphysema and chronic bronchitis can exist without evidence of clinically significant obstruction or functional limitations. However, by the time that the patient presents to the healthcare provider with symptoms, extensive irreversible lung damage is present. COPD results in a limitation of airflow. The lumen size of the bronchioles is decreased because of smooth muscle proliferation and contraction and because of bronchial edema resulting from inflammation. With the loss of the lung parenchyma, there is a reduction in the elastic recoil of the airways, leading to dilatation of the distal airways and early airway closure. The end result of these changes in structure within the lungs is an increase in the ease with which air can enter the lungs during inspiration, which is referred to as an increase in compliance. Unfortunately, the changes also result in the closure or collapse of the fragile airways upon exhalation, leading to air becoming trapped in the distal respiratory bronchioles and acini. This presents clinically as hyperinflation of the lung. The hyperinflation causes shortening of the inspiratory muscles and a flattening of the diaphragm. This leads to compensatory changes in the chest wall called barrel chest deformity, which is an increase in the anterior–posterior dimension and rib angle. These musculoskeletal changes lead to a decline in the mechanical effectiveness of the diaphragm and other respiratory muscles to support the increased demands of ventilation.

The clinical presentation of patients with COPD includes dyspnea, an increase in the work of breathing and a cough. Upon auscultation, there are diminished normal breath sounds and wheezing, particularly associated with exertion. There is an elongated expiratory phase because the patient tries to slow down the change in airway pressure during expiration to minimize the degree of air trapping or obstruction. Accessory respiratory muscles are commonly hypertrophied and there is a decrease in the excursion of the diaphragm. On percussing over the intercostal spaces, there is hyper-resonance. With exertion, there is a marked increase in muscle recruitment, both for inspiration and expiration. Shortness of breath is the leading cause of exercise intolerance.

Patients who have a mismatch between ventilation and perfusion have the clinical presentation of desaturation because of the disruption of gas exchange. There may be areas of the lung where there is good blood flow through the pulmonary capillaries but poor ventilation. There may also be areas with an increase in the dead space in patients with COPD, which means that there is sufficient ventilation occurring in areas of the lungs where the capillary bed has been destroyed or pruned. This mismatch between ventilation and perfusion leads to hypoxia and the retention of carbon dioxide.

Examination of pulmonary function tests in patients with COPD reveals a classic pattern. Patients have a marked reduction in the ability to expel air rapidly, measured by the forced expiratory volume in 1 s (FEV_1) and forced vital capacity (FVC). The decline in FEV_1 is associated with the degree of dyspnea or shortness of breath. Exercise

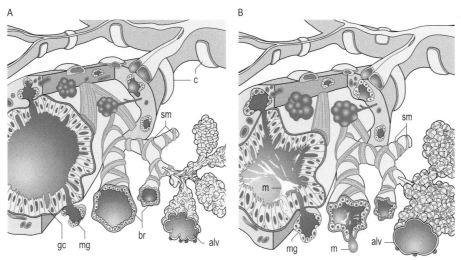

Figure 47.2   Comparison of a normal airway (A) with a chronic bronchitic airway (B). alv, alveoli; br, bronchi; c, cartilage; gc, goblet cell; m, mucus; mg, mucus gland; sm, smooth muscle. (From Des Jardins T 1984 Clinical Manifestations of Respiratory Disease. Year Book Medical Publishers, Chicago, IL, with permission. Redrawn by Kenneth Axen.)

limitations because of dyspnea are associated with a FEV_1 of less than 50% of the predicted value for age, height and weight. When the patient is dyspneic at rest, the FEV_1 will be as low as 25% of the predicted value. There is also a marked increase in the total lung capacity and the residual volume, which clearly represents the increased compliance of the lung and the degree of air trapping or obstruction (see Fig. 47.3).

Although the majority of patients with COPD have mixed features of both emphysema and chronic bronchitis, there are certain clinical signs and symptoms that are associated more with emphysema than with chronic bronchitis. With emphysema, there is a long history of dyspnea on exertion and little sputum production. These patients favor a posture of forward trunk flexion; this is to fixate their upper extremities so that accessory muscle recruitment is increased and the influence of gravity is decreased. The patient with emphysema is more likely to practice pursed lip breathing or grunt during expiration to keep the airways open. The patient will present with an elevated minute ventilation (respiratory rate × tidal volume), which aids in maintaining a sufficient arterial oxygen concentration at least through the early to mid-stages of the disease. In addition, a patient who suffers predominantly from emphysema will have an underweight to cachectic appearance (Hogg 2004).

In contrast, a patient who suffers predominantly from chronic bronchitis usually presents with a long history of a chronic and productive cough. Initially, the productive cough may only occur during the winter months; however, as the disease progresses in duration, frequency and severity, there is excessive sputum production and mucopurulent infections. By the time the patient experiences exertional dyspnea, there is a severe degree of airway obstruction. These patients have a tendency to be overweight and cyanotic, with a lower minute ventilation than patients with emphysema (Hogg 2004).

As these diseases progress to end-stage, there will be further declines in lung function. The destruction of the respiratory bronchioles and acini lead to additional difficulties with proper ventilation, an increased airway resistance and a significant increase in the work of breathing. The disruption of the capillary bed within the lung causes a rise in pulmonary pressure and places a strain on the right ventricle. Over time, the patient will develop cor pulmonale, or right heart failure, which is associated with peripheral pitting edema, ascites and enlargement of the liver, jugular vein distension and anorexia.

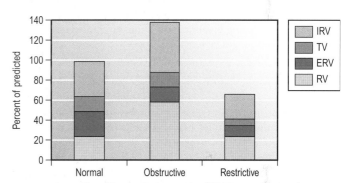

Figure 47.3   The effects of obstructive (COPD, emphysema) and restrictive (pulmonary fibrosis) pulmonary diseases on lung volumes. ERV, expiratory reserve volume; IRV, inspiratory reserve volume; RV, residual volume; TV, tidal volume.

Therapeutic intervention

Smoking cessation is instrumental in the care of patients with COPD. Cessation leads to a decrease in the rate of loss of FEV_1. Importantly, cessation also means the avoidance of people or places where there is the risk of exposure to second-hand smoke. Behavioral modification training should also focus on weight management, developing coping strategies to minimize anxiety attacks, controlling responses to stress and learning breathing strategies to control dyspnea.

Beyond behavioral modifications, there are many pharmacological options to assist in the management of the disease and the associated symptoms. Short- and long-acting β2-agonists or bronchodilators such as albuterol can be used to minimize bronchospasm and decrease wheezing and airway resistance. Anticholinergic drugs, such as atrovent, can block bronchoconstriction; xanthine-derived medications, such as theophylline, also produce bronchodilation and accelerate the mucociliary transport system and limit the inflammatory response. Corticosteroids, such as prednisone or flovent, are used for their anti-inflammatory benefits. It is critical for patients with lung disease to receive a flu shot annually to decrease the risk of infection. When a patient has a history of recurrent infections, antibiotics play a critical role not only in the treatment of a recurrent infection but also as part of prophylactic care. These patients may also benefit from chest physical therapy including postural drainage, percussion and assistive breathing techniques, or the use of an oscillating device to mobilize secretions. Finally, supplemental oxygen is used to correct hypoxemia and minimize secondary pulmonary hypertension. Oxygen therapy has been shown to reduce the level of dyspnea, decrease pulmonary hypertension, reduce the incidence of cardiac arrhythmias and improve quality and quantity of life. In the patient who presents with hypercapnia and respiratory insufficiency, bilevel positive airway pressure (BiPAP) ventilation has become recognized as an effective device in the management of patients with progressive disease. The ventilator provides positive airway pressure to decrease the work of inspiration and minimize the air trapping, which can reduce the retention of carbon dioxide.

Pulmonary rehabilitation has become a widely accepted intervention in the care of patients with COPD, with the ultimate goal of improving quality of life. The therapy program should consist of a comprehensive educational program to address such issues as nutrition, weight management, pathology and medical management, including the proper use of medications, work simplification and coping strategies. The program should stress and progress aerobic tolerance and include weight training to improve the muscular strength and endurance of the upper body; this will increase the effectiveness of the accessory respiratory muscles and antigravity muscles in maximizing breathing and promoting functional mobility. The exercises should be functional and weight-bearing in nature to aid in the management of osteopenia and osteoporosis, which are very common in this patient population. Oxygen saturation should be monitored closely and supplemental oxygen adjusted to provide sufficient perfusion to support aerobic training. With training, the majority of patients with COPD will improve their exercise capacity, and there is a decrease in the perception of dyspnea, an increase in self-control and a marked improvement in quality of life (Salman et al 2003, Anonymous 2004).

There are surgical options for the treatment of emphysema and chronic bronchitis. In the presence of a large bulla, which is a large airspace that is no longer contributing to gas exchange and is compressing adjacent tissue, surgical resection of this tissue (bullectomy) can be performed. Volume reduction surgery is an option for patients with emphysema, in which about 20% of dysfunctional lung tissue is surgically removed to decrease hyperinflation and improve ventilation and perfusion. Finally, lung transplantation has become a viable option for patients with end-stage COPD who have maximized medical therapy (Nathan et al 2004).

The prognosis for patients with COPD varies depending upon the degree of obstruction, the presence of hypercapnia, the level of hypoxemia, functional mobility, body mass index and the recurrence of infections. It is generally accepted that a FEV_1 of less than 25% is associated with a 50% mortality rate within 2 years. In chronic bronchitis, the prognosis is dependent upon age, smoking and the degree of airway obstruction. The 10-year mortality rate is 60% in smokers but only 15% in nonsmokers. Mortality rates based on FEV_1 for patients with chronic bronchitis are similar to patients with emphysema (White et al 2003, Pinto-Plata et al 2004).

PULMONARY FIBROSIS

Pulmonary fibrosis is the name for the hundreds of pulmonary pathologies that result in a restriction of the lungs. The ability of the patient to increase the volume of air in the lungs, or lung compliance, diminishes as the disease progresses; the compliance of the chest wall also decreases because of the decrease in range of motion. Pulmonary fibrosis can be caused by autoimmune diseases, such as rheumatoid arthritis, lupus and scleroderma, or can result from occupational exposure, such as farmer's lung, silicosis and black lung. Pulmonary trauma, fat embolism and infection are associated with the development of acute respiratory distress syndrome. Other diseases, for example interstitial pulmonary fibrosis, are idiopathic in nature.

Occupational disease

There is a subset of pulmonary interstitial disorders that result from the inhalation of inorganic dusts (pneumoconioses), organic particles (hypersensitivity pneumoconioses) and industrial gases, fumes and smoke. These occupational lung diseases are associated with a chronic inflammatory process (Kushner & Stark 2003, Ross 2003).

Pneumoconioses involves the permanent deposition of inorganic material (coal, asbestos, silica, beryllium, etc.) within the pulmonary system. The risk of developing pulmonary fibrosis is related to the duration and intensity of exposure and the size and water solubility of the particles. There is a long latency between exposure and disease, sometimes as long as 20–40 years, which may place the onset of disease in the fifth to seventh decades of life.

If the inorganic materials are able to get beyond the ciliary structures of the nasal passage and mucociliary blanket, they may cause an inflammatory process within the air spaces and interstitium, resulting in lung injury. Hyperplasia and proliferation of pulmonary epithelial cells characterize the immune response, which is accompanied by fibroblastic proliferation and collagen and protein deposition.

Hypersensitivity pneumonitis, or external allergic alveolitis, is an immunologically mediated disease that is typically associated with sensitivity from repeated exposure to an antigen. Further exposure results in an inflammatory response that involves the distal airways and alveoli. There are numerous agents that can be the impetus for developing hypersensitivity pneumonitis; these include moldy hay or grains, fungi from water reservoirs, bird serum, feathers and excreta, mining dust and pharmacological products such as gold, amiodarone and minocycline. The inflammatory response persists beyond the exposure time and leads to permanent lung damage. There is infiltration of macrophages and lymphocytes and epithelioid granuloma formation, which eventually leads to obliteration of the bronchioles because of scarring. If the disease progresses into the chronic phase, the granulomas disappear and are replaced by fibrotic tissue formation and destruction of the architecture of the lung.

Acute respiratory distress syndrome

Acute respiratory distress syndrome (ARDS) is an acute lung injury that results in pulmonary infiltrates, severe refractory oxygenation and an increase in lung stiffness (i.e. a decrease in compliance). It has been suggested that ARDS is the severest form of pulmonary edema, in which diffuse alveolar involvement proceeds to promote further injury. In total, 22% of trauma cases that are complicated with ARDS will involve a lung contusion. In addition, 50% of aspiration cases will progress to ARDS, with 85% of the cases showing signs of ARDS within 72 h.

This heterogeneous disorder changes over time. The initial phase (exudate phase) is characterized by pulmonary edema, hemorrhage and hyaline membrane formation. Clinically, there is a rapid onset of respiratory failure that is refractory to supplemental oxygen. The second phase involves cellular proliferation, with an elevation in the number of neutrophils and other inflammatory cells. This phase is characterized by diffuse alveolar disease (DAD); this is associated with cellular necrosis, epithelial hyperplasia and further inflammation, which leads to destruction of the delicate structures of the lung. The third phase is fibroproliferation, which is the result of chronic inflammation whereby injured lung tissue is replaced with fibrotic tissue. Beyond the destruction of terminal bronchioles and alveoli, there is also obliteration of the pulmonary capillaries, leading to pulmonary hypertension and, eventually, right heart failure (Blaivas 2004, Piantadosi & Schwartz 2004).

Idiopathic pulmonary fibrosis

The onset of idiopathic pulmonary fibrosis (IPF) occurs in mid to late life with usual interstitial pneumonia (UIP) characterized by patchy, non-uniform and variable destruction of interstitial tissue. There is a minimal inflammatory component to this disease, involving collagen deposition that thickens the alveolar septum. Desquamative interstitial pneumonia (DIP) is another form of IPF that presents with little fibrosis but a significant inflammatory response, with an accumulation of alveolar macrophages within the alveolar spaces and interstitium. The initial injury appears to damage the alveolar and epithelial cells, causing inflammatory cells to release cytokines, tumor necrosis factor and platelet-derived growth factor. These inflammatory chemicals result in smooth muscle proliferation, degradation of the alveoli and the proliferation of fibroblasts and an increase in collagen deposition (Swigris et al 2005).

Clinical manifestation

Despite the range of etiologies that result in pulmonary fibrosis, patients present with a similar clinical picture of a slowly progressive decline, exertional dyspnea, a nonproductive cough that worsens with exertion and severe cyanosis. Along with severe dyspnea, patients generally experience severe desaturation with exertion. There is a decrease in normal breath sounds and the development of rales and clubbing of the nail beds. The breathing pattern is typically shallow with an elevated rate and there is a reduction of rib cage mobility, leading to a marked increase in the work of breathing. Anorexia, malaise and muscle weakness are also common clinical signs. Finally, pulmonary fibrosis is commonly associated with pulmonary hypertension and right heart failure.

Conventional chest radiography reveals diffuse infiltrates, and honeycombing develops in the later stages of pulmonary fibrosis. When pulmonary function tests are examined, there is a decrease in lung volume, especially vital capacity (VC) and total lung capacity (TLC), a decrease in the gas exchange ability of the respiratory system [diffusion capacity; measured using the diffusing capacity of the lung for carbon monoxide (DLCO) test] and a decreased pulmonary compliance with a normal FEV_1–FVC ratio (see Fig. 47.3). A ventilation–perfusion mismatch occurs as ventilation declines and this is associated with severe hypoxia (Lindell & Jacobs 2003).

Therapeutic intervention

The best defense against pneumoconioses is prevention; this is achieved with the use of proper respiratory filter devices and proper ventilation in the work area. Management includes the use of corticosteroids to minimize the inflammatory response and monitoring the progression of the disease with radiological studies, pulmonary function tests and exercise testing. Other medications that inhibit the immune response are also utilized in the treatment of IPF. Cyclophosphamide impairs the function of neutrophils, eventually decreasing fibroblast and collagen proliferation. Azathioprine and cyclosporin (ciclosporin) suppress the production and maturation of T and B cells involved in the immune response. With the progression of the disease, medical care may include the use of supplemental oxygen and prostacyclin drugs for the treatment of right heart failure resulting from pulmonary hypertension. Mechanical ventilatory support may be helpful to decrease the work of breathing, improve oxygen delivery and allow for rest periods. In the presence of isolated pulmonary fibrosis, lung transplantation should be considered on a case-by-case base.

Pulmonary rehabilitation can also be beneficial for patients with pulmonary fibrosis. Once again, the ultimate goal is to improve the quality of life. An educational and exercise program, similar to that described in the COPD section, should be provided for this patient population but the clinician should expect the progress to be much slower than with COPD patients. It is important that the exercise program includes stretching exercises to maintain chest wall mobility and, in the presence of pulmonary hypertension, interval exercises. Prescribed rest times are essential to decrease the strain on the right ventricle. These patients typically require high levels of supplemental oxygen to prevent severe hypoxia. The disease progression is generally aggressive, so work simplification training is also valuable.

The prognosis is generally poor for patients with pulmonary fibrosis because of refractory hypoxemia, right heart failure and the increased risk of bronchogenic carcinoma in patients who smoke and those with occupational exposure pulmonary fibrosis. In ARDS, the mortality rate is as high as 60%, with a higher death rate in older patients because of respiratory failure. In general, the mean survival time in cases of pulmonary fibrosis is 3–6 years but this will vary based on the aggressiveness and type of disease, duration of symptoms and responsiveness to therapy (Lindell & Jacobs 2003, Khalil & O'Connor 2004).

PULMONARY HYPERTENSION

Secondary pulmonary hypertension can be the sequela of a congenital heart defect, collagen vascular disease, lung disease with hypoxia, thromboembolic disease and left heart failure resulting from cardiomyopathy and valvular disease. As pulmonary disease progresses to the point where the pulmonary capillary bed becomes affected, pulmonary pressure begins to rise. Pulmonary hypertension can be defined as a mean pulmonary arterial pressure that is greater than 25 mmHg at rest and greater than 30 mmHg during exercise.

A significant amount of the lung parenchyma must be involved to cause pulmonary hypertension because the reserve capacity of the lungs is so vast. As the intrinsic obstructive lung disease progresses, the disruption of capillary beds and destruction of the gas exchange area of the parenchymal tissue leads to hypoxia and vasoconstriction, producing pulmonary hypertension. Precapillary arteries and arterioles also become less distensible and constricted. With pulmonary fibrosis, for example in collagen vascular disease, the scarring of the airways and capillaries causes a decrease in compliance and arterial hypertension. The consequences of abnormal and chronic vasoconstriction include intimal proliferation, smooth muscle hypertrophy and changes in the endothelium that lead to a decrease in the diameter of the arterial lumen and vascular remodeling.

If the pulmonary pressure is not relieved, the pulmonary vascular system becomes less distensible and blood is shunted to the larger vessels, which causes a ventilation–perfusion mismatch. To compensate for the elevated pulmonary vascular resistance and to maintain cardiac output, the right ventricle hypertrophies. Over time, the myocardium dilates and is unable to maintain efficient blood flow through the lungs for gas exchange, leading to heart failure.

Clinical manifestation

The progression of dyspnea and the early onset of fatigue are typically the first symptoms of pulmonary hypertension, although many patients associate this with aging and deconditioning. Patients may begin to complain of presyncopal symptoms or may experience syncope. Chest pain, muscle fatigue, hypoxemia and hemoptysis are other common symptoms related to pulmonary hypertension. As the patient develops cor pulmonale, the signs and symptoms of right heart failure become present, which include jugular vein distension, peripheral edema and hepatic congestion.

Upon examination, the right ventricle may be palpable in the lower left sternal or subxiphoid area and abnormal heart sounds are present, including S4 gallop and a split S2 sound. As the disease progresses, S3 gallop can be heard, indicating advanced right heart failure. Abnormal valvular heart sounds may also be audible including a systolic ejection click and tricuspid murmur. The electrocardiogram (ECG) is consistent with right ventricular hypertrophy and changes in the T wave. As the disease progresses, there will be clear signs of right heart failure in most cases including jugular vein distension, hepatic congestion, peripheral edema, ascites and systemic hypotension (Higenbottam 2005).

Therapeutic intervention

The treatment of pulmonary hypertension involves treating the primary cause of the hypertension. Drugs to decrease the strain on the right side of the heart, such as digitalis and diuretics, and supplemental oxygen therapy to treat the hypoxemia may be effective. Continuous intravenous prostacyclins, for example Flolan, may decrease pulmonary hypertension by vasodilation when infused into the pulmonary arterial system. The most common positive effects of the intravenous use of prostacyclins are an improvement in exercise tolerance and a decrease in symptoms experienced at rest and with exertion. Anticoagulation medications may be used to decrease the risk of thromboembolic events because of polycythemia, which may develop as a compensatory mechanism to offset hypoxemia.

Rehabilitation for patients with pulmonary hypertension typically focuses on functional mobility. It is also important to review job simplification and energy conservation in these patients. Patients typically tolerate an interval aerobic program, particularly a walking program. Exercises that isolate muscle groups, such as cycling, are usually less well tolerated because of local muscle fatigue. It is important that the therapist prescribe an exercise intensity that is sufficient for the patient to experience the benefits of exercise without causing abnormal responses to exertion. These patients should be monitored closely for signs of chest discomfort, lightheadedness or excessive fatigue. The therapist should also educate the patient about the adverse signs and symptoms that indicate distress and progression of the disease. It is also vital that the therapist works directly with the physician to establish safe parameters for functional mobility activities (see Box 41.4 and Tables 41.4 and 41.6 for guidelines).

PULMONARY EMBOLISM

Pulmonary embolism is closely linked to the presence of blood clots or thrombi in the peripheral venous system, known as deep vein thrombosis (DVT). Typically, the source of the embolism originates from a DVT in the upper legs or pelvis. Small emboli may present little compromise to a healthy individual but may cause severe respiratory failure in an elderly individual with a reduced reserve of the cardiopulmonary systems. In the elderly, there are several risk factors that should be part of the clinician's screening process including previous DVT or pulmonary embolism, surgery, malignancy, hormonal therapy, obesity, venous stasis, immobility, cerebrovascular accident (CVA) and heart failure (Charlebois 2005).

Clinical manifestation

The most pronounced clinical presentation in cases of pulmonary embolism includes unexplained dyspnea of rapid onset and pleuritic chest pain. The presence of hemoptysis indicates pulmonary hemorrhage or infarction.

During the process of evaluation, it is important to develop a differential diagnostic list and proceed with testing to enable a clinical diagnosis to be formulated. The differential diagnosis may include the following conditions: acute myocardial infarction (MI), asthma, pneumothorax, congestive heart failure (CHF), acute pulmonary edema, pleurisy, pericarditis, musculoskeletal trauma to the chest wall, sepsis, tamponade and aortic dissection.

Upon physical examination, there may be a low-grade fever, cyanosis, tachycardia, jugular vein distension, tachypnea and hypotension. Upon auscultation, there may be a pleural rub and split of the S2 heart sound may be heard over the pulmonic valve. The degree of respiratory compromise is dependent on the size of the pulmonary embolism and the preexisting cardiopulmonary reserves. An echocardiogram may be suggestive of right heart strain or ischemia and the ECG may demonstrate T-wave inversion.

Clinical intervention

The key to appropriate medical care is the identification of patients that are at high risk and the implementation of effective prophylactic treatment. Treatment includes early mobilization and the use of graduated compression devices and TED stockings. The use of intermittent pneumatic compression stockings provides peripheral pumping to encourage venous return and reduce venous stasis. Many patients will be prescribed anticoagulants for the prevention and treatment of DVT formation. In patients who cannot take anticoagulants, an inferior vena cava filter may be placed to decrease the risk of a pulmonary embolism occurring from a lower extremity or pelvic thrombus. Finally, thrombolytic therapy has also been used successfully to break down the DVT or pulmonary embolism, but is associated with a risk of hemorrhage.

The prognosis for a patient suffering from a pulmonary embolism is dependent upon the size of the pulmonary embolism, the underlying compromise of the cardiopulmonary system and the promptness of medical care.

PULMONARY INFECTIONS

Pneumonia

The pulmonary system has two primary mechanisms to manage the presence of foreign matter that may precipitate a pulmonary infection. The upper airway warms and humidifies the air and the mucociliary cells aid in the entrapment of particles in this conductive system of the lungs. If particles enter the lung, there is an immune response that attacks the foreign material and removes it. When one or both of these mechanisms is impaired, there is an increased risk of developing a pneumonia, which is defined as an acute inflammation of the lungs, causing the small bronchioles and alveoli to become plugged with fibrous exudate.

Pneumonias can be classified based on several parameters: (i) by the etiology underlying the infection, including bacterial, viral and fungal sources; (ii) as typical or atypical, based on the incidence of the infection in a given population or location; and (iii) by the site in which the infection occurs, with acquired pneumonias referring to infections obtained in the community and nosocomial pneumonias defined as infections that occur during the hospitalization of the patient. With the increase in admissions to such facilities as long-term care or nursing homes, acquired infections may be subdivided into community-acquired and institutionally acquired pneumonia. However the infection is classified, there are common risk factors that contribute to the susceptibility of developing pulmonary infections (see Box 47.1)

Box 47.1   Risk factors associated with pulmonary infections

- Age
- Health of the immune system
- State of the pulmonary system
- Ability to protect airway
- Mechanical ventilation
- Medications
- General health status
- Atelectasis
- Aerosolized breathing
- Functional mobility status
- Level of alertness
- Hospitalization (intensive care unit)
- Gastroesophageal reflux disease
- Smoking
- Strength and motor control

When a pathogen enters the respiratory system and is able to multiply and overwhelm the preventive function of the immune system, an infection begins and the inflammatory process is activated along with a further response from the immune system. This vicious cycle continues, leading to the progression of edema and the aggregation of red and white blood cells, which begins to interfere with the ability of the lungs to ventilate and participate in diffusion.

Clinical manifestation

The typical clinical presentation for pneumonia includes fever and a productive cough with sputum that is usually yellowish-green or a rust color. In most cases, there is also an elevation in the white blood cell count and a positive sputum culture identifying the infectious agent. The patient may report an increased level of fatigue and weight loss. If a substantial amount of lung tissue is involved, the patient may also present with dyspnea, tachycardia and tachypnea, and hypoxemia with desaturation upon exertion. The elderly patient may present with atypical signs and symptoms. Consequently, the clinician needs to monitor the patient's vital signs as well as be aware of any unexplained changes in mental status, an increased incidence of falls, decreased appetite, incontinence and decreased functional mobility and activity tolerance.

The diagnosis of pneumonia is based on a series of clinical findings, including a positive chest radiograph showing infiltration or consolidation of the infected segment along with clinical symptoms. The clinician should also be aware of the patient's oral motor control. In patients with poor motor control, hypotonic state of the musculature of the face and neck, poor phonation and difficulty with motor

planning and execution, the clinician should have a heightened concern for aspiration pneumonia.

Clinical intervention

The primary focus of care should be prevention, which includes proper cleaning of rooms and equipment and compliance with good hand washing. Emphasis should be placed on mobilizing patients to decrease the incidence of atelectasis and muscle atrophy. In patients that cannot participate in some form of exercise or mobilization, methods to increase the minute ventilation, a program of assisted repositioning and assisted breathing and coughing techniques should be employed. Proper seating should be achieved to minimize aspiration. Good dental hygiene is important and all high-risk patients should receive an annual flu vaccine.

Once the diagnosis of pneumonia has been made, treatment should include the administration of the correct medications based on the suspected pathogen. Typically, the patient is placed on a widespectrum antibiotic. If the signs and symptoms do not resolve or become recurrent, a sputum culture should be tested. Chest physical therapy or other techniques to promote the mobilization of sputum, increase lung volumes and assist in effective cough should be implemented. Mobilizing the patient is also vital to increase ventilation and diffusion of the lungs and to promote increases in minute ventilation.

Prognosis is dependent upon may factors including age and the presence of other comorbidities such as smoking, COPD, diabetes mellitus, heart failure and decreased mental status. The need for mechanical ventilation only increases mortality rates. The pathogen's sensitivity to medication will affect the outcome, including the patient's level of function.

Mycobacterium tuberculosis

With the increase in the number of patients who are living with an impaired immune system because of human immunodeficiency virus (HIV) infection and acquired immunodeficiency syndrome (AIDS), transplantation, a general increase in life expectancy, substance abuse and homelessness with malnutrition, mycobacterium tuberculosis is on the rise.

As a primary infection, mycobacterium tuberculosis is an airborne-acquired infection of the lungs. It is spread when a person has sufficient exposure to an infected individual and is commonly transmitted through coughing or sneezing. The risk of infection is dependent on exposure, concentration of the mycobacterium and the health of the immune system. The incubation period is 2–12 weeks. The disease can be reactivated or a secondary infection can occur when the patient's immune system is further compromised because of illness or aging. The site of infection can be the lungs or elsewhere in the body (Zevallos & Justman 2003).

Clinical manifestation

During the primary infection, most patients are asymptomatic. If there are signs and symptoms, they are similar to the clinical presentation of pneumonia, with a nonproductive cough and fever. Lymph nodes are enlarged and the patient may experience chest wall or pleuritic pain if the pleural lining is involved. Rales may be heard in the area of infection over the infected segments of the lungs, along with bronchial breath sounds if there is consolidation. Radiographs are abnormal, showing atelectasis and usually cavitations in the upper lobes. There is scarring of the lungs, with a loss of tissue function.

Secondary infections are associated with a cough that becomes increasingly productive as the disease progresses, night sweats, weight loss, low-grade fever and sometimes pleuritic pain. There are subtle inspiratory rales, a decrease in tactile fremitus and breath sounds over areas of pleural thickening and cavitation. The signs and symptoms of extrapulmonary disease are dependent upon the particular tissue that is infected.

Clinical intervention

The best intervention is again preventative, including the use of universal precautions, general healthcare for high-risk groups and screening. If a skin test is positive, individuals should undergo a year of treatment to minimize the risk of a secondary infection. During the primary infection, respiratory isolation is important to minimize the spread of the disease and clinicians should comply with the use of personal protective equipment. Patients are usually given rifampin and isoniazid for 1 year to suppress the infection. Further medical or surgical intervention will depend on the site and severity of the extrapulmonary infections.

PULMONARY ONCOLOGY

Lung cancer is a leading cause of cancer-related deaths in the US despite the advances in diagnostic and medical therapies. As part of the medical workup, it is important to obtain an accurate history of tobacco use and occupational exposures that increase the risk of developing lung cancer.

Lung carcinomas are divided into small cell and non-small cell cancers. Small cell carcinomas are linked to smoking and there is a high incidence of metastasis at the time of diagnosis, either to bone or the brain. The non-small cell carcinomas include squamous cell cancer, adenocarcinoma and large cell cancer. Non-small cell cancer constitutes more than three-quarters of lung cancer diagnoses. The lung can be the primary site of the cancer or secondary to metastatic cancer from another site, such as breast or colorectal cancer (Institute NC 2003).

Clinical manifestation

In many instances, the diagnosis of lung cancer is made during routine testing for another elective procedure. In other cases, the patient may seek medical attention because of a persistent cough, hemoptysis, dull ache in the thorax, fatigue and progressive shortness of breath. A thorough interview may reveal sleep disturbances, night sweats and unintentional weight loss. Diagnosis is made by abnormal findings on radiographic studies and is confirmed with a biopsy.

Clinical intervention

As for many of the diseases briefly discussed in this chapter, prevention is the first line of treatment. Smoking cessation and decreasing exposure to chemicals and particles is vital. Routine medical screening, such as mammograms and colonoscopies, has had a huge impact on the early detection and treatment of cancer in general. Medical management may include radiation, chemotherapy or surgical resection. The treatment that is offered to the patient will depend on the type and staging of the tumor. Prognosis is improving but, once again, is dependent on the type of cancer, time of detection and responsiveness to medical therapies. Therapy may involve a spectrum of care, including general strength and conditioning, pain management, functional mobility restoration after surgery and end-of-life issues.

CONCLUSION

This chapter briefly discussed the three major categories of intrinsic lung disease that can impair activity tolerance and diminish quality of life. Clinically, these diseases present with a constellation of signs and symptoms that facilitate diagnosis and management. In the elderly, emphysema is so prevalent after the fifth decade of life that it is important for the therapist to be very familiar with the clinical characteristics of both emphysema and chronic bronchitis, and the management of obstructive lung disease. Rehabilitation involving education, strengthening and aerobic exercise is an effective intervention for patients with obstructive disease. The therapist should also be able to modify the rehabilitation process for patients with pulmonary fibrosis and pulmonary hypertension. The ultimate goal of a comprehensive plan of care is to improve functional mobility and quality of life.

References

Anonymous 2004 Effects of pulmonary rehabilitation on dyspnea, quality of life and health care cost in California. J Cardiopulm Rehabil 24(1):52–62

Blaivas A 2004 Available: www.nlm.nih.gov/medlineplus. May 5 2004

Charlebois D 2005 Early recognition of pulmonary embolism: the key to lowering mortality. J Cardiovasc Nurs 20(4):254–259

Higenbottam T 2005 Pulmonary hypertension and chronic obstructive pulmonary disease. Proc Am Thoracic Soc 2:12–19

Hogg J 2004 Pathophysiology of airflow limitation in chronic obstructive pulmonary disease. Lancet 364:709–721

Institute NC 2003 Available: http://nihseniorhealth.gov/lungcancer/toc.html. March 2003

Khalil N, O'Connor 2004 Idiopathic pulmonary fibrosis: current understanding of the pathogenesis and the status of treatment. Can Med Assoc J 171(2):153–160

Kushner W, Stark P 2003 Occupational lung disease, part 2: discovering the cause of diffuse parenchymal lung disease. Postgrad Med 113(4):81–88

Lindell K, Jacobs S 2003 Pulmonary fibrosis: new guidelines for diagnosing and managing the disease. Demand a fresh approach to nursing care. Am J Nurs 103(4):33–42

Nathan S, Edwards L, Barnett S, Burton N 2004 Outcomes of COPD lung transplant recipients after lung volume reduction surgery. Chest 126(5):1569–1574

Piantadosi C, Schwartz D 2004 The acute respiratory distress syndrome. Ann Intern Med 141:460–470

Pinto-Plata V, Cote C, Cabral H et al 2004 The 6-minute walk distance: change over time and value as a predictor of survival in severe COPD. Eur Respir J 23:28–33

Ross R 2003 The clinical diagnosis of asbestosis in this century requires more than a chest radiograph. Chest 124(3):1120–1128

Salman G, Mosier M, Beasley B, Calkens D 2003 Rehabilitation for patients with chronic obstructive pulmonary disease: meta-analysis of randomized controlled trials. J Gen Intern Med 18(3):213–221

Swigris JJ, Kushner WG, Kelsey JL, Gould MK 2005 Idiopathic pulmonary fibrosis: challenges and opportunities for the clinician and investigator. Chest 127:275–283

White A, Gompertz S, Stockley R 2003 Chronic obstructive pulmonary disease: the aetiology of exacerbations of chronic obstructive pulmonary disease. Thorax 58:73–80

Zevallos M, Justman J 2003 Tuberculosis in the elderly. Clin Geriatr Med 19: 121–138

UNIT 6

Blood vessel changes, circulatory and skin disorders

Chapter 48

Diabetes

Dominique Noë Long, Carol Probst, David E. Kelley and Emily L. Germain-Lee

CHAPTER CONTENTS

INTRODUCTION

Diabetes mellitus is a prevalent disease, especially among the elderly. In the last 10 years alone, the prevalence of diagnosed diabetes cases has increased by 50%, mostly because of the increase in obesity. Age-related changes involving decreased insulin sensitivity in the peripheral tissues and reduced insulin control of hepatic glucose output, coupled with physical inactivity and increased obesity, contribute to higher incidences of abnormal glucose tolerance in the older population.

It is estimated that the prevalence of diabetes for all age groups worldwide was 2.8% in 2000 and will be 4.4% in 2030. The total number of people with diabetes in 2000 was 171 million and it has been estimated that this number will rise to 366 million in 2030. The increasing proportion of individuals who are older than 65 years of age is an important demographic influence (Wild et al 2004).

Diabetes is more prevalent in certain populations, for example American Indians/native Alaskans, Hispanic/Latino Americans and African–Americans. Approximately 18.2 million people in the US, or 6.3% of the total US population, have diabetes mellitus. Of those aged 60 or above, 8.6 million, or 18.3%, have diabetes. It is estimated that one-third of these individuals are unaware of their disease state. Further, it is estimated that 41 million adults aged between 40 and 74 have impaired glucose tolerance (IGT), a condition that often precedes diabetes mellitus. Diabetes mellitus is a serious disease that causes a wide range of complications. In 2002, the total cost of diabetes in the US was US$132 billion, US$40 billion of which resulted from indirect costs because of disability, work loss or premature mortality (National Diabetes Fact Sheet 2003).

CLASSIFICATION AND DIAGNOSIS OF DIABETES MELLITUS

In 2003, the American Diabetes Association (ADA) modified the diagnostic criteria for the classification of impaired fasting glucose (IFG) and diabetes. There are four clinical classes of diabetes including type 1, type 2, other specific types of diabetes (genetic defects in β-cell function or insulin action, disease of exocrine pancreas, drug- or chemically-induced diabetes) and gestational diabetes mellitus (GDM). An elevated fasting glucose is one of several risk factors that are known to increase an individual's risk of developing heart disease, stroke and diabetes. These risk factors, grouped together, are called the 'metabolic syndrome' or 'syndrome X' and will be discussed later in this chapter (see under Medical treatment). For the purposes of this chapter, discussion will focus on type 1 and type 2 diabetes (see Table 48.1).

There are three ways to diagnose diabetes, each of which must be confirmed on a subsequent day unless there are definitive symptoms of hyperglycemia, such as excess thirst and urination (polydipsia and polyuria), and unexplained weight loss accompanied by increased or normal food intake. The criteria for the diagnosis of diabetes include the following: (i) symptoms of diabetes and a random plasma glucose $\geq 200 \, \text{mg/dL}$ (11.1 mmol/L); (ii) fasting plasma glucose (FPG) $\geq 126 \, \text{mg/dL}$ (7.0 mmol/L) (fasting is defined as no

Table 48.1 Comparison of type 1 and type 2 diabetes

	Type 1 diabetes	Type 2 diabetes
No. of diabetics (%)	2–5	90–95
Onset of disease	Abrupt	Insidious
Age of onset	<35 years	>35 years
Symptoms at onset	Often ketoacidosis	May be asymptomatic
Requiring insulin	Yes	In 25% of cases
Risk for ketoacidosis	Yes	Rare
Body type	Thin or normal	80% are overweight
Suspected cause	Autoimmune reaction with islet cell destruction	Insulin resistance/ poor insulin secretion
Genetic predisposition	Yes	Yes

caloric intake for at least 8 h); and (iii) 2-h plasma glucose ≥200 mg/dL (11.1 mmol/L) during an oral glucose tolerance test (OGTT) with 75 g of glucose. FPG is the preferred test for diagnosing diabetes in nonpregnant adults. Other common presenting symptoms of diabetes include poor wound healing, fatigue, vaginal yeast infections and blurred vision (American Diabetes Association 2005).

Hyperglycemia that is not sufficient to meet the diagnostic criteria for diabetes is categorized as either IFG or IGT. IFG is defined as a FPG between 100 mg/dL (5.6 mmol/L) and 125 mg/dL (6.9 mmol/L). IGT is defined as a 2-h plasma glucose between 140 mg/dL (7.8 mmol/L) and 199 mg/dL (11.0 mmol/L). IFG and IGT are also called 'prediabetes' (American Diabetes Association 2005).

TYPES OF DIABETES MELLITUS

Type 1

Type 1 diabetes is caused by autoimmune destruction of the insulin-producing β-cells of the pancreatic islets; as a result, these patients have an absolute need for insulin therapy. The age of onset of type 1 diabetes is most commonly during childhood or young adulthood, although it can begin at any age. In the absence of insulin replacement, patients with type 1 diabetes develop severe hyperglycemia and metabolic acidosis, which results from the excess production of ketones, a by-product of fat breakdown in the absence of insulin. Diabetic ketoacidosis (DKA) is a medical emergency.

Type 2

Of all individuals with diabetes, 90–95% have type 2 diabetes. This is most commonly a disease of adults and its incidence increases with each decade of aging. However, type 2 diabetes is increasingly being diagnosed in children and adolescents. Type 2 diabetes is associated with obesity, a family history of diabetes, a previous history of gestational diabetes, IGT, physical inactivity and the physical finding of acanthosis nigricans. Other factors associated with type 2 diabetes are race/ethnicity, with African–Americans, Hispanic/Latino Americans, native Americans and some Asian–Americans and other Pacific Islanders being at particularly high risk. Type 2 diabetes is regarded as being a metabolic disorder that is linked to a modern lifestyle involving stress, excess caloric intake (particularly fat) and inadequate physical activity. From a metabolic perspective, these patients generally have the twin defects of sluggish secretion of insulin following meals (leading to poor overall insulin production with long duration) and peripheral insulin resistance (reduced cellular uptake and utilization of insulin).

THERAPEUTIC INTERVENTION

Newly diagnosed diabetes

Patients newly diagnosed with diabetes mellitus have a special need for comprehensive education. Diabetes self-management education is an integral component of medical care. The onset of diabetes can be precipitated by physical and emotional stress and other illnesses and, usually, the diabetic state persists. In addition, certain medications, most notably oral or parenteral steroid therapy, can trigger the onset of diabetes mellitus or upset metabolic control in a previously diagnosed patient.

Medical treatment

Diet and exercise are the cornerstones of the treatment of type 2 diabetes mellitus and many individuals with diabetes can control their blood glucose by following a careful diet and exercise program, losing excess weight and taking oral hypoglycemic agents (medications that lower plasma glucose levels). Generally, it is not necessary to increase food intake before exercise of short duration or low intensity. Exercise of moderate intensity (e.g. 1 h of tennis) may be preceded by consuming 10–15 g of carbohydrate, although this is often unnecessary.

Among adults with diagnosed diabetes, about 12% take both insulin and oral medications, 19% take insulin only, 53% take oral medications only and 15% take neither insulin nor oral medications.

Glycemic control in patients with type 1 and 2 diabetes is most often measured using levels of blood glycosylated hemoglobin, or hemoglobin A_{1c} (HbA_{1c}), in addition to self-monitoring of blood glucose. The HbA_{1c} level reflects the mean blood glucose concentration over the previous 6–12 weeks. The ADA's current glycemic goal for nonpregnant adults is a value of <7.0% (compared with a normal nondiabetic range of 4–6%).

As many as one in six Americans over the age of 50 may have the 'metabolic syndrome', a pathophysiological condition that increases the risk of heart disease, stroke and diabetes. The criteria for metabolic syndrome are met by having any three of the following risk factors, which have been recently defined by the American Heart Association: (i) an elevated waist circumference (abdominal obesity), (ii) an elevated triglyceride level of ≥150 mg/dL, (iii) a reduced high-density lipoprotein (HDL; good cholesterol) level of <40 mg/dL for men and <50 mg/dL for women, (iv) an elevated blood pressure of 130/85 mmHg or higher; and (v) an elevated fasting glucose of ≥100 mg/dL.

Although it is clear that each of the above risk factors does increase an individual's cardiovascular risk, the ADA recently stated that the metabolic syndrome has been vaguely defined and should not be designated as a syndrome until more research is completed (American Diabetes Association Statement 2005). The ADA recommends that blood pressure in patients with diabetes should be <130/80 mmHg. Lipid goals for patients with diabetes include a low-density lipoprotein (LDL) level of <100 mg/dL (<2.6 mmol/L), tri-glyceride level <150 mg/dL (<1.7 mmol/L) and HDL level >40 mg/dL (>1.1 mmol/L) (American Diabetes Association 2005).

Insulin therapy for type 1 diabetes

Therapy for individuals with type 1 diabetes always includes insulin. Insulin is given by subcutaneous injection or with an insulin pump, which also delivers insulin subcutaneously. Combinations of rapid-, short-, intermediate- or long-acting insulin are used, such as Humalog, Regular, NPH and glargine respectively. In most centers, patients with type 1 diabetes are treated with two or three doses per day of rapid- or short-acting insulin combined with intermediate-acting insulin. However, many patients require more frequent insulin injections to obtain good glycemic control. Cross-sectional studies have not documented improved control with an increasing number of insulin injections per day, showing that the number of injections alone is not sufficient to achieve optimal glycemic control. The method of using long-acting insulin (glargine) combined with rapid-acting insulin (Humalog), given before meals and snacks, provides greater flexibility but requires a knowledge of carbohydrate counting and the use of an insulin–carbohydrate ratio. Because blood glucose can fluctuate widely in patients with type 1 diabetes, it is recommended that blood glucose be monitored several times a day, before meals and bedtime, and insulin doses adjusted accordingly.

The Diabetes Control and Complications Trial (DCCT) demonstrated that the risk of progression of diabetic microvascular disease (retinopathy, nephropathy and neuropathy) and possibly the occurrence of macrovascular disease (cardiovascular) in patients with type 1 diabetes can be significantly reduced with improved glycemic control.

Treatment of type 2 diabetes

Treatment options for patients with type 2 diabetes are diverse. Control can be achieved with diet and exercise therapy, especially if weight loss is achieved in an overweight patient. However, most type 2 patients also require some pharmacological treatment, either oral hypoglycemic medication or insulin. Oral medications include the sulfonylureas (e.g. glyburide, glipizide, chlorpropamide) and meglitinides, which increase insulin release; thiazolidinediones (rosiglitazone, pioglitazone), which increase target tissue sensitivity to insulin; metformin, which increases glucose utilization and decreases glucose production by the liver; acarbose, which slows down the absorption of carbohydrate through the intestine; and prandial glucose regulators (repaglinide), which are taken with meals and help to increase insulin release. These medications can be used alone or in combination.

The United Kingdom Prospective Diabetes Study (UKPDS) showed that good glycemic control in patients with type 2 diabetes results in a reduction in the risk of microvascular disease. Specifically, a 1% fall in HbA_{1c} was associated with a 35% reduction in microvascular complications (retinopathy, nephropathy and neuropathy). The risk reduction of macrovascular disease was less clear. Based on the results of the UKPDS, normoglycemia is now the goal for most patients with type 2 diabetes. Although insulin may be considered for initial therapy in type 2 diabetes, especially if the patient presents with a very elevated HbA_{1c} level, it is most often used when hyperglycemia persists despite the use of oral hypoglycemic agents. The dose of insulin needed to control glucose levels in obese patients with type 2 diabetes can be extremely large.

Hypoglycemia

The main adverse effect of insulin or oral therapy is hypoglycemia (low blood glucose). In a patient with diabetes, symptoms of hypoglycemia generally have a rapid onset and occur when blood glucose is less than 70–80 mg/dL (Table 48.2). A severe reaction can occur below 60 mg/dL. A patient may complain of shakiness and sweating or other symptoms caused by increased epinephrine (adrenaline) release, such as tachycardia and anxiety. Deprivation of glucose in the central nervous system causes blurred vision, weakness, confusion, slurred speech and, potentially, seizure and coma, with permanent neurological damage. Symptoms of hypoglycemia may be blunted in a patient with long-standing diabetes, especially the early warning signs of nervousness, tremor and sweating. The initial symptom in patients with long-standing diabetes mellitus may be confusion.

In a diabetic patient, hypoglycemia occurs because of too much insulin (or oral medications), insufficient food intake (relative to

Table 48.2 Comparison of diabetic complications

	Complication		
	Hyperglycemia with diabetic ketoacidosis (DKA)	Hyperglycemia, hyperosmolarity, nonketosis, coma	Hypoglycemia
Precipitating factors	Absence of insulin	Illness, infections, steroid use, burns	Excessive exogenous insulin, decreased oral intake, stress
Onset	Gradual	Gradual	Abrupt
Initial effect	Lethargy	Lethargy	Agitation, shakiness
Skin	Hot, dry	Warm	Clammy, diaphoretic
Serum glucose levels	>300 mg/dL	>300 mg/dL	<70 mg/dL
Hydration	Increased thirst, polyuria, dehydration	Rapid volume depletion with increased thirst; initial polyuria progressing to decreased urine output	Unchanged
Cardiopulmonary symptoms	Rapid deep breathing		Tachycardia
Early CNS symptoms	Headache		Headache, blurred vision, slurred speech
Late CNS symptoms	Confusion, coma, death	Confusion, coma, death	Confusion, coma, rarely death
Metabolic acidosis	Elevated serum acetone and ketone bodies in urine, fruity breath	No	No
GI symptoms	Abdominal pain	Abdominal pain	Hunger
Intervention required	Insulin, fluid and sodium bicarbonate replacement	Insulin, fluid and electrolyte replacement	4 oz (120 mL) juice, half a nondiet soda, two glucose tablets or two to four hard candies

CNS, central nervous system; GI, gastrointestinal.

insulin or medication dose) or increased physical activity (again, relative to insulin dose). Treatment of hypoglycemia must be prompt. Mild hypoglycemia can usually be quickly reversed by ingesting something containing sugar. Handy sources of sugar include 4 oz (120 mL) of orange juice, half a nondiet soda, a few hard candies, two glucose tablets or two packets of sugar. Patients with a hypoglycemic episode should monitor their blood sugar carefully in the hours following the episode. Severe hypoglycemic reactions can require intravenous glucose or an intramuscular glucagon injection; these are also necessary if the patient is obtunded and cannot safely be given oral glucose because of the risk of aspiration. A therapist who has treated a patient for a severe hypoglycemic reaction should always notify the physician. Hypoglycemia caused by sulfonylureas can be prolonged and has a higher risk of mortality than that caused by insulin; patients can require short-term hospitalization.

Exercise and diabetes

Individuals without diabetes can maintain stable blood glucose levels during exercise. However, physical activity can have a marked effect on blood glucose in a person with diabetes. Exercise increases glucose use by muscles and improves muscle sensitivity to insulin. A regular program of exercise may lower the requirements for insulin or oral medication. These are desirable effects but it should be recognized that exercise can increase the risk of hypoglycemia. About 30 min of interval or continuous exercise can decrease blood glucose regardless of fitness level.

Glucose control does not always improve with exercise, so the effect must be evaluated for each patient. Patients should increase their blood glucose self-monitoring during exercise. This is especially important for patients on insulin or oral medications. At the beginning of an exercise program, particularly with type 1 diabetic patients, blood glucose levels should be checked before exercise, every 15–30 min during exercise and after stopping exercise. Blood glucose should continue to be checked frequently, as levels can continue to fall for up to 24 h after exercising. Blood glucose self-monitoring data can be used to assess a patient's response to physical activity and improve performance.

Hyperglycemia

In type 1 diabetes, exercising during insulin insufficiency can promote a hyperglycemic response and place the individual at risk for metabolic acidosis. Additional insulin may have to be administered and exercise deferred if the glucose level is higher than 250 mg/dL and ketones are present in the urine. Caution should be used if blood glucose is >300 mg/dL and no ketosis is present. Patient's with type 1 diabetes should ingest additional carbohydrate if glucose levels are below 100 mg/dL. With type 2 diabetes, the upper value for deferring exercise is higher (300 mg/dL) because ketosis if far less common and is unlikely to be provoked by exercise. Occasionally, especially in elderly type 2 individuals, a medical crisis of severe hyperglycemia and cellular dehydration may develop, often in response to the physiological stress of infection, burns or illness. These individuals may progress to a hyperglycemic, hyperosmolar, nonketotic coma. Because of the absence of ketosis, the diagnosis may be overlooked and, in this population, treatment delay can easily result in mortality (see Table 48.2). Proper hydration during exercise is essential.

If exercise substantially lowers blood glucose, particularly if it drops into the range where hypoglycemia is a risk, then some of the following strategies should be considered. The most fundamental options are either to reduce insulin (or the oral medication dose) on

Table 48.3   Precautions to take during exercise if diabetic

Physical feature	Precaution
Hypoglycemia	Exercise 45–60 min after eating; may need to increase dietary intake before and during exercise; keep sugar supplements handy; be aware of delayed onset (up to 24 h)
Insulin levels	Exercise 1 h after injections; monitor glucose levels carefully; avoid exercise during peak insulin activity; use caution when injecting insulin over an exercising muscle
Cardiovascular functioning	Be aware that vital signs may not be an accurate indicator of exercise tolerance; utilize perceived exertion scale and note dyspnea with exertion; do not exercise with resting claudication
Proliferative retinopathy	Keep systolic blood pressure <170 mmHg; avoid isometrics, Valsalva maneuvers, head-jarring
Autonomic nervous system dysfunction	Be alert to signs of cardiac denervation syndrome (heart rate unresponsive to activity level); orthostatic hypotension; inability to perceive presence of angina or myocardial infarction; distal anhidrosis; poor heat compensation
End-stage renal disease	Stay hydrated; avoid systolic blood pressure >170 mmHg
Peripheral neuropathy	Wear proper footwear; avoid repetitive stresses; monitor distal extremities closely

exercise days or to take a supplemental snack before exercise (Table 48.3). One approach is to reduce the insulin dose by approximately 20%; the glucose response to exercise will provide additional information when making this decision. If weight loss is a goal, it is desirable to avoid supplemental caloric intake. It is also important to consider the timing of exercise with respect to the timing of insulin or oral medication administration and meals. Exercise should be done at least 1–2 h after meals and vigorous exercise should be undertaken when insulin levels are near the lower range. This might be in the morning, before injection or 4 or more hours after injection of regular insulin. Also, consideration should be given to the site of the insulin injection. Insulin injected over an exercising muscle is absorbed more quickly and this translates into more potent glucose-lowering effects. Because of this, if exercising within 30 min of injection, a patient should be advised to use the abdomen, not the arm or thigh, for the subcutaneous injection of insulin (Table 48.3). Exercise should include a standard warm-up and cool-down period as in nondiabetic individuals.

It is common for a patient initially referred for rehabilitation to have a relatively low fitness level that requires a cautious and gradual introduction to exercise. Before increasing the usual patterns of physical activity or starting an exercise program, patients with diabetes should undergo a detailed medical evaluation and, if indicated, appropriate diagnostic studies such as an electrocardiography, graded exercise test or radionuclide stress testing. The presence of micro- and macrovascular complications should be screened for as some may be worsened by the exercise program. Identification of areas of concern will allow the formulation of an individualized exercise program that can minimize the patient's risk.

Table 48.4   Diabetes timeline

Complication	Incidence	Prevention	Screening
Progression from IGT (prediabetes) to diabetes		Lifestyle changes (diet, exercise, behavior modification), pharmacological intervention (metformin, acarbose, troglitazone)	Consider FPG or 2-h OGTT in those ≥45 years with BMI ≥25 kg/m² and those <45 years if overweight and have other risk factors for diabetes. Repeat screen every 3 years
Nephropathy	Occurs in 20–40% of patients with type 2 diabetes; develops slowly over 15–25 years; may be noted early in disease in type 2 diabetes	Optimize blood glucose control (goal HbA$_{1c}$ of <7%); lower blood pressure	Annual test for microalbuminuria after ≥5 years duration of type 1 diabetes and after diagnosis in type 2 diabetes using spot urine microalbumin–creatinine ratio. If found, treat with an ACE inhibitor or an ARB. May require protein restriction
Retinopathy	Occurs in 80% of diabetics after 15 years' duration; occurs in 10–20% at diagnosis with type 2 diabetes	Optimize blood glucose control (goal HbA$_{1c}$ of <7%); lower blood pressure	An initial dilated and comprehensive eye examination within 5 years of onset of type 1 diabetes and shortly after diagnosis in type 2 diabetes. Repeat examination annually
Neuropathy/ delayed wound healing	Occurs in 60–70% of patients with diabetes; symptoms such as numbness and tingling occur 10–20 years after diabetes has been diagnosed; increased risk of foot ulcer or amputation in diabetes of ≥10 years' duration	Optimize blood glucose control (goal HbA$_{1c}$ of <7%)	Annual foot examination to identify high-risk foot conditions. Examination involves a Semmes–Weinstein 5.07 monofilament examination, tuning fork, palpation and visual examination
Cardiovascular disease	60–75% of diabetics die from cardiovascular causes: incidence of CVD is two to three times higher in diabetic men and three to four times higher in diabetic women, after adjusting for age and other risk factors	Optimize blood glucose control (goal HbA$_{1c}$ of <7%); lower blood pressure; treat dyslipidemia if present; with or without aspirin, and smoking cessation	Frequent blood pressure monitoring. Intervention with lifestyle modifications if systolic pressure ≥130 mmHg and diastolic pressure ≥80 mmHg. If systolic pressure ≥140 mmHg or diastolic pressure ≥90 mmHg, should receive drug therapy with ACE inhibitors, ARBs, beta blockers, diuretics or calcium-channel blockers, along with lifestyle changes. Lipids should be checked at least annually (goal: LDL, 100 mg/dL; TG < 150 mg/dL; and HDL > 40 mg/dL)

ACE, angiotensin-converting enzyme; ARB, angiotensin receptor blocker; BMI, body mass index; CVD, cardiovascular disease; FPG, fasting plasma glucose; HbA$_{1c}$, hemoglobin A$_{1c}$; HDL, high-density lipoprotein; IGT, impaired glucose tolerance; LDL, low-density lipoprotein; OGTT, oral glucose tolerance test; TG, tryglycerides.

DIABETIC COMPLICATIONS

Diabetes is a systemic disorder and the function of every organ system in the body can be affected (Table 48.4). The following discussion emphasizes the diabetic complications that have particular relevance to rehabilitation (see Table 48.3).

As mentioned previously, several recent trials, including the DCCT and the UKPDS, have shown that improved glycemic control in patients with type 1 and type 2 diabetes mellitus significantly reduces the risk of development or slows the progression of the microvascular complications of diabetes (retinopathy, nephropathy and neuropathy). The risk of microvascular complications is highest if the HbA$_{1c}$ is above 12% but is also increased at all values above the non-diabetic range.

The data on the effect of glycemic control on the development of macrovascular disease in patients with type 2 diabetes are less clear. However, a recent meta-analysis of 13 prospective cohort studies showed that, for every one percentage point increase in HbA$_{1c}$, the relative risk for any cardiovascular event is 1.18 (Selvin et al 2004).

Clinically, this means that patients with poor glycemic control, as reflected by elevated HbA$_{1c}$ levels, have a higher risk of having a cardiovascular event than someone with better glycemic control, as reflected by a lower HbA$_{1c}$ level.

Cardiovascular functioning

In total, 60–75% of deaths among individuals with diabetes are due to heart disease or stroke (National Diabetes Fact Sheet 2003). Diabetic patients who are at high risk for underlying cardiovascular disease include those above 35 years of age, those above 25 years of age with type 2 diabetes of more than 10 years duration, those above 25 years of age with type 1 diabetes of more than 15 years' duration, those with additional risk factors for coronary disease and those with microvascular disease, peripheral vascular disease or autonomic neuropathy. Diabetic patients who are at high risk for underlying cardiovascular disease may need to undertake a graded exercise test if they are about to begin a moderate to high intensity physical activity program. Patients who have nonspecific ECG changes in response to exercise, or who have nonspecific ST- and T-wave changes on the resting ECG, may require additional tests such as radionuclide stress testing. Clinical judgment must be used when assessing the need for exercise stress testing in patients planning to participate in low intensity forms of physical activity such as walking (American Diabetes Association 2004).

Delayed wound healing

Delayed wound healing is a complication of diabetes that is related to poor metabolic control, arterial insufficiency, neuropathy and other factors. In total, 5–10% of diabetic patients have had past or have present foot ulceration. Individuals at greatest risk are men who have had diabetes for more than 10 years, who have poor glucose control or who have cardiovascular, retinal or renal complications. Diabetic foot ulcers are a principal cause of the high rate of lower extremity amputations in diabetics, which is 1–3 times higher than in nondiabetic individuals. Prevention of foot ulcers is the best therapy, and prevention starts with a careful foot and lower extremity examination along with an aggressive program of patient education. Patients must be taught to monitor closely for blisters and other potential damage to their feet, both before and after exercise. Proper footwear is important, especially for patients with peripheral neuropathy. The use of silica gel or air midsoles, as well as polyester or blend socks to prevent blisters and keep feet dry, may minimize trauma to feet during exercise (Larsen et al 2003, American Diabetes Association 2005).

Neuropathy

Neuropathy is found in approximately 60–70% of individuals with diabetes, with sensory loss being more prevalent than motor loss (see Chapters 34 and 35) (National Diabetes Fact Sheet 2003). Sensory loss typically presents in a stocking/glove pattern. Patients who are unable to perceive the touch of a Semmes–Weinstein 5.07 monofilament on the plantar surface of the foot are at high risk for ulceration. Decreased proprioceptive input may cause balance and motor deficits that typically affect the smaller intrinsic muscles of the feet, thus altering foot structure and pressure dynamics. Patients with insensitive feet (see Chapter 51) are at increased risk for callus or blister formation and this can be the trigger event that leads to serious infection (see Chapter 52), ulcer formation (see Chapter 50) and loss of limb or life (see Chapter 49). The education of patients should include recommendations against walking barefoot and suggestions that water temperatures be tested with the elbow and daily foot inspections be made. Although walking is the form of exercise that many older people prefer, with the considerable advantage of being low in intensity and cost, a diabetic patient with a marked neuropathy or foot deformity may be exposed to an increased risk of foot ulceration with a walking program. These individuals may benefit more from a nonweight-bearing type of exercise, such as cycling or swimming. Prescription footwear with orthotics may alleviate some of the risk. Medicare has authorized payments for podiatry visits and specialized footwear for diabetic individuals. When a transtibial amputation does occur, 60% of diabetic patients lose the remaining leg within 5 years. Smoking significantly compounds the problem (American Diabetes Association 2004).

Physical therapists who are treating orthopedic problems should document a concomitant diagnosis of diabetes, as this may help to justify extended interventions. The healing of a foot ulcer can take weeks to months and a multidisciplinary approach is necessary to optimize conditions.

Vascular complications

Vascular complications are the leading cause of death among individuals with diabetes, as they are at an increased risk for coronary artery disease, stroke and peripheral vascular disease (PVD) and often have coexisting hypertension and dyslipidemia. An examination of the feet of a diabetic should assess for the presence of cold feet, a decrease or absence of the dorsalis pedis and posterior tibial pulses, atrophy of subcutaneous tissues and hair loss, all of which are suggestive of PVD. An ankle brachial pressure index (ABPI) can also be obtained. A positive ABPI indicates the need for further vascular assessment.

Symptomatic PVD often presents as intermittent claudication resulting in a burning cramping sensation, usually in the calf, that is caused by activity-induced ischemia. These symptoms can be difficult to distinguish from painful diabetic peripheral neuropathy. Some patients may have significant arterial disease yet remain asymptomatic because of low levels of activity, and the demands of rehabilitation may unmask these problems. Physical rehabilitation should emphasize a graded program of exercise to encourage collateral circulation to the limbs. This entails encouraging patients to exercise the involved muscles to the point of pain but to avoid persisting once ischemia begins. For calf claudication, heel lifts, toe taps, toe raises and ankle circles may be good exercises. It usually takes about 3 months for symptomatic relief through collateral circulation to occur. If the PVD has progressed to the point of constant pain and resting claudication in the foot, all lower extremity exercises are contraindicated. This is because such individuals are at risk for limb loss and require surgical revascularization. Whenever PVD is present, individuals should consult with a physician before using any over-the-counter medications for the foot (American Diabetes Association 2004).

Autonomic neuropathy

In total, 60–70% of individuals with diabetes have mild to severe nervous system damage (National Diabetes Fact Sheet 2003). Autonomic neuropathy develops in the sympathetic and parasympathetic nervous systems of 20–40% of those with long-term diabetes. Exercise programs for diabetic patients with autonomic neuropathy should proceed cautiously. Autonomic neuropathy can result in distal anhidrosis, leading to poor heat dissipation as a result of the decreased sweating in the extremities. Patients with this symptom should avoid overheating when exercising. Genitourinary autonomic dysfunction leads to impotence and the risk of urinary infections. Gastrointestinal disturbances include constipation and diarrhea.

Some individuals with autonomic involvement may present with significant cardiac autonomic neuropathy. These individuals do not perceive anginal pain and may be at risk for 'silent' myocardial infarction. Cardiac arrhythmias are not uncommon. Cardiac denervation syndrome (also referred to as cardiac autonomic neuropathy), a result of autonomic dysfunction, produces a heart rate that is typically around 80–90 beats per minute and is unresponsive to activity levels, beta blockers and antiarrhythmics. If a sustained grip, holding one's breath or a Valsalva maneuver produces no changes in vital signs, cardiac denervation syndrome may be present. The inability of the cardiovascular system to augment cardiac output places such individuals at risk for postural hypotension. Orthostatic problems (a fall in systolic blood pressure of >20 mmHg on standing) superimposed upon cerebral arteriosclerotic changes may precipitate transient ischemic attacks. Whenever cardiac autonomic changes are present, monitoring vital signs to assess exercise tolerance may not always produce accurate information. Individuals in this state should have thorough cardiac workups before increasing activity levels, including stress or resting thallium myocardial scintigraphy to look for the presence and extent of macrovascular coronary heart disease. If cardiac neuropathy is present, during exercise, emphasis should be placed on perceived exertion rates, dyspnea and other observed symptoms of distress and not simply on pulse and blood pressure. Exercise warm-ups and cool-downs should be stressed. Patients prone to orthostatic changes may benefit from minimizing changes in position during rehabilitation, wearing compressive stockings and ensuring an adequate fluid intake (American Diabetes Association 2004).

Retinopathy

Retinopathy is a frequent complication of diabetes. About 80% of type 1 diabetics will have some diabetic retinopathy after 15 years of disease, and 60% of patients with type 2 diabetes will develop some degree of retinopathy after 20 years. Further, 20% of type 2 diabetics have some degree of retinopathy at diagnosis (Larsen et al 2003). Although most cases of retinopathy are of the nonproliferative variety (with only mild background changes in vision), some patients progress to proliferative retinopathy, which is the leading cause of blindness in adults aged from 20 to 74. Using the Joslin Clinic experience, the degree of diabetic retinopathy has been used to stratify the risk of physical activity and to discourage certain activities based on this stratification. For example, in patients with active proliferative diabetic retinopathy (PDR), strenuous activity may lead to vitreous hemorrhage or tractional retinal detachment. Patients with active PDR should avoid physical activity that involves straining, jarring, jogging, high-impact aerobics or Valsalva-like maneuvers. Patients with moderate to severe nonproliferative diabetic retinopathy (NPDR) should also limit activities such as heavy lifting, Valsalva maneuvers, boxing and highly competitive sports. Systolic blood pressure should be kept below 170 mmHg during exercise (American Diabetes Association 2005).

Nephropathy

Diabetic nephropathy occurs in 20–40% of patients with diabetes and is the leading cause of end-stage renal disease, accounting for 43% of new cases (National Diabetes Fact Sheet 2003). The earliest sign of diabetic nephropathy in type 1 diabetes is persistent albuminuria in the range of 30–299 mg over 24 h (microalbuminuria). Microalbuminuria is also a marker for the development of nephropathy in type 2 diabetes, as well as a marker for increased cardiovascular disease risk. Controlling blood pressure has been shown to reduce the development of nephropathy; blood pressure should be carefully monitored during exercise. The ADA has not developed specific physical activity recommendations for patients with microalbuminuria or overt nephropathy. Patients with nephropathy may have a reduced capacity for physical activity leading to self-limitation of activity level. High intensity and strenuous physical activity should probably be discouraged in these individuals unless blood pressure is carefully monitored (Larsen et al 2003, American Diabetes Association 2005).

In 2000, a total of 129 183 people with diabetes underwent dialysis or kidney transplantation (National Diabetes Fact Sheet 2003). For patients on dialysis therapy, fluid replacement is a crucial issue that must influence the scheduling of exercise and rehabilitation. In addition, patients are given heparin during infusions and any wound care that is performed within 24 h of dialysis should minimize aggressive debridement. Exercise programs should incorporate anticoagulant precautions, such as guarding against skin trauma caused by weights, hand placement or jarring, especially at intravenous sites, and there should be renewed vigilance against falling.

CONCLUSION

Diabetes is a common and chronic disease that includes multisystem involvement. Many patients with diabetes mellitus need medical and rehabilitative care because of complications resulting from the diabetes or from other illness. It is important that the healthcare provider be aware of the significant influence that diabetes has on rehabilitation.

References

American Diabetes Association (ADA) 2004 Physical activity/exercise and diabetes. Diabetes Care 27(suppl1):S58–62

American Diabetes Association (ADA) 2005 Standards of medical care in diabetes. Diabetes Care 28(suppl1):S4–36

American Diabetes Association Statement 2005 The metabolic syndrome: time for a critical appraisal. Diabetes Care 28(9):2289–2304

Larsen PR, Kronenberg H, Melmed S, Polonsky K (eds) 2003 Williams Textbook of Endocrinology, 10th edn. Elsevier

National Diabetes Fact Sheet 2003 Available: www.diabetes.org/diabetes-statistics/national-diabetes-fact-sheet.jsp)

Selvin E, Marinopoulos S, Berkenblit G et al 2004 Meta-analysis: glycosylated hemoglobin and cardiovascular disease in diabetes mellitus. Ann Intern Med 141(6):421–431

Wild S, Roglic G, Green A et al 2004 Global prevalence of diabetes: estimates for the year 2000 and projections for 2030. Diabetes Care 27:1047–1053

Chapter 49

Amputations

Joan E. Edelstein

INTRODUCTION

Amputation is the removal of a body segment. Peripheral vascular disease, with or without diabetes, is the leading cause of amputation in the US and Europe; however, dysvascular amputations are likely to increase (Fletcher et al 2002). Trauma, congenital anomalies and cancer are other possible etiologies. Elderly patients are much more likely to have lower than upper limb amputations. Older individuals with amputations resulting from any cause usually have years of experience in accommodating their lifestyles to cope with the interference that amputations impose on walking and other daily activities. Nevertheless, insidious musculoskeletal, neuromuscular, integumentary and cardiopulmonary changes associated with aging are troublesome to older adults with amputations. This is because of the added stress that a limb anomaly and prosthesis impose on remaining tissues (see Chapter 71 for details about evaluating the patient and prescribing prostheses).

CLASSIFICATION OF AMPUTATIONS

Amputations can be classified by anatomical location. Partial foot amputations are very common among those with peripheral vascular disease. The different levels of amputation include phalangeal, ray and transmetatarsal. Removal of one or more of the phalanges compromises late stance. If an entire toe is absent, including the proximal phalanx, the longitudinal arch of the foot will flatten because the insertion of the plantar aponeurosis is disrupted. A ray pertains to a metatarsal and its phalanges. Ray amputation interferes with late stance and the longitudinal arch; in addition, the foot will be narrowed. Transmetatarsal amputation has major negative effects on late

stance, foot support and balance; the patient tends to lean backwards on the heel. In all cases of partial foot amputation, the patient should be fitted with a shoe that has a rocker sole to aid late stance and an arch support. The shoe insert for an individual with a ray amputation must have a longitudinal insert to prevent the narrowed foot from sliding in the shoe.

Syme's amputation involves surgical removal of the entire foot except for the calcaneal fat pad. The fat pad is sutured to the distal tibia and fibula. The patient should be given a Syme's prosthesis, which replaces the shape and basic function of the foot. Syme's and partial foot amputations provide good support and sensory feedback because the patient can stand on the distal end of the amputation limb (end-bearing).

Transtibial (below-knee) amputation is the most common site for major lower-limb amputation (i.e. proximal to the ankle) (Fletcher et al 2002). Retaining the anatomic knee enables the individual to sit and walk reasonably well. Geriatric patients with transfemoral (above-knee) amputation have poorer functional capacity and generally rely on a wheelchair for long-distance community travel. Ankle, knee and hip disarticulations are uncommon, particularly among older adults.

The older individual with bilateral amputations resulting from vascular disease generally undergoes one amputation before the other. The presence of diabetes accelerates the loss of the contralateral limb, so individuals with an amputation resulting from diabetes must be taught the proper care of the residual and contralateral limbs (Thornhill et al 1986, Eneroth & Persson 1992) (see the discussion on education and prevention in Chapter 48, Diabetes).

CONDITIONS RELATED TO AMPUTATION

Individuals who sustain dysvascular amputations often have other evidence of vascular disease, including cardiovascular disease, which compromises their ability to tolerate vigorous exercise. Severe cardiovascular disease, in which the patient has dyspnea at rest, contraindicates fitting of a prosthesis. Cerebrovascular disease is a frequent concomitant condition. Hemiparesis, usually ipsilateral, is also not uncommon. Paresis does not preclude prosthetic use, particularly if the amputation predated the stroke. When peripheral vascular disease in one limb is severe enough to lead to amputation, circulation in the opposite limb is also compromised. Individuals may complain of intermittent claudication after a short walk; prosthetic fitting reduces stress on the remaining limb. The remaining foot is vulnerable to pressure ulcers, which can lead to amputation. Vigilant foot inspection and hygiene, as well as suitable footwear, are essential.

Peripheral vascular disease associated with diabetes is often accompanied by obesity, visual impairment, proprioceptive and tactile loss and renal dysfunction, all of which complicate the use of prostheses. Severe arthritis in the lower limbs or the hands also hampers the fitting and wearing of a prosthesis.

TESTS IN PATIENTS WITH AMPUTATION

In addition to tests of the peripheral vascular system, including angiography, pulse oximetry and Doppler ultrasound, the patient with an amputation should be investigated for sensory diminution. Tactile sensation may be graded with a 5.07-g filament, whereas proprioception can be judged with balance testing. Heart rate and blood pressure should be monitored to enable the rehabilitation program to be kept at a challenging level without overstressing the patient.

The amputation limb requires daily inspection to identify any incipient ulceration. A patient who has had a recent amputation should have the surgical scar examined to ascertain whether healing is proceeding satisfactorily. Amputation limbs at or above the transtibial level are measured longitudinally and circumferentially. The longer the amputation limb, the more efficient the gait. The proximal circumferential measurement of the transtibial limb is taken at the fibular head. For the transfemoral limb, the measurement is taken at a fixed distance below the greater trochanter. Additional distal measurements are taken at 4-cm intervals. Consistent circumferential measurements indicate that edema has subsided and the patient is ready for a permanent prosthesis.

Motor power and joint excursion in all limbs and the trunk should be assessed periodically. Weakness interferes with the ability to maintain sitting balance, transfer from bed to wheelchair, stand and manage a prosthesis. Hip- and knee-flexion contractures compromise prosthetic alignment and the patient's ability to stand and walk with a prosthesis. The clinician should ask the patient about the presence and intensity of phantom (awareness of the missing body part) sensation and pain, which is highly prevalent (Ephraim et al 2005). Phantom sensation is likely to present permanently, whereas phantom pain can be expected to subside within the first year after surgery. Many modalities, such as ultrasound, transcutaneous electrical nerve stimulation (TENS) and massage reduce pain intensity.

The initial evaluation should also include an inquiry about the individual's functional level before surgery. An individual with a bilateral amputation who was not able to use a unilateral prosthesis is unsuitable for bilateral prostheses. Cognitive assessment is also essential because the presence of dementia contraindicates prosthetic fitting. Other factors that influence rehabilitation include environmental features, such as the number of steps at the entrance to and within the home, and the patient's vocational and avocational interests. For example, an individual who enjoyed playing golf before surgery may benefit from a prosthetic foot that can accommodate the sloping terrain of a golf course.

CLINICAL RELEVANCE: MOBILITY AND REHABILITATION

Preprosthetic rehabilitation involves measures designed to improve the health of the amputation limb and interventions that increase the individual's independence. The goals of treating the amputation limb are to reduce postoperative pain, foster healing, stabilize limb volume and prevent complications, particularly contractures and skin disorders. The patient should be guided towards increasing self-care including dressing, grooming, personal hygiene, maneuvering in bed and various transfers, such as from bed to wheelchair, wheelchair to toilet and standing. Some older people with unilateral amputation can negotiate short distances with a walker or a pair of crutches and the remaining leg. These activities should not be performed unless the patient is wearing a clean sock and a well-fitting shoe on the intact foot.

Most individuals with unilateral amputation or bilateral transtibial amputation receive prostheses (see Chapter 71, Prosthetics). Rehabilitation aims to enable the individual to don and use the prosthesis safely, either as the sole mode of locomotion or as an alternative to wheelchair mobility, particularly indoors. A preparatory prosthesis for balance during transfers or for cosmetic value may be considered. The clinical team, consisting of physician, physical therapist and prosthetist, should select the prosthetic components that will provide the patient with the best opportunity for accomplishing meaningful activities and that are within the person's functional capacity. The following Medicare guidelines for prosthetic prescription (Health Care Financing Administration 2001) are based on predicting the function of an individual with unilateral amputation:

- *Level 0*: patient does not have the ability or potential to ambulate or transfer safety, with or without assistance, and a prosthesis does not enhance the quality of life or mobility.

- *Level 1*: patient has the ability or potential to use a prosthesis for transfer or ambulation on level surfaces at fixed cadence; a typical limited or unlimited household ambulator.

- *Level 2*: patient has the ability or potential for ambulation with the ability to traverse low-level environmental barriers such as curbs, stairs or uneven surfaces – a typical community ambulator.

- *Level 3*: patient has the ability or potential for ambulation with variable cadence; a typical community ambulator with the ability to traverse most environmental barriers and who may carry out vocational, therapeutic or exercise activities that demand prosthetic use beyond simple locomotion.

- *Level 4*: patient has the ability or potential for prosthetic ambulation that exceeds basic ambulation skills, exhibiting high impact, stress or energy levels typical of the prosthetic demands of the child, active adult or athlete.

THERAPEUTIC INTERVENTIONS

Early care

Reducing postoperative edema has the triple benefit of diminishing pain, fostering healing and stabilizing limb volume by promoting resorption of interstitial fluid. An elastic bandage or other modality is often used until limb girth stabilizes. Most patients can learn to apply an elastic bandage to a partial foot, Syme's or transtibial amputation limb but it is exceedingly difficult for a person of any age to wrap a transfemoral amputation limb. Regardless of amputation level, the elastic bandage loosens as the patient moves in bed or transfers into and out of a wheelchair. Consequently, the bandage must be reapplied several times a day. Elastic shrinker socks are easier to apply and can be used at the transtibial and transfemoral levels, although suspension on the thigh is difficult to maintain. As limb volume reduces, successively smaller socks are needed.

Elastic bandages and shrinker socks are the least effective ways of controlling edema. A rigid plaster dressing applied at the time of surgery is a much more effective way to control edema, particularly for transtibial amputation (Van Velzen et al 2005). Unless signs of infection are evident, the dressing is left in place until the time of suture removal. An aluminum or plastic pylon and a prosthetic foot can be attached to the rigid dressing to create an immediate postoperative prosthesis, although this modification is rarely used with older patients. Unfortunately, plaster dressings are more difficult to apply, require suspension from a waist belt and usually prevent inspection of the operative wound. Sometimes, the distal portion of the dressing over the scar is cut, so that the plaster can be removed for wound inspection and then easily replaced. Alternatively, a removable rigid dressing can be used, which also allows the wound to be viewed. Removal of the plaster requires a cast cutter.

An Unna semirigid dressing is comprised of zinc oxide, calamine, gelatin and glycerin in a gauze bandage. It is easy to apply and remove, adheres to the skin and thus requires no waist belt, and promotes healing; it is well suited to amputations at every level, including transfemoral (Wong & Edelstein 2000). The dressing remains on the limb until the sutures are removed. The semirigid dressing by itself cannot support a pylon and foot. After removal of the rigid or semirigid dressing, most patients wear a shrinker sock to resolve residual edema.

Additional care

In addition to stabilizing amputation limb volume, other interventions that focus on the amputation limb are those that reduce phantom pain, including ultrasound, TENS, bilateral resistive exercise and percussive massage. An educational program and peer support may help the patient accept the phenomenon of phantom sensation (Carroll & Edelstein 2006). Contractures can be prevented by encouraging the patient to use alternative positions rather than remain seated. A bivalved plaster or a canvas knee splint and a wheelchair knee support retard development of a knee-flexion contracture. Resistive exercises should emphasize hip and knee extension. Once the scar has healed, it can be massaged to prevent adherence.

Interventions that enable the patient to resume self-care and mobility foster independence (Lusardi & Nielsen 2006). Most patients receive a wheelchair; the wheelchair should promote good sitting posture and the seat should have a firm foundation and a proper cushion to distribute pressure. A lumbar support to overcome the slingback effect of a flexible backrest is helpful. The brakes must be operative. Leg amputation shifts one's center of gravity posteriorly. Consequently, either a special model of wheelchair should be obtained that has posteriorly offset wheels or a pair of adapters should be bolted to the rear wheels of a standard wheelchair. The wheelchair will then have an increased base of support, preventing upset of the wheelchair and its occupant when ascending steep ramps. An individual with a unilateral amputation should have a wheelchair with swing-out footrests so that the remaining foot and the prosthesis can be supported. The individual with bilateral amputations who is not a candidate for prostheses will have a less difficult time transferring if the wheelchair does not have footrests. Removable armrests facilitate transfers.

The physical therapist should demonstrate the safest way of transferring into and out of the wheelchair and the most efficient ways of maneuvering it. The home may require modification to accommodate the wheelchair, such as rearranging furniture to create a pathway and removing throw rugs and saddle boards at doorways to enable the wheelchair to be rolled with ease. If the wheelchair cannot fit through the bathroom door, a commode and alternative bathing facilities will be needed.

Exercises that improve the flexibility, coordination and strength of the hands, shoulders and trunk are important. All patients with unilateral amputation should be taught how to inspect and clean the remaining foot and the need for a suitable sock and shoe. Peer support can help many patients and their families cope with the emotional and practical problems associated with amputation.

Rehabilitation

Prosthetic rehabilitation begins with assessment to ascertain whether the prosthesis fits well and that all components function properly. The basic program emphasizes correct donning of the prosthesis, transfer into and out of chairs, balance when standing, and walking, as well as instruction in care of the amputation limb and the prosthesis. Some older adults are able to climb stairs and ramps, drive a car and engage in a wide range of recreational activities once they become used to the prosthesis.

Applying a partial foot prosthesis generally involves slipping the prosthesis into the shoe, donning the appropriate sock, making sure that it is not wrinkled and, finally, inserting the foot into the shoe. The sequence for dressing with the usual transtibial prosthesis is to put the sock and shoe on the prosthetic foot, drape the trouser around the prosthesis, don the amputation limb sock, insert the amputation limb into the socket and secure any straps or other fastenings. Some people prefer to don the amputation limb sock and the socket liner and then enter the socket. The entire sequence can be performed while sitting. If the prosthesis has distal pin suspension, the patient applies a silicon sheath to the amputation limb, along with one or more socks, and then inserts the covered amputation limb into the socket, matching the pin in the sheath to its hole at the base of the socket.

Donning of the transfemoral prosthesis can begin while sitting. The patient applies the amputation limb sock, bringing its proximal margin to the groin, removes the suction valve from the prosthetic socket and then places the thigh in the socket. At this point, the patient stands and pulls the distal end of the sock through the valve hole in order to smooth superficial tissues into the socket. The patient tucks the sock end into the socket, installs the valve and fastens the belt around the torso. If the prosthesis has total suction suspension, the easiest method is to lubricate the thigh, insert it into the socket while sitting or standing and install the valve.

Teaching the patient to move safely from various chairs to the standing position and back again is the most critical aspect of prosthetic rehabilitation in the older adult. Regardless of amputation level, it is easiest for the patient to stand from an armchair with a firm seat, such as a wheelchair. Both feet should be on the floor, with the sound foot placed slightly posteriorly. Initially, the patient may use the armrests to assist in rising.

Balancing with a prosthesis may begin at the parallel bars or at the side of a sturdy table. The latter approach prevents the individual from forming the habit of pulling, rather than pushing, on the supporting structure. The therapist should guide the patient in shifting from side to side, forward and backward, and diagonally while maintaining upright posture. Eventually, the patient should be able to shift their weight without holding onto a support. Advanced balancing exercises include stepping onto a low stool with the sound foot, thus prolonging weight-bearing on the prosthesis.

Gait training may involve the use of a cane, forearm crutch or a walker, depending on the patient's ability to masterbalance exercises. Proper adjustment of the assistive device and instruction in its use are essential to promote safe walking. The two-wheeled walker enables a faster gait than a four-wheeled aid (Tsai et al 2003). The goals of gait training are safety, symmetrical step length and equal time spent on each leg. Older adults who wear transfemoral prostheses walk faster when the knee unit is locked, even though the appearance of the gait is abnormal, assuming the alternative knee unit has no stance contral mechanism (Devlin et al 2002). Patients should practice walking on various surfaces, such as smooth flooring, carpets and grass.

Individuals who are able to walk safely on level surfaces should be given an opportunity to climb stairs and ramps. The easiest task is ascending stairs that have a handrail on the contralateral side. Most individuals with transtibial or more distal amputations ascend and descend in a foot-over-foot manner, alternating feet on each step. In contrast, those with transfemoral prostheses ascend leading with the sound foot and descend leading with the prosthesis. A few exceptionally agile individuals learn to descend in a foot-over-foot pattern. Stair climbing by those who wear bilateral transfemoral prostheses is exceedingly rare. They may choose to ascend and descend seated on the buttocks. Maximal assistance is often necessary. Two handrails may be facilitative or an electric stair glide may be appropriate. Ramps pose a problem for those who wear prostheses because most prosthetic feet have limited ranges of dorsiflexion and plantarflexion. Diagonal (sideways) climbing may be more practical for older adults (Smith et al 2004).

There are two concerns with driving a car, namely transferring into and out of the car and operating the vehicle. An individual with a right-side amputation will find it easier to enter the car on the passenger side. With a left prosthesis, the patient should first sit sideways on the passenger seat and then lift the prosthesis to the forward-facing position while pivoting on the buttocks. Operating an automobile that has automatic transmission is easier for an individual with a left-side amputation. An individual with a right prosthesis may choose to cross the left leg so that the sensate left foot moves the accelerator and brake pedals. Alternatively, it is possible to install an extension to the accelerator so that the left foot can reach it comfortably. Individuals with transtibial amputation often require no special adaptation or equipment for driving.

CONCLUSION

Amputation in an aging adult usually results from peripheral vascular disease. Key assessment factors include sensory evaluation and measurement of joint excursion and motor power. Preprosthetic care should focus on controlling edema of the amputation limb and fostering resumption of self-care. Prosthetic training begins with assessment of the fit and function of the prosthesis. Basic care includes teaching the patient to transfer from one seat to another and to stand, as well as walk with or without assistive devices. Environmental modifications facilitate household ambulation. Some older patients with amputations resume full independence, including driving a car and participating in recreational activities.

References

Carroll K, Edelstein JE (eds) 2006 Prosthetics and Patient Management: A Comprehensive Clinical Approach. Slack, Thorofare, NJ

Devlin M, Sinclair LB, Colman D et al 2002 Patient preference and gait efficiency in a geriatric population with transfemoral amputation using a free-swinging versus a locked prosthetic knee joint. Arch Phys Med Rehabil 83:246–249

Eneroth M, Persson BM 1992 Amputation for occlusive arterial disease: a prospective multicenter study of 177 amputees. Int Orthop 16:383–387

Ephraim PL, Wegener ST, MacKenzie EJ et al 2005 Phantom pain, residual limb pain, and back pain in amputees: results of a national survey. Arch Phys Med Rehabil 86:1910–1919

Fletcher DD, Andrews KL, Hallett JW et al 2002 Trends in rehabilitation after amputation for geriatric patients with vascular disease: implications for future health resource allocation. Arch Phys Med Rehabil 83:1389–1393

HCFA Common Procedure Coding System 2001 US Government Printing Office, Washington, chapter 5.3

Lusardi MM, Nielsen CC (eds) 2006 Orthotics and Prosthetics in Rehabilitation, 2nd edn. Elsevier, Philadelphia, PA

Smith D, Bowker JH, Michael JW (eds) 2004 Atlas of Limb Prosthetics: Surgical, Prosthetic, and Rehabilitation Principles, 3rd edn. American Academy of Orthopaedic Surgeons, Chicago, IL

Thornhill HL, Jones GD, Brodzka W, VanBockstaele 1986 Bilateral below-knee amputations: experience with 80 patients. Arch Phys Med Rehabil 67:159–163

Tsai HA, Kirby RL, MacLeod DA, Graham MM 2003 Aided gait of people with lower-limb amputations: comparison of 4-footed and 2-wheeled walkers. Arch Phys Med Rehabil 84:584–591

Van Velzen AD, Nederhand MJ, Emmelot CH, Ijzerman MJ 2005 Early treatment of trans-tibial amputees: retrospective analysis of early fitting and elastic bandaging. Prosthet Orthot Int 29:3–12

Wong CK, Edelstein JE 2000 Unna and elastic postoperative dressings: comparison of their effects on function of adults with amputation and vascular disease. Arch Phys Med Rehabil 81:1191–1198

Chapter 50

Wound management

Richard Mowrer and Pamela G. Unger

INTRODUCTION

The integument (the skin) is a vital organ. When a person sustains an injury to the integument, a break has occurred in the protective barrier between the organs/underlying tissues and the outside environment. This principle is crucial to the survival of the elderly. It is fairly common knowledge that chronic dermal wounds occur most frequently in the elderly (Wong 2000). The body's ability to heal is altered by various health problems – diabetes mellitus, circulatory problems, hypertension and chronic obstructive pulmonary disease (COPD). Normal age-related changes in the skin also affect the rate and quality of healing (see Chapter 52, Skin Disorders), and there may be additional risk factors including inadequate nutrition, limited mobility and muscle atrophy.

WOUNDS AND THE HEALING PROCESS

The normal healing process has three phases (Stillman 2005). In phase one, the inflammatory response is activated, which is the body's natural response to injury. This inflammatory response extends from injury to 4–6 days after injury. The process follows a normal sequence of events including vasoconstriction, fibrin clots, vasodilation and the presence of neutrophils and macrophages that remove bacteria and debris. Initially after injury, transudate leaks out of the blood vessels to fill the interstitial space, leading to localized edema and, thus, slowing the bleeding. Next, blood vessels reflexively constrict to assist with reducing blood loss. Platelets aggregate and become 'sticky'; this plugs up the lymphatic tissue, causing greater edema. The platelets release growth factors that control cell growth, differentiation and metabolism. Finally, chemotactic agents are released to attract cells that are necessary to fight infection and repair the wound. As the chemotactic agents attract new healing cells, the vasoconstriction changes to vasodilation, allowing these cells to reach the site of the injury. Vasodilation results in localized redness, swelling and warmth, which are characteristics of inflammation. Fluid seeping from the wound, containing macrophages, white blood cells (WBC) and neutrophils, is called exudate; it is yellow/cream colored and more viscous than transudate. Pain is also usually present (Mowrer 2004).

Phase two, the proliferative phase, occurs approximately 7 days after injury. This phase includes the utilization of growth factors, endothelial cells, fibroblasts, new blood vessels and collagen. The growth factors also generate keratinocytes, which are involved in re-epithelialization. The inflammatory and proliferation phases usually overlap, with no definitive marker for when one ends and the other begins. There are four crucial events of the proliferative stage:

1. Angiogenesis is the formation of new capillaries; these capillaries tie into loops that bring nutrition and blood to the injured site (this does not happen in areas of ischemia).

2. Granulation tissue is formed as dead tissue is removed and the capillary network 'fills in' the space. This tissue serves as a latticework for new epithelium to grow on.

3. Fibroblasts lay down a fibrous network in which myofibroblasts (complete with actin) begin to pull the edges of the wound together.

4. The wound contracts: keratinocytes begin to migrate across the wound bed and growth factors act to produce proliferation of new epithelial growth, also known as re-epithelialization.

In phase three, the remodeling phase, there is no longer an open wound. During this phase, the connective tissue becomes better aligned and tensile strength increases. After the re-epithelialization process has completely covered the wound surface, the maturation phase begins; this means that the 'new skin' begins to thicken and mature. The new skin is primarily scar tissue that is formed by randomly laid down collagen. This collagen will eventually need to be 'remodeled' so that it can work in conjunction with the surrounding tissue, i.e. move or become mobile. This process can take up to 2 years to complete (Stadelmann et al 1998).

Wound classification

Wounds are generally classified according to the predominant underlying cause. Common categories include arterial insufficiency, venous insufficiency, pressure ulcers, neurotrophic ulcers, traumatic wounds and burns. There are several wound classification systems.

Table 50.1   Wound classification systems

Wound type	Classification	Characteristics
Pressure ulcers	Stage I	Nonblanchable erythema of intact skin, the heralding lesion of skin ulceration
	Stage II	Partial-thickness skin loss involving epidermis and/or dermis; ulcer is superficial and presents clinically as an abrasion, blister or hollow crater
	Stage III	Full-thickness skin loss involving damage or necrosis of subcutaneous tissue that may extend down to, but not through, underlying fascia; ulcer presents clinically as a deep crater, with or without undermining of the adjacent tissue
	Stage IV	Full-thickness skin loss with extensive destruction, tissue necrosis or damage to muscle, bone or supporting structures (e.g. tendon or joint capsule)
Burns	First-degree	Involves the superficial epidermal layer; skin is pink or red, dry and painful, and sheds within a week without residual scar
	Second-degree	Involves the epidermis and the dermis; wound is immediately blistered and wet, local edema is present; if superficial, will heal within 2–3 weeks and will not scar if not infected or unduly traumatized; if deep, may require skin grafting to achieve optimal healing
	Third-degree	Involves the entire thickness of the skin; wound varies in color from white to black and may present with dark networks of thrombosed capillaries that do not blanch with pressure; surface is usually dry, but may be wet; these wounds require skin grafting for closure if more than 1in (2.54 cm) in diameter
		Burns are also designated, at times, by partial- and full-thickness; first- and second-degree burns are synonymous with partial-thickness. Full-thickness burns are those in which the entire epidermis has been destroyed. Parts of the dermis may also be destroyed, along with injury into the subcutaneous structures
Venous, arterial, and traumatic wounds	Partial-thickness	Penetration into the epidermis or into the beginning of the dermis
	Full-thickness	Penetration into the subcutaneous tissue, muscle or bone

Table 50.1 presents the classifications systems for pressure ulcers (Agency for Health Care Policy and Research, AHCPR 1992), burns, and venous, arterial and traumatic wounds that are not included in the other classifications. The Wagner (1981) system is another important assessment tool for the classification of ulcer stages (Table 50.2).

EVALUATING THE PATIENT

The evaluation of a patient with a wound should be completed by a multidisciplinary team (physician, nurse, physical therapist and social worker). A nutritionist may also be involved if no other member of the team assesses these needs. The physical therapist on the wound-care team plays an important role and must have expertise in dealing with the integumentary system. This should not only include expertise in the active range of motion of all joints, strength, bed mobility, transfers and gait status but also the classification of wounds. This information can then be processed to establish a plan of care that optimizes wound homeostasis and healing. It is important to remember to treat the patient, not the wound.

When initiating the evaluation, the following elements should be included (see Forms 50.1, 50.2 and 50.3):

- Obtain a thorough medical history; a patient's past medical history may predispose them to a nonhealing wound (e.g. diabetes mellitus or peripheral vascular disease).
- Encourage the patient's primary care physician to evaluate the patient's medical status extensively (e.g. assess blood sugars, albumin, hemoglobin, wound cultures, if necessary, and medications).

Table 50.2   Wagner classification system of ulcer stages

Stage	Description
0	Intact skin
1	Superficial ulcer involving skin only
2	Deep ulcer involving muscle and, perhaps, bone and joint structures
3	Localized infection; may be abscess or osteomyelitis
4	Gangrene, limited to forefoot area
5	Gangrene of the majority of the foot

- Assess the patient's physical mobility; contractures may predispose a patient to pressure ulcers and immobility limits a patient's ability to change positions in bed or a chair.
- Assess the integument. Is it well hydrated? Is there good turgor?
- Assess nutrition. What and how much is the patient eating?
- Assess the patients support surface. What type of bed, chair and shoes does the patient use regularly?
- Review the patient's personal care (hygiene).
- Assess peripheral pulses, i.e. ankle brachial pressure index (ABPI) (see Table 50.3).
- Assess the wound:
  - specific location of the wound;
  - size of the wound (length, width, depth);
  - wound classification;
  - wound odor;

Form 50-1 Sample form for taking a patient history

Physical History

Name: _____ Date: _____

Brief history: _____

_____

_____

_____

Past medical history:

Major illness:

Cardiovascular:	Coronary disease _____	Angina _____	Malignancies: _____
	Congestive heart failure_____	Arrhythmia _____	_____
	Myocardial infarct _____	Hypertension _____	_____
	Hypercholesterol _____	_____	
	Other _____		Operations: _____
Pulmonary:	COPD_____	Pneumonia _____	_____
	TB _____	Asthma_____	
	Other_____		Injuries: _____
Diabetes mellitus:	Insulin-dependent_____	_____	
	Noninsulin-dependent_____	_____	Hospitalizations: _____
Vascular:	Claudication _____	Rest pain_____	_____
	Varicose veins _____	DVT_____	_____
	Other _____		_____
Musculoskeletal:	Arthritis _____	Muscle weakness _____	Medications: _____
	Fractures _____		_____
Gastrointestinal:	Peptic ulcer disease _____	Cirrhosis_____	Allergies: _____
	Bleeding _____	Hepatitis _____	_____
	Pancreatitis _____	Other _____	
Genitourinary:	Kidneys _____	_____	Social history:
	Bladder _____	_____	Occupation_____
	Other_____		Smoking_____
Hematology:	Anemia _____	Bruisability _____	Alcohol_____
	Sickle cell anemia _____	_____	Drugs_____
	Bleeding tendency_____	_____	Family history:_____
Neurological:	TIA _____ Stroke _____	RIND_____	_____
	Other_____	_____	_____

Family physician:_____

Other physicians_____

_____

COPD, chronic obstructive pulmonary disease; DVT, deep vein thrombosis; RIND, reversible ischemic neurological deficit; TB, tuberculosis; TIA, transient ischemic attack.

– percentage of necrotic tissue, slough and granulation tissue;
– drainage (amount, odor, color, consistency);
– presence of undermining or tunneling;
– wound color;
– periwound condition;
– girth measurements (when applicable).

ABPI procedure

ABPI is measured using Doppler ultrasound, a hand-held device that utilizes sound waves to determine blood flow, and a blood pressure cuff. This is a quantitative way to measure blood flow without invasive testing. With the Doppler ultrasound, a whooshing sound is

Form 50-2 Sample physical assessment form

Physical Assessment

General:

    Alert_____   Oriented_____   Height_____   Weight_____

Vital signs:

    Temperature_____   Pulse_____   Respiration_____   BP _____

    RN_____

HEENT:

    Normal_____   Abnormal_____   _____

Neck:

    JVD_____   Node_____   Bruits_____   Thyroid_____

Heart:

    Regular_____   Irregular_____

Lungs:

    Clear_____   Rhonchi_____   Rales_____   Wheezes _____

Abdomen:

    Tenderness_____   Masses_____   Hernias_____   Organs_____

Extremities:

    Edema _____   Cyanosis_____   Clubbing _____

    Other_____

Pulses (0–4+):

    (R)   Radial _____ Femoral _____ Popliteal _____ Dorsalis pedis _____ Post-tibial _____

    (L)   Radial _____ Femoral _____ Popliteal _____ Dorsalis pedis _____ Post-tibial _____

Description of wound: _____

_____

_____

_____

Impression: _____

_____

_____

_____

Plan: _____

_____

_____

_____MD

BP, blood pressure; HEENT, head, ears, eyes, nose, throat; JVD, jugular vein distension; L, left; R. right.

heard, either biphasic (two sounds) or monophasic (one sound). The ultrasound device should be held at a 45-degree angle to the artery, against the direction of flow (gel will need to be utilized). The blood pressure of the brachial artery is taken as 'normal' and the maximum cuff pressure at which the pulse can just be heard with the Doppler ultrasound is recorded. This is repeated on the lower extremity (usually the dorsalis pedis). The blood pressure of the lower extremity is divided by that of the upper extremity to give the ABPI. In the presence of diabetes mellitus, the arteries may be calcified, therefore the measurements will be altered and unreliable. If this is the case, an arterio-gram is indicated. If Doppler ultrasound is not available, pulses will need to be assessed using palpatory skills or vascular studies.

Types of ulcers

In order to intervene appropriately in the treatment of ulcers, it is crucial to be able to distinguish between the various different types (Table 50.4).

Venous

Venous insufficiency is defined as a disturbance in the forward flow of blood in the lower extremities that may progress to increased hydrostatic pressure, venous hypertension and, ultimately, dermal ulceration (Fig. 50.1). Signs and symptoms of venous disease are hemosiderin staining, a purple hue that covers the skin (Fig. 50.2),

Form 50-3 Sample wound evaluation form

Name: _____

Date: _____

Pulses: (R) Post-tibial _____ Dorsalis pedis _____ Popliteal _____

        (L) Post-tibial _____ Dorsalis pedis _____ Popliteal _____

Location: _____

_____

Type of wound: _____

_____

_____

Stage: _____

Partial/full thickness: _____

_____

Size/depth: _____

_____

Exposed tendon: _____

Exposed bone: _____

Color: _____

_____

Percent of necrosis: _____

_____

Drainage: _____

_____

Odor: _____

_____

Undermining: _____

_____

Periwound condition: _____

_____

_____

Assessment: _____

_____

_____

_____

Plan: _____

_____

_____

_____

_____

coupled with a 'heavy feeling' in the legs and edema. Venous wounds are usually found in the lower leg in the proximity of the medial malleoli. These wounds present with large surface areas and have shallow edges. Many patients will complain of increased pain with prolonged lower extremity dependence, such as standing or sitting, with relief upon elevation of the involved limb.

The wound bed will be wet with a mixture of viable and nonviable tissues. An ABPI of >0.8 will present in the venous wound, as will palpable pulses. Palpating pulses in the edematous lower extremity can be difficult. In this instance, it may be beneficial to seek a noninvasive vascular study through the patient's referring physician or the medical director.

Patients with venous insufficiency are frequently significantly overweight. Therefore, it is important to include a weight loss program or consult a dietician for the comprehensive management of venous disease.

The etiology includes valvular incompetence of lower extremity veins, obstruction of the deep venous system, congenital absence or malformation of valves in the venous system and regurgitation from the deep to the superficial venous system via the venous perforators

Table 50.3   Interpretation of ABPI values

ABPI	Interpretation	Possible vascular interventions
1.1–1.3	Vessel calcification	ABPI not valid measure of tissue perfusion
0.9–1.1	Normal	None needed
0.7–0.9	Mild to moderate insufficiency	Conservative interventions normally provide satisfactory wound healing
0.5–0.7	Moderate arterial insufficiency with intermittent claudication	May perform trial of conservative care, physician may consider revascularization
<0.5	Severe arterial insufficiency, rest pain	Wound is unlikely to heal without revascularization, limb-threatening arterial insufficiency
<0.3	Rest pain and gangrene	Revascularization or amputation

From Myers (2004), with permission.

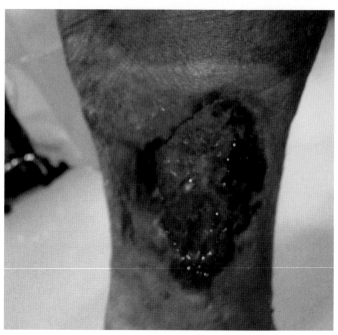

Figure 50.1   Venous wound: medial calf, large wet granular wound.

Table 50.4   Clinical typing of ulcers

	Pressure	Venous	Arterial	Neuropathic
Location	Bony prominences	Medial aspect lower leg/ankle; superior to medial malleolus	Between toes, tips of toes; around lateral malleolus; over phalangeal heads	Plantar aspect of foot; metatarsal heads; heels; altered pressure points; site of repetitive trauma
Wound appearance	Presence of redness, tunneling/undermining, maceration, induration, pain and odor; necrotic tissue may be present	Irregular wound margins; ruddy base (color); shallow depth; moderate to heavy exudate; granulation present	Pale or necrotic base; granulation absent or minimal; minimal exudate; gangrene/necrosis; infection	Even, well-defined wound margins; variable depth; variable exudate; variable extent of necrotic tissue; granulation present
Surrounding skin	Erythema; possible induration	Erythema; possible induration; cellulitis; hemosiderin stains	Erythema; possible induration; cellulitis	Erythema; possible induration; cellulitis; callus frequently present
Pain	Frequent pain	Minimal unless infected or desiccated	Frequently painful	Usually painless
Prevention	Education; identify at-risk patients; improve tissue tolerance; protect against pressure	Patient education; no smoking; adequate nutrition; skin care; optimize venous return; take medications; constant compression	Patient education; no smoking; take medications; diabetes control; avoid leg crossing, cold, moisture; professional foot care; well-fitting footwear; pressure reduction	Patient education; no smoking; take medications; control diabetes; avoid cold, moisture, extreme temperatures, external heat; daily foot care; appropriate footwear

that connect the deep and superficial venous systems. Inadequate pulmonary function will augment the problem because of a weak 'pulmonary pump'. The pulmonary pump functions via deep breathing, forcing the diaphragm against the abdominal cavity and increasing the pressure on the venous system, which increases the flow of blood. Additionally, the deep veins are surrounded by calf muscles that act as pumps by squeezing the veins and forcing the blood proximally. Paralysis or atrophy (possibly caused by a sedentary lifestyle) will impair this pump. This demonstrates the importance of exercise, specifically aerobic exercise, for patients with open wounds. Failure of the muscle pump is usually coupled with venous dysfunction, i.e. the veins fail to function and/or the one-way valves stop working. The veins become distended, with the increased internal pressure from the backflow of blood and subsequent increase in pressure in the capillaries leading to a 'cuff-like' pressure around the wound that limits oxygen and nutrients reaching the tissues. Proteins and fluids migrate out of the vein walls and flood the interstitial tissues, leading to edema and hemosiderin staining

The treatment of venous insufficiency involves four major areas: (i) control of underlying medical and nutritional disorders; (ii) education of the patient; (iii) control of edema; and (iv) topical therapy to reduce bacterial load, control drainage and promote granulation tissue formation.

Arterial

Arterial insufficiency is defined as insufficient arterial perfusion of an extremity or particular location (Fig. 50.3). It may be caused by arteriosclerosis, trauma, rheumatoid arthritis, diabetes mellitus, Buerger's disease or atherosclerosis. The ABPI will be <0.8, signifying arterial involvement. Any edema is localized or can be associated with an infection.

Pain is a significant symptom associated with arterial insufficiency. The pain may be described as intermittent claudication, which is pain during fast/prolonged ambulation or cramping of the muscles of the lower extremity on climbing many steps. This results from inadequate blood flow to the musculature of the lower extremity; the muscles begin to cramp, secondary to loss of oxygen perfusion and subsequent fuel usage. Ischemic rest pain is another type of problem that is positional in nature, i.e. during sleeping, when the legs are flat on the bed, blood flow is decreased, leading to pain. Often patients will describe a 'pain in my feet (or legs) that wakes me up, I need to walk around for a little while before it goes away'. Often, these patients will sleep with their legs dangling over the side of the bed or even in a recliner to allow gravity to assist with circulation. A final type of pain that is reported by patients is an intractable pain that is not managed or decreased in response to analgesia.

There are a few simple tests that can be used to assess perfusion: (i) check to see whether peripheral pulses are absent or diminished (the ABPI is a useful measure); (ii) check for a decrease in skin temperature; (iii) check for a delayed capillary refill time (more than 3 s); and (iv) check color; is there pallor on elevation or rubor?

The treatment of arterial insufficiency involves seven major focuses: (i) control any underlying medical and nutritional disorders; (ii) educate the patient on controlling risk factors, such as smoking, high blood pressure and cholesterol management, as well as utilization of proper footwear; (iii) manage the pain; (iv) control edema; (v) encourage ambulation and/or exercise to tolerance; (vi) use of topical therapy; and (vii) daily skin checks of sensitive areas, especially toes and feet.

Ulceration and gangrene (Fig. 50.4) are physical representations of significant peripheral vascular disease (PVD). These types of wounds require vascular surgery to bypass the blockages in the lower extremity arterial system and increase blood flow. A physician may prescribe anticoagulants and other medications to increase blood flow to the lower extremities; however, this may only be a temporary solution to the underlying problem.

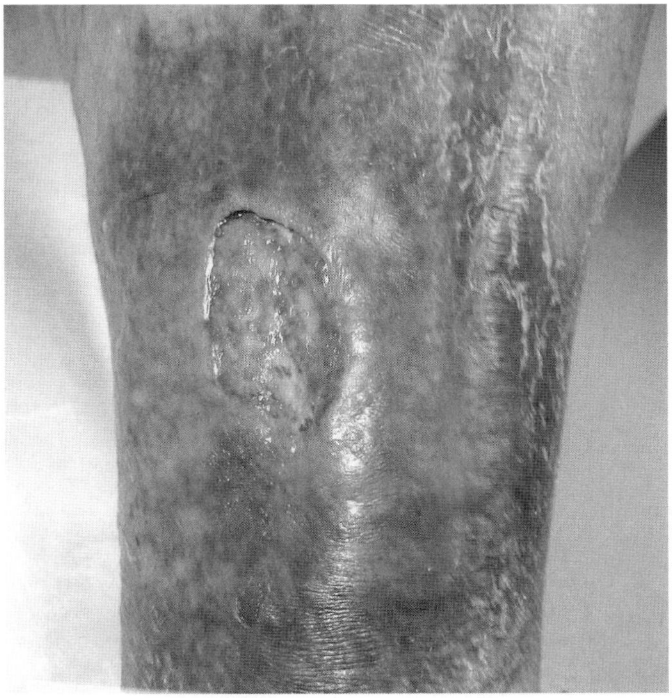

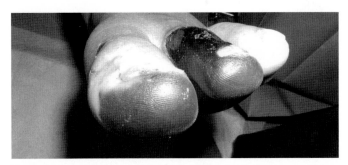

Figure 50.3   Arterial wound: note capillary occlusion in great toe and line of demarcation at the base of the second toe.

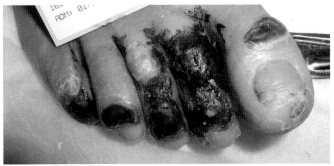

Figure 50.4   Arterial wound: significant necrotic tissue involved in all toes. This resulted in a transmetatarsal amputation.

Figure 50.2   Venous wound: significant hemosiderin staining and edema.

Neuropathic

Neuropathic ulcers (also referred to as neurotrophic or diabetic ulcers) have a direct correlation with peripheral neuropathy. peripheral neuropathy is defined as an altered function in the extremities that may involve a diminished or absent sensation in response to touch, pain or temperature, an absence of sweating, foot deformities and altered gait and weight-bearing.

Causes of peripheral neuropathy include damage to sensory, motor and autonomic nerves of the lower extremities. Gradual paralysis of the intrinsic muscles of the foot leads to muscle imbalances, atrophy and instability of the foot during stance. This, in turn, leads to increased pressure and shearing forces on the metatarsal heads of the feet. The foot itself can also change in shape, leading to hammer toes, hallux valgus or hyperextension of the great toe, all of which change the weight-bearing forces on the plantar aspect of the foot. Patients begin walking on bones and skin that have never been weighted and/or do not have sufficient padding to withstand the shearing/pressure forces they are subjected to.

Additionally, autonomic neuropathy increases the risk of ulceration secondary to impaired sweating mechanisms, increased callus formation and impaired blood flow. Impaired sweating mechanisms decrease the elasticity of skin, leading to greater 'overgrowth' of skin or callous formation and increased pressure at the point of 'overgrowth'. In turn, the callous formation develops a reduced or altered blood flow, decreasing the body's ability to heal itself. This affects the bones, resulting in a loss of calcium from the bone and fractures because of bone softening. The foot changes shape, often resulting in the appearance of a 'rocker bottom foot' or Charcot's foot (Figs 50.5 and 50.6)

The physical examination of the patient should include (i) palpation of peripheral pulses; (ii) notation of skin temperature; (iii) notation of skin color; (iv) assessment of capillary refill (less than 3 s); and (v) assessment of motor, sensory and autonomic neuropathy. Clinicians must also determine if the neuropathic ulceration has exposed (or tunnels down to) bone. In these instances, radiographic studies will be needed to rule out osteomyelitis. As already noted, ABPI assessment of the diabetic patient may be unreliable because of calcification of the arteries.

The treatment of neuropathic ulcers involves six major areas: (i) control of underlying medical and nutritional disorders; (ii) patient education; (iii) cessation of smoking; (iv) good control of diabetes; (v) off-weighting of the affected area coupled with good wound care to assist in wound healing; and (vi) use of innovative ointments and procedures to assist with wound healing including growth factors, synthetic skin grafting and hyperbaric oxygen. At this stage, a referral may be needed to a prosthetist/orthotist for custom-molded shoes or inserts. Keeping the callus thin by filing or sharp debridement will maintain good skin integrity in the periwound skin and promote contraction of wound edges. Keeping the wound moist, free from bacterial colonization and devoid of nonviable tissue are fundamental for the care of diabetic/neuropathic wounds.

Pressure

Pressure ulcers are a serious problem that can affect patients regardless of their usual living environments. Pressure ulcers lead to pain, longer hospital stays and slower recovery. They are defined as lesions that usually develop over bony prominences and are caused by unrelieved pressure, resulting in damage to the underlying tissue. The four main risk factors for developing pressure ulcers are shear, moisture, impaired mobility and malnutrition.

The staging system for pressure ulcers classifies the degree of tissue damage. It is important to note that pressure ulcers do not necessarily progress from stage I to stage IV, and they do not heal from stage IV to stage I, i.e. documenting reverse staging is a misnomer. Reverse staging implies that the tissue reforms with all of its original components. New tissue formation is scar tissue and not the normal epidermis/dermis organization. The treatment of pressure ulcers involves six major areas: (i) control of underlying medical and nutritional disorders; (ii) management of tissue loads; (iii) ulcer care; (iv) topical therapy, i.e. enzymatic/autolytic debridement;

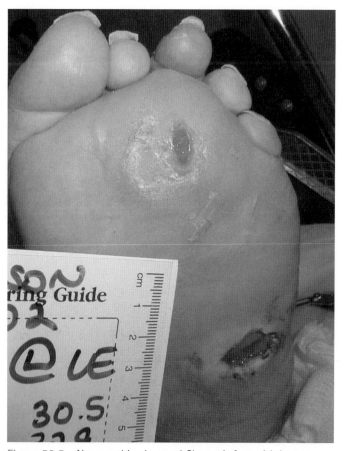

Figure 50.5 Neuropathic ulcer and Charcot's foot with hammer toes and pes planus deformity or 'rocker bottom'.

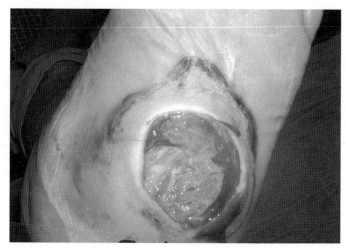

Figure 50.6 Neuropathic ulcer with 'rocker bottom foot'.

(v) management of bacterial colonization and infection; and (vi) education. In terms of the management of tissue loads, it is paramount in the treatment of pressure ulcers to keep pressure off the wound bed. This may seem simple; however, some patients may have difficulty with this concept, for example patients who are active, must work a full-time job or have significant infirmities may not be able to effectively relieve pressure over their wounds. Patients with heel ulcerations (Fig. 50.7) will benefit from pressure relief provided by many different types of off-weighting boots, such as the multipodus splint and/or the RIK boot™ (KCI Products, Boulder, CO). Paralyzed patients will need consistent weight-shifting when sitting and lying, as well as proper cushioning in wheelchairs and mattresses (Fig. 50.8).

Wounds with significant nonviable tissue covering cannot be assessed for depth or undermining. Therefore, they are documented as 'depth undetermined, secondary to nonviable tissue, covering wounds'. Individuals with limited mobility should always be assessed for additional factors that increase the risk of developing pressure ulcers. These factors include immobility, incontinence, nutritional factors and altered levels of consciousness. The multidisciplinary team should adopt a validated risk assessment tool such as the Braden Scale or the Norton Scale (Forms 50.4 and 50.5). The results recorded on these scales should be documented and used periodically to reassess the patient's risk.

THERAPEUTIC INTERVENTION

A wide variety of interventions are used by physical therapists to treat patients with chronic dermal wounds (Tables 50.5 and 50.6). When physical therapy intervention is utilized, the two primary goals are (i) to directly amplify the body's natural healing processes, and (ii) to eliminate factors that block the activity of the body's natural healing processes.

Hydrotherapy is the oldest known modality of physical therapy and its use is crucial for the cleansing of wounds. Over the years, hydrotherapy has taken various forms, such as whirlpools, water piks and pulsatile lavage. The combination of water, heat and agitation is successful in cleansing, softening necrotic tissue, assisting with the debridement process and removing residues left after the application of topical agents (see Table 50.6).

Compression therapy is the primary modality used to control edema (Stillman 2005). Edema is a major factor in the lack of healing of lower extremity ulcers complicated by venous insufficiency. Compression devices assist in decreasing interstitial fluid. The pressure shift encourages the movement of fluid and proteins from the interstitial spaces into the veins and lymphatics. Compression therapy also increases the efficiency of the muscle pump, as well as physically approximating the valves of the veins. Compression therapy can be provided by a variety of devices including intermittent/ sequential compression pumps, custom-made elastic stockings, Unna boots, elastic bandages and ready-made elastic stockings. The goal is to provide sufficient compression to stimulate fluid resorption. The compression found in elastic garments ranges from 8 mmHg to 60 mmHg. Numerous multilayer and multiday (usually 5–7 days) compression bandages, with a compression approaching 40 mmHg, are on the market today. The challenge for the patient with these dressings is not to get them wet, i.e. the patient must cover the leg for showering. Pressures greater than 40 mmHg may occlude blood flow, so caution is necessary if arterial insufficiency is suspected and the use of compression on arterial wounds is dependent upon the ABPI

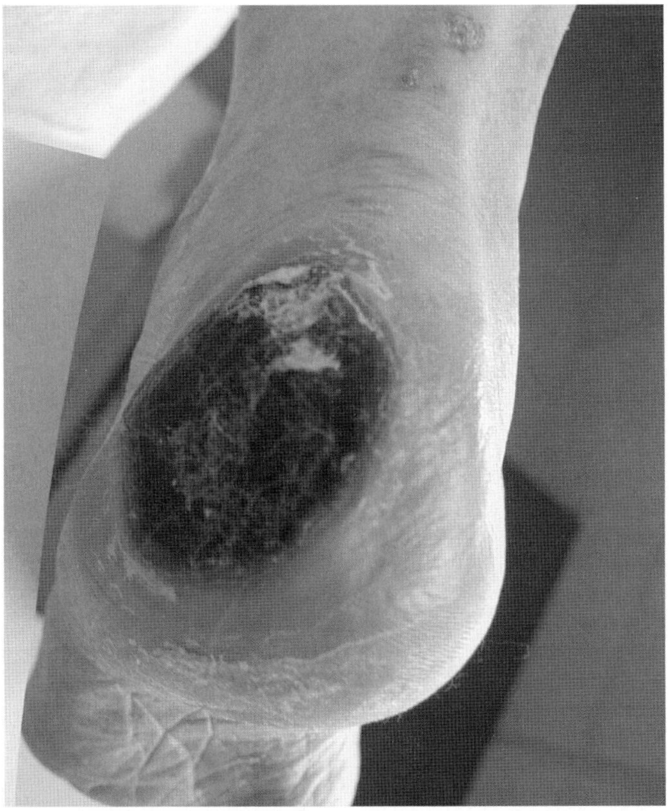

Figure 50.7   Left posterior/lateral heel ulcer. Note the 100% nonviable tissue (necrotic) covering.

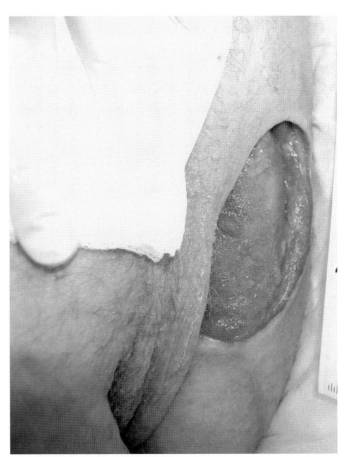

Figure 50.8   Right ischial tuberosity pressure ulcer, full thickness.

Form 50-4 Braden Scale for predicting pressure-sore risk

Patient's name: _____ Evaluator's name: _____ Date of assessment: _____

	1	2	3	4
Sensory perception: ability to respond meaningfully to pressure-related discomfort	**1. Completely limited:** unresponsive (does not moan, flinch or grasp) to painful stimuli because of diminished level of consciousness or sedation OR a limited ability to feel pain over most of body surface	**2. Very limited:** responds only to painful stimuli; cannot communicate discomfort except by moaning or restlessness OR has a sensory impairment that limits the ability to feel pain or discomfort over half of the body	**3. Slightly limited:** responds to verbal commands but cannot always communicate discomfort or need to be turned OR has some sensory impairment that limits ability to feel pain or discomfort in one or two extremities	**4. No impairment:** responds to verbal commands; has no sensory deficit that would limit ability to feel or avoid pain or discomfort
Moisture: degree to which skin is exposed to moisture	**1. Constantly moist:** skin is kept moist almost constantly by perspiration, urine etc; dampness is detected every time patient is moved or turned	**2. Moist:** skin is often, but not always, moist; linen must be changed at least once a shift	**3. Occasionally moist:** skin is occasionally moist, requiring an extra linen change approximately once a day	**4. Rarely moist:** skin is usually dry; linen changed only at routine intervals
Activity: degree of physical activity	**1. Bedfast:** confined to bed	**2. Chairfast:** ability to walk severely limited or nonexistent; cannot bear own weight and/or must be assisted into chair or wheelchair	**3. Walks occasionally:** walks occasionally during day but for very short distances, with or without assistance; spends majority of each shift in bed or chair	**4. Walks frequently:** walks outside the room at least twice a day and inside room at least once every 2 h during waking hours
Mobility: ability to change and control body position	**1. Completely immobile:** does not make even slight changes in body or extremity position without assistance	**2. Very limited:** makes occasional slight changes in body or extremity position but unable to make frequent or significant changes independently	**3. Slightly limited:** makes frequent, though slight, changes in body or extremity position independently	**4. No limitations:** makes major and frequent changes in position without assistance
Nutrition: usual food intake pattern	**1. Very poor:** never eats a complete meal; rarely eats more than one-third of any food	**2. Probably inadequate:** rarely eats a complete meal and generally eats only about one-half of any food offered;	**3. Adequate:** eats over one-half of most meals; eats a total of four servings of protein (meat, dairy products) each day;	**4. Excellent:** eats most of every meal; never refuses a meal; usually eats a total of four or more servings of meat and dairy

	1	2	3	4
	offered; eats two servings or less of protein (meat or dairy products) per day; takes fluids poorly; does not take a liquid dietary supplement OR is NPO and/or maintained on clear liquids or IV for more than 5 days	protein intake includes only three servings of meat or dairy products per day; occasionally takes a dietary supplement OR receives less than optimum amount of liquid diet or fed by tube	occasionally refuses a meal but will usually take a supplement if offered OR is on a tube feeding or TPN regimen, which probably meets most of nutritional needs	products; occasionally eats between meals; does not require supplementation
Friction and shear	1. **Problem:** requires moderate to maximum assistance in moving; complete lifting with-out sliding against sheets is impossible; frequently slides down in bed or chair, requiring frequent repositioning with maximum assistance; spasticity, contractures or agitation leads to almost constant friction	2. **Potential problem:** moves feebly or requires minimum assistance; during a move, skin probably slides to some extent against sheets, chair, restraints or other devices; maintains relatively good position in chair or bed most of the time but occasionally slides down	3. **No apparent problem:** moves in bed and chair independently and has sufficient muscle strength to lift up completely during move; maintains good position in bed or chair at all times	
				Total score

From Braden BJ, Bergstrom N 1987 A conceptual schema for the study of the etiology of pressure sores. Rehabil Nurs 12:8–12, with permission. IV, intravenously; NPO, nothing by mouth; TPN, total parenteral nutrition.

Form 50-5 Norton Scale

	Physical condition		Mental condition		Activity		Mobility		Incontinent		Total score
	Good	4	Alert	4	Ambulant	4	Full	4	No	4	
	Fair	3	Apathetic	3	Walks with help	3	Slightly limited	3	Occasionally	3	
	Poor	2	Confused	2	Chairbound	2	Very limited	2	Usually (urine)	2	
	Very bad	1	Stupor	1	Bed	1	Immobile	1	Doubly	1	

Name: Date:

From Norton D, McLaren R, Exton-Smith AN 1962 An investigation of geriatric nursing problems in the hospital. National Corporation for the Care of Old People (now the Centre for Policy on Ageing), London, with permission.

Table 50.5 Therapeutic interventions

Treatment	Used for	Clinical applications	Physiological response
Hydrotherapy/pulsatile lavage	Neurotrophic, venous, arterial, pressure and diabetic ulcers; burns; acute trauma	Cleanse; debride; soak off dressings	Superficial heat/cold; micromassage; increased moisture
Ultrasound	Neurotrophic, venous, arterial and diabetic ulcers	Debride; promote clean wound bed	Increase microcirculation; edema absorption; superficial/deep heat
Compression	Venous, arterial and diabetic ulcers; burns	Reduce edema	Decrease venous hypertension; increase venous return
Electrical stimulation	Neurotrophic, venous, arterial, pressure and diabetic ulcers; burns; acute trauma	Debride; decrease infection and pain; increase circulation; promote closure	Increase circulation; bactericidal effects; increase fibroblast activity; decrease edema
Pulsed electromagnetic fields	Venous, arterial, pressure and diabetic ulcers; acute trauma	Reduce pain and edema	Edema reduction; increase transport of cutaneous oxygen

and the amount of edema. An ABPI should also be performed to rule out concomitant arterial issues. In general practice, the compression stocking is donned before getting out of bed and removed before bedtime. One common problem in the geriatric population is the inability to pull on the compression stocking. In these cases, compression pumps are a great help in fluid resorption. Compression stockings should be replaced every 9–12 months, depending upon wash/wear times, because they tend to lose their compressive qualities over time. Patients tend to neglect replacing them (usually because of cost) and this can lead to reoccurrence.

Ultrasound (non-thermal) has been found to be effective in enhancing wound healing, particularly when venous insufficiency is a major factor. The 3-MHz unit has been proposed to be the most effective frequency because most energy is absorbed by the superficial tissues. Ultrasound has been found to enhance the body's ability to move from the inflammatory to the proliferative phase of wound healing. It has also been associated with less dense and more resilient scar tissue. Ultrasound must be administered through a medium such as a hydrogel or a hydrogel sheet. The treatment can be administered either along the periphery or directly over the wound bed (see Table 50.6 for parameters).

Electrical stimulation has been advocated over the years for the enhancement of wound healing, regardless of the underlying cause. Numerous studies have shown the effectiveness of electrical stimulation in enhancing wound healing (Baker et al 1997, Kloth 2002). In many studies, high voltage electrical stimulation has been shown to alter the pH of wound chemistry and facilitate a decrease in inflammation. Current protocols result in removal of nonviable tissue from the wound bed. Unfortunately, the ideal parameters have yet to be defined and it is therefore best to choose parameters based upon the desired treatment effect. An alternative protocol, proposed by Sussman (1998), utilizes the following parameters:

- Settings for the inflammatory phase of healing:
  - negative polarity;
  - 100–128 pulses per second (pps);
  - 100–150 V;
  - 60 min for 5–7 days/week.

- Settings for the epithelialization phase of healing:
  - alternating current: 3 days positive, 3 days negative etc.,
  - 64 pps;
  - 100–150 V;
  - 60 min for 5–7 days/week.

Utilization of a hydrogel-impregnated or saline-soaked gauze as a wound contact conductor is optimal. Petrolatum-based products will impede the efficacy of electrical stimulation. The dispersive pad (which should be larger than the wound-contact pad) should be

Table 50.6 Treatment suggestions

Hydrotherapy	
Whirlpool	10–20 min per treatment session (daily); temperature 92–99°F
Pulsatile lavage	10–30 min in entirety, periodic placement of tube throughout the wound; room-temperature saline solution
Ultrasound 3 MHz pulsed (partial-thickness wounds) and 1 MHz (full-thickness wounds)	0.5–1.5 W/cm^2 for 1 min/cm^2 of wound; pulsed, 20–40% duty cycle; use hydrogel medium or conductive gel; use over the wound or around the wound periphery
Compression Sequential/intermittent	Ideally, patient is supine with lower extremity elevated; use a pressure at least 20 mmHg below the diastolic reading of the blood pressure taken in the treatment position; treat for a minimum of 1 h; treat in morning if possible; follow with static compression wrap
Static	Wrap bandage from metatarsophalangeal joints to two fingers below the fibula head; be certain to apply equal pressure; overlap bandage by at least two-thirds with each wrap; cover with protective stocking or additional elastic wrap
Electrical stimulation (high-voltage pulse current)	Initially (−) polarity, 50–80 pps, 100–150 V; after five visits (or when wound is clean), (+) polarity, 80–100 pps, 100 V; electrode placement: dispersive pad proximal, foil electrode with saline-soaked or conductive hydrogel pad placed directly into the wound
Pulsed electromagnetic fields Thermal	5-min warm-up (5/10 cycle); 20-min treatment (10/12 cycle); 5-min cool down (5/10 cycle); treat once per day
Nonthermal Acute wound	30-min cycle, cycle 6
Chronic wound	45-min cycle, cycle 4; treat once per day

placed proximal to the wound surface. The pads should be placed close together for shallow wounds and further apart for deeper or undermining/tunneling wounds.

Pulsed electromagnetic fields are a relatively new entity in wound care. Solid-state equipment generates radio waves into the tissues, creating an electrical charge. The specifications include using radio waves with a frequency of 27.12 MHz. To date, conclusive scientific evidence for the efficacy of pulsed electromagnetic fields in wound care has not been established, although several clinical trials have been completed in the US (see Table 50.6 for parameters).

Total contact casting is used primarily in the treatment of patients with neuropathic plantar ulcers that are classified as grades I and II. The goal of this treatment is to remove weight-bearing forces from inflamed tissues and immobilize them so that healing can occur. Following the application of a total contact cast, a patient must be instructed in partial weight-bearing with an appropriate assistive device. Generally, these patients have altered sensation, which makes an exact fit of the cast crucial. The cast is generally reapplied every 1–2 weeks; however, loosening of the cast, large amounts of drainage or damage to the cast requires premature removal. In some cases, a bivalve cast is appropriate. The patient must understand that the bivalve cast is not to be removed until bedtime.

Currently, there are many skin substitutes available on the market for increasing the wound healing rate. These skin substitutes have all of the components of normal skin, including all 21 growth factors, except for hair follicles and sweat glands. They are applied by a physician and are accompanied with strict protocols for dressing changes.

Additional products on the market for the treatment of neuropathic ulcers are specific mediums containing the dominant skin growth factor (Stillman 2005). These prostaglandin growth factors play a large role in wound healing. There are currently a few products available, such as Regranex™ (Ortho-McNeil, Somerville, NJ), that use topical application of growth factors. This gel-type medium is an expensive product but has been successful in speeding up the closure of different types of wounds. A clean granulating wound bed is necessary to increase the effectiveness of the gel. Regranex™ has biological activity similar to that of endogenous platelet-derived growth factor, which includes promoting the chemotactic recruitment and proliferation of cells involved in wound repair and enhancing the formation of granulation tissue.

The wound VAC® (vacuum-assisted closure) device has significantly decreased the healing time for pressure ulcerations. In this technique, a special sterile sponge-type dressing is cut slightly smaller than the diameter of the wound. This is covered with an occlusive dressing and hooked to a suction unit with a canister/reservoir to collect wound fluid. The wound VAC is then used to wick all of the air and fluid away from the wound bed. Blood flow at the wound surface is increased and the wound edges are pulled together. This author has found it a very effective adjunct to traditional wound-healing methods (see www.kci1.com for further information).

All members of the wound-care team should be aware of the importance of nutrition and recognize that adequate calories and protein; vitamins A, C and E; zinc; glucosamine (MacKay & Miller 2003, Stillman 2005); and the amino acids arginine and glutamine (MacKay & Miller 2003) are important for proper wound healing.

THE ROLE OF EXERCISE IN WOUND CARE

Therapeutic exercise, specifically aerobic exercise, has been found to have a positive effect on wound healing. Emery et al (2005) found that 1 h of aerobic exercise at 70% of the maximum heart rate, three times a week, increased wound healing in healthy individuals. The mean healing time was 29.2 days in the exercise group compared with 38.9 days in the nonexercise group. The authors theorized that exercise may increase blood flow to the skin and skin oxygen tension. The subjects in this report were healthy older men and women; the authors admit that further studies need to be performed on patients with comorbidities.

Finally, it is important for physical therapists/physical therapist assistants and all medical care providers to treat the patient as a whole. It is likely that the patient's wound has had other physiological, musculoskeletal or biomechanical effects that require expertise. It is important to treat the entire patient, not just the open wound area. This is ethically correct as well as financially sound.

CONCLUSION

Effective intervention for wound care requires a thorough examination and evaluation and an individualized treatment plan established by a multidisciplinary team. The team must coordinate a plan that focuses on removing the factors that contribute to the nonhealing status and choosing an intervention that will foster healing. This plan may require multiple revisions before healing is achieved. When healing has been attained, the patient, family and caregivers must be educated in continued care and prevention. Clinicians who frequently treat open wounds must continually keep up-to-date on new products, dressings and techniques for the effective healing of wounds.

References

Agency for Health Care Policy and Research (AHCPR) 1992 Pressure Ulcers in Adults: Prediction and Prevention. Clinical Practice Guideline no.3. Public Health Service, US Department of Health and Human Services, Rockville, MD

Baker LL, Chambers R, DeMuth SK, Villar F 1997 Effects of electrical stimulation on wound healing in patients with diabetic ulcers. Diabetes Care 20(3):405–412.

Emery CF, Kiecolt-Glaser JK, Glaser R et al 2005 Exercise accelerates wound healing among healthy older adults: a preliminary investigation. J Gerontol 60:1432–1436

Kloth L, McCulloch J, Feeder J 2002 Wound Healing: Alternatives in Management, 3rd edn. FA. Davis, Philadelphia, PA

MacKay D, Miller A 2003 Nutritional support for wound care. Altern Med Rev 8:359–377

Mowrer R 2004 Wound Care for Older Adults: Implications for the Physical Therapist Assistant. American Physical Therapy Association, La Crosse, WI, p 14–15

Myers B 2004 Wound Management: Principles and Practice. Prentice Hall, Pearson Education, Upper Saddle River, NJ, p 211

Stadelmann W, Digenis A, Tobin G 1998 Physiology and healing dynamics of chronic cutaneous wounds. Am J Surg 176(suppl2A):26–38

Stillman RM 2005 Wound Care. Available: htpp://www.emedicine. com/med/topic2754.htm. Accessed 3 April 2006

Sussman C 1998 Electrical stimulation. Available: www.medicaledu.com/estim.htm. Accessed June 30 2006

Wagner F 1981 The dysvascular foot: a system for diagnosis and treatment. Foot Ankle 2:64–122

Wong R 2000 Chronic dermal wounds in older adults. In: Guccione A (ed) Geriatric Physical Therapy, 2nd edn. Mosby-Year Book, St Louis, MO

Chapter 51

The insensitive foot

Jennifer M. Bottomley

INTRODUCTION

Insensitivity of the foot is the usual end result of numerous pathological conditions that affect the elderly. Chronic diseases, such as diabetes mellitus, Hansen's disease, peripheral vascular disease, Raynaud's disease, deep vein thrombosis, spinal cord injury (e.g. spinal stenosis, tumors), peripheral nerve injuries, hormonal imbalances and vitamin B-complex deficiencies, result in breakdown of the microvascular structures and diminution of sympathetic nerve endings and somatic sensory receptors, leading to neuropathic conditions of the foot. These pathologies lead to a decrease in circulatory and peripheral nerve integrity, which results in edema, discoloration, diminished skin status, increased pain, absence of sensation and, ultimately, a decrease in functional mobility (Bottomley & Herman 1992, McGill et al 1996, Birke et al 2002).

Typical warning signs such as changes in gait patterns and pain associated with foot pathologies are absent in the insensitive foot. Repetitive stress, coupled with the loss of protective sensation, is a primary cause of foot ulcerations. The lack of a warning system for pain and abnormal stress on the plantar surface of the foot predisposes the neuropathic foot to injury and ulceration (Birke & Sims 1988). However, if the mechanism of injury and the risk factors are recognized (Table 51.1), foot ulcerations are preventable and treatable injuries (Bottomley 2003).

Neuropathic changes in the insensitive foot are a heterogeneous mixture of disorders that includes progressive distal polyneuropathy, ischemic mononeuropathy, amyotrophy and neuroarthropathy (Birke & Sims 1988). A combination of sensory, autonomic and motor neuropathies of the foot results in symmetrical or asymmetrical loss of perception of pain and temperature. Sympathetic denervation can lead to a progressive mixed-fiber neuropathy with a loss of light touch and vibratory sensation and motor loss in the intrinsic muscles of the foot (McGill et al 1996, Birke et al 2002). Characteristic foot deformities such as hyperextension of the metatarsophalangeal joints, clawing of the toes and distal migration of the fibroadipose cushions under the

Table 51.1 Risk factors in the neuropathic foot

Risk factor	Possible injury
Loss of protective sensation	Absence of pain-warning input
High plantar pressures	Ulcers occurring at peak pressure sites
Autonomic neuropathy	Dehydrated inelastic skin
Previous ulceration or amputation	Concentration of stress over scar or lesion
Foot deformities	Increased local pressures
Neuropathic fractures	Increased plantar pressures and foot instability
Abnormal foot function	Abnormal load application
High activity level	Increased cumulative stress
Vascular disease	Devitalized tissue susceptible to injury, poor healing
Inadequate footwear or foot care	Decreased protection, instability, poor hygiene
Visual loss	Inappropriate assessment of environment, inability to inspect feet
Poor insulin regulation	Complications of diabetes

heel and metatarsal heads result in abnormal weight-bearing patterns and increased plantar pressures (Lemaster et al 2003). Tissue damage to the insensitive foot may result from continuous pressure that causes ischemia or from concentrated high pressure, heat or cold, repetitive mechanical stress or infection of the tissues (Bottomley & Herman 1992).

Amyotrophic changes result from a lack of nourishment to the musculature. There is a progressive weakening and wasting of muscles accompanied initially by an aching or stabbing pain and resulting in the total loss of muscle function because of atrophy, paresthesia, paralysis and loss of sensory input (McGill et al 1996).

Neuropathic arthropathy results from joint erosions, unrecognized fractures and demineralization and devitalization of the bones and articulations of the foot. Typically, these changes are caused by routine weight-bearing activities in the absence of normal protective proprioceptive and nociceptive functions of the peripheral sensory system. In the limb with intact sensation, pain inhibits functional activities and further trauma to the joints so that the hypertrophic or reparative phases of callus formation can commence. In the insensate limb, however, the injured part is repeatedly traumatized, leading to increased hyperemia and resorption of damaged bone (McGill et al 1996).

Loss of sensation in the joints and bones of the foot predisposes the neuropathic foot to bony destruction. Midtarsal fractures or dislocations and hypertrophic bone formation may lead to a Charcot's deformity, which is the collapse of the foot into a severe rocker bottom foot deformity. Charcot's fracture is evidenced by swelling and increased temperature in the area of bone involvement (Armstrong et al 2003). Clinically, neuropathic fractures should be suspected in all patients with signs of inflammation in the absence of an open wound. The differential diagnosis includes osteomyelitis as well as cellulitis, pyarthrosis and reflex sympathetic dystrophy.

EVALUATION OF THE NEUROPATHIC FOOT

Regular and comprehensive screening of the neuropathic foot is essential for early identification of risk factors that may predispose an elderly individual to injury (Form 51.1). The foot screening evaluation is a brief examination to identify the history of any previous ulceration, motor weakness, sensory dysfunction or deformity that might predispose the foot to local areas of high stress. Circulatory status, color, temperature, general condition and the presence of edema or skin lesions should be assessed. Based on the foot screening evaluation, the relative risk of foot complications can be determined for each individual (Bottomley 2004). A risk classification scheme (Box 51.1) identifies individuals most likely to benefit from protective footwear and education.

Box 51.1   Risk classification

0 No loss of protective sensation
1 Loss of protective sensation with no deformity or history of ulcer
2 Loss of protective sensation with deformity but no history of ulcer
3 Loss of protective sensation with history of ulceration

Evaluating sensation and neurological involvement

The level of sensory loss that places an individual at risk for foot injury is referred to as loss of protective sensation. The use of nylon monofilaments calibrated to bend at 10g of force (Semmes–Weinstein monofilaments) is a precise method of determining loss of sensation. The inability to feel a monofilament of 5.07g has been determined to be the level at which loss of protective sensation occurs (Birke et al 2002). The Semmes–Weinstein monofilaments have been found to be a reproducible and accurate way to test sensation, and can reliably predict which individuals are at risk for ulceration because of the loss of protective sensation. The Carville group, of the G.W. Long Hansen's Disease Center in Carville, LA, measured protective sensation using the Semmes–Weinstein monofilaments and found that individuals who could not feel the 5.07-g monofilament were at greater risk for skin breakdown than

those who could. Standardization of sensory testing is crucial in evaluation so that adequate protective measures can be taken to prevent feet that are at risk from developing ulcers (Birke et al 2002, Coleman et al 2003). Specific evaluation of the entire plantar surface of the foot determines areas of sensory loss that are vulnerable to breakdown (Birke & Sims 1988, Birke et al 2002). Vibratory and temperature sense are diminished very early in the process of peripheral vascular disease, which compromises proprioception, kinesthesia and awareness of temperature gradients.

The neurological examination requires a reflex hammer, a tuning fork (128 cycles per second) and Semmes–Weinstein filaments. Testing for vibratory, proprioceptive, temperature and protective sensation should be done with the patient's eyes closed. The boundaries of any hyper- or hypoesthesias should be distinguished and it should be determined whether these patterns are symmetrical or asymmetrical. The absence or presence of sweating should also be noted. Reflexes to be tested include the patellar reflex and the ankle jerk. As the ankle jerk is increasingly difficult to elicit with increasing age, it may appear to be absent. To aid this reflex, gently pronate and dorsiflex the foot to put tension on the Achilles tendon and gently tap the tendon. The Babinski reflex can be tested to determine whether there is a superficial plantar response. To determine if there is clonus, forcibly dorsiflex the foot at the ankle. To test for loss of balance, the stance of the individual with eyes closed and feet close together should be compared with that when the eyes are open (Romberg's sign) (Bottomley & Schwartz 1995).

Muscle strength should be tested in all lower extremity muscles using a graded manual muscle test. Again, symmetry should be noted. Gait evaluation is a helpful adjunct to muscular evaluation to determine unsteady gait patterns, foot-drop or the presence of a 'steppage' gait. Range of motion and joint mobility should be evaluated and any deformities (e.g. Charcot joints, hammer, claw or mallet toes, hallux abductus valgus) should be noted; these abnormalities are usually indicative of intrinsic foot muscle weakness. Trophic nail changes should also be evaluated (Bottomley & Herman 1992).

Evaluating circulatory status

Vascular evaluation should include the palpation and grading of the femoral, popliteal, dorsalis pedis and posterior tibial pulses and the observation of other clinical signs and symptoms indicating vascular compromise in the lower extremities. These include intermittent claudication, foot temperature (i.e. cold feet), nocturnal pain, rest pain, nocturnal and rest pain relieved by dependency, blanching on elevation, delayed venous filling time after elevation, dependent rubor, atrophic skin, absence of hair growth and presence of gangrene. Any lesions or areas of hyperkeratosis or discoloration should be observed and documented (Bottomley 2003).

To differentiate an organic disorder, such as blockage of the lumen of the vessel, from a vasospastic condition, temporary dilation of the vessel in question is a useful vascular test. This is accomplished by using an arterial tourniquet for 3 min and then releasing it. The perfusion distal to the tourniquet should increase if the condition is caused by vasospasm (Bottomley & Schwartz 1995).

A determination of blanching and filling times is accomplished using the Buerger–Allen vascular assessment (see Forms 51.2–51.4). A stopwatch is used to measure the time it takes the veins in the dorsum of the foot to fill with blood after they have been drained by elevating the leg; this is a means of appraising the general circulation in the foot. The arterial blood being pumped into the dependent leg diffuses into the arterioles, the capillaries and the venules and then into the veins of the foot. The time of venous filling is subject to several variables: the

Form 51.1   Foot-screening evaluation guide

Date: _____

Name:_____

Address:_____

Phone: ( )_____

Sex: _____ Date of birth _____

Language or communication problems: No   Yes   (describe) _____

Primary doctor/podiatrist: _____

Address:_____

Phone: ( )_____

Subjective data

Medical history: _____
_____

1. Do you have:
   - Arthritis _____
   - Circulatory problems _____
   - Heart disease _____
   - Diabetes mellitus _____
   - Kidney problems _____
   - High blood pressure _____
   - Foot problems _____
   - Eye problems _____
   - Thyroid problems _____
   - Hearing problems _____
   - Vertigo _____
   - Dizziness _____
   - Fractured (Fx) hip _____

2. Did you have an injury in the:

		Left leg		Right leg	
		Sprain	Fx	Sprain	Fx
No					
Yes	Hip				
	Knee				
	Ankle				
	Foot				
	Back				

3. Are you experiencing any leg pain?

		Left leg	Right leg
No			
Yes	Hip		
	Knee		

4. Are you experiencing any foot pain?

		Left leg	Right leg
No			
Yes	Aching		
	Burning		
	Stabbing		
	Nail pain		
	Shoe pain		
	Metatarsal heads		
	Toes		

(*Continued*)

Pain increased:

	Left leg	Right leg
When standing		
When walking		
When wearing shoes		
In the morning		
In the afternoon		
At other times (describe)		

Objective data

1. Ambulates without assistance? No Yes
2. Ambulates with assistive devices? No Yes

Cane	
Walker	
Crutches	
Other	

3. Falls? No Yes Describe_____

4. Distance ambulated? Home One block Two blocks Five blocks 1 mile Unlimited
5. Regular exercise? No Yes
6. Examination of feet (remove shoes and stockings)

	Left foot		Right foot	
	Unacceptable	Acceptable	Unacceptable	Acceptable
Cleanliness of foot?				
Socks/stockings a good fit?				
Proper fitting shoes?	Short		Short	
	Long		Long	
	Narrow		Narrow	
	Worn down		Worn down	
Shoe wear: Heel				
Sole				
Lateral counter				

7. Problems

- Bunions

	Left foot	Right foot
HAV		
Taylor		

		Left foot					Right foot				
		I	II	III	IV	V	I	II	III	IV	V
• Calluses	Spin										
	Pinch										
	IPK										
	Sub										
	Shear										
• Corns	Metatarsal heads										
	Heloma molle										
	Heloma duram										
• Involuted nails											
• Ingrown toenails											
• Nail trophic changes											

(Continued)

- Circulatory problems

	DPP: 0		PTP: 0			DPP: 0		PTP: 0		
	1+		1+			1+		1+		
	2+		2+			2+		2+		
	3+		3+			3+		3+		
• Toe clubbing										
• Toe deformities: Hammer										
Claw										
Mallet										
Overlap										
Hallux										
	I	II	III	IV	V	I	II	III	IV	V

	Left leg	Right leg
• Foot/ankle deformities		
• Dermatitis (PI) fungus infection		
• Dry scaly skin		
• Edema Foot		
Ankle		
Extremity		

- Infection (describe): _____
- Other: _____

Foot screening evaluation

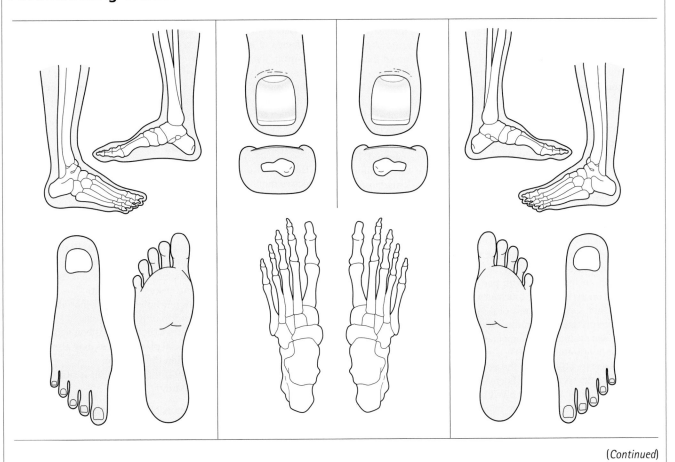

(*Continued*)

Comments:
_____
_____
_____

Assessment
_____
_____
_____

Recommend:
- None
- Refer to orthotics clinic   date: _____   Time: _____
- Refer for shoes
- Refer to pediatrist
- Refer to podiatrist
- Educated in: _____
- Orthotics fabricated: Date: _____   Time: _____

- 2-month follow-up: Date: _____   Time: _____
- 6-month follow-up: Date: _____   Time: _____

DPP, distal pedal pulse; HAV, hallux abductus valgus; IPK, interphalangeal keratosis; IP, interphalangeal; PTP, posterior tibial pulse

arterial blood pressure, the caliber of the arteries, the volume of blood reaching the capillary bed of the foot with each thrust of the heart and the rate of venous return. A filling time of up to 20 s indicates reasonably good collateral circulation. A venous filling time of longer than 20 s is indicative of a compromised peripheral vascular system and venous insufficiency (Bottomley 2003).

The rubor of the skin should be noted. Dependent rubor is the reddish-blue color of the toes and forefoot caused by reduced blood flow in the capillaries. When there is diminished arterial flow, the peripheral resistance drops with arteriocapillary dilatation and maximum oxygen extraction by the tissues and, with dependency, this is exaggerated. The actual degree of rubor can be noted when measuring venous filling time. Maximum rubor is usually evident within 2–3 min; it manifests as a dusky red color when severe ischemia is present (Peters et al 2001).

The evaluation of skin temperature and circumferential measurements are two other means of assessing circulatory insufficiency and determining whether inflammation and infection are present. Skin temperature measurements are useful if the circulatory problem is asymmetrical, although test results may be variable because of ambient temperature. In an individual with peripheral vascular disease, the extremities are often cool to the touch and, in the presence of infection, there may be hot spots. The use of a skin temperature monitoring device to obtain precise temperature measures is helpful, although the therapist can also evaluate skin temperature by touch, rating it as cold, cool, warm or hot (Bottomley 2003). Circumferential measurements of the lower leg and foot also aid in the assessment of an individual with peripheral vascular pathology. Edema is often present when the peripheral vascular system is involved because of the inability of the vessels to efficiently remove waste materials from the interstitial tissues. This edema will increase in the dependent position because of gravity. Determination of circumference can be accomplished using Jobst measurement tapes (free from local vendor) to measure around the metatarsal heads, the midfoot, in a figure of eight around the

ankle, and in 3 in (7.62 cm) increments up the lower leg, from the malleolar level to the subpatellar level. Another means of determining the degree of edema is by volume displacement; this is achieved by measuring the amount of water that is displaced upwards when the lower extremity is submerged in a bucket of water (using a ruler taped to the inside of the bucket). This method provides an objective and reproducible means of assessing edema in the lower extremity (Bottomley & Schwartz 1995).

Evaluating wound status

In the presence of foot lesions, it is helpful to grade the lesion for objective monitoring. Wagner's classification grades the risk of ulceration as a result of sensory loss as follows:

Grade 0 foot: the skin is without ulceration; no open lesions are present but potentially ulcerating deformities, such as bunions, hammer toes and Charcot's deformity, may be present; healed partial-foot amputations may also be included in this group.

Grade 1 foot: a full-thickness superficial skin loss is present; the lesion does not extend to bone; no abscess is present.

Grade 2 foot: an open ulceration is noted, deeper than that of grade 1; it may penetrate to the tendon or joint capsule.

Grade 3 foot: the lesion penetrates to bone and osteomyelitis is present; joint infection or plantar fascial plane abscess may also be noted.

Grade 4 foot: gangrene is noted in the forefoot.

Grade 5 foot: gangrene involving the entire foot is noted; this is not salvageable by local procedures.

In the presence of an ulceration, objective documentation of wound size is best accomplished by tracing the wound on sterilized X-ray film or by photographing it on line-graphed film. This is helpful in the monitoring of any improvement or decline in wound status (McGill et al 1996).

Form 51.2 Buerger—Allen Initial Evaluation form[a].

PATIENT:_____ AGE: _____ SEX: _____ RM no.: _____

DIAGNOSIS: _____ Physician: _____

DATE INITIAL EVALUATION: _____ Therapist: _____

Signature

	RIGHT LEG	LEFT LEG
APPEARANCE:	_____	_____
SKIN INTEGRITY:	_____	_____
SKIN TEMPERATURE:	_____	_____
EDEMA PRESENT:	0☐ +1☐ +2☐ +3☐	0☐ +1☐ +2☐ +3☐

CIRCUMFERENTIAL:		Right	Left
	☐ Metatarsal heads	_____	_____
	☐ Arch	_____	_____
	☐ Ankle	_____	_____
	☐ Supramalleolar	_____	_____
	☐ Mid-calf	_____	_____
	☐ Subpatellar	_____	_____

PULSES:			
	Dorsal pedalis	0☐ +1☐ +2☐ +3☐	0☐ +1☐ +2☐ +3☐
	Post-tibialis	0☐ +1☐ +2☐ +3☐	0☐ +1☐ +2☐ +3☐
	Popliteal	0☐ +1☐ +2☐ +3☐	0☐ +1☐ +2☐ +3☐
	Femoral	0☐ +1☐ +2☐ +3☐	0☐ +1☐ +2☐ +3☐

SENSORY TESTING:	Vibratory sense:	☐ PRESENT ☐ DIMINISHED ☐ ABSENT	☐ PRESENT ☐ DIMINISHED ☐ ABSENT

Protective sensation:

1 = 0.1 g (4.17 for normal)
2 = 10 g (5.07 protective sense)
3 = 75 g (6.10 loss protective sense)
4 = No protective sensation

	Right	Left
Dorsum:	1☐ 2☐ 3☐ 4☐	1☐ 2☐ 3☐ 4☐
Plantar digit 1:	1☐ 2☐ 3☐ 4☐	1☐ 2☐ 3☐ 4☐
Plantar digit 3:	1☐ 2☐ 3☐ 4☐	1☐ 2☐ 3☐ 4☐
Plantar digit 5:	1☐ 2☐ 3☐ 4☐	1☐ 2☐ 3☐ 4☐
Metatarsal head 1:	1☐ 2☐ 3☐ 4☐	1☐ 2☐ 3☐ 4☐
Metatarsal head 3:	1☐ 2☐ 3☐ 4☐	1☐ 2☐ 3☐ 4☐
Metatarsal head 5:	1☐ 2☐ 3☐ 4☐	1☐ 2☐ 3☐ 4☐
Proximal head 3:	1☐ 2☐ 3☐ 4☐	1☐ 2☐ 3☐ 4☐
Arch:	1☐ 2☐ 3☐ 4☐	1☐ 2☐ 3☐ 4☐
Heel:	1☐ 2☐ 3☐ 4☐	1☐ 2☐ 3☐ 4☐

STRENGTH:

	Right		Left
	Anterior tibialis:		
	Extensor hallucis longus:		
	Flexor hallucis longus:		
	Posterior tibialis:		
	Peroneus longus:		
	Gastrocnemius/soleus:		
	Intrinsics (strong/weak/atrophied)		

DEFORMITIES:	Right	Left
Hammer/claw:	____	____
Bony prominence:	____	____
Drop-foot:	____	____
Charcot's foot:	____	____
Hallux limitus:	____	____
Rear/forefoot varus:	____	____
Plantar flexed first:	____	____
Equinus:	____	____
Amputation:	____	____

FOOTWEAR: ☐ Standard ☐ Special Describe _____

☐ Adequate ☐ Inadequate Describe _____

Blanching/filling times: _____ Elevated _____ Horizontal _____ Dependent _____

TREATMENT RECOMMENDATIONS:[b]

☐ Buerger–Allen exercises Cycles _____ Times/day_____ Modified Yes/no

☐ Patient education ☐ Skin care ☐ Footwear ☐ Orthotics

[a] Buerger–Allen evaluation form created by: Jennifer M. Bottomley, PT, MS, PhD © 1996
[b] Refer to Buerger–Allen treatment flow sheet for initial blanching/filling times etc.

Form 51.3 Buerger–Allen Follow-up Evaluation form[a].

PATIENT:_____ AGE: _____ SEX: _____ RM no.: _____ MD: _____

DIAGNOSIS: _____ Initial evaluation: _____ F/U evaluation:_____

TOTAL NO. TREATMENTS: _____ Therapist: _____

Signature

	RIGHT LEG	LEFT LEG
APPEARANCE:	_____	_____
SKIN INTEGRITY:	_____	_____
SKIN TEMPERATURE:	_____	_____
EDEMA PRESENT:	0☐ +1☐ +2☐ +3☐	0☐ +1☐ +2☐ +3☐

CIRCUMFERENTIAL:

	Right	Left
☐ Metatarsal heads	_____	_____
☐ Arch	_____	_____
☐ Ankle	_____	_____
☐ Supramalleolar	_____	_____
☐ Mid-calf	_____	_____
☐ Subpatellar	_____	_____

PULSES:

	Right	Left
Dorsal pedalis	0☐ +1☐ +2☐ +3☐	0☐ +1☐ +2☐ +3☐
Post-tibialis	0☐ +1☐ +2☐ +3☐	0☐ +1☐ +2☐ +3☐
Popliteal	0☐ +1☐ +2☐ +3☐	0☐ +1☐ +2☐ +3☐
Femoral	0☐ +1☐ +2☐ +3☐	0☐ +1☐ +2☐ +3☐

SENSORY TESTING:

Vibratory sense:

	Right	Left
	☐ PRESENT	☐ PRESENT
	☐ DIMINISHED	☐ DIMINISHED
	☐ ABSENT	☐ ABSENT

Protective sensation:

1 = 0.1 g (4.17 for normal)
2 = 10 g (5.07 protective sense)
3 = 75 g (6.10 loss protective sense)
4 = No protective sensation

	Right	Left
Dorsum:	1☐ 2☐ 3☐ 4☐	1☐ 2☐ 3☐ 4☐
Plantar digit 1:	1☐ 2☐ 3☐ 4☐	1☐ 2☐ 3☐ 4☐
Plantar digit 3:	1☐ 2☐ 3☐ 4☐	1☐ 2☐ 3☐ 4☐
Plantar digit 5:	1☐ 2☐ 3☐ 4☐	1☐ 2☐ 3☐ 4☐
Metatarsal head 1:	1☐ 2☐ 3☐ 4☐	1☐ 2☐ 3☐ 4☐
Metatarsal head 3:	1☐ 2☐ 3☐ 4☐	1☐ 2☐ 3☐ 4☐
Metatarsal head 5:	1☐ 2☐ 3☐ 4☐	1☐ 2☐ 3☐ 4☐
Proximal head 5:	1☐ 2☐ 3☐ 4☐	1☐ 2☐ 3☐ 4☐
Arch:	1☐ 2☐ 3☐ 4☐	1☐ 2☐ 3☐ 4☐
Heel:	1☐ 2☐ 3☐ 4☐	1☐ 2☐ 3☐ 4☐

STRENGTH:

	Right	Left
Anterior tibialis:		
Extensor hallucis longus:		
Flexor hallucis longus:		
Posterior tibialis:		
Peroneus longus:		
Gastrocnemius/soleus:		
Intrinsics (strong/weak/atrophied)		

DEFORMITIES:

	Right	Left
Hammer/claw:		
Bony prominence:		
Drop-foot:		
Charcot's foot:		
Hallux limitus:		
Rear/forefoot varus:		
Plantar flexed first:		
Equinus:		
Amputation:		

FOOTWEAR: ☐ Standard ☐ Special Describe _____

☐ Adequate ☐ Inadequate Describe _____

TREATMENT RECOMMENDATIONS:[b]

☐ Buerger–Allen exercises Cycles _____ Times/day_____ Modified Yes/no

☐ Patient education ☐ Skin care ☐ Footwear ☐ Orthotics

[a] Buerger–Allen evaluation form created by: Jennifer M. Bottomley, PT, MS, PhD © 1996
[b] Refer to Buerger–Allen treatment flow sheet for initial blanching/filling times etc.

Form 51.4 Buerger–Allen Treatment Flow Sheet[a] DB17

Patient _____ Age _____ Sex _____ Rm no.: _____ Therapist initials _____

Diagnosis _____ Diabetes _____ □ Cardiac □ Htn

Wound: □ Present □ Not present □ Describe □ Pvd □ Amputee

Buerger–Allen protocol: Cycles _____ Times/day _____ Modified _____

Parameter	Initial evaluation	Follow-up	Follow-up	Follow-up	Notes
Date/therapist initials					
Resting heart rate (supine)					
Blood pressure (supine)					
Respiratory rate (supine)					
Plantar skin temperature	L: _____ R: _____	L: _____ R: _____	L: _____ R: _____	L: _____ R: _____	
Dorsal pedalis pulse left	0□ +1□ +2□ +3□	0□ +1□ +2□ +3□	0□ +1□ +2□ +3□	0□ +1□ +2□ +3□	
Dorsal pedalis pulse right	0□ +1□ +2□ +3□	0□ +1□ +2□ +3□	0□ +1□ +2□ +3□	0□ +1□ +2□ +3□	
Post-tibialis pulse left	0□ +1□ +2□ +3□	0□ +1□ +2□ +3□	0□ +1□ +2□ +3□	0□ +1□ +2□ +3□	
Post-tibialis pulse right	0□ +1□ +2□ +3□	0□ +1□ +2□ +3□	0□ +1□ +2□ +3□	0□ +1□ +2□ +3□	
Edema (supine)	0□ +1□ +2□ +3□	0□ +1□ +2□ +3□	0□ +1□ +2□ +3□	0□ +1□ +2□ +3□	
Circumferential measures					
Metatarsal heads	L: _____ R: _____	L: _____ R: _____	L: _____ R: _____	L: _____ R: _____	
Arch	L: _____ R: _____	L: _____ R: _____	L: _____ R: _____	L: _____ R: _____	
Ankle (figure of eight)	L: _____ R: _____	L: _____ R: _____	L: _____ R: _____	L: _____ R: _____	
Supramalleolar	L: _____ R: _____	L: _____ R: _____	L: _____ R: _____	L: _____ R: _____	
Mid-calf	L: _____ R: _____	L: _____ R: _____	L: _____ R: _____	L: _____ R: _____	
Subpatellar	L: _____ R: _____	L: _____ R: _____	L: _____ R: _____	L: _____ R: _____	
Blanching time elevated					
Filling time horizontal					
Filling time dependent					

[a]Jennifer M. Bottomley, PT, MS, PhD © 1996.
Pvd, peripheral vascular disease; Htn, hypertension.

THERAPEUTIC INTERVENTIONS

Preventive management

A management plan for the neuropathic foot patient is based on the risk classification scheme (Box 51.1). Patients in risk categories 1–3 are educated in foot inspection, skin care and selection of footwear. Footwear recommendations depend on the level of risk and the specific needs of each individual. For example, patients in category 1 benefit from shoes with leather (or other compliant material) uppers and a toe-box that accommodates the shape of the foot. A cushioned insole may be added. Patients in categories 2 and 3 may need customized insoles and shoe modifications that are appropriate for their deformities (Bottomley & Herman 1992). Once a patient is assigned a level of risk through the screening process, a program of routine follow-up is recommended: once a year for category 0 patients, biannually for category 1 patients, every 3 months for category 2 patients, and monthly for those in category 3.

Treatment of plantar ulcers

The treatment of choice for plantar ulcers is the total contact cast (Coleman et al 1984). In this casting technique, foam padding encloses the toes; felt pads provide protection over the malleoli, tibial crest, posterior heel and navicular tuberosity; and local padding provides relief at the ulcer site. The initial cast should be changed within the first week as edema resolves, to prevent injury because of an improper fit. The effectiveness of walking casts in healing diabetic and non-diabetic foot ulcers has been demonstrated in numerous studies. Walking casts promote plantar wound healing by (i) reducing plantar pressures, (ii) reducing leg edema, and (iii) protecting the area from traumatic reinjury (Bottomley & Herman 1992, Coleman et al 2003, Lemaster et al 2003, Bottomley 2004).

Not every patient will accept, or is a candidate for, a walking cast. Infection and fragile skin are contraindications to casting and, in these cases, alternatives should be used. A walking splint is a posterior cast secured to the leg by an elastic wrap. The shell is made of plaster reinforced by fiberglass taping, and relief for the posterior heel and plantar lesion is provided by adhesive backed padding (Coleman et al 2003). The ulcer-relief (cut-out) sandal is another device that can be used as an alternative to casting. The foot bed of molded plastazote is cut out or cut in relief to reduce pressure beneath the plantar lesion (Coleman et al 2003).

Prevention and treatment

A major challenge is to prevent re-ulceration. The patient must be provided with temporary protective footwear at the time of healing and be given protective footgear following the healing of the ulceration. The patient is gradually allowed to resume activities, avoiding those that may have contributed to the ulcer formation. A sandal molded from thermoplastic materials is an acceptable device during this critical period. Individuals who resume activity too quickly after a period of casting or other immobilization with protective footwear are at risk of developing a neuropathic fracture. The best way to monitor infections is by comparing the temperature between the involved and uninvolved foot. Temperatures increase by as much as 1°F(17.22°C) because of stress-induced inflammation. A skin-surface temperature monitor can by employed to evaluate differences in temperature between the inflamed area and the non-inflamed areas of the foot. The patient must be aware that the first evidence of injury to the bones of the foot is swelling and warmth (Birke et al 2002, Bottomley 2003).

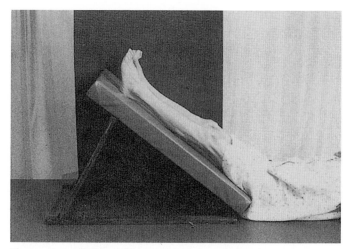

Figure 51.1 Buerger–Allen protocol: legs elevated.

When the ulcer site is fully healed, footwear is progressed to modified shoes fitted with accommodative orthotics. With mild deformities, molded insoles are added to extra-depth shoes or sneakers. For healed forefoot ulcers, a rocker sole is applied to the sole of the shoe to assist with push-off. If the foot is significantly shortened or deformed, custom shoes may be required. Custom shoes are made by pedorthists or orthotists over plaster models of the patient's feet, and extra depth is incorporated into the shoe to accommodate a soft molded interface beneath the foot (Bottomley & Herman 1992, Praet & Louwerens 2003).

Charcot fractures often result in serious deformities of the foot. Acute Charcot fractures may require surgery or long periods of immobilization in a cast; temperature monitoring is also required. The length of time of casting and immobilization depends on the individual rate of healing. Custom shoes are prescribed when there is no longer a difference in skin temperature between the fractured and the uninvolved foot (Coleman et al 2003).

Buerger–Allen exercise protocol

Buerger–Allen exercises are performed according to the protocols displayed in Figs 51.1–51.3 (Bottomley 2003).The individual lies supine with the legs elevated at an angle of 45 degrees until blanching occurs or for a maximum of 3 min (Fig. 51.1). Active pumping and circling of the feet and isometric quadriceps and gluteal contractions are performed for the first minute or more in the elevated position. Once the blanching has occurred, the subject sits up and hangs the lower leg over the edge of the bed (Fig. 51.2). While the legs are in the dependent position, the individual is encouraged to actively plantarflex, dorsiflex and circle the foot. This position is maintained for a minimum of 3 min or until rubor has occurred. Finally, the individual lies supine with the lower extremities flat for 3 min (Fig. 51.3). Again, active contraction of the leg muscles is performed for at least 1 min in this position. It is important to note that, in the presence of severe physiological compromise of the cardiovascular system, it is recommended that the supine position be assumed between the elevation and dependent phases, as well as between the dependent and elevation phases, to prevent the consequences of orthostatic hypotension. The entire sequence is repeated three times in each session. Buerger–Allen exercises should be performed twice a day for maximum benefit. If peripheral neuropathy is present and active muscle contraction is not possible, the clinician can passively plantarflex and dorsiflex the foot in each of the respective positions to increase blood flow, which is facilitated by the

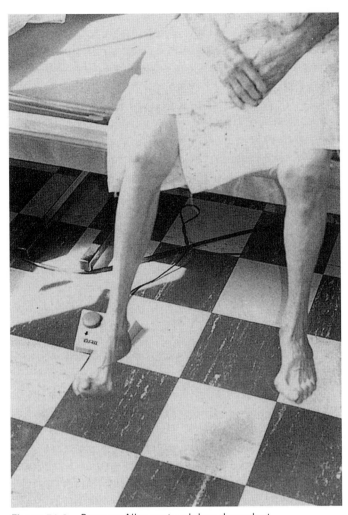

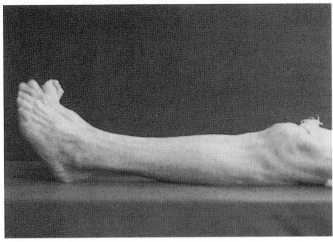

Figure 51.3   Buerger–Allen protocol: legs horizontal.

pumping action of the surrounding musculature. High-frequency electrical stimulation can be employed to elicit threshold muscle contractions in the lower extremities of elderly patients with peripheral neuropathy.

CONCLUSION

The insensitive foot, which results from various pathological conditions, is very common and problematic in aging individuals. The key to good care is a proper evaluation, which leads to appropriate therapeutic intervention. Several evaluation tools have been presented and the interventions of total-contact casting, protective footgear and the Buerger–Allen exercise routine described. In conjunction with patient education, which is crucial for prevention, effective care can mitigate the deleterious effects of the insensitive foot.

Figure 51.2   Buerger–Allen protocol: legs dependent.

References

Birke JA, Sims DS 1988 The insensitive foot. In: Hunt GC (ed) Physical Therapy of the Foot and Ankle. Churchill Livingstone, New York, p 133–168.

Birke JA, Pavich MA, Patout Jr CA, Horswell R 2002 Comparison of forefoot ulcer healing using alternative off-loading methods in patients with diabetes mellitus. Adv Skin Wound Care 15(5):210–215

Bottomley JM 2003 Neuropathic plantar ulcer in a patient with diabetes who is homeless: diabetic case study. PT Magazine, APTA, April 2003. Available: Website; www.apta.org

Bottomley JM 2004 Footwear: the foundation for lower extremity orthotics. In: Lusardi MM, Nielsen CC (eds) Orthotics and Prosthetics in Rehabilitation, 2nd edn. Butterworth-Heinemann, Boston, MA

Bottomley JM, Herman H 1992 Making simple, inexpensive changes for the management of foot problems in the aged. Top Geriatr Rehabil 7:62–77

Bottomley JM, Schwartz N 1995 The diabetic foot. In: Donatelli R (ed) The Biomechanics of the Foot and Ankle, 2nd edn. FA Davis, Philadelphia, PA, p 223–251

Coleman WC, Brand PW, Birke JA 1984 The total contact cast: a therapy for plantar ulceration on insensitive feet. J Am Podiatr Med Assoc 74:548–552

Lemaster JW, Reiber GE, Smith DB et al 2003 Daily weight-bearing activity does not increase the risk of diabetic foot ulcers. Med Sci Sports Exerc 35(7):1093–1099

McGill M, Collins P, Bolton T, Yue DK 1996 Management of neuropathic ulceration. J Wound Care 5(2):52–54

Peters EJ, Lavery LA, Armstrong DG, Fleischli JG 2001 Electric stimulation as an adjunct to heal diabetic foot ulcers: a randomized clinical trial. Arch Phys Med Rehabil 86(6):721–725

Praet SF, Louwerens JW 2003 The influence of shoe design on plantar pressures in neuropathic feet. Diabetes Care 26(2):441–445

Chapter 52

Skin disorders

Randy Berger and Barbara A. Gilchrest

INTRODUCTION

As the skin ages, many structural and functional changes take place. These alterations include a flattening of the dermal–epidermal junction and, in the epidermis, a 20–50% decrease in the number of Langerhans cells, which are responsible for immune recognition, a decrease in the number of melanocytes, which are responsible for protective pigmentation, and a variation in the size and shape of keratinocytes (Yaar & Gilchrest 2001). The dermis is characterized by a decrease in thickness cellularity, a decrease in vascularity and a degeneration of elastic fibers. Photoaging, which results from chronic exposure to ultraviolet radiation, potentiates the average 20% age-related loss of dermal thickness. The numbers of mast cells, fibroblasts and specialized nerve endings are also diminished. Between the ages of 10 and 90 years, about one-third of the cutaneous sensory nerve-end organs are lost, which may contribute to a 20% increase in the cutaneous pain threshold. In general, the hair follicles and sebaceous glands, as well as eccrine glands, decrease in number. During adulthood, there is a 15% loss of eccrine glands and a diminished output by the remaining glands, which, compounded by the reduced cutaneous vascularity, increases the risk for heatstroke, especially in dry heat. The loss of hair bulb melanocytes accounts for the graying of hair, which is substantial in 50% of individuals by the age of 50. Subcutaneous fat, an insulator that helps with thermoregulation, provides shock absorption and protects the body from trauma, decreases with age. The body's overall proportion of fat, however, usually increases and is redistributed to the thighs and abdomen (Merck 2000).

Functional changes in aging skin include altered permeability, diminished sebum production, decreased inflammatory and immunological responsiveness, and attenuated thermoregulation with decreased sweating. Wound healing and sensory perception are impaired, elasticity is reduced and vitamin D production is decreased. In addition to these normal changes, known as intrinsic aging, additional changes take place in response to cumulative ultraviolet irradiation; this is called photoaging. These changes include atrophy of the epidermis, epidermal dysplasia and atypia, a further decrease in the number of Langerhans cells, increased and irregular distribution and activity of melanocytes, dermal elastosis (deposits of abnormal elastic fibers) and further decreases in inflammatory and immunological responsiveness.

GENERAL PRINCIPLES

When evaluating a patient with a skin disorder, it is important to ascertain which topical home remedies and other products, such as alcohol or detergents, are being applied, as these products often exacerbate the primary skin condition. It is essential to take a full medical history, with particular emphasis on medications. The chronicity of the condition and whether others in the patient's environment have a similar condition may also provide clues to the diagnosis (Fitzpatrick et al 1998).

Management of skin conditions must be tailored to the patient's physical capabilities and circumstances. Limitations in movement of the geriatric rehabilitation patient can make application of topical treatments difficult, and remedies commonly used in younger patients, such as oil in bath water, may be quite dangerous for the elderly. To avoid errors, treatment regimens should be as simple as possible. Moreover, the elderly are two to three times more likely to experience adverse reactions to antihistamines and corticosteroids, drugs frequently used to treat skin disorders. These drugs should be prescribed reluctantly and always with clear written instructions.

Most dermatological agents are applied topically, and the choice of a base for the active ingredient is important. Ointments, greasy preparations containing little water, are most useful for treating conditions in which the skin is dry, scaly or thickened. In general, a medication in an ointment base is better absorbed, and therefore more potent, than the same medication in a cream or lotion vehicle. Creams, semisolid emulsions of water in oil, are more cosmetically appealing but can be drying and are thus useful for treating exudative conditions. However, most creams contain stabilizers or preservatives that can induce allergic sensitization. Lotions, usually suspensions of fine powder in an aqueous base, are useful in the evaporative cooling and drying of the skin and are preferred on hair-bearing areas because of their ease of application. Powders are useful for absorbing moisture from weepy or intertriginous skin. Soaks and compresses, which are very drying as they evaporate, are soothing and thus appropriate for highly exudative and vesicular lesions.

Topical steroid medications are commonly used in the treatment of dermatological conditions. Numerous preparations are available, which are classified by their potency. This chapter offers guidelines as to the appropriate potency of topical steroids to use for the various conditions discussed; however, certain basic principles should be emphasized. Overuse of topical steroids can result in local side effects of skin atrophy, telangiectasia, hypopigmentation and tachyphylaxis. The higher the potency of the drug and the longer the duration of use, the greater the risk. Only mild-potency topical steroids should be used on the face, genitalia and intertriginous areas. Finally, application of topical steroids over a large area of the body results in systemic absorption, which can lead to possible adrenal suppression and other sequelae.

TREATMENT OF INFECTIONS

Viral infections

Herpes simplex

Herpetic infection appears clinically as grouped vesicles on an erythematous base (Elgart 2002). Vesicles can become pustules and eventually crusts and erosions, with a characteristic punched-out appearance. Herpes simplex virus (HSV) infection can be accompanied by pruritus, burning or pain. The diagnosis can be confirmed either by the presence of multinucleated giant cells on a Tzank smear or by viral culture. Herpes simplex eruptions can be either primary or secondary; secondary eruptions can be provoked by stress, infection, trauma or ultraviolet radiation. They are most commonly seen in the perioral and anogenital regions, although they can be seen in any location. Herpetic whitlow is a herpes simplex infection of the finger, classically seen in healthcare workers as a result of inoculation by a patient's lesions. In the immunocompetent host, HSV is a self-limited infection that does not necessarily require treatment; this is often the case with perioral herpes. If treatment is desired, as in genital herpes, 200 mg of oral acyclovir five times a day is effective (treat for 10 days for primary infection, 5 days for recurrent infection). When indicated, acyclovir can be used for the chronic suppression of HSV (400 mg twice a day). A severe herpes simplex infection in an immunocompromised host should be treated with 5 mg/kg of intravenous acyclovir every 8 h until resolution.

Herpes zoster

Otherwise known as shingles, herpes zoster is an acute eruption caused by a reactivation of latent varicella virus in the dorsal root ganglia. Although it may occur at any age, elderly patients are at greater risk (Elgart 2002). Other, often additive, factors that predispose to zoster include immunosuppressive drugs, corticosteroids, malignancies, local irradiation, trauma and surgery. A common sequela of herpes zoster infection is postherpetic neuralgia, for which the incidence, duration and severity increase with age. Other complications include encephalitis, ophthalmic disease when the first branch of the trigeminal nerve is involved, facial paralysis and taste loss when the

second branch of the trigeminal nerve is involved (Ramsay–Hunt syndrome), motor neuropathies, Guillain–Barré syndrome and urinary or fecal retention when sacral nerves are involved.

The clinical presentation of herpes zoster infection is sometimes preceded by prodromal symptoms of pain, pruritus or paresthesia along the affected dermatome. Fever, chills, malaise and gastrointestinal symptoms can also occur. Usually, red papules appear along a dermatome within 3 days. These rapidly progress to grouped vesicles on an erythematous base that may become hemorrhagic vesicles or pustules. After about 5 days, the vesicle formation ceases and crusts form. Gradual healing occurs over the next 2–4 weeks, sometimes resolving with pigmentary disturbances or scarring. Disseminated herpes zoster infection can occur in patients with underlying malignancy or immunodeficiency. This is a potentially life-threatening infection that requires hospitalization and intravenous acyclovir (10–12 mg/kg every 8 h).

Not all cases of herpes zoster require treatment. If treatment is to be instituted, it should be started within 72 h of the onset of symptoms. Two antiviral drugs are currently available: 800 mg of acyclovir five times a day (Beutner et al 1995) for 7–10 days (note that a much higher dose is needed than for herpes simplex) or 500 mg of famcyclovir three times a day for 7 days. Other antivirals are currently undergoing testing. Antiviral therapy has been shown to hasten the resolution of the acute disease; however, its role in decreasing the incidence of postherpetic neuralgia is controversial. In addition, the use of systemic steroids has been in and out of favor in recent years. Certainly, antiviral therapy has a more favorable side-effect profile and, if systemic steroids are prescribed, they must be used with care in the elderly. Topical soaks with an astringent solution such as Burow's solution (aluminum acetate) can help dry up vesicles and soothe the affected area. Analgesics are commonly required. It should be kept in mind that vesicle fluid is contagious to those who have never had varicella and to immunocompromised individuals. Thus, caregivers should wear gloves to avoid direct contact with the lesions and pregnant women should also avoid contact. Once the lesions have crusted over, they are no longer infectious.

Fungal infections

Superficial fungal infections may be caused by yeast or dermatophytes. Deep fungal infections of the skin are rare and occur mainly in severely immunocompromised patients. They will not be discussed here.

Tinea

Tinea, the name given to superficial dermatophyte infection of the skin, is further classified by anatomical location: tinea pedis (foot), tinea cruris (groin), tinea manuum (hand), tinea corporis (body) and tinea unguium or onychomycosis (nails). Tinea cruris characteristically spares the genitalia, as opposed to candidiasis, in which the scrotum and penis in men and the vulva in women are usually involved. Tinea capitis, or fungal infection of the scalp, is rare in older adults. Heat and moisture predispose to fungal infection. Tinea manifests clinically as scaly patches or plaques with annular or serpiginous, often slightly raised, borders. Varying degrees of erythema may be present. Tinea pedis and tinea manuum may present as diffuse scaling of the plantar or palmar surfaces. Often, one hand and two feet are affected. Tinea pedis may also present with toe-web maceration. Nails are also commonly involved, showing thickening and yellow discoloration of the nail plate, onycholysis (separation of the nail plate from the nail bed) and hyperkeratotic debris under the nail plate. Greenish discoloration indicates pseudomonal superinfection of the nail. When fungal infections are mistakenly treated with topical steroids, they initially appear to improve and show diminished scaling and inflammation; however, fungal organisms flourish and infected areas enlarge (tinea incognito). Discontinuation of steroids results in a flare in the affected area. The infection can invade the hair follicle, resulting in a deeper infection known as Majocchi's granuloma.

Diagnosis of a fungal infection is made by culture or by direct microscopic visualization of fungal hyphae in scales after treatment with potassium hydroxide. Most cutaneous dermatophyte infections can be treated with a 4-week course of topical antifungal medication. Affected areas should be kept as dry as possible, particularly the groin and toe-web spaces. The exceptions to topical treatment are tinea unguium, tinea capitis and, often, tinea manuum and Majocchi's granuloma, which require oral antifungal agents. Until recently, the only agent approved for the treatment of cutaneous dermatophyte infection was griseofulvin, which is quite effective for infections of the scalp and skin. A dose of 3.3 mg/kg/day of ultramicrosized griseofulvin, given once or twice a day for 4–6 weeks, is usually curative. Nails, however, are best treated with itraconazole. Because the drug is retained in the nail plate for extended periods, controlled trials support a pulsed regimen of 200 mg twice a day for 1 week of each month; however, current Food and Drug Administration (FDA) guidelines recommend a dose of 200 mg/day for 3 months. Other agents undergoing FDA review for use in onychomycosis include fluconazole and terbinafine. In patients with both tinea pedis and onychomycosis, recurrence of tinea pedis is common if the nails are not also treated, often necessitating indefinite topical treatment.

Candidiasis

Candida albicans, the most frequent cause of candidiasis, thrives in warm moist areas such as the groin, the axilla and the inframammary regions. Diabetic and immunosuppressed patients, as well as those receiving systemic antibiotic therapy that reduces competing surface bacteria, are at increased risk for infection. The organism may be carried asymptomatically in the bowel, mouth and vagina. Cutaneous candidal infection is characterized by beefy red, often moist, plaques with satellite pustules and papules. As mentioned above, unlike tinea cruris, candidiasis involves the skin of the genitalia. Oral candidiasis, or thrush, presents as creamy white plaques on the tongue, palate or buccal mucosa that can be easily scraped off. Perleche, or angular cheilitis, is a candidal infection of the corners of the mouth characterized by erythema, fissuring and a white exudate. Predisposing factors are dental malocclusion, poorly fitting dentures and deep folds at the corners of the mouth, with consequent retention of saliva and food particles in the affected area. Candida paronychia is an infection of the skin proximal and lateral to the nails, characterized by erythema, tenderness and swelling, with separation of the nail plate from the adjacent nail folds. This condition is chronic and should be distinguished from acute paronychia, which is usually bacterial in origin. Frequent immersion of the hands in water is a predisposing factor.

Confirmation of cutaneous candidal infection is by culture or potassium hydroxide preparation. Topical antifungal medication is usually curative, and attempts should be made to keep affected areas clean and dry.

Bacterial infections

Impetigo

Impetigo is a superficial bacterial infection of the skin that is most commonly caused by either *Staphylococcus aureus* or group A streptococci (Elgart 2002). Vesicles or pustules in the early stages break down to form golden-colored crusts that often adhere to the underlying skin. The infection can occur on previously normal intact skin or it can present as a superinfection of a primary skin disorder (e.g. eczema, neurodermatitis, herpes zoster), in which breaks in the cutaneous barrier allow bacteria to penetrate.

In managing impetigo, a skin swab should be sent for culture and to determine sensitivity. Single or localized lesions can be treated topically with mupirocin ointment applied three times a day, but more extensive impetigo requires systemic antibiotics, such as 250–500 mg of dicloxacillin four times a day for 7–10 days. Wet lesions can be soaked in an astringent such as Burow's solution that also has antimicrobial properties.

Folliculitis

Infection of the hair follicle is manifested by follicularly based erythematous papules and pustules. Lesions can be either superficial or deep (Elgart 2002). Areas of predilection are the scalp and extremities, although the eruption can occur anywhere. Sweating and occlusion, such as under a splint, predispose to folliculitis; however, as long as therapy has been initiated, exercise and splints are not contraindicated in patients with this condition. The most common causative organism is *S. aureus*. However, Gram-negative organisms (such as *Pseudomonas*, which causes hot-tub folliculitis), candida and *Pityrosporum* yeast can also be pathogenic. Because of the variety of potentially causative organisms, it is advisable to send pustule contents for culture and determination of sensitivity. However, given that most cases are caused by *S. aureus*, it is reasonable to start antistaphylococcal treatment, such as 250–500 mg of dicloxacillin four times a day for 1–2 weeks, pending culture results. Mild cases can be treated with topical antistaphylococcal antibiotics, such as erythromycin, clindamycin or mupirocin. Antibacterial soaps, such as Hibiclens, pHisoHex and Lever 2000, help to maintain a lower bacterial count on predisposed hosts. The treatment of candidal infection has already been discussed. *Pityrosporum* folliculitis occurs mainly on the trunk and is often associated with diabetes mellitus, antibiotic therapy or immunosuppression. Treatment is with a 2-week course of selenium sulfide 2.5% lotion applied daily for 10 min and then washed off. Topical antifungal creams are also effective (Table 52.1).

Erysipelas

Erysipelas is a superficial infection of the skin caused by group A or group C hemolytic streptococci. The organism may enter the skin through minor cuts, wounds or insect bites. Lesions of erysipelas are characterized by warm edematous erythematous plaques with well-defined, often rapidly advancing, margins. Vesicles and bullae may

Table 52.1 Examples of antifungal preparations[a]

Compound	Formulation
Clotrimazole	Cream or lotion 1.0%
Ketoconazole	Cream 2.0%
Nystatin	Cream or powder[b]
Terbinafine hydrochloride	Cream 1.0%[c]

[a]Many equally effective compounds and formulations are not listed.
[b]Effective against candida but not dermatophytes.
[c]Fungicidal against dermatophytes (others are fungistatic), thus allowing shorter duration of treatment; activity against candida is variable.

be present and can even be hemorrhagic. Fever, malaise and lymphadenopathy accompany cutaneous infection. The face is the most common location for erysipelas but infection can occur anywhere. Treatment is with oral or intravenous antistreptococcal antibiotics such as penicillin or erythromycin (in penicillin-allergic patients). A typical outpatient regimen is 250–500 mg four times a day for 2 weeks. Clinical judgment and continuous evaluation of the clinical course determine the treatment setting and route of administration of antibiotics. Because infection continues to spread during the first 12–24 h of oral therapy, patients with facial lesions often require hospitalization and intravenous antibiotics to prevent the complication of cavernous sinus thrombosis.

Cellulitis

Cellulitis is a deeper infection of the skin, most commonly caused by group A streptococci and occasionally by *S. aureus* or Gram-negative organisms (Merck 2000). It can occur as a complication of an open wound, a venous ulcer or tinea pedis, or it can develop on intact skin, particularly on the legs. Clinically, it presents as erythema, tenderness, swelling and warmth. Fever and lymphadenopathy may also occur. Treatment is with oral or intravenous antibiotics, depending upon the severity of infection and the background health of the patient. Streptococcal cellulitis is best treated with penicillin, as outlined above; however, if *S. aureus* is suspected or the causative agent is unclear, broader coverage antibiotics, such as 250–500 mg of dicloxacillin or cephalexin four times a day, should be instituted and adjusted according to the clinical response. Patients with diabetes mellitus or peripheral vascular disease will probably need close monitoring and intravenous therapy. Diabetic patients are more likely to have Gram-negative, anaerobic and mixed microbial infections. The treatment of any underlying predisposing condition should also be undertaken. If the cellulitis does not respond to antimicrobial therapy, Gram-negative or resistant organisms or an alternative diagnosis should be considered.

Swelling, pain and open lesions may necessitate modification or temporary suspension of physical rehabilitation; however, cellulitis is not a frank contraindication to physical exercise. Clinical judgment must be used and the effects of disuse weighed against the need for rest. It is important to avoid aggravating the condition.

TREATMENT OF INFESTATIONS

Scabies

Scabies is an intensely pruritic eruption caused by the *Sarcoptes scabiei* mite. The female mite burrows into the skin and deposits eggs, which hatch into larvae in a few days. Scabies is easily transmitted by skin-to-skin contact and can be readily spread between residents of the same household, nursing home or institution. Pruritus is caused by a hypersensitivity reaction, so infestation has usually been present for weeks before it manifests clinically. Pruritus is severe and often worse at night. The hallmark of scabies is the burrow, which is a linear ridge, often with a tiny vesicle at one end; however, these lesions may be obscured by scratching. Other cutaneous signs of scabies are papules, nodules and vesicles. Lesions are characteristically found in the interdigital web spaces, the flexor aspects of the wrists, the axilla, the umbilicus, around the nipples and on the genitalia. The skin is almost always excoriated and lesions are susceptible to secondary impetiginization. In elderly and physically or mentally disabled patients, scabies may present less typically because of the inability to scratch and is often a long-standing infestation. The condition may mimic eczema or exfoliative dermatitis and widespread hyperkeratotic and crusted lesions may be present.

The diagnosis is confirmed by observation of the scabies mite, eggs or excretions in a skin scraping placed in mineral oil and examined under a microscope. A typical patient has only 10–12 adult female mites at one time, so confirmation of scabies is not always possible and diagnosis is often presumptive. Several antiscabitic creams and lotions are effective in treating scabies. The two most commonly used today are 5% permethrin cream and 1% lindane lotion or cream. Lindane, particularly if overused, can have neurotoxic side effects, including headaches, dizziness, nausea and, rarely, seizures. Permethrin is thought to be a safer treatment for infants and pregnant women. Successful treatment requires the treatment of all close personal contacts. In an inpatient or residential facility, all clinical staff, patients, selected visitors and their household contacts should be treated. As mentioned earlier, the infestation can be subclinical for weeks, so infested contacts may be asymptomatic. The medication should be applied to the entire body, from the neck down (the head is also treated in infants). Particular attention should be paid to applying the cream or lotion under the fingernails and to the external genitalia. The medication should be washed off 8 h later and, at that time, all clothing and linens should be washed in hot water, dry-cleaned or placed in a hot dryer. This process should be repeated 1 week later, to kill any newly-hatched larvae. Unlike lindane, permethrin has the advantage of killing scabies eggs as well as the mites and larvae, so, in theory, only one application is necessary; however, two applications are usually performed to ensure cure. It must be kept in mind that, as pruritus is caused by allergic sensitization and not viable organisms, it may continue for 1–2 weeks after successful treatment. This can usually be controlled with mild- to mid-potency topical steroids (Table 52.2) and oral antihistamines. Itching that continues beyond a few weeks may indicate treatment failure, reinfestation or an incorrect diagnosis (Elgart 2002).

Table 52.2 Examples of topical corticosteroid preparations[a]

Potency	Compound	Formulation
Very high	Clobetasol proprionate	Cream or ointment 0.05%
	Halobetasol proprionate	Cream or ointment 0.05%[b]
High	Betamethasone diproprionate	Cream or ointment 0.05%
	Betamethasone valerate	Ointment 0.1%
	Fluocinonide	Cream or ointment 0.05%
	Halcinonide	Cream or ointment 0.1%
Medium	Betamethasone valerate	Cream 0.1%
	Fluocinolone acetonide	Cream or ointment 0.025%
	Hydrocortisone valerate	Cream or ointment 0.2%
	Triamcinolone acetonide	Cream, ointment or lotion 0.1% or 0.025%
Low	Hydrocortisone	Cream, ointment or lotion 2.5% or 1.0%

After Gilchrest BA 2000 Skin changes and disorders. In: Beers MH and Berkow R (eds) The Merck Manual of Geriatrics, 3rd edn. Merck & Co, Whitehouse Station, NJ, p 1247, with permission.
[a]Many equally effective compounds and formulations are not listed.
[b]Ointments are more potent than creams containing the same corticosteroid in the same concentration because of their enhanced penetration.

Pediculosis

Three species of lice infest humans: *Pediculus humanus* var. *capitis* (head lice), *Pediculus humanus* var. *corporis* (body lice) and *Phthirus pubis* (pubic lice, also known as crab lice). Transmission is by close person-to-person contact or by sharing clothing, hats or combs. Elderly individuals who have poor personal hygiene or who live in an overcrowded environment are at risk for head and body lice. *Pediculosis capitis* presents with scalp pruritus, which can progress to eczematous changes with impetiginization. Localized lymphadenopathy can occur. Examination reveals small, gray-white nits (ova) adherent to hair shafts. Adult lice can occasionally be found. *Pediculosis corporis* should be considered in a patient who presents with generalized pruritus. Again, secondary eczematous changes, excoriation and impetiginization can occur. Lice and nits are usually not found on the body but rather in the seams of clothing. *Phthirus pubis* is usually spread by sexual contact but may also be transmitted via clothing or towels. The bases of pubic hairs should be examined for lice and nits in a patient complaining of pubic pruritus.

Head lice are treated with 1% lindane shampoo, which is applied for 4 min and then washed off. Treatment should be repeated in 7–10 days. Close contacts should also be examined and treated. Combs and brushes should be soaked in lindane shampoo for 1 h. The presence of nits after appropriate treatment does not signify treatment failure. They can be removed from the hair with a fine-tooth comb dipped in vinegar.

Body lice are treated by washing the affected clothing in hot water, dry-cleaning them or placing them in a hot dryer and then ironing the seams. Alternatively, the clothing can be disinfected with an insecticidal powder such as DDT 10% or malathion 1%. If lice or nits are found on the skin, the patient can wash with lindane shampoo as above. Pubic lice are treated identically to head lice, with local application of lindane shampoo. In all forms of infestation, pruritus and dermatitis can be treated with emollients and topical steroids, and impetiginization may require antibiotics.

TREATMENT OF INFLAMMATORY SKIN CONDITIONS

Pruritus

Pruritus, or itching, is a common complaint. It can occur in the presence or absence of objective cutaneous findings; associated skin eruptions may be causative (primary) or secondary. Patients who complain of pruritus should be examined for inconspicuous primary skin lesions because some pruritic skin diseases, such as bullous pemphigoid and scabies, may show little, if any, cutaneous signs initially. Systemic disorders that are associated with generalized pruritus without primary skin lesions include liver and renal disease, polycythemia vera, iron deficiency anemia, lymphomas, leukemias, parasitosis (usually of the gastrointestinal tract) and psychiatric disease. Some drugs (e.g. barbiturates, narcotics) can also cause itching without a skin eruption. Disorders rarely associated with itching include diabetes mellitus, hyperthyroidism, hypothyroidism (where pruritus is usually secondary to xerosis) and solid malignancies. The most common cause of pruritus is xerosis (dry skin) and, regardless of cause, most patients complaining of pruritus benefit from treatment for xerosis (see the following section). Antihistamines can be helpful in some cases but should be used cautiously in the elderly.

If no skin disease is evident, patients should be examined for evidence of systemic disorders such as lymphadenopathy, hepatosplenomegaly, jaundice and anemia. Appropriate laboratory tests for screening include a complete blood count, erythrocyte sedimentation rate, electrolytes (including urea nitrogen and creatinine), urine glucose, thyroid function tests and liver function tests. If indicated by history or physical examination, a chest radiograph may be obtained or stools tested for occult blood, ova and parasites. When itching begins suddenly and is severe and unrelenting, an underlying disease should be strongly suspected and laboratory evaluation should be thorough (*Merck Manual of Geriatrics* 2000).

Xerosis

Xerosis is quite common in the elderly and it is the most common cause of pruritus. Symptoms are often worse in the winter when central heating decreases the humidity indoors and the skin is exposed to cold and wind outdoors. Patients should be advised to avoid very hot baths or showers, as well as irritants such as harsh detergents and topically applied alcohol. Emollients should be applied liberally and frequently, especially immediately after bathing when the skin is still moist. Severely dry skin may become inflamed (see Asteatotic eczema, below).

TREATMENT OF DERMATITIS

Often used interchangeably with the term eczema, dermatitis indicates a superficial inflammation of the skin caused by exposure to an irritant, allergic sensitization, genetically determined factors or a combination of these factors. Pruritus, erythema and edema progress to vesiculation, oozing, crusting and scaling. Eventually, the skin may become lichenified (thickened and with prominent skin markings) from repeated rubbing or scratching (*Merck Manual of Geriatrics* 2000).

Allergic contact dermatitis

Allergic contact dermatitis is an immune-mediated, type IV, delayed hypersensitivity reaction. The prototype is Rhus dermatitis, or poison ivy. Acute lesions tend to be vesicular, whereas chronic contact dermatitis appears scaly and lichenified. Clues to an allergic contact dermatitis are a bizarre shape or location or linear arrangement of lesions. Common contact allergens include nickel, fragrance additives, preservatives in cosmetics or medications, rubber, lanolin, chromates (used in tanning leather), topical antibiotics (especially neomycin, which is used, for example, on chronic ulcers) and topical anesthetics (e.g. benzocaine). Treatment consists of identifying and removing the causative agent and applying mid- to high-potency topical steroids (Table 52.2). Soaks such as Burow's solution dry acute vesicular lesions, whereas emollients soothe dry chronic lesions and resolving acute lesions. Pure petrolatum has no fragrances or preservatives and is advised when a fragrance or preservative allergy is suspected or when the allergen is unknown. If a contact dermatitis is suspected and a causative agent is not apparent by history and physical examination, patch-testing, usually performed by a dermatologist, can aid in making a diagnosis. All cutaneous allergies should be documented on the patient's chart because systemic exposure (e.g. via oral medication) to chemically related compounds may result in severe systemic allergic reactions.

Irritant contact dermatitis

Unlike allergic contact dermatitis, irritant contact dermatitis is not immune mediated. Given enough contact with an irritant, any patient will develop a dermatitis. Common irritants are soaps and detergents.

Although the elderly have a less pronounced inflammatory response to most irritants than younger patients, chronic irritant dermatitis is a common occurrence in the elderly. Clinical manifestations are identical to those of allergic contact dermatitis and treatment is similar.

Atopic dermatitis

Atopic dermatitis, commonly referred to as eczema, is a chronic pruritic condition that is commonly associated with other atopic features, such as asthma, allergic rhinitis and xerosis. Atopic dermatitis is often referred to as 'the itch that rashes', highlighting pruritus as the hallmark of this condition. Atopic dermatitis rarely begins in adulthood and usually improves with age. However, it can be exacerbated by environmental factors, for example the dry environment that occurs in winter as a result of central heating, woolen clothing, harsh detergents and prolonged bathing. Treatment centers around altering habits to avoid these factors and aggressively using emollients and mid-potency topical steroids.

Lichen simplex chronicus

Also known as neurodermatitis, lichen simplex chronicus is a localized pruritic eruption that results from chronic scratching and rubbing, eventuating in a scratch–itch–scratch cycle. Clinically, lesions appear erythematous or hyperpigmented, lichenified and scaly. High-potency topical steroids are often required to break the cycle. Steroid-impregnated tape, such as flurandrenolide (Cordran), applied at bedtime or after bathing and left in place up to 24h, also protects the lesions from being scratched. When symptoms improve, the potency can be reduced. Topical doxepin relieves pruritus and also helps to break the scratch–itch–scratch cycle, but systemic absorption and drowsiness sometimes limit its use. If applicable, lesions can be covered with dressings such as an Unna boot to prevent the patient from scratching. More nodular lesions are termed prurigo nodularis.

Asteatotic eczema

When skin becomes excessively dry and scaly, fissures and excoriation allow environmental irritants to penetrate and further worsen the condition, adding inflammation to dryness. This commonly occurs on the lower legs and is characterized by scaly erythematous plaques with a 'cracked porcelain' appearance, which are caused by superficial fissures and scalecrust; this condition is referred to as eczema craquele. Treatment consists of the aggressive use of emollients and, initially, the additional use of a low- to mid-potency topical steroid ointment.

Stasis dermatitis

Stasis dermatitis, commonly seen in the aging population, occurs in the context of chronic venous hypertension. Scaling and erythema are seen on a background of edema, varicosities, and hemosiderin hyperpigmentation. At times, stasis dermatitis may be confused with cellulitis, but it is usually chronic and bilateral. When severe *and* chronic, the condition may induce sclerosis, beginning at the ankles and progressing proximally (termed lipodermatosclerosis). Another complication of severe venous stasis is ulceration. Successful treatment of stasis dermatitis is contingent upon treating the underlying venous hypertension with leg elevation and compression therapy, if not contraindicated by concomitant arterial disease. Low-potency topical steroids and emollients relieve the dermatitic component and

the frequently associated pruritus. Potential contact allergens, such as neomycin, should be avoided (*Merck Manual of Geriatrics* 2000).

Seborrheic dermatitis

Seborrheic dermatitis is a common scaly erythematous eruption of the central part of the face (particularly eyebrows, glabella, eyelids and nasolabial folds), postauricular and beard areas, body flexures and scalp, where it is known in lay terms as dandruff. The central chest and interscapular areas can also be affected. Seborrheic dermatitis affecting the eyelids causes blepharitis and, sometimes, associated conjunctivitis. Seborrheic dermatitis is especially prevalent among patients with neurological conditions, particularly Parkinson's disease, facial nerve injury, poliomyelitis, syringomyelia and spinal cord injury. Neuroleptic drugs with parkinsonian side effects can also bring about seborrheic dermatitis. More recently, severe seborrheic dermatitis has been found with increased frequency in human immunodeficiency virus (HIV)-infected individuals. Although still a controversial theory, an inflammatory response to an overgrowth of the normally resident lipophilic yeast *Pityrosporum ovate* is thought to be the cause. Treatment focuses on suppressing inflammation by means of a mild-potency topical steroid such as hydrocortisone or on killing the yeast with a topical antifungal such as ketoconazole. Topical ketoconazole also exerts some anti-inflammatory effects. Seborrheic dermatitis of the scalp responds to shampoos containing selenium sulfide, zinc pyrithione, salicylic acid and tar. Ketoconazole shampoo and mild topical steroid solutions can also be helpful.

Intertrigo

Intertrigo is an inflammation of intertriginous skin, resulting from irritation, friction and maceration. It appears as moist, erythematous and, sometimes, scaly areas in the flexures. Patients may complain of pruritus or soreness. Contributing factors include obesity, poor hygiene, hot weather, irritating or occlusive products applied locally and clothing made of synthetic fabrics that do not breathe. Secondary candidal or dermatophyte infection is common and should be treated with an antifungal cream. Treatment should focus primarily on eliminating the contributing factors mentioned above. The affected areas should be kept as dry as possible. A low-potency topical steroid such as hydrocortisone is used initially to decrease inflammation and allow restoration of an intact skin barrier. Lotrisone, a commonly prescribed combination antifungal and topical steroid cream, should not be used for this condition because the steroid that it contains (betamethasone diproprionate) is too strong for use in intertriginous locations.

TREATMENT OF PSORIASIS

Psoriasis is a common chronic papulosquamous condition that follows an unpredictable waxing and waning course. It usually occurs in individuals from 16 to 22 years of age or later, in the sixth decade of life (van Voorhees et al 2001). The cause of psoriasis is not known, although a genetic predisposition has been noted. Clinically, it is characterized by well-demarcated pink plaques with adherent thick 'silvery' scales. Areas of predilection are the extensor surfaces of both upper and lower extremities, the scalp, the gluteal cleft and the penis. Psoriatic plaques commonly occur in areas of trauma, such as scars or burns. This is referred to as the isomorphic response or Koebner's phenomenon. Nails are often involved, with pitting of the nail plate, areas of yellowish discoloration known as oil spots, onycholysis (separation of the nail plate from the nail bed) and subungual debris. Psoriatic arthritis accompanies skin lesions in 5–8% of patients. Factors that exacerbate psoriasis include stress, streptococcal infection, cold climate and certain medications, for example beta blockers, antimalarials, nonsteroidal anti-inflammatory drugs, lithium and alcohol. Systemic steroids should be used with care and tapered slowly in a psoriatic patient, as a severe flare can occur with discontinuation. Psoriatic variants include inverse psoriasis of intertriginous areas, guttate psoriasis, pustular psoriasis and erythrodermic psoriasis.

Treatment is suppressive rather than curative and, in the elderly, is aimed at keeping the patient comfortable and functional (van Voorhees et al 2001). The most commonly used medications are the topical steroids. In general, mid- to high-potency steroids are needed. The vitamin D-derived calcipotriene (Dovonex) ointment is often effective and lacks the side effects of atrophy, tachyphylaxis and (rarely) adrenal suppression resulting from systemic absorption that are associated with topical steroid use. A maximum of 100 g can be used per week and it is contraindicated in patients with hypercalcemia, vitamin D toxicity or renal stones. Tar-containing bath additives, shampoos and ointments are good adjunctive therapy, although they can be messy and baths are often not feasible for the elderly or disabled. Treatment of a coexisting streptococcal infection often results in improvement of the psoriasis. Emollients should be used liberally. Other treatment modalities used by dermatologists include anthralin, phototherapy, oral retinoids and methotrexate.

TREATMENT OF DRUG ERUPTIONS

Drug eruptions can present in a wide variety of clinical manifestations. Adverse drug reactions are found in 10–20% of all hospitalized patients and are the cause of hospitalization in 3–6% of admissions (Sullivan & Shear 2002). They typically appear 1–10 days after starting a drug and last for up to 14 days after discontinuation of the drug. A rechallenge results in more rapid development of a rash. Rarely, drug eruptions can occur after weeks, months or even years of using a medication. The drugs most commonly implicated are penicillins, sulfonamides, cephalosporins (10% cross-reactivity with penicillins), anticonvulsants, blood products, quinidine, barbiturates, isoniazid and furosemide (frusemide). However, any medication, including over-the-counter preparations and sporadically used drugs, can cause eruptions (Goldstein & Wintroub 1994).

The most common morphology is the morbilliform, or maculopapular, eruption, which is a symmetrical pruritic eruption of coalescing erythematous macules and papules distributed on the trunk and extending peripherally onto the extremities. Other forms of drug eruptions are urticaria, photosensitivity, lichenoid drug eruption, vasculitis (discussed below) and fixed-drug eruption (a single or a few localized red-to-violaceous round plaques that resolve with hyperpigmentation and recur in the same location with rechallenge). Treatment of a drug eruption requires discontinuation of the culprit drug. Medium-potency topical steroids, antihistamines and antipruritic lotions, such as calamine and Sarna lotion, give symptomatic relief.

Potentially life-threatening drug eruptions requiring hospitalization, especially in the elderly (Sullivan & Shear 2002), are exfoliative erythroderma, anticonvulsant hypersensitivity syndrome, erythema multiforme major (Stevens–Johnson syndrome) and toxic epidermal necrolysis. These are dermatological emergencies, requiring hospitalization and supportive care. Exfoliative erythroderma is characterized by generalized erythema and scaling. The inability to maintain fluids, regulate electrolytes and temperature, and high-output cardiac failure are complications. Anticonvulsant hypersensitivity syndrome is a multiorgan reaction that occurs with phenobarbital, carbamazepine and phenytoin, all of which cross react with each other.

In addition to cutaneous findings, which can be of any type, fever, lymphadenopathy, hematological abnormalities and hepatitis are seen. Other organs can also be affected. In erythema multiforme major, the pathognomonic target lesions, which have red peripheries and cyanotic or bullous centers, are accompanied by erosion of the mucous membranes. This can sometimes be seen on a continuum with toxic epidermal necrolysis, which is characterized by a tender skin eruption that rapidly progresses to blistering and sloughing of skin. Applying lateral force to the skin causes the overlying epidermis to shear off (Nikolsky's sign). This condition, with its 50% mortality rate, is best treated in a burn unit.

TREATMENT OF URTICARIA

Urticaria, or hives, is characterized by pruritic, edematous and, usually, erythematous papules and plaques, often surrounded by a red halo (flare). Angioedema or deeper subcutaneous swellings may accompany urticaria. By definition, individual lesions last no longer than 24 h; if lesions are longer lasting, urticarial vasculitis or other diagnoses should be considered. Urticaria has a variety of causes, the most common of which is an allergic reaction to foods (e.g. strawberries, nuts, shellfish) or drugs (e.g. penicillin, contrast dye). Physical factors, such as cold, pressure or sunlight, emotional stress or infections (e.g. dental abscess, streptococcal upper respiratory infection, parasitic infection), can also induce urticaria. Certain medications, such as aspirin and narcotics, can cause direct nonimmunological degranulation of mast cells, which results in urticaria. Bullous pemphigoid (see below) can initially mimic urticaria. Urticaria usually resolves spontaneously within days to a few weeks; if lesions continue to appear for more than 6 weeks and if no allergen can be identified, a workup for systemic disease is warranted (Sullivan & Shear 2002). Whenever possible, the causative agent should be identified and eliminated. Antihistamines are the mainstay of treatment. In cases of anaphylaxis or laryngeal edema, emergency resuscitation measures should be undertaken, including the administration of epinephrine (adrenaline), support of blood pressure and maintenance of a patent airway.

DIFFERENTIAL DIAGNOSIS AND TREATMENT OF BLISTERS

Bullous eruptions in an elderly patient can range from those caused by benign physical factors to life-threatening immune-mediated bullous disorders. A flattening of the dermal–epidermal junction with aging results in increased skin fragility and susceptibility to blistering. Edematous skin is even more likely to develop blisters. The following is a partial list of diagnoses to consider.

Pressure blisters

Lesions can occur over pressure points such as the heels and maleoli in a patient with a diminished level of consciousness or with sensory deficits. Macular erythema often precedes blistering. Treatment consists of relieving the causative pressure, usually by frequent repositioning, protective cushioning or both.

Burns

Chemical, thermal and ultraviolet-light injury can result in blisters in affected areas. A diagnosis can usually be made after taking a patient history. Treatment is supportive, employing cool soaks for thermal and ultraviolet burns, as well as antibiotic ointments, such as silver sulfadiazene and protective dressings. Nonsteroidal anti-inflammatory drugs, such as aspirin or indomethacin, can also be beneficial in the early treatment of sunburns.

Contact dermatitis

As discussed above, an acute contact dermatitis can result in such serious inflammation and edema that it leads to frank vesiculation. Clues to contact dermatitis are a linear arrangement of vesicles, odd-shaped lesions and sharply demarcated lesions. Treatment is outlined above (see under Dermatitis).

Bullous impetigo

This superficial staphylococcal infection presents as flaccid bullae that easily rupture, leaving yellowish crusts. Treatment is with antistaphylococcal antibiotics, such as 250–500 mg of dicloxacillin four times a day.

Bullous pemphigoid

This is a chronic, immunologically mediated, bullous disorder characterized by tense bullae on normal or erythematous skin. Pruritus is common and mucous membrane involvement occurs in approximately 20–50% of cases. As mentioned above, bullous pemphigoid can have a prebullous phase that presents as urticaria or pruritus without distinct skin lesions. Men and women are equally affected and most patients are over 60 years of age at the onset of disease. Diagnosis is made by skin biopsy followed by routine pathology and immunofluorescence. Immunofluorescence reveals immunoglobulin G (IgG) and complement (C3) deposits at the dermal–epidermal junction of perilesional skin. Traditionally, bullous pemphigoid has been treated with systemic corticosteroids and immunosuppressive therapy. Recently, tetracycline and nicotinamide have been shown to be effective in some patients. Consultation with a dermatologist is strongly advised.

Pemphigus vulgaris

Much less common than bullous pemphigoid, pemphigus vulgaris is another chronic immunologically mediated bullous disease that presents with flaccid, rather than tense, bullae. Often, only ruptured bullae (erosions and crusts) are present. Mucous membranes are almost always affected and may sometimes be the only manifestations of the disease. Again, the diagnosis is made by skin biopsy and immunofluorescence, which shows IgG and C3 deposited on the surface of keratinocytes. Before the advent of corticosteroids, pemphigus vulgaris was universally fatal. Today, it is treated aggressively with corticosteroids and other immunosuppressives, leading to long-lasting remissions.

TREATMENT OF PURPURA

When blood extravasates into cutaneous tissue, purpura results. Purpura can be classified as a disorder of hemostasis, increased fragility of blood vessels and their supporting connective tissue, vasculitis (inflammation of blood vessels) or pigmented purpura.

Disorders of hemostasis

Purpura can be a manifestation of bleeding disorders, such as idiopathic thrombocytopenic purpura, thrombotic thrombocytopenic purpura, disseminated intravascular coagulation, liver disease, thrombocythemia or bone marrow dysfunction secondary to leukemia or drugs. Anticoagulants, such as heparin, coumadin, aspirin or nonsteroidal anti-inflammatory drugs, can also be associated with purpura, usually in response to an injury to the skin. Often in such patients, other dermatitides, such as drug eruptions, can become purpuric. Treatment is directed at the underlying problem.

Fragility of blood vessels

The most common cause of this purpura is actinic (Bateman's) purpura (Merck 2000). The combination of aging and chronic sun damage leads to degeneration of the collagen that surrounds and supports small vessels. Minor trauma, often not even noted by the patient, results in slowly resolving purpuric macules. Chronic corticosteroid administration can produce similar changes.

Vasculitis

Palpable purpuric papules should point to the possibility of vasculitis, although lesions of vasculitis need not always be palpable. Causes of vasculitis include drug allergy, bloodborne infection (e.g. streptococcus, meningococcemia, viral hepatitis, endocarditis), serum sickness, collagen vascular diseases and cryoglobulinemia. Wegener's granulomatosis and polyarteritis nodosa are examples of vasculitis involving larger medium-sized vessels. When vasculitis is present in the skin, it is important to rule out systemic involvement with a urinalysis, renal and liver function tests and a stool guaiac test. Whenever possible, treatment is directed at the underlying condition. Treatment is generally supportive, although some forms of vasculitis, particularly those with systemic involvement, may require treatment with corticosteroids or other antiinflammatory or immunosuppressive drugs.

Pigmented purpuras

In this disorder, there are several idiopathic purpuric eruptions, unrelated to any systemic disease, that primarily affect the lower legs. Lesions may be predominantly red/purple (of recent onset) or brown to golden-brown (chronic hemosiderin deposits). No treatment is necessary and, indeed, none is very effective.

CONCLUSION

Age-related changes occur in the structure and function of the skin. Viral, fungal and bacterial infections of the skin, as well as infestations and inflammatory conditions, can occur; the use of some common treatment interventions can be affected by the advanced age of the patient and so precautions must be taken. The proper care of the skin of an aging individual is confounded by coexisting pathologies; thus, special considerations may be necessary.

ACKNOWLEDGMENT

Tim Kauffman PT, PhD, completed this revision.

References

Beers MH, Berkow R (eds) 2000 The Merck Manual of Geriatrics, 3rd edn. Merck Research Laboratories, Whitehouse Station, NJ

Beutner KR, Friedman DJ, Andersen PL et al 1995 Valaciclovir compared with acyclovir for improved therapy for herpes water in immunocompetent adults. Antimicrob Agents Chemother 39:1546–1553

Elgart ML 2002 Skin infections and infestations in geriatric patients. Clin Geriatr Med 18(1):89–101

Fitzpatrick TB, Eisen AZ, Wolff K et al 1998 Dermatology in General Medicine, 5th edn. McGraw-Hill, New York

Goldstein SM, Wintroub BU 1994 A Physician's Guide: Adverse Cutaneous Reactions to Medication. CoMedia, New York

Merck Manual of Geriatrics, 3rd edn 2000 Merck & Co, Whitehouse Station, NJ

Sullivan JR, Shear NH 2002 Drug eruptions and other adverse drug effects in aged skin. Clin Geriatr Med 18(1):21–42

van Voorhees A, Vittorio CC, Werth VP 2001 Papulosquamous disorders of the elderly. Clin Geriatr Med 17(4):739–768

Yaar M, Gilchrest BA 2001 Skin aging: postulated mechanisms and consequent changes in structure and function. Clin Geriatr Med 17(4):617–630

UNIT 7

Aging and the pathological sensorium

Chapter 53

Functional vision changes in the normal and aging eye

Bruce P. Rosenthal and Michael Fischer

INTRODUCTION

Demographics

Changes in the visual system resulting from the normal aging process, as well as those caused by pathological eye diseases, dramatically increase after the age of 60. In light of the worldwide increase in longevity, the number of individuals affected is significant, especially in developed nations. At age 60, for example, life expectancy is 18 years for men and 23 years for women in developed nations (United Nations 2001). Estimates for the number of individuals over the age of 70 and 80 are continuing to grow rapidly (Table 53.1), and there are also greater numbers of people living well into the ninth, as well as tenth, decades of life (US Census 2004).

The dramatic upward demographic shift in aging translates into greater numbers of individuals who will experience changes in vision as a result of the normal aging process. These changes range from a decrease in the ability to focus on the printed page, to the reduction in the production of tear fluid, to a need for greater illumination when reading. By 2020, there will also be a considerable number who will experience a significant loss of vision because of pathological eye conditions such as macular degeneration, diabetic retinopathy, glaucoma and cataract (Table 53.2).

Vision–related healthcare costs

The escalation of health costs combined with increased longevity will have immediate as well as long-range implications for healthcare planning. Important issues range from deciding on the number of doctors to train to the cost of healthcare delivery to the millions of people in need of treatment. An analysis of the economic costs of treating visual disorders shows that these costs have more that quadrupled in the past 25 years (Table 53.3).

Terminology

Specialists in geriatric medicine should be aware of the terminology used by those involved in the care of the partially sighted. Such

Table 53.1 Estimates of Americans with visual system changes

Age	Population
60+	48 883 408
65+	36 293 985
85+	4 859 631

From US Census Bureau, July 1 2004 estimates.

Table 53.2 Eye disease prevalence and projections

	Current estimates (in millions)	2020 projections (in millions)
Advanced age-related macular degeneration (with associated vision loss)	1.8[a]	2.9
Glaucoma	2.2	3.3
Diabetic retinopathy	4.1	7.2
Cataract	20.5	30.1

From Congdon N, O'Colmain B, Klaver CC et al 2004 Causes and prevalence of visual impairment among adults in the United States. Arch Ophthalmol 122:477–485; 2004 Arch Ophthalmol 122:444 (Special Issue: Blindness), with permission.
[a]Another 7.3 million people are at substantial risk for vision loss from AMD.

information is useful for understanding medical records and eye reports, as well as understanding any implications that there may be regarding disability benefits. The most commonly used terms are low vision, blindness, visual impairment, functional vision, visual disability and visual handicap. Definitions are provided in the glossary at the end of this chapter.

Disability evaluation under social security

Health professionals, especially those involved in geriatric rehabilitation, should be aware of any disability benefits available from the Social Security Administration (SSA). These may include benefits for impaired visual acuity, a decrease in the field of vision, a loss of eye muscle function or a loss of visual efficiency (how easily and effectively the visual system processes visual information).

Table 53.3 Economic costs of visual disorders and disabilities in the USA in 1981 and 2003

Category of costs	Economic costs (in millions of US dollars)	
	1981	2003
Direct costs		
Visits to ophthalmologists	924.5	6663.8
Visits to other MDs	115.5	832.5
Eye surgery (MD fees)	1134.0	8173.9
Optometrists' services and materials	2061.9	14 862.2
In-patient hospital care	762.7	3655.6
Nursing home care	1517.2	8846.8
Ophthalmic drugs and optical goods[a]	1185.7	5050.9
Rehabilitation services and equipment	178.1	656.5
Total	**7 879.6**	**48 742.2**
Indirect costs		
Days lost from work (acute episodes)	109.8	332.8
Individuals unable to work	4636.9	14 054.4
Women unable to keep house	973.5	2950.7
Institutionalized persons	438.7	1329.7
Waiting time for eye care	75.9	230.1
Total	**6234.8**	**18 897.7**
Grand total	**14 114.4**	**67 639.9**

From the National Eye Institute October 2004. Available: http://www.nei.nih.gov/eyedata/hu_estimates.asp#table1).
[a]Drugs constituted approximately 10% (US$118m) of this cost category in 1981, with the remaining 90% (US$1067.7m) being for optical goods.

The normal aging eye: presbyopia – the first sign of aging in the visual system

Many normal changes take place in the aging eye, on a physiological as well as a functional level. As noted above, there is also a sharp increase in the incidence of ocular disease in the seventh, eighth and ninth decades of life. It is therefore important to understand the changes that occur in the visual system of the normal aging eye in order to differentiate them from the more serious changes resulting from ocular pathology.

The earliest signs of change in the aging visual system are the subtle changes that take place in the focusing ability of the eye (known as accommodation). The mechanical system that regulates accommodation consists of the lens, the ciliary body and the zonules or tiny guy wires connecting the lens to the ciliary body (Fig. 53.1).

The crystalline lens of the eye normally changes its shape and becomes more convex when viewing an object nearby. In most individuals, the accommodative ability of the eye begins to decrease around the age of 40; this eventually leads to the need for prescriptive reading glasses to make up for the lack of accommodative flexibility. This gradual loss of elasticity of the lens is known as presbyopia, which, translated literally, means 'the eyesight of the aged'.

A reading prescription will facilitate the ability to resolve newspaper-size print. However, vision at intermediate distances may also be affected by aging. Regardless of one's age, computers are an accepted part of modern day life and are used for everything from work-related activities to email. Although the computer screen has a lower demand for accommodation than reading at a distance of 13–16 in (33–40 cm), most people will eventually require prescriptive lenses to avoid 'computer fatigue'.

The symptoms of presbyopia generally include blurring of print, headaches and the inability to comfortably sustain reading. Arm length is one of the variables that influence the age of onset of presbyopia. The onset of the first symptoms may appear earlier in life in individuals who are short in stature because the accommodative demand is greater when the print is held closer to the eye. For example, an individual of 6' 6" (2 m) may only have to exert +1.00 diopter (United Nations 2001) of accommodation at age 40, whereas a person of 5' (1.5 m) may have a greater accommodative demand

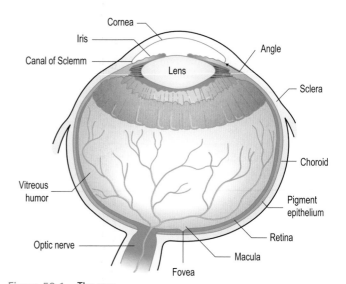

Figure 53.1 The eye.
(From the National Eye Institute, National Institutes of Health, ref no. NEA01.)

(e.g. +1.50 diopters) and may therefore require a reading prescription at an earlier age.

At the age of 75, the 'maximum' reading prescription, determined by the optometrist or ophthalmologist during a refraction, is generally assumed to be from +2.50 diopters (focal distance 16 in/40 cm) to +3.00 diopters (focal distance 13 in/33 cm). Reading corrections may be prescribed as single vision lenses, bifocals (combination of distance and reading lenses), contact lenses, monovision lens (contact lens in one eye for distance or near) or trifocals. New surgical restorative methods are being developed for presbyopia by ophthalmologists who specialize in the anterior segment (the front portion of the eye).

VISION FUNCTION AND ASSESSMENT

Visual function consists of a number of components including visual acuity, visual field and contrast sensitivity. Glare sensitivity, metamorphopsia, stereoacuity, color perception, dark adaptation and photopsia may also be manifested in the presence of eye disease but are not usually as important as visual acuity, visual field or contrast sensitivity deficits. However, they can seriously affect an individual's performance.

Visual acuity

Visual acuity is a single aspect of vision but perhaps the most synonymous with visual health because it is the standard measurement for vision testing in the USA. Visual acuity is the ability to distinguish object details as well as a measure of the clarity of vision. Static visual acuity is the standard type of visual acuity measurement and is one of the primary measurements used in clinical eye trials in the USA. In general, static visual acuity declines very little with age other than what can be accounted for by miosis (reduction in pupil size) or by the increased density and yellowing of the lens.

Clinical assessment of visual acuity is commonly performed using a projected Snellen eye chart (Fig. 53.2) or the ETDRS (Early Treatment of Diabetic Retinopathy Study) eye chart (Fig. 53.3) (Ferris & Sperduto 1982, Ferris et al 1982).

Visual acuity or the 'acuteness' of vision has been measured for centuries. However, Dr Herman Snellen is credited with introducing the modern system in 1862 that, for the most part, remains in place to this day. It is based on the ability of an individual to resolve the detail of a target: the Snellen fractions 20/20, 20/30 and 20/200 relate to the ability to identify a letter (optotype) of a certain size at a specific distance. The numerator or top of the Snellen fraction indicates the test distance. The fraction 20/ × (6/ ×) indicates that the test was performed at a distance of 20 feet (6 m) from the eye. The 20-foot test distance was selected because it is considered to be optical infinity and no focusing (accommodation) is required for an object placed at this distance from the eye. The denominator of the fraction is the distance at which a letter would subtend 5 minutes of arc at the retina. For example, the fraction 20/20 (6/6) indicates that someone has the ability to resolve or see a target that is 1 minute of arc at a distance of 20 feet (6 m) from the eye. A person who is only able to see a letter (or groups of letters) that is twice as large as an individual having 20/20 vision would be recorded as having 20/40 vision. The letters on the 20/200 line are 10 times larger than those on the 20/20 line; they are used to indicate legal blind status when this is the best visual acuity that an individual has when wearing glasses or contact lenses.

When vision is decreased because of ocular pathology, visual acuity may be measured at closer distances (2 m, 10 feet or less). For example, 10/200 is equivalent to 20/400; 1/40 is equivalent to 20/800. When possible, the low vision clinician will record a functional acuity and avoid notations such as CF (counts fingers) or HM (hand motion). Light perception indicates the ability to see a light source, whereas light projection indicates the position of the projected light.

As noted above, in the USA, visual acuity is one of the parameters used in the definition of legal blindness to determine eligibility for disability benefits as well as entitlement to income tax benefits (US Census 2004). Individuals who satisfy the definition of legal blindness are also entitled to talking books from the Library of Congress, operator-assisted service, handicapped parking privileges and, in some areas of the country, access-a-ride.

Visual fields and assessment

Visual field testing is another measure of visual function that provides information about motion detection and peripheral vision, as well as playing an important role in mobility. Visual field testing determines the extent and distribution of the patient's sensitivity to light. It involves measuring the extent of the visual field in all directions while the eye is fixating in the straight-ahead position. The normal

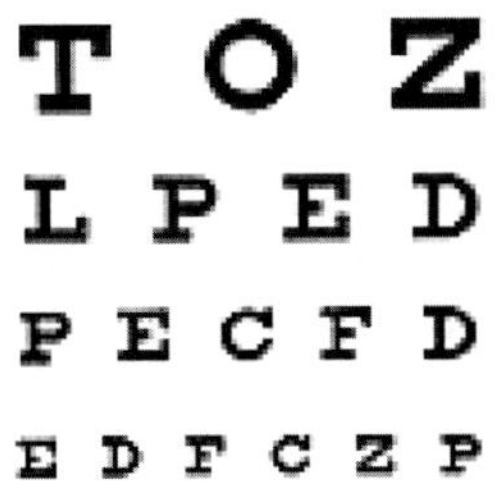

Figure 53.2   Snellen eye chart.
(From the National Eye Institute, National Institutes of Health, ref no. EC01.)

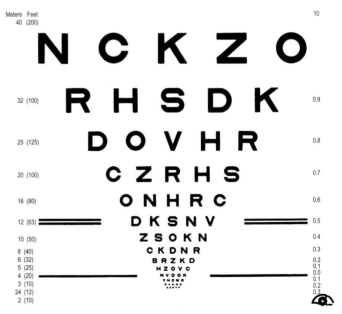

Figure 53.3   ETDRS eye chart.
(From the National Eye Institute, National Institutes of Health, ref no. EC05.)

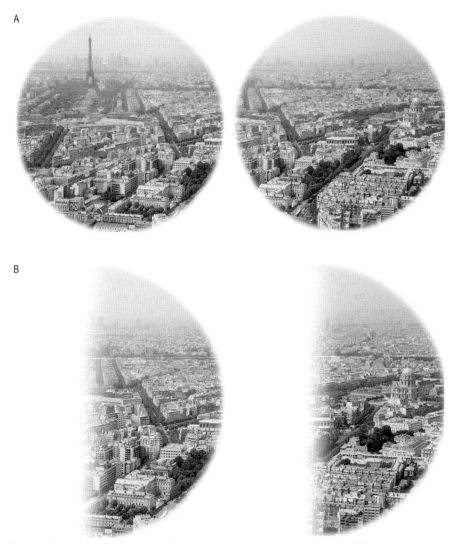

Figure 53.4   Normal visual field (A) and left homonymous hemianopia (B).

visual field for each eye when looking in the straight-ahead position is approximately 60 degrees to the nasal side, 90 degrees to the temporal side, 50 degrees superior and 70 degrees inferior.

Measurement of visual fields will help to reveal any depression in sensitivity, constriction or scotomas (areas of no vision). Loss of visual fields may be relative (sensitive to certain stimuli but not others) or absolute (demonstrate no sensitivity to a stimulus). Visual field measurements will also locate and define the shape of the scotoma, as well as any sector or field cut.

Visual field losses may vary according to the etiology. For example, peripheral field losses are primarily the result of two major pathologies that may severely affect mobility: glaucoma and retinitis pigmentosa. Central visual loss may be caused by conditions that affect the macula of the eye, including macular degeneration, central retinal artery occlusion and central retinal vein occlusion. Stroke, as well as brain tumors, may result in disabling visual field loss and may be manifested as homonymous hemianopsia (total loss of the visual field on one side in both eyes) (Fig. 53.4) or as a quadranopsia (loss of a quarter of the visual field). Patients with hemianopic field loss may bump into objects on the side of the field loss when moving around and may have difficulties with near activities, such as reading or finding things at the dinner table. Some patients also demonstrate visual neglect

after a stroke and may not even be aware that they are missing half of their visual world (Wikipedia).

Methods used to determine the extent of visual field involvement include observational assessment, the confrontation test (the ability to detect a moving object in the field while fixating straight ahead) or the use of a precision quantitative device, such as the Goldmann or automated perimeter. The automated perimeters are rigorously utilized in the management of conditions such as chronic open-angle glaucoma and have programs that can measure the extent of the visual field using targets that can be varied in size and density, as well as position.

Measurement of the visual field following a stroke may require modification or simplification of the testing procedure to obtain the extent of the visual field involvement. The Amsler grid (Fig. 53.5) is the most commonly used assessment tool for the analysis of the central 20 degrees of the visual field in age-related macular degeneration. Changes in the retina may be reflected on the grid as distortions, decreased sensitivity or scotomas (Fig. 53.6). The grid is also used as a home procedure to detect any changes such as bleeding or fluid leakage that may warrant immediate intervention. The confocal scanning laser ophthalmoscope is another precise way of measuring the involvement of the visual field in age-related macular degeneration

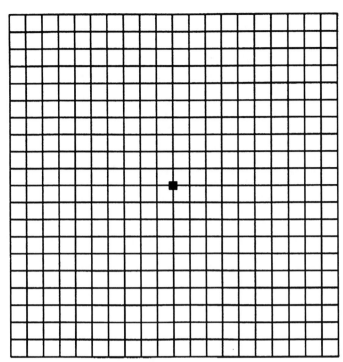

Figure 53.5   Amsler grid.
(From the National Eye Institute, National Institutes of Health, ref. no. EC03.)

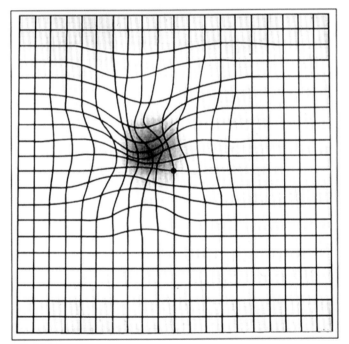

Figure 53.6   Distorted Amsler grid.
(From the National Eye Institute, National Institutes of Health, ref. no. EC04.)

but is generally limited to institutional settings because of cost (Fletcher 1994).

Contrast sensitivity

Contrast sensitivity is a measure of how much a pattern must vary in contrast to be seen (compared with visual acuity, which measures

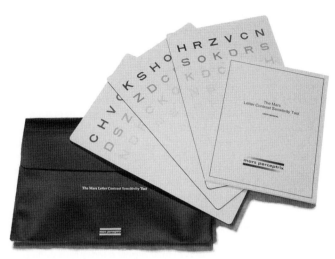

Figure 53.7   Mars contrast sensitivity chart (www.marsperceptrix.com/).

how big an object must be to be seen). Contrast sensitivity is increasingly recognized as an important factor influencing the quality of vision. A decrease in the contrast sensitivity function can lead to a loss of spatial awareness and mobility and increase the risk of accidents. Reduced contrast sensitivity may also affect the ability to walk down steps, recognize faces, drive at night or in the rain, find a telephone number in a directory, read instructions on a medicine container or navigate safely through unfamiliar environments. Reading is also compromised, for example letters may be almost invisible if the print is too light. Environmental modifications, such as high-contrast colors or strips on the first and last steps of staircases, contrasting colors on door frames and the use of contrast on electrical outlets, can all improve patient safety.

Decreasing contrast sensitivity function is associated with ocular pathological conditions such as a cataract, age-related macular degeneration, diabetic retinopathy, glaucoma and optic nerve degenerations. Various charts have been designed for the measurement of the contrast sensitivity function. See the Mars contrast sensitivity chart in Fig. 53.7.

Glare sensitivity

Glare sensitivity is generally classified as either discomfort glare or disability glare. Disability glare is the common type of glare encountered from an oncoming headlight at night and may result from the formation of a cataract as well as an uncorrected refractive error. Discomfort glare may be experienced, for example, when the sun is too bright.

Older individuals are generally more sensitive to glare and often take longer to recover when exposed to a glare source (Paulson & Sjostrand 1980). It is important that they be aware of this inability to quickly adapt to varying light levels when moving from an area of low-light level to one of high-light level. The failure to adapt quickly can result in a serious fall (McMurdon & Gaskell 1991).

Color vision

Macular degeneration and other retinal diseases affecting the macular region may also decrease color sensitivity. This is because color receptors (cones) are densely packed in the macula and color perception will be seriously affected when there is damage to the retinal receptor layer. Changes in color perception may affect the ability to see traffic lights and distinguish colors when dressing, for example, as well as distinguishing whether fruit is ripe or food is cooked.

It has been established that the ability to see color declines with age because of changes in the absorption of light by the ocular media such as the lens, as well as a reduction in pupil size (Aston & Maino 1993). Acquired color vision loss in older individuals differs from congenital (present at birth) defects, in which altered characteristics of cone photopigments lead to color confusion. One way of classifying acquired color defects is Köllner's law, which describes the location of the color vision loss. This law states that lesions in the outer retinal layers give rise to blue–yellow defects, whereas lesions in the inner retinal layers and optic nerve give rise to red–green defects.

Individuals with cataracts that have only a nuclear yellowing commonly have a blue–yellow defect, as do individuals with age-related macular degeneration. Other individuals with optic neuritis (inflammation of the optic nerve) may report a red–green defect.

Individuals who are taking medications or combinations of drugs may also experience a change in the perception of color. Drugs that affect color perception are sedatives, antibiotics and antipsychotics.

Dark adaptation

It becomes progressively more difficult for many individuals, especially those with retinal disease, to adjust to a new level of illumination, for example when going from the outdoors to the indoors. Individuals with eye diseases such as age-related macular degeneration may actually have to wait until their eyes become adjusted to the indoor lighting. As noted above, poor adaptation to changes in light level is also more common in the elderly and may result in falls. Absorptive lenses are often indicated to minimize the adaptation time as well as enhance the contrast.

Stereoacuity vision

Stereoacuity loss may often result in the vision being much poorer in one eye. This disparity between the two eyes may manifest itself in such tasks as threading a needle or tying shoelaces.

PHYSIOLOGICAL CHANGES IN THE AGING EYE

Various physiological changes can occur in the aging eye that may result in decreased vision. Structural changes in the eyelids with age sometimes result in damage to the cornea. Ectropion is an in-turning of the lower eyelid and is caused by atrophy and loss of tonicity, as well as elasticity. There is a sensation of discomfort, which is the result of the eyelashes rubbing against the front surface (epithelial layer) of the cornea. One of the many consequences of ectropion is that the nasal lacrimal duct (drainage canal in the eyelid) cannot handle the profuse tearing, resulting in tears running down the cheek. A more serious effect, however, is the possibility of exposure keratitis (inflammation of the cornea).

Blepharoptosis is a drooping of the upper eyelid and generally results in a narrowing of the palpebral fissure (space between the eyelids) when the eyelid is open. This results in a reduction in the amount of light entering the eye because the pupillary aperture is obscured. Treatment involves supporting the upper lid by surgical means, as well as physically holding the lid up with a 'ptosis' crutch or tape. Precautions must be taken to protect the corneal surface from extensive exposure by supplementation with artificial tears.

Additional age-related physiological changes include the thinning and yellowing of the conjunctiva (Michaels 1993). The corneal surface tends to dry out as tear production by the lacrimal gland decreases and tear film loses stability during the aging process (Horn & Maino 1993). The tear film, composed of oil and mucus, protects and lubricates the eye. The use of artificial tears is often indicated to avoid irritation, as well as possible damage, to the cornea. The cornea itself does not appear to be affected as much by the aging process, although there is an increase in light scatter as well as an overall flattening.

Between the ages of 20 and 80 there is a decrease of about 2.5 mm of the size of the pupil (Morgan 1986). The decrease in pupillary aperture size can be clinically significant under low levels of illumination. In addition, mobility at night and reading (e.g. the menu in a restaurant) may be affected by the resulting loss of light because of the decrease in pupil size.

The density and weight of the crystalline lens increases with age. The lens becomes yellowed and demonstrates fluorescence. Other physiological changes include a decrease in the number of retinal pigment epithelial (RPE) cells in the posterior pole of the eye (Dorney et al 1989).

IMPACT OF VISUAL LOSS ON ACTIVITIES OF DAILY LIVING AND EMOTIONAL STATUS

Visual loss may have a severe impact on activities of daily living, such as driving a car, reading and crossing the street, and seeing traffic signs, the temperature on the oven and steps. This, in turn, may result in clinical depression. Scott et al (2001) found that patients with retinal disease had a 59.3% prevalence of emotional stress compared with 2% in the control group.

A low-vision evaluation, as well as a vision rehabilitation team, may help to enable an individual to return to many of the activities that were previously enjoyed before the loss of vision. This will often lead to an improvement in the quality of life and the development of new strategies for coping with everyday activities.

The low-vision evaluation

The low-vision evaluation is carried out by an optometrist or ophthalmologist who specializes in the care of the partially sighted. The evaluation includes a detailed functional history, measurement of visual acuity, an external evaluation, subjective and objective evaluations and tests of visual function, as well as a prescription of distance, intermediate and near-vision lenses or low-vision devices.

The case history (Faye 1984, Rosenthal & Cole 1991) provides information on patient objectives as well as the need for medical counseling, mobility rehabilitation and training or surgical intervention. The medical history provides the ocular history of any surgery, laser treatment, eye medications or other treatments; a general health history; and an analysis of tasks. The task analysis will explore activities of daily living in detail, for example the ability to see the microwave dials, the food on the plate, the label on a prescription bottle and the numbers on the telephone; the ability to travel independently; other distance and near tasks; lighting considerations; and job activities. Near tasks are especially important and may include the ability to read a newspaper, see prices and labels, fill a syringe or write a check. By the end of the case history, the clinician should have an impression of the patient's objectives and goals and whether or not they are realistic, the patient's reaction to the vision loss and how much time to spend with the patient (i.e. sense what can and cannot be covered during the initial evaluation without fatiguing the patient).

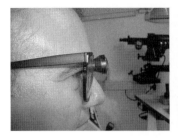

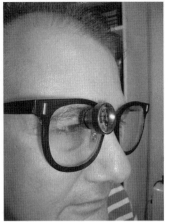

Figure 53.8   Telescopic systems.

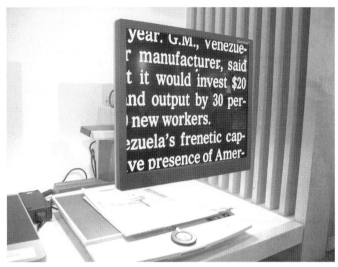

Figure 53.10   CCTV.
(From Lighthouse International, with permission.)

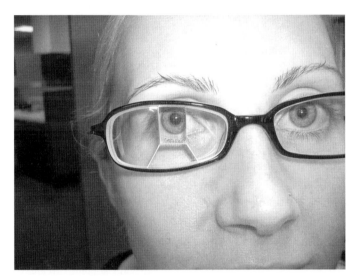

Figure 53.9   Visual field enhancing lens.

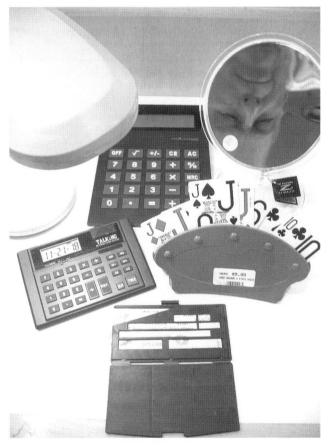

Figure 53.11   Non-optical low vision.
(From Lighthouse International, with permission.)

As discussed above, distance and near visual acuity are evaluated using specialized charts (Bailey & Lovie 1976, Bailey 1978, NAS–NRC Committee on Vision 1980) The external evaluation, which follows visual acuity measurement, should include pupillary position, size and responses, and position of the lids, eyes and orbits, and nystagmus. Refraction is essential in determining the best correction for the patient at distance and near.

The low-vision evaluation also determines the appropriate low-vision devices to achieve the patient objectives. These include high-plus reading lenses, hand and stand magnifiers, hand-held and spectacle-mounted telescopic systems (Fig. 53.8), filters and absorptive devices (Fig. 53.9), electronic magnification and closed-circuit television (CCTV) (Fig. 53.10), as well as non-optical devices such as a bold-line pen (Fig. 53.11).

MAJOR PATHOLOGICAL CHANGES ASSOCIATED WITH AGING

As previously noted, there is a marked prevalence in eye disease with increasing age, especially after the age of 80. It is estimated that 68.3% of individuals over the age of 80 will have cataracts, 35.4% will have some form of macular degeneration and 7.7% will have glaucoma (Table 53.4).

Cataracts

A cataract is clouding or a change in the clarity of the crystalline lens of the eye. The lens consists of a central nucleus surrounded by the

Table 53.4   Summary of eye disease prevalence data

Age (years)	Cataract		Advanced AMD		Intermediate AMD		Glaucoma	
	No.	%	No.	%	No.	%	No.	%
40–49	1 046 000	2.5	20 000	0.1	851 000	2.0	290 000	0.7
50–59	2 123 000	6.8	113 000	0.4	1 053 000	3.4	318 000	1.0
60–69	4 061 000	20.0	147 000	0.7	1 294 000	6.4	369 000	1.8
70–79	6 973 000	42.8	388 000	2.4	1 949 000	12.0	530 000	3.9
=80	6 272 000	68.3	1 081 000	11.8	2 164 000	23.6	711 000	7.7
Total	20 475 000	17.2	1 749 000	1.5	7 311 000	6.1	2 218 000	1.9

From The Eyes Diseases Prevalence Research Group, Prevalence of cataract, age-related macular degeneration, and open-angle glaucoma among adults 40 years and older in the United States. Arch Ophthalmol 122:564–572, 532–538; Vision problems in the US Report (Prevent Blindness America 2002, National Eye Institute).

cortex, which is enclosed in a sac. Cataracts are the most common cause of visual loss after the age of 55 years. The prevalence dramatically increases with age, ranging from 74% between the ages of 65 and 74 to 91% between the ages of 75 and 84.

Cataracts may lead to a variety of signs and symptoms (Faye et al 1995) including problems with glare, blurred vision or difficulties in seeing the printed page (www.nei.nih.gov/ health/cataract/web-cataract.pdf). Streaks or rays of light, especially at night, may seem to be emitted from light sources such as car headlights or traffic lights. Fluorescent lights, especially, may also be a source of glare for many individuals. The person subjected to glare tends to shade their eyes from the sun or wear a wide-brimmed hat to eliminate the annoying glare.

Functionally, cataracts may be the causative factor in falls because of impaired depth perception and the inability to judge distances. Cataracts may also reduce the ability to see stair edges and curbs.

Risk factors, evaluation and intervention

Risk factors for cataracts include smoking and alcohol consumption, systemic diseases (e.g. diabetes), drugs (especially long-term use of steroids), malnutrition, trauma to the eye, hypercholesteremia, elevated triglycerides and exposure to sunlight. New studies have begun to link cataracts with specific genes. For example, a major locus involved in age-related cortical cataracts was found to lie on chromosome 6p12–q12 in the Beaver Dam Eye Study (Congdon et al 2004, Iyengar et al 2004).

Cataract surgery is indicated when the loss of visual function affects everyday activities (e.g. driving) and the quality of life. Preoperative testing, for example a case history, visual acuity measurements, contrast sensitivity and glare testing will provide information on visual function, such as the presence of significant glare outdoors. Ultrasonic measurements of the length of the eyeball are performed to help determine the power of the intraocular lens (IOL) implant that will be inserted when the cataract is removed. Predictive tests of the postoperative visual potential may also be carried out. Contraindications to surgical cataract extraction include a history of complications after previous surgery on the other eye, for example hemorrhaging or postsurgical macular edema.

Therapeutic intervention involves removal of the cataract and insertion of an IOL implant. One of the most common techniques employed in the surgical removal of cataracts, phacoemulsification, involves suctioning out most of the old lens and leaving the posterior capsule. The new IOL is placed in the posterior portion of the capsule. However, the capsule may opacify over time, necessitating a simple YAG laser posterior capsulotomy, which is a procedure used to open up the cloudy membrane that may develop following cataract extraction.

Reading glasses are generally required following surgery because the IOL implant that is inserted generally corrects for distance vision. Newer corrective approaches make use of diffractive and refractive technology to create IOL implants that are similar in function to a bifocal lens.

Age-related macular degeneration

The macula is the area of the retina (located in the posterior pole of the eye) containing the most acute vision, ranging from 20/20 to 20/200. Despite its importance, the macula only subtends an area of 20 degrees of the visual field. Therefore, any changes in the macula may affect the ability to, for example, resolve letters on a sign, read a newspaper, see a computer monitor or see actors in a play.

Age-related macular degeneration (AMD) may be classified as either dry (atrophic) or wet (exudative). Approximately 85–90% of individuals have the dry type, with the remainder having the more aggressive wet type. The symptoms of AMD include reduced visual acuity, reduced contrast sensitivity function, scotomas, metamorphopsia or image distortion, reduced stereoacuity, decreased color perception and the formation of visual hallucinations (Charles Bonnet syndrome).

Activities of daily living may also be affected. For example, there may be difficulties in performing tasks such as threading a needle or tying shoelaces, distinguishing the colors of traffic lights and decorating the home. The loss of vision may lead to individuals losing their independence because they are not able to perform tasks such as preparing food. Referral for vision rehabilitation services, such as orientation and mobility, is indicated when there is concern for an individual's safety as well as their independence.

The possible risk factors for AMD include genetics, cataracts, smoking, hypertension, sun exposure, farsightedness, light skin or eye color and a diet low in vitamins, minerals and antioxidants.

One of the earliest signs of AMD is the presence of hard or soft deposits in the retina known as drusen. A significant amount of research has been carried out to determine the composition of drusen;

new evidence is pointing to a protein common in extracellular deposits associated with atherosclerosis, amyloidosis and Alzheimer's disease (Mullins et al 2000). Research has also been carried out on how to prevent these waste products from being deposited in the retina.

Diagnosis of the wet form of macular degeneration, also known as choroidal neovascularization, involves the use of fluorescein angiography. A small catheter is placed into a large vein and a dye is injected into the vein. A series of photos are taken of the retina through a special filter to identify the presence of any choroidal neovascularization. Optical coherence tomography (OCT) is another tool used to evaluate the progression of AMD, as well as the efficacy of treatment. OCT is an interferometric, noninvasive imaging technique (Huang et al 1991).

There have been significant changes in the treatment of AMD. Until 2000, thermal laser was the predominant method used to treat the wet form of the condition. This technique is now used in less than 5% of individuals with wet AMD because of the destruction of collateral tissue that occurs when the thermal laser is used to seal off the leaky blood vessel. Photodynamic therapy (PDT, also known as Visudyne therapy) was approved by the Food and Drug Administration (FDA) in 2000 to treat one form of the wet condition, known as predominantly classic choroidal neovascularization. It uses a medication to destroy the abnormal blood vessels, which is activated using a cold laser.

Another treatment for the wet form of AMD involves the use of pegaptanib sodium (Macugen), an RNA aptamer (an RNA molecule that can act like an antibody) (Gragoudas et al 2004). It was approved by the FDA in 2004 for the treatment of the classic, minimally classic and occult forms of AMD. Vascular endothelial growth factor (VEGF) is involved in the pathogenesis of choroidal neovascularization (Ferrara 2000), and basic and clinical scientific evidence links excessive VEGF production to retinal angiogenesis. Macugen is known to be an anti-VEGF agent because of its ability to bind to the 165-amino acid isoform of extracellular VEGF (FDA news 2004) and essentially stop the growth of new destructive porous blood vessels in the retina. New therapies are being directed towards all isoforms of extracellular VEGF.

Glaucoma

It is estimated that 2 million people in the USA have glaucoma and that 80 000 of these individuals are registered as legally blind because of the disease. Among African–Americans, glaucoma is now recognized as the leading cause of blindness (www.nei.nih.gov/neitrials/viewStudyWeb.aspx?id=24). The Ocular Hypertension Treatment Study (OHTS) also revealed that the prevalence of glaucoma is much higher among African–Americans.

Glaucoma is recognized as a group of diseases that generally involves an increase in the intraocular pressure of the eye. The optic nerve, as well as the visual field, may be severely affected if the pressure is left unchecked. The OHTS revealed predictors for the development of primary open-angle glaucoma that include older age, race (African–American), sex (male), larger vertical cup–disc ratio of the optic nerve, larger horizontal cup–disc ratio of the optic nerve, heart disease and thinner central cornea measurements.

Left untreated, primary open-angle glaucoma will result in permanent visual field loss as well as a loss of night vision. Severe visual field loss requires the help of a mobility specialist to learn how to renavigate in the environment and may require the use of a cane or guide dog if the impairment is profound.

Normal intraocular pressure ranges from 10 to 20 mmHg (Gordon et al 2002, Higginbotham et al 2004). However, normal pressure may be as high as 23 mmHg in some patients and they never develop glaucomatous changes. As noted, observation of the optic nerve head is very important in the management of glaucoma. Damage is assessed by looking at the loss of the nerve fibers as well as the visual field loss.

The tests used in the evaluation of glaucoma include measuring the intraocular pressure with a Goldmann tonometer, visual field analysis with an automated perimeter, evaluation of the optic nerve with indirect ophthalmoscopic observation and the use of OCT for optic nerve head analysis. The use of OCT enables the creation of a contour map of the optic nerve and optic cup. Other tests include an analysis of the retinal nerve fiber layer (RNFL) thickness with scanning laser polarimetry and confocal scanning laser ophthalmoscopy. Pachymetry is another routine test that evaluates the thickness of the cornea.

Therapeutic intervention may include drug therapy with cholinergic, anticholinesterase and β-adrenergic agents, carbonic anhydrase inhibitors, hyperosmotic agents and prostaglandins. However, there are some side effects associated with these medications that must be taken into account with geriatric patients. For example, the use of beta blockers may result in bradycardia, hypotension, altered lipid profiles and atrial tachycardia.

Surgical procedures to control eye pressure include trabeculectomy, trabeculoplasty and iridotomy. These procedures are performed to facilitate the outflow of aqueous fluid from the eye.

Diabetic retinopathy and other conditions

Other retinal pathologies, especially diabetic retinopathy, necessitate comanagement by a team of specialists including a diabetologist, ophthalmologist, physical therapist and low-vision optometrist or ophthalmologist. Patients with insulin-dependent diabetes may experience significant vision loss from hemorrhaging as well as from exudates in the retina.

The most common diabetes-related eye symptoms are changes in refraction, variable vision or focus, blurred or hazy vision, sensitivity to glare, faulty color vision and blindness.

Treatment may include cataract extraction, laser treatment (panretinal photocoagulation) or vitrectomy (removal of the vitreous humor). Low-vision devices are also important to enable the patient to monitor blood sugar levels and administer the correct dosage of insulin.

Because vision can vary with fluctuations in blood glucose levels, an ophthalmologist or optometrist should carry out a careful refraction test and eye examination at intervals to check for presbyopia, secondary myopia, cataract or retinopathy (www.visionconnection.org/Content/YourVision/EyeDisorders/DiabetesRelatedEyeDisease/DiabetesVisionLossandAging.htm).

Other prevalent retinal conditions in the elderly include retinal tears, macular holes and retinal detachments. Treatment for these conditions includes laser, cryosurgery and surgery. Macular holes and epiretinal membranes may also be treated with a vitrectomy or with membrane peeling.

THE FUTURE

The field of genomics is beginning to play a major role in the understanding and improvement in the management of ocular disease of the aging eye. The incidence of severe and late-stage eye disease will begin to drop with the implementation of new approaches to control the mechanisms that presently precipitate irreversible damage to the eye. Improved control of comorbidities, such as diabetes and hypertension, will also result in a further reduction of significant vision loss.

However, with the changes in nutritional habits being adopted by the younger generation throughout the world, there is also the potential for a significant increase in the incidence of visual loss in the future. In fact, diabetes will become the number one cause of systemic and visual problems worldwide. With the increase in life expectancy, there will also be a significant rise in the number of elderly individuals with visual impairments worldwide.

One of the last frontiers will be the development of artificial vision, including 'replacement' vision. Clinical studies have already begun into the efficacy of implanting chips on the retina and in the visual cortex for individuals with no usable vision. The world of stem cell research also holds great promise for the restoration of visual function.

Governments and non-governmental agencies around the world must begin planning and enhancing strategies for training personnel, as well as increasing resources to handle the expected geriatric and visual impairment explosions.

GLOSSARY

Blindness: the term blindness has two generally accepted definitions:

1. Blindness can be used for total loss of vision and for conditions in which individuals have to rely predominantly on vision substitution skills. In this context, blindness indicates no useable vision.
2. Blindness has a different connotation when used in 'blindness' statistics (synonymous with legal blindness). In the USA, the definition of legal blindness is a visual acuity of 20/200 (6/60) or worse in the better-seeing eye (Fig. 53.8) or a visual field of 20 degrees or less in the widest meridian with the best correction.

Functional vision: used to describe a person's ability to use vision in activities of daily living. Presently, many of these activities can be described only qualitatively.

Low vision: there are many definitions of low vision; one common one is having a visual acuity of <20/40 (United Nations 2001).

Table 53.5 Prevalence of blindness and low vision among adults 40 years and older in the USA

Age (years)	Blindness		Low vision		All vision-impaired	
	No.	%	No.	%	No.	%
40–49	51 000	0.1	80 000	0.2	131 000	0.3
50–59	45 000	0.1	102 000	0.3	147 000	0.4
60–69	59 000	0.3	176 000	0.9	235 000	1.2
70–79	134 000	0.8	471 000	3.0	605 000	3.8
> 80	648 000	7.0	1 532 000	16.7	2 180 000	23.7
Total	937 000	0.8	2 361 000	2.0	3 298 000	2.7

From http://www.nei.nih.gov/eyedata/pbd_tables.asp, October 2004.

Partially sighted: another term for low vision, which means having reduced visual function but still usable vision (i.e. not totally blind).

Visual disability: the lack, loss or reduction of an individual's ability to perform certain tasks (e.g. reading a medication label, traveling safely in the environment).

Visual handicap: the societal and economic consequences of a visual disability.

Visual impairment: used when the condition of vision loss is characterized by a loss of visual function (e.g. visual acuity, visual field, contrast sensitivity, color vision, etc.) at the organ level. Many of these functions can be measured quantitatively.

The prevalence of blindness and low vision increases significantly among adults of 40 years and older in the USA (Table 53.5).

References

Aston SJ, Maino JH 1993 Clinical Geriatric Eyecare. Butterworth-Heinemann, Boston, MA, p 58–59

Bailey IL, Lovie JE 1976 New design principles for visual acuity letter charts. Am J Optom Physiol Optics 53:740–745

Bailey IL 1978 Visual acuity measurement in low vision. Optom Monthly 69:418–424

Congdon N, Broman KW, Lai H et al 2004 Nuclear cataract shows significant familial aggregation in an older population after adjustment for possible shared environmental factors. Invest Ophthalmol Vis Sci 45(7):2182–2186

Dorney CK, Wu G, Ebenstein D et al 1989 Cell loss in the aging retina. Invest Ophthalmol Vis Sci 30:1691–1699

Faye E 1984 Clinical Low Vision, 2nd edn. Little, Brown, Boston, MA, p 28

Faye EE, Rosenthal BP, Sussman-Skalka CJ 1995 Cataract and the aging eye. Lighthouse National Center for Vision and Aging, New York

FDA news 2004 Available: http://www.fda.gov/bbs/topics/news/2004/new01146.html

Ferrara N 2000 Vascular endothelial growth factor and the regulation of angiogenesis. Rec Prog Horm Res 55:15–36

Ferris F, Sperduto R 1982 Standardized illumination for visual acuity testing in clinical research. Am J Ophthalmol 94:97–98

Ferris F, Kassoff A, Bresnick G, Bailey E 1982 New visual acuity charts for clinical research. Am J Ophthalmol 94:91–96

Fletcher D 1994 Scanning laser ophthalmoscope macular perimetry and applications for low vision rehabilitation clinicians. Ophthalmol Clin North Am 7:257–265

Gordon MO, Beiser JA, Brandt JD et al for the Ocular Hypertension Treatment Study Group 2002 The Ocular Hypertension Treatment Study: baseline factors that predict the onset of primary open-angle glaucoma. Arch Ophthalmol 120:714–720

Gragoudas ES, Adamis AP, Cunningham ET et al 2004 Pegaptanib for neovascular age-related macular degeneration. N Engl J Med 351:2805–2816

Higginbotham EJ, Gordon MO, Beise JA et al for the Ocular Hypertension Treatment Study Group 2004 The Ocular Hypertension Treatment Study: topical medication delays or prevents primary open-angle glaucoma in African–American individuals. Ophthalmology 122:813–820

Horn MJ, Maino JH 1993 Normal vision problems in the elderly. In: Aston SJ, Maino JH (eds) Clinical Geriatric Eyecare. Butterworth-Heinemann, Boston, MA

Huang D, Swanson EA, Lin CP et al 1991 Optical coherence tomography. Science 254:1178–1181

Iyengar SK, Klein BEK, Klein R et al 2004 Identification of a major locus for age-related cortical cataract on chromosome 6p12-q12 in the Beaver Dam Eye Study. Proc Natl Acad Sci USA 101:14485–14490

McMurdon ME, Gaskell A 1991 Dark adaptation and falls. Gerontology 37(4):221–224

Michaels DD 1993 Ocular disease in the elderly. In: Rosenbloom AA, Morgan MW (eds) Vision and Aging. Butterworth-Heinemann, Boston, MA

Morgan MW 1986 Changes in visual function in the aging eye. In: Rosenbloom AA, Morgan MW (eds) Vision and Aging. Fairchild Publications, New York, p 121–134

Mullins RF, Russell SR, Anderson DH, Hageman GS 2000 Drusen associated with aging and age-related macular degeneration contain proteins common to extracellular deposits associated with atherosclerosis, elastosis, amyloidosis, and dense deposit disease. FASEB J 14:835–846. Available: http://www.fasebj.org/cgi/content/full/14/7/835

NAS–NRC Committee on Vision 1980 Recommended standard procedures for the clinical measurements and specification of visual acuity. Adv Ophthalmol 41:103

Paulson LE, Sjostrand J 1980 Contrast sensitivity in the presence of a glare light. Invest Ophthalmol Vis Sci 19:401–406

Rosenthal BP, Cole RG 1991 The low vision history. In: Eskridge JB, Amos J, Bartlett I (eds) Clinical Procedures in Optometry. JB Lippincott, Philadelphia, PA, p 749–761

Scott IU, Schein OD, Feuer WJ et al 2001 Emotional distress in patients with retinal disease. Am J Ophthalmol 131:584–589

Social Security Administration. Available: http://www.ssa.gov/disability/professionals/bluebook/2.00-SpecialSensesandSpeech-Adult.htm#2.02%20Impairment%20of%20Central%20Visual%20Acuity

US Census 2004

United Nations 2001 World Population Ageing: 1950–2050. United Nations, New York

Wikipedia: The Free Encyclopedia. Available: http://en.wikipedia.org/wiki/Visual_field

Chapter 54

Functional changes in the aging ear

Stephen E. Mock

Aging is a gradual process. It does not happen suddenly but rather in such a way that most people sense a slow deterioration of sensory and motor skills over time. The aging process causes both structural and functional changes to occur in the body. Twentieth and twenty-first century science and technology have led to many advances that have improved both quality of life and life expectancy, thus enabling the average human to live longer and better. If a person lives through the sixth or seventh decade of life or longer, they must anticipate that modifications of mind and body will occur. Areas such as cognition, circulation, coordination and vision can be affected. Another area that is frequently affected by aging is the inner ear.

AGING AND THE INNER EAR

The bilateral inner ear structures contain organs for both hearing and balance. Fluid-filled cavities, located within the temporal bones of the skull, receive airborne and mechanically transmitted stimuli from both the environment and conductive aspects of the hearing mechanism. The hair cell structures within the inner ears transform these conductive signals into electrical impulses that are sent via nerve conduction to the brain and central nervous system for inter-pretation and utilization. The inner ear is composed of three major parts: (i) the semicircular canals; (ii) the vestibule; and (iii) the cochlea. The first two structures are primarily involved with balance and equilibrium, whereas the cochlea is the sensory organ for hearing sensitivity. Unfortunately, all three of these inner ear structures can be adversely affected by the aging process. In fact, according to several studies, hearing loss associated with the aging process may begin in some individuals between the ages of 30 and 35 years. This incidence increases with age so that by the age of 65, approximately one-third of all individuals, both male and female, will suffer from significant hearing loss; this figure rises to almost two-thirds in those over the age of 80 (National Center for Health Statistics 1987, Christensen et al 2001). In addition to these auditory changes, the inner ear balance structures can also be adversely affected by age.

DIZZINESS AND AGING

According to Desmond and Touchette (1998), dizziness is the most common reason for primary care physician visits for patients over the age of 75, and almost 80% of these visits were found to be directly related to inner ear dysfunction. Dizziness, or the loss of orientation of the body in space, can be an extremely frightening experience to the older adult. Individuals are used to being in control of their bodies and doing what they want, when they want; however, the dizzy patient may no longer be able to control spatial orientation. In addition, the person's fright may be complicated by concern that the dizziness is a symptom of a serious problem, such as a heart attack or stroke. However, the potential causes of dizziness may be many and varied and it is therefore imperative that a comprehensive examination be completed to determine the correct paths for evaluation and treatment of any condition.

The historical perspectives presented by the patient are the most important aspects of the vestibular evaluation. According to a study by Kroenke et al (1992), and supported by Desmond and Touchette (1998), when performed by an experienced examiner, the case history is effective in presenting a valid hypothesis for diagnosis and treatment of the dizzy patient more than 75% of the time. The intake should cover such areas as a description of the sensation, both at time of onset and at present; the frequency and duration of the episodes; precipitating factors; associated factors; and past medical and social history (Roberts et al 2005). However, the results of the historical intake are not the only avenues of evaluation available to the clinician. A broad range of other evaluative procedures have been developed to aid in the diagnosis and treatment of the dizzy patient (Eggers 2003). These procedures may include mechanisms such as electro- or videonystagmography, which measure voluntary and involuntary eye movement or nystagmus; rotational testing, which permits pre-cise measurements of the vestibulo-ocular reflex (VOR), the reflex that allows an individual to maintain balance in the presence of move-ment; and dynamic or platform posturography, which aids in the identification of the presence or absence of both sensory and motor aspects that are important for balance. The results of these evaluations may provide recommendations for treatment and/or appropriate referral. Whereas in the past, many patients were advised that dizzi-ness was a condition that they would 'have to live with', rehabilitative treatment is now available for the vast majority of dizzy patients. These treatments may include medical therapy, vestibular rehabilitation therapy, physical therapy and surgical intervention.

One specific cause of dizziness should be highlighted. Benign paroxysmal positional vertigo (BPPV) is the most common type of dizziness in individuals over the age of 60 (Herdman 2000). BPPV can be an extremely frustrating or even debilitating condition; however, it can now be effectively treated more than 90% of the time by a simple maneuver called the Epley maneuver (Gans 2000). Although not all conditions of dizziness can be so effectively cured, progress continues to be made in many areas and, through appropriate treatment, most patients suffering from a vestibular condition can experience an improved quality of life.

TINNITUS

Tinnitus, another inner ear-related difficulty, affects millions of people in the USA alone (Morgenstern 2005). Sindhusake et al (2004) reported that as many as one in three older individuals may be affected by this condition. Tinnitus is commonly described as a ringing or other noise in one or both ears or sometimes within the skull itself. In most instances, tinnitus is a subjective sensation and, therefore, audible only to the individual suffering from the condition. However, in rare instances, tinnitus can be termed 'objective', in that the noise can be audible to others. According to House (1981), more than 80% of patients who suffered from inner ear hearing loss also experienced an associated tinnitus condition. It should be noted that tinnitus is not a disease itself, but rather a symptom of a hearing deficit. Although most instances of tinnitus are classified as a 'nuisance', some individuals may suffer from tinnitus conditions that may be debilitating in nature. These individuals may be subjected to both physiological and psychological ramifications that can significantly affect their quality of life. At present, most tinnitus treatment strategies focus on alleviating the severity of the symptoms of the condition, rather than improving the condition itself. A wide variety of tinnitus treatment strategies have been proposed over time, yet none has been totally successful. A number of 'home remedies' or anecdotal treatments have also been introduced over the years. Unfortunately, these reports are often embraced by vulnerable people who are desperate in their search for tinnitus relief. It is the duty of the hearing specialist to be aware of the current evaluations, strategies and treatments that are available and to serve as both a guide and a counselor to those patients suffering from intractable tinnitus conditions. An excellent resource for both patients and professionals who express a desire to learn more about tinnitus is the American Tinnitus Association (www.ata.org).

PRESBYCUSIS

Hearing loss associated with aging is commonly referred to as presbycusis (from the Greek: *presby* = elder; *akouein* = hearing). Although some think of presbycusis as being a factor of age alone, it is actually the outcome of several variables that can occur within an individual's lifespan (Rosenhall 2001). These variables may include, but are not limited to, metabolic, vascular or renal diseases, inflammations and infections, medications, head trauma, nutritional deficiencies and hereditary factors. However, the most common factor related to inner ear hearing damage is exposure to intense noise levels. In a classic study published in 1962 by Rosen et al, individuals living in a relatively noise-free environment in the Sudan showed significantly less hearing loss than people living in industrialized societies. As a result of this and other studies, attempts have been made to educate people about the

effects of noise on hearing. Although some progress has been made in protecting industrial workers from hearing loss, recreational noise (associated with such pastimes as automobile racing, hunting or shooting) and intense music continue to be unregulated and, thus, will continue to contribute to presbycusis for generations to come.

The hearing loss associated with presbycusis is usually insidious and is initially noted as a problem in clarity or understanding of speech, rather than as a true hearing deficit. Sound may be distorted secondary to inner ear hair cell damage. Many patients with presbycusis will present with the complaint of, 'I hear but cannot understand'. This initial complaint is usually a result of a decrease in hearing within the high frequency range of the inner ear cochlea. At birth, the normal human ear is thought to be functional within a frequency range of 20–20000 Hz. However, as the individual ages, the cochlear hair-cell function begins to diminish, especially in the higher frequencies. The cochlear change deprives the inner ear of a critical connection to the cerebral cortex. If the auditory signal is unable to reach the brain, interpretation will be lacking, resulting in a deficit or loss of auditory function. The greater the amount of hair-cell damage, the greater the amount of hearing loss and the greater the handicap imposed on the individual. Unfortunately, no medical or surgical treatments are presently available to remediate the vast majority of inner ear hearing loss. Although ongoing laboratory studies present hope in such areas as hair-cell regeneration and temporal bone transplant, it will probably be many years before such dramatic innovations are readily available. At present, the best hope for alleviation of inner ear hearing loss lies with electroacoustic devices that can assist the hearing impaired. The most common of these is the hearing aid.

EVALUATION OF THE HEARING–IMPAIRED ADULT

No rehabilitative process can be effective without a comprehensive identification program. The current protocol for initial auditory evaluation is based upon both traditional and modern procedures. The purposes of a hearing evaluation include to diagnose conductive versus inner ear lesions, determine the need for medical or surgical referral, create a course of rehabilitation, determine the need for a site-of-lesion evaluation and determine the extent of disability. The two professions primarily involved in inner ear evaluation and treatment are otolaryngology and audiology. The otolaryngologist, or ear, nose and throat specialist, is a physician who is skilled in the medical treatment of auditory disease or dysfunction. Over the years, many auditory conditions that were once thought to be permanent have been found to be treatable through medical or surgical techniques. Although reversal of inner ear aging patterns has not yet been accomplished, ongoing research, including genetic modification practices, shows promise for the regeneration of hair-cell tissue or recovery of hair-cell damage.

The audiologist is a non-medical specialist involved with the evaluation, diagnosis and treatment of hearing and balance problems that cannot be managed medically. It is usually the realm of the audiologist to initiate and complete the comprehensive testing process necessary to identify any problem and develop a course of realistic treatment. The initial aspect of the auditory evaluation includes such time-tested measures as otoscopic examination and tuning-fork testing. These procedures can act as a screening mechanism to allow the professional audiologist to determine, within a reasonable degree of certainty, whether a hearing loss is present and whether it can be localized within the conductive or inner ear mechanism.

Following these initial screening procedures, the audiologist uses two other traditional hearing measures: pure-tone audiometry and speech audiometry. In pure-tone audiometry, hearing thresholds are obtained at several frequencies. In pure-tone air-conduction testing, the entire auditory system is evaluated, whereas in pure-tone bone-conduction testing, only the inner ear reserve is evaluated. By comparing air conduction thresholds with bone conduction thresholds, the clinician can determine, among other things, if medical referral is indicated.

The pure-tone test results are supplemented by speech audiometry. Using speech signals to evaluate the auditory system is a tradition that has been ongoing since the earliest days of auditory testing. Speech testing can not only be used to validate and confirm the reliability of pure tones but also to estimate the presence or absence of any distortion that may be present within the auditory system, secondary to hair-cell damage.

Other diagnostic measures that are routinely applied include acoustic immittance testing, which is an objective measure of the peripheral auditory system and which can provide efficient information regarding that system. Pure tone, speech and acoustic emittance evaluations coupled with otoscopy and tuning-fork testing are considered the bedrock of the auditory evaluation. However, these tests can be supplemented with other measures, such as auditory brainstem response testing, otoacoustic emission evaluation and electrocochleography, to provide additional diagnostic data and site-of-lesion information. When performed by a licensed physician or audiologist, these diagnostic services are recognized and covered for reimbursement by Medicare and most third-party insurances.

REMEDIATION OF HEARING LOSS

Hearing loss is a disability that is experienced not only by the affected individual but also by all those who attempt to communicate with that individual. In addition, it is not uncommon for hearing loss to be considered by both patient and physician alike as a somewhat benign condition that is a recognized by-product of the aging process. Some feel that, although conversation may be difficult, the hearing loss does not pose a significant threat to the overall health of the patient. However, in a breakthrough study by Bess et al (1989), it was dramatically demonstrated that hearing loss in the elderly can have significant ramifications in both physical and psychosocial function. Hearing loss is communicatively isolating, and an individual suffering from such a handicap may be deprived of social relationships, occupational opportunities and quality-of-life

factors that make living worthwhile. For the elderly individual, hearing loss may also come to symbolize the physical and emotional changes that occur with age.

At one time, when patients were advised to 'get a hearing aid', they were usually fitted with a large unsightly device that was cosmetically challenging and that also amplified the wrong sounds. Fortunately, with the integration of computer technology, today's hearing aids are not only more cosmetically acceptable but are also capable of artificially processing speech signals to a degree never before possible. However, despite these technological advances, it is important to note that today's hearing instruments continue to be an 'aid' and not a 'cure' for hearing loss; even with the use of a hearing aid, there will be times when speech may be unclear or distorted. Although hearing aids are not a panacea, they are capable of providing a significant improvement in hearing ability when fitted by a competent professional.

The improvement in hearing provided by hearing aids can be even further enhanced by an assortment of rehabilitative devices that are available to help the hearing-impaired individual. These devices are usually classified into four functional categories: (i) sound-enhancement technology; (ii) television-enhancement technology; (iii) telecommunication technology; and (iv) signal/alerting technology. For the severely hearing-impaired individual, cochlear implantation, in which surgically implanted electrodes provide direct stimulation of the auditory nerve, has become an acceptable, beneficial and widely available procedure. As technology continues to evolve, additional beneficial devices will be developed. The future for the treatment of the hearing impaired continues to be bright (see Chapter 55 for further suggestions on how to enhance communication with the elderly).

CONCLUSION

The aging process frequently results in changes to the inner ear structures of hearing and balance. These changes may present significant quality of life issues, not only to affected individuals but also to their families. Although evaluation of these patients may be challenging, both traditional and advanced technology methods are now available to aid in differential diagnosis. Remediation procedures are progressing; however, few 'cures' for inner ear damage are available at this time. Ongoing research efforts continue to provide hope for a future in which hearing and balance disorders can be eradicated.

References

Bess FH, Lichetenstein MJ, Logan SA et al 1989 Hearing impairment as a determinant of function in the elderly. J Am Geriatr Soc 37:123–128

Christensen K, Frederiksen H, Hoffman HJ 2001 Genetic and environmental influences on self-reported reduced hearing in the old and oldest old. J Am Geriatr Soc 49(11):1512–1517

Desmond AL, Touchette DT 1998 Balance Disorders. Micromedical Technologies, Chatham, IL

Eggers SDZ 2003 Evaluation of the dizzy patient: bedside examination and laboratory assessment of the vestibular system. Semin Neurol 23(1):47–58

Gans RE 2000 Overview of BPPV: treatment methodologies. Hearing Rev 7:34–38

Herdman SJ 2000 Vestibular Rehabilitation. FA Davis, Philadelphia, PA

House JW 1981 Management of the tinnitus patient. Ann Otol 90:597–601

Kroenke K, Lucas CA, Rosenberg ML et al 1992 Causes of persistent dizziness: a prospective study of 100 patients in ambulatory care. Ann Intern Med 117(11):898–904

Morgenstern L 2005 The bells are ringing: tinnitus in their own words. Perspect Biol Med 48(3):396–407

National Center for Health Statistics (NCHS) 1987 Current estimates from the National Health Interview Survey: United States, 1987. Vital and Health Statistics, Series 10. Public Health Service, Government Printing Office, Washington, DC

Roberts R, Gans R, Kastner A et al 2005 Prevalence of vestibulopathy in benign paroxysmal positional vertigo patients with and without prior otologic history. Int J Audiol 44(4):191–196

Rosen S, Bergman M, Plester D et al 1962 Presbycusis study of a relatively noise-free population in the Sudan. Transcripts Otologic Soc 50:135–152

Rosenhall U 2001 Presbyacusis – hearing loss in old age. Lakartidningen 98(23):2802–2806

Sindhusake D, Golding M, Wigney D et al 2004 Factors predicting severity of tinnitus: a population-based assessment. J Am Acad Audiol 15(4):269–280

Chapter **55**

Considerations in elder patient communication

Carolyn Marshall

INTRODUCTION

For healthcare professionals to deliver the best possible treatment to their older patients, some special considerations must be discussed. In order to understand patients' expectations regarding proposed treatment or procedures, and their ability to follow through with prescribed self-care, both during and after treatment, a mutually understandable, accurate and satisfying communication between practitioner and patient should be established.

The healthcare provider and staff have to identify what communication skills are necessary to reach each older individual. They must be familiar with the patient's physical assessment so that they can be aware of any hearing or visual deficits. Knowledge of a patient's educational level and reading ability is also necessary to determine how to most effectively present information concerning treatment and self-care. It has become increasingly recognized that knowledge of the level of a patient's health literacy is critical because inadequate health literacy is common among elderly patients, particularly inner-city minorities. However, many articulate, well-groomed individuals may also have limited health literacy. Such patients often have an array of communication problems that may affect treatment outcome. Williams et al (2002) recommend that relatives should be encouraged to participate in patient interviews or education sessions to ensure that patients have understood essential information. Creative alternatives to pamphlets and other written patient education materials should be used. Cultural differences should also be considered.

If there is a question concerning the patient's status, simple evaluation tools can be used. If a barrier does exist, how is it determined whether there is a short-term confusional state or long-term dysfunction? Executive dysfunction and its implications for treatment is another important aspect to consider. Specific communication techniques can be used with patients who exhibit executive dysfunction.

CULTURAL CONSIDERATIONS

Healthcare professionals must consider how those receiving care should be informed in order to reduce future risk. To understand and reach a patient, it is necessary to look at each individual's physical and genetic history (Hispanic, African–American, Asian, Anglo, etc.), as well as cultural beliefs, myths and customs concerning diet and health. The patient's attitude toward the specific healthcare setting can strongly affect their interactions with caregivers.

For example, how can one convince a patient who holds healthcare professionals in great respect or awe that it is proper to ask questions or even to ask for another opinion at times? No matter what the culture, the accepted health professional/patient relationship can usually be described as one of dependence. In the Mexican–American culture, with which the author is most familiar, *respeto* (respect) is valued highly. Health professionals are greatly respected and are not usually questioned, even if the patient does not understand the explanation of the illness or the treatment prescribed.

Health professionals who do not understand the Mexican–American culture often mistake the polite smile and nod of the head for understanding when patients are asked if they comprehend what has been explained. In fact, it may mean that the patient does not want to admit lack of understanding, either for fear of insulting the provider of the information by implying that a poor explanation has been given or for fear of being considered ignorant. When patients do not follow a prescribed treatment regimen, they are described as being 'not compliant'. Compliance is understood to mean the act of conforming or yielding, a tendency to yield readily to others, especially in a weak or subservient way. 'Adherence', a term much preferred by this author and used by others concerned with healthcare and effective adult patient education, is defined as 'a mutually agreed-upon course of action'. A person is more likely to make behavioral changes if situations are explained in a manner that can be understood both intellectually and emotionally. The possible or probable outcomes are put forward by the healthcare provider and the expectations of both provider and patient can be discussed. Then, the mutually agreed-upon course of action is clear and the patient assumes a measure of control and responsibility for the outcome.

Similarly, how should an issue as culturally sensitive and culturally based as diet be addressed in cases in which a patient is to follow a specific diet? In addressing the role of diet and the importance of nutrition in healthcare, Payne (1980) says that nutritional considerations are not yet an integral part of most provider/patient office experiences. This is in spite of the fact that no custom is more universally shared then the ritual of eating a meal together. This ritual symbolizes family traditions, close relationships, friendships and sentiments, and results in definite dietary and cultural habits, which are passed on from generation to generation. Attitudes about food and dietary practices within cultural groups can often be related to attitudes and beliefs that influence diet and consequently have an impact on health. Therefore, although a clinician may not be fully armed with knowledge of the intricacies of the diet of a particular cultural group, there should be at least some awareness of cultural dietary practices when managing a patient whose culture is different from the clinician's own.

To answer some of the preceding questions, a practitioner must go beyond the traditional methods of patient education used in most settings and look at each person as an individual.

LITERACY

The unabridged edition of *The Random House Dictionary of the English Language* (1973) defines 'literate' as (i) being able to read and write; (ii) having an education; and (iii) having or showing knowledge of literature, writing, and so forth. The same reference defines 'illiterate' as (i) being unable to read and write; (ii) lacking education; and (iii) showing lack of culture, especially in language and literature.

The preceding definitions make it necessary to define the words 'culture' and 'knowledge', as they are used in the context of this chapter. 'Culture' can be defined as (i) a particular form or stage of civilization, that of a certain nation or period; and (ii) the sum total of ways of living built up by a group of human beings and transmitted from one generation to another. 'Knowledge', on the other hand, is defined as (i) acquaintance with facts, truths or principles, as from study or investigation; (ii) the body of truths or facts accumulated by humankind in the course of time; and (iii) the sum of what is known.

Although the ability to read is probably assumed when literacy is mentioned, the preceding definitions of culture and knowledge do not depend on that ability. When considering the concept of literacy, it is important to realize that, of the tens of thousands of languages spoken during human history, only 106 have ever produced literature and most have never been written down at all. Of the 3000 spoken languages that exist today, only 78 have a literature (Greenlaw 1987).

Although the generally held concept is that lack of reading ability means that an individual cannot produce abstract thought, this notion is emphatically wrong. The inability to read is often the result of the circumstances in which the individual has lived and is not an indicator of lack of intelligence. For example, Mexican–American elders have worked in a predominately literate (reading) world where another language is the norm. Most did not have the opportunity to go to school on a regular basis but have supported and reared children who probably live in a cultural world that is different from their own.

Most people would be hard-pressed to function in today's world without the ability to read and write. Yet, despite the fact that their health status is generally lower than that of the Anglo population, Mexican–American elders see themselves as competent and functional members of their culture and the world in which they live (Smith 1989).

Educators and healthcare providers must approach older individuals in a way that honors their culture. For any culturally sensitive population, instructional materials should validate the life experiences and coping skills that have been developed in order to survive without the ability to read. To produce materials that are relevant to a particular culture, the developers must always pay close attention to detail and learner analysis, be aware of limited abilities and be sensitive to cultural norms (Kearney 1984).

WORLD VIEW

World view, as described by Kearney (1984), is the way that human societies look at reality and make sense of their world. A world view consists of basic assumptions that may or may not be accurate, but are more or less coherent. Geertz (1973) identified a world view as 'their picture of the way things in sheer actuality are; their concept of nature, of self, of society'. For example, according to Kearney, every society has a time orientation. For the dominant Anglo culture in the USA, the orientation is a future orientation; however, for most Mexican–American elders and many other cultures, the orientation is that of the timeless present. This has implications because the changes that practitioners often recommend are seen as applying to something that might occur in the future. The concepts of chronic disease, risk factors and the prevention of complications are based in a future orientation.

An article by Hamadeh (1987) describes an excellent example of a practitioner of Western medicine who recommended going beyond what some consider to be customary practice in order to understand his patient and the patient's situation. He used what he described as the Ecological Framework approach to generate hypotheses about the patient's responses. Hamadeh described several levels of analysis: (i) the individual level, in which psychological problems, stress and depression may all be factors that contribute to a poor response; (ii) the family level, in which the factors affecting the patient's illness include family myths and beliefs about disease and the family's experience with the medical profession; and (iii) the cultural level, in which factors affecting illness behavior may be misunderstood by healthcare providers unless they are aware of the larger context of the patient's background; this background includes knowledge of the economic, social and religious factors affecting the patient's life.

Hamadeh's article concludes with a list of pertinent questions to be asked when a healthcare provider is new to a community and wishes to understand the patients (Hamadeh 1987).

1. What is the community's understanding of good health?
2. When is a member considered to be ill?
3. What are common explanations for causes of illness in the community?
4. What usual modes of treatment and alternative healthcare systems are available?
5. How much is the patient responsible for illness, cure or prevention?
6. Who is the medical decision-maker in the family?
7. What are the attitudes towards death and dying?

To understand and treat elders who have lived a traditional life within their particular culture, healthcare professionals of all disciplines should learn about their traditions and relate to them with understanding and acceptance. The way in which educators and healthcare providers approach individuals must honor their culture. Is it ethical to keep on insisting on behavioral change when individuals demonstrate that they understand the intentions of the caregiver but they do not wish to change? The attitude of the provider can have a great impact on the acceptance of a course of action, depending on whether rigid compliance is expected or whether a course of action toward change is recommended and mutually agreed upon (adherence). The attitude of the provider can greatly affect the likelihood that a change in behavior or lifestyle will occur.

Because each individual who presents for treatment brings with them a unique and complex background, it is important to consider that each also has a unique personality and may respond to treatment situations in a different manner. There are three issues that may have an effect upon the treatment experience: self-efficacy, learned helplessness and authentic happiness. Self-efficacy is described by Rowe & Kahn (1998) as the can-do factor and is the individual's belief in an ability to handle most situations. These authors report that research has shown this kind of self-esteem leads to improved performance of many kinds. Individuals who do not exhibit self-efficacy falsely conclude that even small age-related losses in physical ability must result in drastic reductions in activities.

Learned helplessness was researched and reported by Seligman (1975) and can be described as the opposite of self-efficacy. Several of the symptoms parallel that of depression. Seligman describes some of the symptoms as: (i) being isolated and withdrawn, preferring to be alone; (ii) having a slow gait and behavior; (iii) feeling unable to act and make decisions; and (iv) giving the appearance of an 'empty' person who has given up. Seligman suggests that learned helplessness, as well as reactive depression, lies in the individual's belief that valued outcomes are uncontrollable.

The issue of authentic happiness looks at the contrast between the pessimist and the optimist (Seligman 2002). Pessimistic individuals have what he describes as a 'pernicious' way of looking at setbacks and frustrations; they view them as being personal and permanent, undermining everything and being the fault of oneself. On the other hand, optimistic individuals have a resilience or strength that allows them to view setbacks as surmountable, relating to a single situation and resulting from temporary circumstances or other people.

It is probable that the optimist and the pessimist will view treatment and outcomes in a different light. Seligman's research over 20 years has shown that pessimists are eight times more likely to become depressed when bad events occur, and have worse physical health and shorter lives.

The reasoning behind this discussion is that most health professionals are likely to encounter individuals that fit into each of these categories. If they come to know their patients' strengths and weaknesses, understand their personalities and listen to them and their family and caregivers, positive treatment outcomes are more likely. Rowe & Kahn (1998) warn, however, that not all supportive actions have the intended effect and that it is possible to provide 'too much of a good thing' to some elders. There can be a fine line between instrumental support (instrumental activities of daily living) and the generally positive relationship between emotional support and physical performance. Providing the best-intentioned support, if not needed, can reduce an individual's self-efficacy and actually lower physical performance. This leads full circle to learned helplessness.

Current research suggests that executive dysfunction or impairment is common in patients with medical illnesses. Schillerstrom et al (2005) believe that most nonpsychiatric clinicians are unaware of the importance of executive impairment in medical conditions. Patients with chronic diseases such as hypertension, chronic obstructive pulmonary disease and diabetes may particularly exhibit executive deficits that are independent of psychiatric conditions.

Most medical and surgical services commonly use the Mini-Mental State Examination (MMSE) or other instruments that are not sensitive to executive function. Executive function is important in many aspects of patient care because impaired patients are more likely to resist care, are less likely to follow medical regimens, for example proper inhaler use, and do not have the capacity to consent to treatment.

PHYSICAL AND COGNITIVE CONSIDERATIONS

Hearing impairment

When considering the cultural setting in which providers observe patients, it is important to remember the physical and cognitive barriers that can stand in the way of good communication. Hearing impairment or loss may have a major impact on rehabilitation (this problem is described in detail in Chapter 54). In elderly individuals, the negative effects of a hearing loss may lead to disengagement and paranoia if impairments are severe and continue for any length of time. Additionally, loss of hearing may create a sense of loneliness and isolation, and result in emotional distress because of anxiety or depression. Certain behavioral compensations by a patient may lead a healthcare provider to suspect a hearing loss. These compensations are listed in Box 55.1.

> **Box 55.1   Behavioral compensations indicative of hearing impairment**
>
> - Leaning closer to the speaker
> - Cupping an ear
> - Speaking in a loud voice
> - Positioning the head so that the 'good' ear is near the speaker
> - Asking for phrases to be repeated
> - Answering questions inappropriately
> - Looking blank
> - Being inattentive
> - Isolating self or refusing to engage in conversation
> - Having a short attention span
> - Not reacting
> - Showing emotional upset

Visual impairment

An additional sensory impairment that leads to communication difficulties is the loss of vision (presbyopia and various visual pathologies are described in Chapter 53). Simple compensations can be used to assist individuals with visual loss, for example increasing print size and using bold print in all printed materials, including medical and personal history forms. Glare should be minimized and bold primary colors used for all written materials, especially instructions.

It is not uncommon for older individuals to have both hearing and visual loss, which leads to typical behaviors such as squinting, frowning or grimacing during conversation. Often, individuals with this type of impairment rely more on touch for reassurance. At times, they appear to be distrusting or withdrawn. Additionally, they may worry about being awkward and may exhibit a reluctance to communicate. This may lead to fearful behavior, even during normal activities. Methods that help in communication with patients who have visual or hearing impairments or both are shown in Box 55.2.

Short-term cognitive dysfunction

In addition to the sensory impairments and cultural problems that lead to communication barriers between healthcare providers and elderly patients, there are a host of short-term confusional states that can impede effective communication during rehabilitation. These include distortion of time and space cues, meaning that the patient becomes confused as a result of being in an unfamiliar room and having no familiar objects in view. The hospital schedule is often totally asynchronous with the individual's normal schedule.

Hospital conditions may lead to depersonalization; the individual loses a sense of self. A patient may simply become 'the woman in

are able. The patient should always be informed of what has happened and what will be happening next. An attempt should be made to include individuals in major decisions while avoiding giving them unnecessary details.

It is important to recognize that everyone is an important member of the team, including the patient. Family and friends should be educated about the nature of the aphasic individual's problems and the ways in which they can be helpful. A tendency for family and friends to prescribe therapy for the aphasic patient should be guarded against. The needs and feelings of the caregiver must not be confused with those of the patient, nor should the caregiver – or the family – expect the patient to appreciate all of their efforts.

It is of the utmost importance to avoid letting the lives of other people revolve around the needs of the individual patient. For family members, particularly, the best counsel is that they should take care of their own physical and emotional health. Taking care of themselves means that they will be in the best possible position to help their loved ones, the patients (Boone 1983).

Executive cognitive function

Dr Donald R. Royall has proposed that dementia might be better understood as a syndrome of executive dyscontrol: 'The executive control functions are the cognitive processes that orchestrate relatively simple ideas, movements, or actions into complex goal-oriented behaviors (such as cooking a meal) (Box 55.3). They help maintain goal-directed behavior in the face of both internal and external distractions. Without them, behaviors important for independent living can be expected to break down into their component parts. Direction and purpose are lost, undermining the independence of demented patients. This situation can lead to problem behaviors in a variety of settings' (Royall 1994a).

room 410, bed one'. The loss of continuity with life history may also lead to some short-term confusional states. This occurs because an individual's cohorts have all died or been institutionalized, so that there is no one to whom they can say 'Do you remember…?' Also, an individual may be living alone and the loss of human companionship can result in withdrawal and disengagement from social activities. Furthermore, hyperthermia and hypothermia, electrolyte imbalance and certain medications may lead to acute short-term states of confusion.

Long-term cognitive dysfunction

In the presence of cognitive dysfunction, communication takes on a whole new meaning. There are various common reasons for long-term cognitive dysfunction in aging patients, including stroke, dementia, head injuries resulting from falls or other accidents and developmental disabilities.

When working with a patient with cognitive dysfunction or aphasia, verbal and nonverbal behavior that makes the individual feel guilty for not speaking should be avoided. It is important to accept individuals at their particular level of function and build on that. It is crucial to point out progress so that the patient grasps the idea that gains are being made. The healthcare provider should ask questions using verbal and nonverbal communication and encourage patients to answer them to the best of their ability. If an individual cannot find the proper words and becomes frustrated, it is important to express empathy and understanding; however, it is unwise to for the caregiver to pretend to understand something that has not been comprehended. The provider should get the patient's attention before speaking and should speak according to their ability, avoiding long sentences, rapid speech or difficult and uncommon words. It is helpful to communicate one idea at a time, using clear short sentences and everyday words, and to avoid speaking in a loud voice unless the individual has suffered a hearing loss. Facing the aphasic individual when speaking and using gestures are also useful practices. In addition, it is wise to avoid asking too many questions at one time or repeating a question immediately.

Sometimes, the use of written language may be a better and more understandable method of communication for a particular individual. A communication board may be of value.

It is crucial that caregivers do not discuss individuals in their presence as if they were not there. Individuals should have every opportunity to hear speech and should be encouraged to participate in social activities in the home and community at whatever level they

Many problem behaviors can be construed as examples of disordered executive cognitive function (ECF).

Treatment outcomes and function are indirectly affected by ECF impairment. Patients are often given responsibilities that are goal-directed and require executive control. Diabetic patients are often required to self-administer insulin based on the outcome of glucose monitoring. Psychologists call this a 'go/no-go' paradigm; it is especially sensitive to ECF impairment in humans. Synthesis is required to bring all the pieces together and administer the correct dosage.

In patients with ECF impairment, the ability to synthesize or to sequence all of the necessary pieces of a plan together to reach a specific goal is simply not there. Even those patients who have successfully completed the MMSE (see Chapter 30) may not be properly diagnosed with ECF dysfunction and may appear simply to fail to follow their insulin regimen or their dietary restrictions. Royall (1994b) has stated that, 'Poor adherence to prescribed diet or medication is a well-known cause of poor outcomes in chronic medical conditions such as diabetes or congestive heart failure.'

For patients to keep appointments made weeks in advance or to remember to refill prescriptions or file for insurance requires ECF behaviors. Therefore, executive impairment that goes unrecognized interferes with treatment, expected outcomes, access to care and follow-up.

There is no single comprehensive test for executive function. Dr Royall and his colleagues have developed the EXIT25 and the CLOX instruments in an attempt to operationalize ECF testing at the bedside. With training, lay personnel can administer EXIT25. EXIT25 and CLOX have demonstrated ECF impairment in a variety of conditions, including in association with problem behaviors.

When there is a diagnosis of ECF dysfunction, or if a patient is unable to go from step one to step two in a procedure in which proper instruction has been given, the family or formal caregiver must be taught the procedure. Instructing a caregiver allows the patient to maintain a feeling of control and self-worth.

Including the caregiver in treatment planning has many positive features: 'Studies indicate that caregiver descriptors are stronger predictors of functional status and level of care than the severity of the patient's dementia or problem behavior. Early in dementia, a patient's executive control allows for his or her participation in decision-making. Once executive control is lost, the caregiver's role in these decisions becomes more important. The maintenance of adequate supervision, a safe environment, treatment adherence, and the avoidance of unwitting cues for inappropriate behavior are all under the caregiver's control. Ritualizing the patient's daily routine early in the course of the dementia may help the caregiver as the disease progresses' (Royall and Mahurin 1990).

In the home or in any other treatment setting, the following suggestions can help those who care for patients with ECF:

- work to establish a daily ritual;
- use new routines to develop new habits and to break old habits:
  - build good new habits through repetition;
  - listen to what the patient's environment is 'saying' to the patient;
- use social and environmental cues to the patient's advantage;
- remove or alter cues that seem to trigger problem behaviors.

CONCLUSION

By focusing on adherence and not compliance, all healthcare disciplines can develop techniques to help patients learn to take personal responsibility for planning and implementing their own care. It is important to work with the whole family within its cultural framework and to determine who is the medical decision-maker. Healthcare professionals must consider the expectations of outcome of the individuals being served rather than their own outcome expectations.

The personal touch is needed. It takes more time but it is very important when working with patients from other cultures, especially older individuals who may also have problems seeing and hearing. It is often overlooked that some older individuals do not read in any language. Technology is a necessary part of modern healthcare; however, it is up to all practitioners to treat those with whom they work with patience and respect. To treat all elders, especially those of other cultures and ethnicities, as a homogeneous group makes no more sense than treating all children from birth to the age of 18 as a unit of similar individuals. The best role for the caregiver is one of patient advocacy and support. Listening and observation should be common practice.

References

Boone DR 1983 An adult has aphasia: for the family; the management and treatment of the aphasic patient. Interstate Printers & Publishers, Danville, IL

Geertz C 1973 Ethos, world view, and the analysis of sacred symbols. In: Geertz C (ed) The Interpretation of Cultures. Basic Books, New York, p 126–141

Greenlaw MJ 1987 The Quest for Literacy (Report no. CS-009-II). US Department of Education (ERIC Document Reproduction Service no. ED 290129), Washington, DC

Hamadeh G 1987 Religion, magic, and medicine. J Fam Pract 25:561–568

Kearney M 1984 World View. Chandler & Sharp, Novato, CA

Payne ZA 1980 Diet and folk remedies: the influence of cultural patterns on medical management. Urban Health 9:24–28

Rowe JW, Kahn RL 1998 Successful Aging. Pantheon Books, New York

Royall DR, Mahurin RK 1996 Executive cognitive functions: neuroanatomy, measurement, and clinical significance. In: Dickstein LJ, Oldham JM, Riba MB (eds) Rev Psychiatr 15: 175–294

Royall DR 1994a Cognitive Dysfunction and Need for Long-Term Care: Implications for Public Policy. American Association of Retired Persons, Washington, DC

Royall DR 1994b Précis of executive dyscontrol as a cause of problem behavior in dementia. Exp Aging Res 20:73–94

Schillerstrom JE, Horton MS, Royall DR 2005 The impact of medical illness on executive function. Psychosomatic 46:508–516

Seligman MEP 1975 Helplessness: On Depression, Development, and Death. Freeman, San Francisco, CA

Seligman MEP 2002 Authentic Happiness: Using the New Positive Psychology to Realize your Potential for Lasting Fulfillment. Free Press, New York

Smith F 1989 Overselling literacy. Phi Delta Kappan 70:353–359

Williams MV, Davis T, Parker RM et al 2002 The role of health literacy in patient-physician communication. Fam Med 34(5):383–389

UNIT **8**

Specific problems

UNIT CONTENTS

Practice problems

Chapter **56**

Dysphagia

Lisa Tews and Jodi Robinson

For most individuals, eating is a pleasurable and social event that is often considered an important part of the quality of life. However, for individuals with dysphagia, the task of eating may be difficult and even lead to serious medical consequences such as dehydration, malnutrition and aspiration pneumonia.

DEFINITION

Dysphagia, or swallowing disorder, is the medical term used when an individual experiences difficulty, discomfort or pain when swallowing.

PREVALENCE

Dysphagia affects millions of individuals; however, there is variability in the literature regarding its prevalence. Figures tend to differ by the type of healthcare setting, the patients sampled and the sampling methodology. In the general population:

- Approximately 10 million Americans with dysphagia are evaluated every year.
- It is estimated that swallowing disorders affect 1 out of 17 people.
- Some studies have found the prevalence to be as high as 22% in adults over the age of 50, whereas other studies indicate that approximately 7–10% are affected. This variation may result from the fact that many patients with dysphagia do not seek medical care.

In specific settings, it has been determined that dysphagia is present in:

- 61% of adults admitted to acute trauma centers;
- 41% of patients in rehabilitation settings;
- 30–75% of nursing home residents;
- 25–30% of patients admitted to hospitals.

It is known that individuals with swallowing disorders have higher rates of mortality and morbidity. In patients with acute stroke, one study estimated that 10% of deaths that occur within 30 days of admission to a hospital are a result of aspiration pneumonia. Further, for every 11 patients in whom pneumonia can be prevented, an estimated one death may be avoided (American Speech-Language-Hearing Association 2006).

ETIOLOGY

Dysphagia can be caused by a multitude of disorders, diseases and surgical procedures. In many cases, it is a side effect of medication (Box 56.1). It is important to understand each etiology and the impact it can have on the swallowing process.

For elderly individuals, in particular, a swallowing problem may be triggered when the body is weak and in a deconditioned state, such as after a major surgery. Moreover, any condition or medication that reduces saliva production, muscle strength, coordination or alertness level may have a negative impact on the swallowing function.

NORMAL SWALLOWING PHYSIOLOGY

The act of deglutition can be divided into four phases: (i) the oral preparatory phase, when food is manipulated in the mouth and masticated if necessary; (ii) the oral or voluntary phase of the swallow, when the tongue propels food posteriorly until the swallowing reflex is triggered; (iii) the pharyngeal phase, when the reflexive swallow carries the bolus through the pharynx; and (iv) the esophageal phase, when esophageal peristalsis carriers the bolus through the cervical and thoracic esophagus into the stomach.

Box 56.1   Conditions that may affect the swallowing process

1. Neurological/neurogenic
   - Pseudobulbar palsy
   - Bulbar palsy
   - Cerebrovascular accident
   - Traumatic brain injury
   - Neurovascular disease
   - Acute encephalitis
   - Acute meningitis
   - Seizure disorder
   - Peripheral neuropathy
   - Transient ischemic attack
   - Metastatic cancer (advanced stages)

2. Congenital/progressive neurological
   - Polio
   - Postpolio syndrome
   - Multiple sclerosis
   - Parkinson's disease
   - Amyotrophic lateral sclerosis
   - Huntington's chorea
   - Myasthenia gravis
   - Myotonic dystrophy
   - Guillain–Barré syndrome
   - Cerebral palsy
   - Tardive dyskinesia

3. Cognitive/psychological
   - Globus hystericus
   - Right hemisphere dysfunction
   - Dementia

4. Structural
   - Head and neck cancer
   - Laryngectomy
   - Glossectomy
   - Esophagectomy
   - Hiatal hernia
   - Zenker's diverticulum
   - Congenital or acquired anomalies
   - Burns
   - Tracheostomy
   - Focal tumors
   - Laryngeal trauma/vocal fold injury

5. Skeletal and connective tissue
   - Lupus
   - Scleroderma
   - Inflammatory myopathy
   - Cervical rheumatoid arthritis
   - Cervical osteophyte
   - Osteoarthritis
   - Cervical spinal cord injury
   - Fractures (facial, spinal)
   - Contractures

6. Respiratory
   - Chronic obstructive pulmonary disease
   - Asthma
   - Emphysema

7. Medical/other
   - Esophageal reflux
   - Decline in functional status/deconditioning
   - Radiation therapy (head and neck)

8. Surgical procedures
   - Laryngectomy
   - Anterior cervical spine surgery
   - Carotid endarterectomy

9. Medications
   - Antipsychotics
   - Anticonvulsants
   - Antihistamines
   - Neuroleptics
   - Barbiturates
   - Antiseizure

For a normal swallow to occur, there must be oral propulsion of the bolus into the pharynx, airway closure, upper esophageal sphincter opening, and tongue base to pharyngeal wall propulsion to transport the bolus through the pharynx into the esophagus (Logemann 1998). During the pharyngeal stage of deglutition, when airway closure is achieved, respiration halts until the swallow is completed. In essence, swallowing and respiration are reciprocal functions. When any one or a combination of the stages of swallowing is atypical, there is an increased potential for aspiration to occur. Aspiration (entry of material into the airway below the level of the true vocal cords) may be considered a hallmark of dysphagia, but there are numerous other complaints or observations that can signal a swallowing disorder, as shown in Box 56.2.

Although the presence of a dysphagia is not necessarily life-threatening, the presence of aspiration, if left untreated, can result in serious medical complications. It is important to recognize overt signs and symptoms of aspiration and report them to the patient's nurse, physician or the speech-language pathologist as quickly as possible (Box 56.3).

The symptom of gagging is listed in Boxes 56.2 and 56.3. Although the absence of a gag reflex has often been associated with an inability to swallow, there are no data to support this premise. In fact, studies show that an estimated 13–37% of normal individuals have a reduced or absent gag reflex when stimulation is applied to the posterior pharyngeal wall. This is especially true in the elderly (Murray 1999).

In most cases, the patient's family, physician or nurse will be the first to identify the warning signs of dysphagia. However, they may also be discovered by other members of the interdisciplinary team who work with the patient in activities of daily living. The occupational

Box 56.2   Examples of dysphagia symptoms

- Coughing or choking on liquid
- Coughing or choking on food
- 'Holding' food in the mouth
- Difficulty chewing or avoiding foods that require mastication
- Pocketing food in the cheek
- Drooling
- Loss of food or fluid from the mouth
- Slow eating, especially with solid foods
- Gagging
- Food sticking in the throat
- Excessive mucus
- Regurgitation
- Weight loss

Box 56.3   Possible signs of aspiration

- Eyes watering
- Reddening of the face
- Change in rate of respiration
- Difficulty or inability to breathe
- Change in lung sounds
- Audible breathing
- Facial grimacing
- Coughing
- Gagging
- Throat clearing
- Gurgly vocal quality
- Chest pain
- High or low back pain
- Inability to produce voice or speaks only in a whisper

therapist may observe problems during feeding skills or the dietician may find that the patient prefers ground meats instead of solids. Regardless of which team member identifies the problem, it is appropriate and necessary that a referral be made to the speech-language pathologist. It is the role of the speech-language pathologist to evaluate the patient, make the appropriate diagnosis and treat the dysphagia, if warranted.

DYSPHAGIA ASSESSMENT

The swallow is most commonly evaluated in one of two ways: using a clinical (or bedside) swallow examination or an instrumental examination.

Bedside examination

After a thorough case history is obtained, the speech-language pathologist performs a bedside exam. Upon completion, it is determined whether the patient is a candidate for oral feeding and the appropriate diet is recommended. If a swallowing problem is suspected in the pharyngeal stage of the swallow or the patient demonstrates clinical signs of aspiration, an instrumental exam is necessary and nothing by mouth (NPO) is generally recommended. It is important to note that the presence of 'silent aspiration' cannot be detected at the bedside. Approximately 50% of individuals who aspirate do not cough when material enters the airway. Studies have shown that 40% of patients who aspirate will be undetected if evaluated by a bedside exam alone, even when performed by the most experienced clinician (Logemann 1983). Hence, it is crucial that the patient have an instrumental exam to fully assess the physiological function of the swallowing mechanism if aspiration is suspected.

Instrumental examination

The most common types of instrumental examination currently being performed in the USA are the radiographic evaluation (also known as a modified barium swallow, videofluoroscopic swallow evaluation or cookie swallow test) and the fiberoptic endoscopic evaluation of swallowing (FEES). The purpose of the instrumental examination is to identify the presence and cause of aspiration. Once the etiology is determined, appropriate therapeutic techniques can be implemented. In cases of severe dysphagia, in which the patient is unable to safely swallow any consistencies, or if the ability to maintain adequate nutrition is a concern, alternative or supplemental nutrition or hydration may be recommended. Nutrition and hydration may be provided using a temporary method, such as intravenous feeding or a nasogastric (NG) tube. If recovery is anticipated to be more long term, a gastrostomy tube (G-tube) or jejunostomy tube (J-tube) is placed. When possible, the efficacy of parenteral nutrition should be discussed with the patient, family and physician. Recently, individuals have become more autonomous when making healthcare decisions; this means that there may be patients who do not agree to the insertion of artificial means of nutrition. If a patient chooses not to comply with recommendations, it is the role of the healthcare team to educate the individual regarding the risks of aspiration pneumonia and other medical sequelae. In knowing that there may always be patients who continue oral nutrition despite the risks, some facilities have adopted the practice of 'pleasure eating' and 'free water protocols' (Franceschini 2002).

DYSPHAGIA TREATMENT

Treatment for a swallowing disorder is specific to the individual. Based on the findings of the assessment, diet modification may be required. Table 56.1 shows some common diet recommendations. Each institution typically has its own diet hierarchy in place.

In addition to diet texture modifications, postural changes such as a chin down position or head rotation may be required during the swallow. The force of gravity on food flow through the pharynx can be altered when a change in posture is applied (Table 56.2).

Dysphagia rehabilitation also typically includes muscular strengthening, range of motion (ROM) exercises and specific swallowing maneuvers. In conjunction with traditional therapy exercises, surface electromyographic (sEMG) biofeedback may also be employed. Research has shown that this noninvasive procedure is useful in providing general information about the duration and amplitude of muscle activity during the swallow. It can also be used to assess aspects of the oropharyngeal swallow, as peak electromyographic

Table 56.1 Dysphagia diet progression

Liquids	Thin liquid Nectar consistency Honey consistency Pudding consistency
Level I	Dysphagia pureed (pureed, smooth and cohesive foods that require very little chewing ability)
Level II	Dysphagia mechanically altered (soft, moist, cohesive semisolid foods that require some chewing and can easily be formed into a bolus; meats are ground or finely chopped)
Level III	Dysphagia advanced (foods that are naturally soft and near regular texture; hard, dry, sticky or crunchy foods are excluded)
Level IV	Regular (all foods allowed)

Adapted from the National Dysphagia Diet Task Force 2002.

Table 56.2 Effects of posture changes during swallowing

Posture	Effect
Head back	Uses gravity to clear the oral cavity
Chin down	(i) Widens valleculae, narrows airway to prevent bolus entering airway; (ii) pushes tongue base backward towards pharyngeal wall; (iii) puts epiglottis in more protective position
Head rotated to damaged side	(i) Puts extrinsic pressure on thyroid cartilage, increasing adduction; (ii) increases vocal fold closure by applying extrinsic pressure; (iii) eliminates damaged side from bolus path
Lying down on one side	Eliminates gravitational effect on pharyngeal residue
Head tilt to stronger side	Directs bolus down stronger side
Head rotated	Pulls cricoid cartilage away from posterior pharyngeal wall, reducing resting pressure in cricopharyngeal sphincter

Adapted from Logemann JA 1998. Swallowing Disorders.

Table 56.3 Exercise programs and swallowing maneuvers

Stage of the swallow	Exercise program/swallowing maneuver
Oral stage	
Reduced lip closure	Lip exercises (resistance, ROM)
Reduced cheek tension	Manual pressure
Reduced tongue elevation	Tongue exercises (resistance, ROM)
Reduced tongue lateralization, anterior to posterior movement	Tongue exercises (chewing with gauze, manipulation)
Reduced range of jaw movement	Jaw ROM exercises
Oral awareness	Oral stimulation (taste, temperature, pressure, texture)
Apraxia	Increase oral sensation (pressure/cold/sour)
Pharyngeal stage	
Delayed or absent triggering of the pharyngeal swallow	Thermal/tactile stimulation; suck/swallow; quick downward pressure on tongue; sour bolus
Slow pharyngeal transit	Lee Silverman voice treatment
Reduced base of tongue movement	Effortful swallow; super-supraglottic swallow; tongue holding (Masako maneuver); tongue-base retraction exercises (yawn, tongue hold, gargle)
Reduced pharyngeal contraction	Falsetto; effortful swallow; effortful phonation of 'eee'
Reduced laryngeal elevation	Super-supraglottic swallow; falsetto; pitch exercises; Mendelsohn maneuver
Reduced closure at laryngeal entrance	Super-supraglottic swallow; Mendelsohn maneuver
Reduced laryngeal closure at vocal folds	Supraglottic swallow; adduction exercises; Teflon or gelfoam injection
Cricopharyngeal dysfunction	Mendelsohn maneuver; Shaker exercises; recovery; dilatation (if scar tissue); myotomy (only after recovery)

Adapted from Logemann JA 1983.

activity indicates maximal hyolaryngeal elevation during the swallow (Crary & Groher 2000).

The speech-language pathologist develops a program that is tailored to the abnormal phases of the swallowing process (Table 56.3). As with any exercise program, the following factors must be taken into consideration: fatigue, ability to follow directions, cognitive and behavioral status, and compliance.

In addition to the conventional therapeutic techniques already discussed, new treatments are emerging for the management of dysphagia. Examples of these less conventional treatments include electrical stimulation (direct stimulation of the suprahyoid and thyrohyoid muscles using hooked-wire electrodes) and deep pharyngeal neuromuscular stimulation (the use of frozen lemon glycerin swabs to stimulate the pharyngeal swallow at specific reflex sites). Interventions such as these are invasive and have been scrutinized by many speech-language pathologists. The research completed thus far is diverse in terms of both quality and results (Freed et al 2001, Leelamanit et al 2002, Burnett et al 2003). As in any profession in which integrity must be upheld, it is vital that evidence-based research be conducted to determine the effects of a treatment on a specific population. In a society in which fads often come and go, it is essential that all team members remain alert. Through practice of the best techniques available and good clinical judgment, patients with dysphagia will be better able to maintain optimal nutrition, health and quality of life.

References

American Speech-Language-Hearing Association (ASHA) 2006 Communication Facts: Special Populations: Dysphagia. Available at: http://www.asha.org/members/research/reports/dysphagia

Burnett TA, Mann EA, Cornell SA et al 2003 Laryngeal elevation achieved by neuromuscular stimulation at rest. J Appl Physiol 94:128–134

Crary M, Groher M 2000 Basic concepts of surface electromyographic biofeedback in the treatment of dysphagia: a tutorial. Am J Speech Lang Pathol 9:116–125

Franceschini T 2002 Issues in Assessment and Treatment of Esophageal and Related Swallow Disorders. Workshop conducted at Trinity Medical Center, Rock Island, IL

Freed ML, Freed L, Chatburn RL et al 2001 Electrical stimulation for swallowing disorders caused by stroke. Resp Care 46:466–474

Leelamanit V, Limsakul C, Geater A 2002 Synchronized electrical stimulation in treating pharyngeal dysphagia. Laryngoscope 112:2204–2210

Logemann JA 1983 Evaluation and Treatment of Swallowing Disorders. Pro-Ed, Austin, TX

Logemann JA 1998 Evaluation and Treatment of Swallowing Disorders, 2nd edn. Pro-Ed, Austin, TX

Murray J 1999 Manual of Dysphagia Assessment in Adults. Singular Publishing Group, San Diego, CA

National Diet Task Force 2002 National Dysphagia Diet: Standardization for Optimal Care. American Dietetic Association, Chicago, IL

Chapter 57

Incontinence of the bowel and bladder

Sandra J. Levi and Scott Paist

INTRODUCTION

Bladder and bowel incontinence among older adults is common and often treatable. Unfortunately, embarrassment and inadequate knowledge of treatment options prevent many older adults from reporting incontinence to healthcare professionals. The social consequences of incontinence are profound, and incontinence often precipitates institutional placement. About 10–40% of community-dwelling older adults report urinary incontinence and up to 10% report fecal incontinence. Among residents of nursing homes, over 50% have urinary incontinence and 16–60% have some problem with fecal incontinence. Both types of incontinence are much more common in women than men but, in the case of fecal incontinence, the gender ratio decreases with increasing age.

INCONTINENCE OF THE BOWEL

Normal control

Incontinence of the bowel is usually defined as an involuntary loss of stool through the anus that is severe enough to cause hygienic or social problems. In older adults, it may occur as an isolated incident in response to an acute event. Chronic fecal incontinence increases with increasing age.

Sensory and motor mechanisms contribute to the control of defecation. Typically, contractions in the proximal colon move feces into the rectum. The rectum stretches to hold the feces. The internal and external anal sphincters, as well as the puborectalis muscle, play especially important roles in preventing leakage. The internal anal sphincter is a 2–3 mm band of smooth muscle surrounding the anus. It is contracted and normally relaxes to allow emptying of the rectum. The external anal sphincter primarily consists of striated muscle; it voluntarily contracts, when needed, to prevent leakage. The puborectalis muscle forms a loop around the posterior aspect of the external sphincter. Contraction of the puborectalis muscle creates an anorectal angle. This angle and the puborectalis muscle assist in preventing defecation.

Defecation is initiated in response to rectal filling. Parasympathetic nerve impulses initiate strong peristaltic waves that move the fecal content along. At the same time, other body actions such as the Valsalva maneuver and upward and outward contraction of the pelvic floor musculature help to move the feces downward and outward. The final response is voluntary relaxation of the external anal sphincter.

With increasing age, pelvic floor musculature may weaken. Age-related loss of strength, as well as possible changes in tissue elasticity, may contribute to a decreased resting tone of the anus, particularly in women (Tariq 2004).

Causes of incontinence

The causes of fecal incontinence in the elderly are shown in Box 57.1. Fecal impaction and diarrhea are the most common causes of fecal incontinence and are often treatable. Leakage of stool may also result from loss of sensation or loss of muscle tone. Finally, stool loss may occur as a result of changes in the cognitive capacity to interpret sensory signals.

Stool leakage around an obstruction is often found in older adults. Most of these individuals have chronic fecal impaction, often as a result of chronic laxative abuse and poor bowel habits. Cancer or a

---

Box 57.1   Etiology of fecal incontinence

- Fecal impaction
- Loss of normal continence mechanism
  - Local neuronal damage (e.g. pudendal nerve)
  - Impaired neurological control
  - Anorectal trauma/sphincter disruption
- Problems that overwhelm normal continence mechanism
- Psychological and behavioral problems
  - Severe depression
  - Dementia
  - Cerebrovascular disease
- Neoplasm (rare)

Adapted from Tariq SH 2004, with permission.

benign polyp will sometimes be the cause. Whatever the cause, liquid stool from higher in the colon will leak past the hard immovable obstruction and drain from the anus, despite the best efforts of the patient.

A patient who has a condition that causes loose stool (drugs, inappropriate diet or infection) may suffer involuntary loss of this watery fecal material. For example, antacids containing magnesium, the consumption of dairy products by a person who is lactose intolerant and Salmonella infection can cause diarrhea. Loose stool may also be seen in bedridden patients who have poor muscle tone. A change of gravitational force may cause additional physiological and social demands on bedridden patients who are starting transfer and gait activities.

Loss of sensation of the perineum results in the patient not sensing the need for rectal emptying until natural forces have done so, leading to involuntary loss. Such perineal anesthesia may result from spinal cord injury, tumor or stroke.

Loss of muscle tone by the muscles of continence may change the balance of forces such that the expulsive force of the colon exceeds any voluntary attempt by the patient to impede such force. Tumor, stroke, spinal cord injury, pudendal neuropathy and surgery frequently precipitate loss of muscle tone.

Patients may lose stool because they lack the cognitive capacity to realize what is happening. Such patients may have forgotten how to properly manage stool (as in dementia) or may not be sufficiently oriented to manage it (as in delirium).

Patients who have a moderate impairment – anatomical, physiological, mental or a combination of these – and who are impeded in some way from establishing a usable stooling position may appear to be incontinent. In addition, individuals with mobility limitations may be prevented from getting to a commode in a timely fashion. Rearranging their environment may make it easier for these patients to manage.

Diagnosis and therapeutic intervention

Diagnosis of fecal incontinence begins by obtaining a careful history from the patient, the nursing staff, the physician and the medical record. The history includes a description of:

- bowel habits, change in habits and fecal consistency;
- bowel frequency, urgency, ability to delay, soiling and ability to distinguish gas from feces;
- emptying difficulties, including straining, incomplete emptying and pain;
- the capacity to access the toilet (communication, cognitive and mobility);
- medication, chronic medical conditions, obstetrical injury, radiation to prostate or cervix and surgeries in the anorectal area;
- any previous treatment.

The physical examination includes palpation of the abdomen to look for colon distention, a rectal examination, a neurological examination and assessment of mobility, hygiene and mental functioning. Diagnostic tests may include stool cultures, blood tests, a barium enema, radiographic procedures, anal manometry, ultrasound and electromyography.

Treatment is guided by the underlying cause and severity of incontinence. Medical management may include dietary management, e.g. increasing fiber intake. Bowel management and training may involve medication (e.g. loperamide can be used to prevent diarrhea) and a toileting schedule. Neuromuscular re-education, including biofeedback, has also shown promising results in some patients. Diarrhea, one of the reversible conditions, should be controlled no matter what its cause. Treatment typically requires multiple approaches.

INCONTINENCE OF URINE

Many of the points already discussed are important when considering urinary incontinence, which is a much more common occurrence. Urinary incontinence is defined as an involuntary loss of urine that is severe enough to cause social or hygienic problems. The consequences of urinary incontinence are listed in Box 57.2. In addition, the direct monetary cost of urinary incontinence has been estimated to be over US $16 billion a year (Wilson et al 2001). The enormity of the problem can be seen by examining the direct and indirect costs as shown in Box 57.3.

Box 57.2   Psychosocial consequences of urinary incontinence for the patient, caregiver and community

Effect on individual

- Psychological strain: shame; anger; depression; embarrassment; loss of confidence; loss of self-esteem
- Social interactions; isolation; disengagement; abandonment
- Diminished sexual interest and activity
- Fear of institutionalization
- Decreased mobility and travel
- Decreased involvement in hobbies and activities
- Diminished interpersonal contact and relationships
- Increased dependence

Effect on caregiver

- Caregiver burden and burnout
- Resentment
- Increased financial burden
- Potential for neglect and abandonment
- Avoidance and diminished interpersonal relationships
- Increased likelihood of placement in long-term institution

Effect on community

- Increased financial burden
- Avoidance behavior
- Feeling of guilt to involved patients
- Feeling of resentment or disdain
- Extrapolating health image to assume individual is demented, debilitated, nonfunctional, incapable of realizing a good quality of life
- Fully dependent

Adapted from Hajjar RR 2004 Psychosocial impact of urinary incontinence in the elderly population. Clin Geriatr Med 20:553–564.

Normal control

Urine is stored in the bladder, which stretches during filling. Urine is held in the bladder as long as the pressure in the bladder remains lower than the urethral resistance. Urination occurs when the bladder

Box 57.3 Costs of incontinence

Diagnostic and evaluation costs

- Diagnostic and evaluation tests
- Physician and health professional services for evaluation and management

Treatment costs

- Behavioral therapy
- Surgery
- Medication

Routine costs

- Pads and protection products
- Hygiene and deodorant products
- Laundry directly related to incontinence

Complications

- Skin irritation
- Urinary tract infections
- Falls

Institutional costs

- Nursing home admissions
- Excess acute hospital days

Adapted from Wilson et al 2001.

---

muscle (detrusor muscle) contracts, forcing urine into the urethra. Muscles surrounding the urethra relax, allowing urine to pass out of the body.

Types of incontinence

Four distinct types of urinary incontinence can be identified, although, in many cases, these presentations are mixed: urge incontinence, stress incontinence, overflow incontinence and functional incontinence.

Urge incontinence occurs when a patient feels the need to empty the bladder but is unable to get to a toilet before urination occurs. In urge incontinence, involuntary loss of urine may be large and post-void residual volume small. Post-void residual volume is measured by having the patient void as completely as possible and then immediately placing a straight catheter into the bladder and measuring the remaining urinary volume. The most common cause of this type of incontinence is an overactive bladder muscle (detrusor instability). It is most prevalent among individuals with diabetes, stroke, Alzheimer's disease, Parkinson's disease and multiple sclerosis.

Stress incontinence occurs when a cough, strain, laugh, sneeze or otherwise-initiated Valsalva maneuver causes involuntary loss of urine. Trunk flexion exercises and, possibly, the sit-to-stand movement may provoke stress incontinence. At such times, a few drops to a few ounces of urine escape from the bladder. Post-void residual

volume is small. This is the most common type of incontinence seen among middle-aged women.

Overflow incontinence occurs when the bladder is overly distended (either because of an outlet obstruction or a bladder anomaly), causing bladder pressure to exceed urethral pressure, no matter what the patient may attempt. Another cause of overflow incontinence is the loss of the bladder sphincter secondary to surgery or injury. Loss of urine occurs in small amounts, but may occur nearly continuously. The post-void residual volume is high (potentially liters). Diabetes, spinal cord injury and an enlarged prostate can all precipitate overflow incontinence.

Functional incontinence occurs when individuals with normal bladder and urethral function have difficulty getting to the toilet before urination occurs. Those with impaired mobility or mental confusion may have this type of incontinence.

Diagnosis and therapeutic intervention

Diagnosis of urinary incontinence begins with a carefully conducted history that includes a description of:

- voiding history;
- urinating difficulties, including straining, decreased flow of stream, intermittent flow, hesitancy;
- irritation symptoms, such as urgency, frequency, urge incontinence;
- communication and cognitive capacity to access a toilet;
- medications, chronic medical conditions, pelvic or spinal surgery, trauma;
- any previous treatment.

The patient should be examined to identify any reversible causes of incontinence, as well as any neurological disease, abdominal mass or pelvic organ prolapse. The DIAPPERS mnemonic shown in Box 57.4

Box 57.4 Reversible causes of urinary incontinence (DIAPPERS)

Delirium or other confusional state
Infection, urinary tract, symptomatic
Atrophic urethritis or vaginitis
Pharmaceuticals
- Sedative/hypnotics, especially long acting
- Alcohol abuse
- Loop diuretics (e.g. Bumex, Lasix, Edecrin)
- Anticholinergic agents (e.g. antipsychotics, antidepressants, antihistamines, antiparkinsonian agents, antiarrhythmics, antispasmodics, opiates, antidiarrheal agents)
Psychological disorders (especially depression)
Endocrine disorders (hyperglycemia or hypercalcemia)
Restriction mobility
Stool impaction

From Clinical Practice Guideline: Urinary Incontinence in Adults. US Department of Health and Human Services, Public Health Service, Agency for Health Care Policy and Research, with permission.

is useful for identifying reversible causes of urinary incontinence. Men should also receive a prostate examination. Diagnostic tests may include post-void residual volume and urodynamic tests, urinalysis and culture, and blood tests.

Treatment is guided by the underlying cause and the severity of incontinence. Some causes of urinary incontinence are reversible and easily treated. Medications may be used to prevent unwanted detrusor muscle contractions or to increase muscle tone. Implants can be used to help close the urethra and reduce stress incontinence. Pelvic floor muscle retraining has been demonstrated to help women with stress and urge incontinence. Bo et al (1999) studied 107 women with stress incontinence, with a mean age of 49.5 years, range 24–70. The mean duration of symptoms was 10.8 years, with a range of 1–45. The group who performed 8–12 repetitions of pelvic floor exercises three times a day and exercise once a week with a skilled physical therapist had significantly improved muscle strength and reduced leakage. These results were superior to those seen in the other treatment groups: the electrical stimulation group, vaginal cones group and control group. Neuromuscular re-education, including biofeedback, has also shown promising results in some patients (Burgio et al 1998).

Treatment typically requires multiple approaches (Wallace et al 2004). Some of the treatment options that are available to physical therapists are listed in Box 57.5.

Box 57.5   Selected treatment options available to physical therapists

- Bladder training including
  - Patient education
  - Scheduled voiding
  - Positive reinforcement
  - Urge-suppression techniques
- Pelvic floor muscle retraining including
  - Biofeedback
  - Strengthening exercises
  - Endurance exercises
- Transvaginal electrical stimulation

CONCLUSION

Constant efforts must be made to find and treat reversible causes of incontinence. It must *never* be assumed that incontinence is a result of aging. Although many people with bowel and bladder incontinence cannot be completely cured, most can be helped significantly if the healthcare team takes the time to think about possible causes and to institute treatment plans based on careful diagnoses.

References

Agency for Health Care Policy and Research 1996 Managing acute and chronic urinary incontinence. Publication no. 96–0686

Bo K, Talseth T, Holme I 1999 Single, blind randomized controlled trial of pelvic floor exercises, electrical stimulation, vaginal cones, and no treatment in management of genuise stress incontinence in women. BMJ 318:487–493

Burgio KL, Locher JL, Goode PS et al 1998 Behavioral vs drug treatment for urge urinary incontinence in older women. JAMA 280:1995–2000

Tariq SH 2004 Geriatric fecal incontinence. Clin Geriatr Med 20:571–587

Wallace SA, Roe B, Williams K, Palmer M 2004 Bladder training for urinary incontinence in adults. Cochrane Database Syst Rev 1:CD001308

Wilson L, Brown JS, Shin GP et al 2001 Annual direct cost of urinary incontinence. Obstet Gynecol 98(3):398–406

Chapter 58

Iatrogenesis in older individuals

John O. Barr, Timothy L. Kauffman and LaDora V. Thompson

INTRODUCTION

Iatrogenesis is defined as any injury or illness that occurs as a result of medical care (Taber's Cyclopedic Medical Dictionary 2005). An iatrogenic condition is a state of ill health or adverse effect caused by medical treatment; it usually results from a mistake made in treatment, and can also be the fault of a nurse, therapist or pharmacist. The risk of iatrogenesis in individuals over the age of 65 is twice as high as that of a younger person (Gurwitz et al 1994).

A host of factors, many of which are hallmarks of aging, increase the risk of the elderly suffering an iatrogenic condition. The presence of multiple chronic diseases potentiates the possibility that the treatment of one problem may have a negative impact on another. For example, the use of a nonsteroidal antiinflammatory medication in the treatment of arthritis may exacerbate heart failure or chronic gastritis. Fragmentation of health delivery into many specialties may lead to changes being made in therapeutic interventions without adequate communication among caregivers.

Hospitalization increases the risk for nosocomial infections, transfusion reactions, polypharmacy and immobility. Mobility is critical for well-being and quality of life in the elderly individual. Surgical and medical interventions may lead to complications because of anesthesia or fluid overload (*Merck Manual of Geriatrics* 2000). Older patients often arrive at hospital without medications or an appropriate list of prescribed drugs, meaning that scheduled doses may be missed for hours or days.

Medical errors can be significant albeit unintentional. The Institute of Medicine (IOM) reported that, in the USA, as many as 44 000–98 000 people of all ages die in hospitals each year as a result of medical errors. These errors occur in all settings and carry a tremendous cost, estimated to be almost US$38 billion each year. The IOM (1999) attributed most errors, not to negligence or misconduct, but to system-related problems. It has even been suggested that the absence of an advanced directive for frail elderly individuals represents iatrogenesis (vonSternberg 1993).

Adverse drug reactions from prescription drugs result from incorrect ordering and administration (Bates et al 1999) and improper dosages (Leape et al 1995). Polypharmacy in the elderly is a confounding issue. Other problematic errors may be based on misreading test results or the ambiguous presentations of symptoms, yet another hallmark of aging (*Merck Manual of Geriatrics* 2000, Lantz 2002, Agency for Healthcare Research and Quality 2004).

In an effort to promote safer healthcare, the US Department of Health and Human Services, the American Hospital Association and the American Medical Association have joined together to develop 'Five Steps to Safer Healthcare', presented in Box 58.1. This fact sheet informs patients about the steps that they can take to ensure safer healthcare.

Box 58.1 Five Steps to Safer Healthcare[a]

1. Ask questions if you have doubts or concerns.
   - Ask questions and make sure you understand the answers.
   - Choose a doctor you feel comfortable talking to.
   - Take a relative or friend with you to help you ask questions and understand the answers.

2. Keep and bring a list of *all* the medicines you take.
   - Give your doctor and pharmacist a list of all the medicines that you take, including nonprescription medicines.
   - Tell them about any drug allergies you have.
   - Ask about side effects and what to avoid while taking the medicine.
   - Read the label when you get your medicine, including all warnings.
   - Make sure your medicine is what the doctor ordered and know how to use it.
   - Ask the pharmacist about your medicine if it looks different than you expected.

3. Get the results of any test or procedure.
   - Ask when and how you will get the results of tests or procedures.

(*continued*)

- Don't assume the results are fine if you do not get them when expected, be it in person, by phone or by mail.
- Call your doctor and ask for your results.
- Ask what the results mean for your care.

4. Talk to your doctor about which hospital is best for your health needs.
- Ask your doctor about which hospital has the best care and results for your condition if you have more than one hospital to choose from.
- Be sure you understand the instructions you get about follow-up care when you leave the hospital.

5. Make sure you understand what will happen if you need surgery.
- Make sure you, your doctor and your surgeon all agree on exactly what will be done during the operation.
- Ask your doctor, 'Who will manage my care when I am in the hospital?'
- Ask your surgeon:
Exactly what will you be doing?
About how long will it take?
What will happen after the surgery?
How can I expect to feel during recovery?
- Tell the surgeon, anesthesiologist and nurses about any allergies, bad reactions to anesthesia and any medications you are taking.

[a]AHRQ 2003 Patient Fact Sheet, Publication no. 03-M007. Agency for Healthcare Research and Quality, Rockville, MD. Available http://www.ahrq.gov/consumer/5steps.htm.

This chapter focuses on iatrogenesis related to adverse drug reactions and immobility, and offers suggestions for proactively preventing these conditions.

ADVERSE DRUG REACTIONS

Polypharmacy is a complex multifactorial issue. Individuals aged 65 and over take 33–40% of all prescription medications in the USA (Lantz 2002) and over 50% of the over-the-counter medicines. Approximately four out of five people in this age group take at least one drug daily (Beyth & Shorr 2002). Zhan and associates (2001) reported that one out of five people aged 65 or older who lived in the community was taking at least one prescription drug that was inappropriate as determined by an expert panel. These researchers recommend that the following medications be avoided in the elderly: barbiturates, flurazepam, meprobamate, chloropropamide, meperidine (pethidine), pentazocine, trimethobenzamide, belladonna alkaloids, dicyclomine, hyoscyamine and propantheline.

Age-related physiological changes affect the absorption, distribution, metabolism and elimination of drugs. Stomach changes, such as increased pH or altered motility, may reduce drug absorption. Decreases in total body water and lean body mass, as well as increases in total body fat, can alter drug distribution. Diminutions of liver mass and blood flow may alter drug metabolism, and reductions in renal plasma flow and glomerular filtration rate (GFR) decrease drug elimination via the kidney (Beyth & Shorr 2002).

A complication of type 2 diabetes mellitus is chronic renal failure. Corsonello et al (2005) reported that chronic renal failure may be unrecognized or 'concealed' and may contribute to an adverse drug reaction (ADR). A standard method for determining renal failure is detection of elevated serum creatinine; however, in the elderly, it may be within the normal range because of the decreased GFR. Thus, renal failure may be 'concealed' and subsequently lead to an ADR, especially in patients using hydrosoluble drugs [sulfonylureas, metformin, digitalis, angiotensin-converting (ACE) inhibitors, insulin, diuretics, antibiotics such as penicillins and cephalosporins, and non-steroidal anti-inflammatory drugs (NSAIDS)]. In their study of 2257 hospitalized patients with type 2 diabetes mellitus, over 16% had concealed renal failure and over 10% of all patients had ADRs.

Individuals with dementia are especially vulnerable to ADRs because of an increased availability of protein-bound agents (because of loss of lean body mass, and reduced albumin) such as antidepressants and antipsychotics (Lantz 2002). Secondary parkinsonism is often caused by medications, including antipsychotics (Merck Manual of Geriatrics 2000). Tardive dyskinesia is a drug-induced movement disorder that is usually caused by antipsychotics such as haloperidol. It is characterized by abnormal involuntary movements involving the tongue and lips, e.g. chewing motions, and produces a feeling of motor restlessness and not wanting to stay still. As with all ADRs, a change of prescription drugs is helpful, if at all possible. Additionally, antipsychotics, as well as beta blockers, carbidopa–levodopa, diuretics and sedative–hypnotics (benzodiazepines), may cause sleep disturbances in elderly individuals.

In recent years, testosterone replacement has been used to treat secondary hypogonadism and the related male problems of sarcopenia and changes in libido, bone mass and visuospatial cognition. Calof et al (2005) performed a meta-analysis of clinical trials to evaluate the risks of ADRs in men over the age of 45 who undergo testosterone replacement. They reported that this medical intervention was significantly associated with higher rates of prostate cancer, elevated prostate-specific antigen and prostate biopsies. Hematocrit was also elevated and warrants monitoring in men taking testosterone. There were no significant differences between the testosterone group and placebo group in the frequency of sleep apnea or cardiovascular events.

Quiceno & Cush (2005) have noted that medication-related iatrogenic events may masquerade as rheumatic disorders. Although rare, myopathic syndromes associated with the use of statins include myopathy, myalgia, myositis and rhabdomyolysis. Drugs that induce lupus include procainamide, hydralazine, methyldopa, quinidine and chlorpromazine. Gout, most commonly produced by underexcretion of uric acid, is associated with ethanol use, diuretics, low-dose salicylate, cyclosporin (ciclosporin), ethambutol, pyrazinamide, levodopa and nicotinic acid. Arthralgias can be the result of antiinfectives (e.g. quinolones and vaccines), biological agents (e.g. interferons and growth factors), supplements (e.g. fluoride and vitamin A), lipid-lowering statins and fibrates, cardiac drugs (e.g. quinidine, propranolol, acetabulol, nicardipine) and hormonal agents (e.g. raloxifene, tamoxifen, letrozole).

The use of medications in the elderly is complex and is associated with iatrogenesis, as noted above. Antidepressant or analgesic medications have also been associated with falls in ambulatory frail elderly individuals (Lipsitz et al 1991). However, medications that carry risks of ADRs may also provide benefits. Won et al (2006) reported that the use of short- or long-acting opioids in nursing home residents was not associated with an increased risk of falls, depression, constipation, delirium, dehydration or pneumonia. They found that the use of pain medications improved functional status and social engagement.

Actions that can be taken to limit drug-related iatrogenesis have been outlined by Stolley and associates (Stolley et al 1991). They include educating patients and staff about drug effects and potential problems; carrying out a formal drug review by a gerontological nurse and pharmacist; and taking an accurate drug history, which includes a thorough assessment of drug allergies, possible drug borrowing and proper drug use by patients.

IMMOBILITY

Many physical, psychological, pathological and environmental factors can result in bedrest or immobility. Box 58.2 summarizes the usual causes of immobility in the elderly; these causes will be discussed below.

Box 58.2   Causes of immobility in the elderly

Musculoskeletal disorders
- Arthritis
- Osteoporosis
- Fractures (especially femur)
- Podiatric problems (bunions, calluses)
- Pain

Neurological disorders
- Stroke
- Parkinson's disease
- Alzheimer's disease

Cardiovascular disease
- Congestive heart failure
- Coronary artery disease (frequent angina)
- Peripheral vascular disease (with frequent claudication)
- Pulmonary disease
- Chronic obstructive pulmonary disease

Environmental causes
- Forced immobility
- Inadequate aids for mobility (canes, walkers, appropriately placed railings)
- Being wheelchair-bound
- Stairs and other architectural barriers

Other
- Fear of falling
- Malnutrition
- Deconditioning
- Drug side effects

As well summarized by Kelley & Mobily (1991), a wide range of factors can contribute to iatrogenic immobility in healthcare settings. These factors include physical and architectural barriers; institutional policies (e.g. related to comprehensive patient assessment, and chemical and physical restraints, etc.); medical regimens (e.g. bedrest, intravenous therapy, indwelling catheters, etc); characteristics of other facility residents and opportunities for socialization; and staff characteristics (e.g. care patterns that promote dependence, inadequate staffing and limited availability of physical and occupational therapists).

Bedrest can be beneficial and necessary during an illness but it can also have negative consequences that complicate the return to independence. It may contribute to iatrogenic complications if activity is not resumed as soon as possible. During a period of immobility, pathophysiological alterations occur in the major organ systems. Box 58.3 outlines the major changes that can occur in the musculoskeletal, cardiovascular, respiratory, integumentary, urinary, gastrointestinal, neurological and metabolic systems. These alterations occur to varying degrees depending on the organ system, the previous level of fitness of the individual and the extent of immobility. Bedrest-induced alterations can begin within the first 24 h and, if immobility continues, can result in new illnesses.

Box 58.3   Pathophysiological alterations of immobility

Musculoskeletal
- Decreased range of motion
- Decreased joint flexibility
- Development of contractures
- Loss of muscular strength (muscular atrophy)
- Loss of muscular endurance (deconditioning)
- Loss of bone mass
- Loss of bone strength

Cardiovascular and respiratory
- Decreased ventilation
- Atelectasis
- Aspiration pneumonia
- Deterioration of the respiratory system
- Increased cardiac output
- Increased resting heart rate
- Increase of orthostatic hypotension

Integumentary
- Development of pressure sores
- Skin atrophy
- Skin tears

Urinary and gastrointestinal
- Urinary infection
- Urinary retention
- Bladder calculi
- Constipation
- Fecal impaction

Neurological
- Compression neuropathies
- Depression
- Perceptual ability
- Social isolation
- Learned helplessness
- Altered sleep patterns, anxiety, irritability, hostility

Metabolic
- Negative nitrogen balance
- Loss of calcium

There are challenges in understanding the consequences of bedrest in older individuals because they have diminished physiological reserves secondary to age-related changes and disease processes. Every organ system is altered when a person is immobile, so it is critical that healthcare professionals recognize the negative consequences of bedrest or immobility for the older individual. The return to independence of elderly individuals can be speeded up if they understand the deleterious consequences of immobility, the relative time frame in which these consequences can develop and the potential value of therapeutic interventions.

Gill et al (2004) examined bedrest in community-dwelling individuals who were at least 70 years old over an 18-month period. Each month, the participants were asked if they had stayed in bed for at least half a day because of illness, injury or other problems. Nearly 60% of the nondisabled volunteers had at least one episode of bedrest, lasting an average of 2.8 months. Bedrest was significantly associated with declines in instrumental activities of daily living and social activity, with trends toward diminished physical activity and mobility also noted.

It is important to ascertain the basis for instituting bedrest. Rest is indeed important for individuals who complain of fatigue and tiredness. However, Avlund et al (2003) determined that community-living individuals who were 'tired' during daily activities at an initial evaluation had greater mobility disability and participated less in strenuous activities at follow-up 18 months later.

Impact of immobility on organ systems and related functions

Musculoskeletal system – joint range of motion

Immobility results in the loss of weight-bearing forces on joints. When joints are unloaded, there is a rapid change in the cellular biochemical and mechanical properties that results in alterations in periarticular and articular structures. The joint capsule becomes thickened and the synovium hyperemic. There is fibrofatty proliferation of connective tissue within the joint space. Collagen becomes denser and develops a more random arrangement, which results in the shortening of tendons. The ligaments of the joint atrophy, which results in a decline of tensile strength. Functionally, there is an increase in joint stiffness, a decrease in the flexibility of joints and a decrease in joint range of motion (ROM). These alterations in the cellular biochemical and mechanical properties can occur within 5 days of immobilization, with measurable losses in joint ROM occurring within a week. Long-term immobilization produces significant reductions in ROM; there can be as much as a 45% decrease after 5 weeks, which can lead to the development of contractures.

All joints are susceptible to the effects of immobilization but the hip, knee and ankle are particularly sensitive. Impairment of the ROM in the hip, knee and ankle can lead to problems with sitting, functional positioning, walking and balance stability. Physical and occupational therapists can counteract joint ROM deterioration secondary to immobilization by enabling continued movement of joints. Decreased ROM (especially in shoulder external rotation, hip extension, knee extension and ankle dorsiflexion), limited joint flexibility and the development of contractures can be counteracted by therapeutic heating. Therapeutic heating increases the compliance of collagen fibers and is followed by ROM exercises, strengthening exercises and stretching. Normal loading of the joints (weight-bearing exercises) may be very important in attenuating the changes in articular cartilage. The objectives of the exercises are to improve mobility and flexibility and to relieve stiffness. The older individual is taught to perform these exercises independently as soon as possible. General body stretching for a period of 15 min increases flexibility. Appropriate positioning, splinting and early ambulation are good therapeutic techniques that assist in maintaining functional ROM of joints. Appropriate resting and night splints can prevent a dropped-foot condition and pressure ulcers.

Musculoskeletal system – muscular strength and endurance

Inactivity causes a significant decline in muscle strength and muscle endurance. The muscles most affected by immobility are the antigravity muscles that facilitate locomotion and assist in maintaining an upright position (quadriceps, glutei, erector spinae and gastrocnemius–soleus muscles). Generally, 10–15% of muscle strength is lost each week; however, as much as 5.5% may be lost for each day of immobility. The greatest loss of strength occurs during the initial period of inactivity. Inactivity-induced loss of muscle strength is not linear; bedrest for 4–5 weeks has been known to decrease the strength of lower-limb extensor muscle groups by 20–25%. In addition to the decrease in physiological and functional muscle strength, muscles atrophy and resting lengths change – shortening leads to loss of motion and lengthening leads to stretch weakness.

As muscle strength decreases, there is a concomitant decline in endurance. The decrease in endurance has a profound influence on the ability to sustain any activity of daily living. Fatigue is a common complaint because of the decreased endurance and diminished exercise tolerance. Adaptations of the muscle system interfere with mobility, performance of the activities of daily living, posture and gait. The amount of strength and endurance lost by the elderly during bedrest is variable.

Rehabilitative services provide essential treatment strategies for disuse atrophy and muscle weakness. Therapeutic exercise is designed to increase muscle strength and endurance. Progressive resistive exercises (isometric and isotonic contractions) are particularly important because they are muscle specific but have crossover effects on other muscle groups. An exercise program that requires the development of maximal muscular contraction intermittently (30- to 60-s contractions) is beneficial in attenuating the decline in muscle strength. Ideally, the exercise program is initiated at 60% of the maximum lift (3–4 sets of 8–10 repetitions per muscle group), with a rest period between each set. The Valsalva maneuver should be avoided because it may elevate blood pressure and jeopardize the cardiovascular response.

Musculoskeletal system – bone mass and strength

Immobility causes a loss of bone mass. With bedrest, there is a decrease in the gravitational forces superimposed on bones, which leads to bone demineralization and a loss of trabeculae volume. Bones become thin, porous and fragile because of a relative increase in osteoclastic activity and greater resorption of bone. Bone loss occurs as early as the third day of immobilization. Bone alterations induced by immobilization predispose the elderly patient to fractures of the hip, spine and extremities. The elderly are especially vulnerable because bone loss resulting from inactivity or limited mobility is compounded by bone loss resulting from age-related osteoporosis. Complications such as urolithiasis and heterotrophic calcification can occur.

Rehabilitative treatment techniques for enhancing bone mass and strength consist mainly of increasing muscle strength, mobility and ambulation as soon as possible. Restoring weight-bearing forces is essential for maintaining bone mass and reversing bone loss. Ambulatory exercise has been found to restore bone mineral at a rate of 1% per month. In addition to early standing and ambulation, isotonic and isometric contractions (muscle-strengthening programs) assist in the prevention of bone wasting.

Cardiovascular system

The cardiovascular system undergoes significant changes during bedrest. Many of the changes are immediate; these are probably the most serious changes. When a patient is in the supine position, approximately 11% of the total blood volume is redistributed from the circulatory system of the lower extremities to the thorax. The increased volume of blood entering the thoracic circulation results in an increase in cardiac output. Thus, there is an increase in the cardiac workload as the heart works harder to circulate the extra volume.

Cardiovascular deconditioning also occurs with bedrest; there is an increase in the resting heart rate and a decrease in maximal oxygen uptake. It has been reported that, after 3 weeks of bedrest, the resting heart rate increases by 20%, with an average increase of one beat for every 2 days of bedrest. Bedrest diminishes physical work capacity by blunting the normal exercise-induced increase in stroke volume and cardiac output. Maximal oxygen uptake goes down, leading to diminished exercise tolerance (manifested by weakness, fatigue and shortness of breath). In young subjects, peak maximal oxygen uptake decreases by an average of 7.5% (range 0.3–26%) after 10–20 days of bedrest.

Orthostatic hypotension is a common cardiovascular complication of immobility. When moving from a supine to a vertical posture, a redistribution of blood occurs. Venous return is reduced and central venous pressure, stroke volume and systolic blood pressure decrease concomitantly. Baroreceptors in the autonomic nervous system typically elicit sympathetic stimulation to counter these effects; however, during bedrest, position changes do not elicit postural vascular responses, resulting in orthostatic hypotension. Orthostatic hypotension can occur in the elderly when they are immobilized for as little as 1 week. Signs and symptoms of orthostatic intolerance include tachycardia, nausea, diaphoresis and syncope. Functionally, orthostatic hypotension can significantly enhance the risk of falls and decrease stability during standing and ambulation. Orthostatic blood pressure changes become more exaggerated after prolonged immobilization, leading to orthostatic intolerance and diminished exercise tolerance.

Recovery from orthostasis is very slow after bedrest. Orthostatic hypotension may not only impair rehabilitative efforts but also predispose the elderly to serious cardiovascular events such as stroke and myocardial infarction.

The development of venous stasis predisposes the patient to the development of both pelvic and peripheral venous thrombosis. Pulmonary emboli can occur as a serious complication of venous stasis. The seated position encourages flexion of the hips, knees and elbows. This position forces the feet to remain dependent and also predisposes the patient to the development of venous stasis.

The Valsalva maneuver, an increase in intrathoracic pressure produced by forceful exhalation against a closed glottis, is common in patients with inactivity. The Valsalva maneuver occurs because of straining when turning in bed, lifting oneself and pushing oneself up etc. With the increase in intrathoracic pressure, venous blood flow is inhibited, resulting in an increase in pulse rate and a transient increase in systemic blood pressure.

Anticoagulants, elastic stockings, changes in position (including sitting) and early rehabilitative intervention can prevent or limit the extent of deconditioning and orthostatic hypotension. Intermittent sitting during the period of immobility attenuates the large decline in maximal oxygen uptake and the development of orthostatic hypotension. Therapeutic exercise consisting of aerobic conditioning is important for preserving cardiopulmonary fitness. Exercise in an upright position or use of a reverse gradient garment prevents or reduces the decrease in maximal oxygen uptake. Both isometric and isotonic exercises incorporating large muscle groups are essential. In the deconditioned patient, therapeutic exercise should be started at a very low intensity. It may be initiated with active and weight-bearing or resistive exercises in the bed or in a chair. For example, adequate sitting tolerance can be established by increasing the frequency and duration of sitting. If orthostatic hypotension is a problem, traditional treatments (elastic hose, elevation of the head of the bed at night and progressive mobility training) are necessary. For the severely deconditioned patient, early mobilization requires close monitoring of the patient's symptoms and vital signs (see Box 41.4, Guidelines for termination of an exercise session). Guidelines for ambulation frequency are not well established but it is reasonable to have the patient walk until mild fatigue is present, three times a day. It is critical to educate patients and their caregivers about the importance of exercise.

Respiratory system

The supine position leads to changes in lung volume and the mechanics of breathing. These changes are significant in the elderly, who already have diminished lung recoil. With immobilization, the vital capacity and tidal volume of the lungs decrease, secretions increase and expectoration decreases. There is insufficient clearance of the airway, which results in the pooling of secretions and increased bacterial growth distal to the obstruction, predisposing the elderly patient to pneumonia and local atelectasis. Atelectasis and pneumonia are common complications of immobility in all patients, and pulmonary embolism and aspiration pneumonitis can also occur. Impaired ventilation–perfusion, the widening of the alveolar–arterial gradient and the decrease in arterial oxygen lead to oxygen desaturation.

Preventive measures include mobility at the earliest possible time and respiratory muscle training, which is taught to patients so that they can practice it independently throughout the day.

Integumentary system

Decubitus ulcers are serious consequences of immobilization. With prolonged compression, skin circulation and skin perfusion decrease over bony prominences, causing infarction of the skin. The skin becomes more vulnerable to the forces of pressure, shear, friction and moisture, and tissue injury results. The extent and duration of immobilization are crucial factors in the development of impaired tissue integrity. If tissue injury does occur, healing is slowed because the body's metabolism is impaired, particularly with respect to nitrogen imbalance. Large decubitus ulcers may lead to even more serious infections such as osteomyelitis.

The older individual is particularly susceptible to the development of pressure sores when immobile. With aging, the skin becomes a less resistant barrier. It is predisposed to injury because of age-related decreases in the amount of subcutaneous adipose tissue, the number of sweat and sebaceous glands and the elasticity of connective tissue (see Chapter 52, Skin Disorders).

Appropriate beds and bed materials (mattresses, e.g. air, fluid, alternating pressure, egg-crate, etc.) that distribute pressure are essential. Changes in position relieve pressure and decrease the risk of pressure sores, so a turning schedule should be instituted. Protective clothing and the incorporation of rehabilitation exercises as soon as possible aid in prevention. All healthcare providers must practice appropriate preventive measures, giving extra attention to patients who have recently had anesthesia or are taking medications that induce relaxation and deep sleep. The effects of these medications increase the risk of pressure sores as do repeated transfers, armrests, foot pedals and the sling effects from a soft pliable chair back or seat.

Urinary system

Elderly hospitalized patients have an increased risk of incontinence (Gill et al 2004). In a recumbent patient, loss of gravitational emptying of the renal pelvis leads to stagnation in the calyces. Impaired renal drainage, changes in urinary calcium levels and the decreased pH of the urine predispose the elderly to calculus formations, aggregation of crystalloids and urinary tract infections. The increased duration of urinary stasis in both the kidney and bladder allows for bacterial growth.

Risks can be lessened by frequent turning, sitting up in a chair and the use of a bedside commode or the bathroom rather than a bed pan. Adequate fluid intake and early mobility can also be beneficial, as can isotonic and isometric exercises performed daily during bedrest to attenuate and stabilize fluid shifts.

Gastrointestinal system

During bedrest, the elderly may have a limited fluid intake, a diminished appetite and alterations in ingestion, digestion and elimination. The ability to digest and use nutrients is interrupted because of the reduction in the cellular exchange of nutrients that occurs with slowed metabolic activity. Constipation and fecal impaction can occur because of the decrease in intestinal motility (peristalsis decreases), inadequate ingestion of fiber and fluid and difficulty in defecating because of weakness. Swallowing may be difficult in a supine position. The disruption of eating habits can cause clinical malnutrition and loss of weight.

Early standing and ambulation are valuable in minimizing declines in gastrointestinal function.

Neurological system

Compression neuropathies can occur with lengthy bedrest. Ulnar, radial, median, sciatic and peroneal nerve compression injuries have been observed. Falling asleep while leaning against the wheelchair armrest can cause a radial nerve injury.

Sleep patterns are altered by immobility and this can cause tiredness, depression and lack of motivation. Distortion of time perception, mood changes, a poorer sense of well-being and learned helplessness can all occur. Loneliness and a longing for recognition have been noted in healthy young individuals during only 3h of immobility. Bedrest causes a decrease in coordination and a marked increase in body sway, resulting in altered balance and stability and an increased risk of falls. Balance decrements occur after 2–3 weeks of bedrest.

Variable high- and low-intensity short-duration isotonic training during bedrest has been shown to assist with sleep patterns and mental concentration. Early mobility, especially standing and ambulation, improve balance.

Metabolic functions

Loss of calcium and the development of a negative nitrogen balance occur during immobility. Hypercalcemia can result and cause further problems such as anorexia, nausea, vomiting, abdominal cramping, constipation, muscle weakness and lethargy. A negative nitrogen balance secondary to muscle breakdown can occur within 5 days of immobilization. Metabolic balance is particularly important if a tissue injury such as a burn or laceration has occurred because the success of repair of damaged tissue is dependent on an optimal metabolic environment. Rehabilitative exercises for mobility and strength attenuate any metabolic imbalances.

SUMMARY OF INTERVENTIONS FOR IMMOBILITY

The longer an individual remains inactive, the more pronounced the negative consequences are and the longer it takes for the body to return to a healthy status. Major physiological changes that occur early in immobility involve the fluid–electrolyte and venous compliance systems, and these changes can be life-threatening. Immobility cannot be avoided but many of its adverse effects can be prevented by means of therapeutic intervention (Box 58.4).

Box 58.4   Strategies for minimizing negative consequences of bedrest

- Minimize duration of bedrest
- Avoid strict bedrest unless absolutely necessary
- Allow bathroom privileges or bedside commode
- Let the patient stand for 30–60s whenever transferring (e.g. bed to chair)
- Encourage the patient to wear street clothes
- Encourage the patient to take meals at a table
- Encourage the patient to walk to hospital appointments
- Encourage patient passes out of the hospital in the evenings and at weekends
- Involve physical therapy, occupational therapy and restorative nursing
- Encourage daily exercises as a basis of good care
- Use protective splinting

Patients' mobility should be assessed and reassessed on an ongoing basis. Optimal management of immobile elderly patients necessitates thorough assessments, specific diagnoses and multimodal treatment by multidisciplinary geriatric consultation teams. Physical and occupational therapists assess and manage immobility and associated functional disabilities and should be consulted as early as possible in cases that involve immobile elderly patients. Even relatively small improvements in mobility can decrease the incidence and severity of complications and improve the well-being of older individuals. When full activity is not possible, limited activity such as movement in bed and intermittent sitting and standing reduce the frequency of some complications of bedrest. Proactive nursing care to prevent the sequelae of bedrest is crucial, as is ongoing nutritional assessment.

Specific rehabilitation objectives include controlling disease activity, decreasing pain, correcting deformities, restoring or improving efficient function and preventing future episodes (Box 58.5).

Box 58.5 Physical therapy in the management of immobile elderly patients

Evaluation
- Assess the need for and teach the use of assistive devices for ambulation and activities of daily living
- Evaluate, maintain and improve joint ROM
- Evaluate and improve strength, endurance, motor skills and coordination
- Evaluate and improve mobility, balance and gait
- Evaluate and improve ability to perform activities of daily living
- Assess mobility: bed mobility, transfers, ambulation

Goals
- Relieve pain
- Restore, maintain and improve the ability to function independently

Interventions
- ROM exercise (active and passive),
- Resistive exercise, including isometric and isotonic
- Heat (hot packs, paraffin, etc)
- Cold
- Hydrotherapy
- Ultrasound
- Transcutaneous electrical nerve stimulation

Therapeutic techniques include pain-relieving and therapeutic exercises to mobilize joints, strengthen muscles and enhance endurance and fitness – ROM exercises, graded strengthening exercises, positioning, mobility skills and transfers to ambulation are all important. The graded strengthening exercise sessions are designed to provide optimal stimulation while allowing sufficient recovery intervals so that excessive fatigue and injury are avoided. Singh (2002) has summarized recommendations for geriatric exercise prescription to counteract iatrogenesis across body systems, including aerobic and balance training, progressive resistance training and high-velocity high-impact loading. Specific goals must be individualized; in some older individuals, these goals will involve preventing the complications caused by immobility and adapting the environment to the individual.

CONCLUSION

Older individuals, especially the frail, are particularly susceptible to the iatrogenic effects of ADRs and immobility. The onset of these negative consequences can occur within the first 24 h and may affect the major organ systems and normal physiological functions. Additionally, immobility caused by an ADR or hospitalization accentuates age-related changes that impair physiological reserve. Management depends on the healthcare provider's awareness of the effects of bedrest and the importance of rehabilitation. Mobility is a critical issue that pertains to all functions and the very quality of life. Members of the rehabilitation team need to be proactive in taking steps to prevent iatrogenesis in older patients.

References

Agency for Healthcare Research and Quality (AHRQ) 2004 Reducing Errors in Healthcare, Publication No. 00-PO58, Agency for Healthcare Research and Quality, Rockville, MD. Available: http://www.ahrq.gov/research/errors.htm. Accessed 18 April 2004

Avlund K, Vass M, Hendriksen C 2003 Onset of mobility disability among community-dwelling old men and women: the role of tiredness in daily activities. Age Ageing 32:579–584

Bates DW, Miller EB, Cullen DJ et al 1999 Patient risk factors for adverse drug events in hospitalized patients. Arch Intern Med 159:2553–2560

Beyth R, Shorr R 2002 Principles of drug therapy in older patients: rational drug prescribing. Clin Geriatr Med 18:577–592

Calof O, Singh A, Lee M et al 2005 Adverse events associated with testosterone replacement in middle-aged and older men: a meta-analysis of randomized, placebo-controlled trials. J Gerentol Med Sci 60A:1451–1457

Corsonello A, Pedone C, Corica F et al 2005 Concealed renal failure and adverse drug reactions in older patients with type 2 diabetes mellitus. J Gerentol Med Sci 60A:1147–1151

Gill T, Allore H, Guo Z 2004 The deleterious effects of bed rest among community-living older persons. J Gerontol Med Sci 59A:755–761

Gurwitz JH, Sanchez-Cross MT, Eckler MA et al 1994 The epidemiology of adverse and unexpected events in the long-term care setting. J Am Geriatr Soc 42:33–38

Institute of Medicine (IOM) 1999 To Err is Human: Building a Safer Health System. National Academy Press, Washington, DC

Kelley LS, Mobily PR 1991 Iatrogenesis in the elderly: factors of immobility. J Gerontol Nurs 17(9):5–11

Lantz M 2002 Problems with polypharmacy. Clin Geriatrics 10:18–20

Leape LL, Bates DW, Cullen DJ et al 1995 Systems analysis of adverse drug events. JAMA 274(1):35–43

Lipsitz L, Jonsson P, Kelley M et al 1991 Causes and correlates of recurrent falls in ambulatory frail elderly. J Gerontol Med Sci 46:114–122

Merck Manual of Geriatrics, 3rd edn 2000 Whitehouse Station, NJ, p 53–74, 432–463, 655–656

Quiceno GA, Cush JJ 2005 Iatrogenic rheumatic syndromes in the elderly. Clin Geriatr Med 21:577–588

Singh MAF 2002 Exercise comes of age: rationale and recommendations for a geriatric exercise prescription. J Gerontol Med Sci 57A(5):M262-M282

Stolley JM, Buckwalter KC, Fjordbak B, Bush S 1991 Iatrogenesis in the elderly: drug-related problems. J Gerontol Nurs 17(9):12–17

Taber's Cyclopedic Medical Dictionary, 20th edn 2005 FA Davis, Philadelphia, PA

vonSternberg T 1993 Iatrogenesis: no advance directive (Letter). J Am Geriatr Soc 41(5):586–587

Won A, Lapane K, Vallow S et al 2006 Long-term effects of analgesics in a population of elderly nursing home residents with persistent nonmalignant pain. J Gerontol Med Sci 61A:165–169

Zhan C, Sangl J, Bierman AS et al 2001 Potentially inappropriate medication use in the community-dwelling elderly. Findings from the 1996 Medical Expenditure Panel Survey. JAMA 286(22):2823–2829

Chapter 59

Hormone replacement therapy

Christine Stabler

INTRODUCTION

Hormone therapy has been riding the roller coaster of public opinion since 1966 when Robert Wilson published Feminine Forever (Wilson 1966). Touted as the fountain of youth, estrogen used in uncontrolled amounts was thought to revitalize and rejuvenate menopausal women. The tidal wave of interest in estrogen replacement therapy came to an abrupt halt 12–15 years later after the publication of an article that provided the first clinical evidence that estrogen therapy may increase a women's risk of endometrial cancer (Mack et al 1976).

Estrogen regained some of its luster 10 years later, with the support of clinical data that demonstrated its efficacy and safety when used in a combined regimen with progesterone. Research demonstrated the protective effects of hormone therapy on the development of osteoporosis, heart disease, Alzheimer's disease and, potentially, colon cancer. These results strengthened support for hormone therapy among clinicians and patients alike (McMichael & Potter 1980, Colditz et al 1987). However, this short-lived respite once again came to a grinding halt in July 2002 when the National Heart, Lung and Blood Institute of the National Institutes of Health (NIH) released the unblinded first arm of the first prospective study into the effects of hormone replacement therapy on postmenopausal women (Petitti 2002).

RESULTS OF THE WOMEN'S HEALTH INITIATIVE

The Women's Health Initiative studied almost 50 000 women receiving hormone replacement therapy after menopause. The women were divided into two groups: those with an intact uterus receiving a combination of estrogen and progesterone and those, posthysterectomy, receiving estrogen alone. The estrogen and progesterone arm was stopped in July 2002 because the apparent risks of hormone replacement therapy outweighed any evident benefits. The estrogen-only arm of the study continued for another 2 years before it,

too, was prematurely discontinued: it failed to show the protective benefit that the study was designed to demonstrate. In total, 7 of the 8 projected years of the study had elapsed and, although with estrogen alone there was no increase in the risk of breast cancer, a significant increase in the risk of heart disease, blood clots and stroke became evident for women receiving hormone replacement therapy (Anderson & Limacher 2004). This information was a wake-up call to physicians to carefully analyze what women need in the menopausal years to maintain health and reduce risk.

The Women's Health Initiative (WHI) was designed to look at the effects of hormone replacement therapy on the risks of breast cancer, heart disease, stroke, blood clotting, osteoporosis and fractures, and colorectal cancers. It did not initially assess the symptoms of menopause, including hot flashes, insomnia, mood changes and genital dryness and atrophy. However, further analysis looked at menopausal quality of life and found that, although women receiving hormone replacement therapy had significant improvements in sleep, physical functioning, body pain, hot flashes and mood swings, overall, there was no significant difference in sexual well-being, mental health or vitality. What the study did show was an increased risk of breast cancer that began after 4 years of clinical use and that raised the relative risk by almost 25% in women receiving estrogen plus progesterone. This extrapolated to eight additional breast cancers per year per 10 000 women receiving hormone replacement therapy. In the women receiving estrogen alone, no such increased risk was evident. Concurrent studies published in the Journal of the American Medical Association reported that breast cancers that developed after hormone replacement therapy were more aggressive and larger than other breast cancers, and that women with a previous history of breast cancer had a higher rate of recurrence when receiving hormone therapy (Anderson & Limacher 2004).

Heart disease was also a major factor in the discontinuation of the WHI (Anderson & Limacher 2004). An increased risk of heart disease was noted in the first year of the study and the relative risk for the development of heart disease rose by 29%, extrapolating to seven more heart attacks per 10 000 women using hormone replacement therapy each year. This seemed to hold true for both women receiving estrogen alone and women receiving estrogen and progesterone in combination. Multiple etiologies for these phenomena have been postulated, including an increase in the levels of C-reactive protein and insulin-like growth factor in women receiving oral estrogen. However, this has yet to be proven definitively (Ridker et al 1999).

The study also found an increased risk of stroke, with an increased relative risk of 41%, which extrapolated to eight more cerebral vascular accidents per 10 000 women taking hormone replacement therapy per year. This risk seemed to hold true for all age groups, regardless of any baseline stroke risk such as hypertension, diabetes, previous coronary disease or use of aspirin or lipid-lowering drugs. A similar and parallel risk was demonstrated for the development of other blood clots: there were approximately eighteen more clots per 10 000 women per year. The risk for the development of blood clots was greatest in the first 2 years of therapy and decreased, but was still significantly elevated, after 4 years of use (Anderson & Limacher 2004).

The Women's Health Initiative Memory Study (WHIMS) was published in May 2003 (Hays et al 2003) and, contrary to previous beliefs supported by the Nurses Health Study, which identified hormone replacement therapy as a major prevention strategy for dementia, demonstrated an increase in dementia among women using hormone replacement therapy over the age of 65. There were an additional 23 cases of dementia per 10 000 women, with no statistical difference in risk regardless of socioeconomic status, educational attainment or use of aspirin. In addition, no protection was afforded for mild cognitive impairment, a less severe form of dementia (Shumaker et al 1999, WHIMS 2006).

There was some good news in the WHI: osteoporotic fracture risk was reduced by 34%, resulting in five fewer fractures per 10 000 women per year. This was the first trial to document a decreased risk of fractures with hormone replacement therapy and not just an improvement in bone density (WHI 2006). A similar reduction in the risk of colon cancer was demonstrated; after 3 years of hormone replacement therapy, the relative risk of the development of colon cancer was reduced by 37%, resulting in six fewer cancers per 10 000 women per year.

Limitations of the Women's Health Initiative

There were some significant limitations to the WHI that may make interpretation of the data difficult. This was a short study; however, breast cancer, colon cancer, osteoporosis and heart disease may take many years to develop. The average age of new participants in the study was 63 years, and many of these women had spent more than 10 years in menopause before beginning hormone replacement therapy.

Subclinical coronary disease, as well as subclinical breast cancer, may have been present before the initiation of therapy, meaning that some so-called healthy participants were, in fact, more ill than the general population. In addition, women with a high risk of developing the symptoms of menopause, such as hot flashes or osteoporosis, were excluded from the study, resulting in an eligibility bias against benefit. Finally, only one in four of the experimental group was actually taking their hormone replacement therapy at the end of the fifth year of study. These limitations make data interpretation a challenge.

ALTERNATIVE MANAGEMENT OF MENOPAUSE

No other menopausal treatment or regimen has undergone this degree of scrutiny. The assumption that alternative treatments for menopause and their effects are safe is unwise (North American Menopause Society 2004). We are therefore faced with an aging population of women who are living more of their life in menopause, and a population of patients who are more educated and more consumer-savvy about healthcare. It is up to clinicians to educate themselves about the management of menopause, to talk to patients and allow them to contribute to decision-making with regard to

menopausal therapies and to continually reassess the risk of adverse outcomes for patients over their lifetime (Carroll 2006).

The Women's Health Initiative has provided physicians with a unique opportunity to join with patients to create a designer approach to their menopause management. No two women have the same experiences, risk and needs. The goal of this partnership is to create a fluid approach that continually evaluates risks, symptoms and comorbidities and addresses the specific needs of women as they enter menopause. Special attention must be given to the prevention of heart disease, osteoporosis, memory loss and sexual dysfunction and the development of menopausal symptoms (WHI 2006).

The modification of heart disease risk requires lifestyle changes. Risk can be reduced by dietary reduction of saturated fats, exercise, smoking cessation, assumption of ideal body weight and reduction of alcohol consumption. Preexisting conditions such as hypertension, diabetes and hyperlipidemia should be optimally controlled to prevent the development of heart disease. The recognition of the gender differences between men and women in the presentation of heart disease is essential for optimal risk reduction.

The prevention of osteoporosis goes beyond hormone replacement therapy. Lifestyle changes such as increasing exercise, smoking cessation, maintenance of an ideal body weight and adequate calcium and vitamin D supplementation will help to prevent osteoporosis. Other therapeutic devices, such as selective estrogen receptor modulators (SERMs) that mimic the effects of estrogen in bone without affecting the cardiovascular system or breasts, have been proven to prevent osteoporosis. Bisphosphonates and calcitonin have been shown to build damaged bone. Unfortunately, natural estrogen analogs have not been found to be as helpful in osteoporosis prevention.

The reduction of menopausal symptoms relies on lifestyle changes such as limiting alcohol and caffeine intake and stress reduction; the wearing of light clothing may also be helpful. Soy supplementation has been shown to reduce mild hot flashes when six to eight servings are taken per day. Selective serotonin reuptake inhibitors, a type of antidepressant, offer moderate relief for women with menopausal symptoms. Estrogen remains the only proven treatment for severe hot flashes and the NIH now recommend short-term use at the lowest effective dose as the ideal treatment for the vasomotor symptoms of menopause.

Urogenital atrophy (vaginal dryness) can be treated with lubricants and feminine moisture replacements. The topical use of estrogen in small doses at infrequent intervals is helpful and may limit systemic exposure and therefore risk. Newer delivery systems, such as the vaginal ring with estrogen, have also proven to be quite successful in the reduction of symptomatology.

The WHIMS demonstrated no benefit of hormone replacement therapy in the prevention of Alzheimer's disease in older women. The improvement of memory as women enter menopause relies upon an active lifestyle and the early recognition and treatment of depression and other forms of pseudodementia that may mimic Alzheimer's dementia (Shumaker 1998).

CONCLUSION

Life after the WHI is more complex for physicians and healthcare providers who care for women as they enter menopause. The designer approach to the management of menopause will require education of the clinician, the continued and ongoing risk assessment of the patient, patient participation and the judicious use of lifestyle changes, nonpharmacological interventions, pharmacological treatments and hormone replacement therapy.

References

Anderson G, Limacher M 2004 The Women's Health Initiative Randomized Control Trial. J Am Med Assoc 291(14):1701–1712

Carroll DG 2006 Nonhormonal therapies for hot flashes in menopause. Am Fam Physician 73:457–467

Colditz GA, Willett WC, Stampfer MJ 1987 Menopause and the risk of coronary heart disease in women. N Engl J Med 316:1105–1110

Hays J, Ockene J, Brunner R et al 2003. Effects of estrogen plus progestin on health related quality of life. N Engl J Med 348(19):1839–1854

Mack TM, Pike MC, Henderson BE et al 1976 Estrogens and endometrial cancer in a retirement community. N Engl J Med 296:1262–1267

McMichael AJ, Potter JD 1980 Reproduction, endogenous and exogenous sex hormones, and colon cancer: a review and hypothesis. J Natl Cancer Inst 65:1201–1207

North American Menopause Society 2004 Treatment of menopause-associated vasomotor symptoms: Position Statement of the North American Menopause Society. Menopause 11:11–33

Petitti DB 2002 Hormone replacement therapy for prevention; more evidence, more pessimism. J Am Med Assoc 288:99–101

Ridker P, Buring J, Cook N et al 2003 C-reactive protein, the metabolic syndrome, and risk of incident cardiovascular events. Circulation 107:391–397

Shumaker SA, Reboussin BA, Espeland MA et al 1998 WHIMS Women's Health Initiative Memory Study. Control Clin Trial 19:604–621. Wilson RA 1966 Feminine Forever. M Evans, New York Available http://www.ncbi.nlm.nih.gov

Wilson RA 1966 Feminine Forever. M. Evans, New York

Women's Health Initiative (WHI) 2006 Findings from the WHI Postmenopausal Hormone Therapy Trials. Available: http://www.nhlbi.nih.gov/whi/. Accessed 14 March 2006

Women's Health Initiative Memory Study (WHIMS) 2006 Estrogen therapy does not reduce dementia risk. Available: http://www.wfubmc.edu/whims/index.html. Accessed 14 March 2006

Chapter 60

Dizziness

Susan L. Whitney

CHAPTER CONTENTS

- Introduction
- Presentation and diagnosis
- Functional deficits
- Therapeutic intervention
- Conclusion

INTRODUCTION

Dizziness is a frequently occurring disorder of older individuals, which can result in serious functional deficits. Older adults often visit their physicians with nonspecific complaints of dizziness; it is the most common complaint of adults over the age of 75 and the third most common complaint to physicians in outpatient settings, regardless of age (Kroenke et al 1992). As dizziness is a subjective experience, it is difficult to determine whether the patient and the examiner agree on what the symptoms are. The most common cause of dizziness is a change in medication.

PRESENTATION AND DIAGNOSIS

Dizziness is interpreted differently by different people and is often difficult to describe. Commonly, people complain of a sense of giddiness, floating, lightheadedness or a sensation of being drunk. Table 60.1 includes other common descriptors associated with dizziness and used by patients to explain their complaints to practitioners.

Some patients who experience dizziness have nystagmus, which is a nonvoluntary rhythmic oscillation of the eyes in either the lateral or the superior/inferior direction, often accompanied by a torsional component. The nystagmus usually manifests with a fast and a slow component to the eye movements, in opposite directions.

Patients also describe having symptoms of vertigo, which is classically defined as an illusion of movement that usually has a rotatory component (Furman & Cass 2003). Individuals who experience vertigo often have a sensation of turning. Vertigo has been described as rotational, translational and as a sense of being tilted. It does not

Table 60.1 Common complaints of individuals experiencing dizziness

Chief complaint	Assessed during the case history	Assessed during the physical exam
Head alignment abnormalities	−	+
Difficulty controlling center of mass within the base of support	+	+
Difficulty orienting body to the vertical	+	+
Difficulty selecting the most appropriate sensory information to make decisions	−	+
Eye movement abnormalities	+	+
Abnormal motion perception	+	+
Physical deconditioning	+	+
Gait abnormalities	+	+
Swimming sensation in the head	+	+
Imbalance	+	+
Blurred vision	+	+
Tinnitus	+	Sometimes
Aural fullness	+	Sometimes
Hearing loss	+	+
Oscillopsia (an illusory movement of the visual world that occurs with high-frequency head movements)	+	+
Confusion, especially in rich sensory environments	+	−
Lightheadedness	+	+

(Continued)

Table 60.1 *(Continued)*

Chief complaint	Assessed during the case history	Assessed during the physical exam
Anxiety	+	Sometimes
Headache	+	–
Fatigue	+	+
Falling	+	Sometimes
Clumsiness	+	Sometimes
Fear of falling	+	–
Neck pain	+	+

Box 60.1 Common causes of dizziness

- Peripheral vestibular disorders
  - Benign paroxysmal positional vertigo
  - Meniere's disease
  - Endolymphatic hydrops
  - Perilymph fistula
  - Vestibular neuritis
  - Labyrinthitis
  - Bilateral vestibulopathy
- Central disorders
  - Cervical vertigo
  - Vestibular ocular dysfunction
  - Traumatic head injury
  - Anterior or posterior inferior cerebellar stroke
  - Post-traumatic anxiety symptoms
  - Transient ischemic attacks
  - Migraines
  - Multiple sclerosis
- Psychiatric disorders
  - Panic disorders
  - Agoraphobia
  - Hyperventilation syndrome
- Other
  - Low blood pressure
  - Medication
  - Presyncope
  - Arrhythmias
  - Vertebral artery trauma
  - Alternobaric vertigo
  - Diabetes mellitus
  - Thyroid dysfunction
  - Renal disease
  - Human immunodeficiency virus
  - Syphilitic labyrinthitis
  - Epstein–Barr virus
  - Brainstem hemorrhage
  - Friedreich's ataxia
  - Recent diplopia

matter whether the patient or their world is spinning, as both are considered to be vertigo. The sensation of vertigo usually indicates an inner ear problem, although occasionally it can be related to an anterior inferior or posterior inferior cerebellar stroke.

Most patients who experience dizziness or vertigo modify their activity levels even when they are not having symptoms. A fear of falling is often associated with the symptoms of dizziness or imbalance in elderly individuals. Such individuals commonly become noticeably less active over time because of the fear of experiencing dizziness or imbalance, especially in unfamiliar environments. This inactivity can start a downward decline in function in older people.

Falls have been related to the most common cause of dizziness, which is benign paroxysmal positional vertigo (BPPV) (Furman & Cass 1999). BPPV can cause people to fall and may also be caused by a fall (Katsarkas 1999). The otoconia within the otolith organs can become dislodged with head trauma (Katsarkas 1999). Several other disease processes or conditions have been associated with BPPV including diabetes, migraine, Meniere's disease and postviral infection. It is also suspected that BPPV in older individuals may be caused by damage to the otolith production area over time. BBPV runs in families (Gizzi et al 1998) and has a recurrence rate of approximately 15% per year, increasing to a 40–50% chance of recurrence 3–4 years after the initial episode (Nunez et al 2000). The spinning is brought on by a change of head position, most commonly when moving from supine to sit first thing in the morning or rolling over in bed at night (Whitney et al 2005). The Epley or the Semont maneuver is commonly used to move the otoconia out of the semicircular canal and back into the otolith organ (Epley 1980, De Vito et al 1987, Semont et al 1988).

There are numerous possible causes of dizziness, as noted in Box 60.1, rendering it impossible to determine the cause without testing. Laboratory and clinical tests that can be performed to diagnose the cause of dizziness are included in Table 60.2. Although thorough testing is crucial to obtain an accurate diagnosis, most physical therapists will not have the benefit of such an extensive workup before seeing a patient. By being aware of the various causes of and tests for dizziness, the physical therapist is more likely to make appropriate clinical decisions about referrals and care (Furman & Cass 1995).

Dizziness history

A complete history of a patient's dizziness is essential to allow the physical therapist to develop the best individualized exercise program. Some of the common questions that should be asked concern the characteristics of the dizziness, how long the patient has had the symptoms, how the first incident would be described, what makes the symptoms worse or better, any associated otological or neurological symptoms and the frequency of the incidents or attacks (Herdman 2000). A thorough history of past and present functional activities is also important. Specific activities of daily living (ADLs) may exacerbate the symptoms. This functional history is helpful in designing a treatment program based on symptoms. The Dizziness Handicap Inventory (DHI) (Jacobson & Newman 1990) provides a numerical score, which ranges from 0 to 100, to describe how handicapped patients perceive themselves to be because of the dizziness (Form 60.1). A 'yes' answer scores 4; 'sometimes' scores 2; and 'no' scores 0. The higher the total score, the greater the dizziness handicap. The DHI has also been used to document a patient's self-rating of improvement or lack of progress. High DHI scores (>60) have been related to reported falls in individuals with vestibular disorders (Whitney et al 2004).

The patient with a chief complaint of dizziness will often receive an antidizziness medication, which can decrease the ability of the

Table 60.2 Common testing provided to older individuals who experience chronic dizziness

Test	Commonly performed by	
	Physician	Physical therapist
Caloric testing	+	
Rotational testing: assesses the vestibulo-ocular reflex independently of vision and can assess the visual/vestibular interaction	+	
Oculomotor testing: smooth pursuit movements, saccades	+	+
Dynamic visual acuity	+	+
Subjective visual vertical	+	+
Vestibular evoked myogenic potentials (VEMPs)	+	
Neurological examination	+	+
Optokinetic screening	+	+
Electronystagmography: a test for vestibulo-ocular asymmetry, which includes caloric testing, positional testing and ocular motor function	+	
Audiogram	+	
Electrocochleography	+	
MRI or CT scan	+	
Brainstem auditory evoked potential	+	
Visual evoked potential	+	
Posturography	+	+
Standing and lying blood pressure measures	+	+
Hallpike maneuver	+	+
Fistula test	+	
Romberg/tandem Romberg test	+	+
Electrocardiogram	+	
Holter monitoring	+	
Cervical spine radiography	+	
Testing for positional nystagmus with Frenzel glasses	+	+
Biochemical metabolic evaluation	+	
Glucose tolerance test	+	
Electroencephalogram	+	

CT, computed tomography; MRI, magnetic resonance imaging.

central nervous system (CNS) to compensate (Peppard 1986). Most antidizziness medications are depressants of the CNS and may limit the ability of the CNS to adapt to change caused by an insult to or dysfunction in the balance mechanism or to respond to physical therapy

intervention. It is best to provide physical therapy when the patient is on a low dose of vestibular suppressants or none at all. However, some patients are unable to function without a vestibular suppressant, so removal may not be possible.

FUNCTIONAL DEFICITS

Dizziness can severely limit a patient's ability to perform ADLs (Cohen et al 1995). Each person's dizziness is unique, but common complaints include having difficulty with transitional movements and with moving quickly. Transitional movements include activities such as rolling, moving from a supine position to sitting, moving from sitting to standing and walking while making certain head movements. Even standing while moving the head can increase symptoms in some patients. Walking while making head movements is often the most difficult activity to perform because the patient is unstable and may feel unsafe.

Often patients complain of having difficulties when movement is perceived within their peripheral vision or when watching television or reading. A patient may have dizziness when driving or when a passenger in a car. Clinically, it is noted that patients report less dizziness when they themselves are driving. For some older adults, losing the ability to drive can cause significant psychosocial dilemmas.

One characteristic symptom in patients with dizziness is having difficulty walking down the aisle of a grocery or department store because of the optic flow inputs (Sparto et al 2004). High-contrast colors and shapes in the older individual's peripheral vision can cause them to become dizzy. The optic flow as one ambulates can be disorienting and can contribute to increased dizziness, nausea and headaches; thus, people with severe dizziness often limit the amount of time they spend out of the home. Indeed, dizziness has been associated with agoraphobia and depression (Jacob et al 1996). Individuals with agoraphobia are not comfortable leaving their homes. This is a problem that can limit function even when the dizziness is not present, for the fear of becoming dizzy in a stressful situation is often enough for some people to limit their activities.

Not all patients with dizziness are easily treated. Patients with unilateral vestibular dysfunction often have the best outcome with exercise programs. Patients with central vestibular dysfunction have more difficulty with exercises because of CNS involvement, and those with fluctuating symptoms have the most difficult time. Some of the fluctuating disorders, such as Meniere's disease and perilymphatic fistulas, may have to be surgically repaired. Dizziness may be decreased or eliminated by surgery; however, some patients continue to experience tinnitus. Tinnitus may be a disabling symptom and has been described as a dull roar or loud noise in the ear. Dizziness can also be caused by multiple sclerosis and stroke; in these patients, dizziness can lessen but may not completely resolve.

People with dizziness often have difficulty explaining their symptoms to family members because there are no obvious external signs of the disorder. Family members can find it hard to comprehend the physical and psychological effects of dizziness and sometimes cannot understand that the patient may be severely disabled by the condition.

THERAPEUTIC INTERVENTION

Not all older patients with dizziness have balance disorders. There appear to be three categories of patients: those with dizziness, those with balance disorders and those with balance disorders and dizziness. Each of these symptom categories should be treated differently.

Form 60.1 Dizziness Handicap Inventory (DHI)[a]

Name: Date:

Instructions: The purpose of this scale is to identify difficulties that you may be experiencing because of your dizziness. Please answer 'yes', 'no' or 'sometimes' to each question. Answer each question as it pertains to your dizziness problem only (Scoring: yes = 4; sometimes = 2; no = 0).

1. Does looking up increase your problem?   _____

2. Do you feel frustrated because of your problem?   _____

3. Do you restrict your travel for business or recreation because of your problem?   _____

4. Does walking down the aisle of a supermarket increase your problem?   _____

5. Do you have difficulty getting into or out of bed because of your problem? _____

6. Does your problem significantly restrict your participation in social activities such as going out to dinner,   _____
   going to the movies, dancing or going to parties?   _____

7. Do you have difficulty reading because of your problem?   _____

8. Does performing more ambitious activities like sports, dancing or household chores, such as sweeping or   _____
   putting dishes away, increase your problem?   _____

9. Because of your problem are you afraid to leave your home without having someone to accompany you?   _____

10. Have you been embarrassed in front of others because of your problem?   _____

11. Do quick movements of your head increase your problem?   _____

12. Do you avoid heights because of your problem?   _____

13. Does turning over in bed increase your problem?   _____

14. Is it difficult for you to do strenuous housework or yard work because of your problem?   _____

15. Are you afraid people may think that you are intoxicated because of your problem?   _____

16. Is it difficult for you to go for a walk by yourself because of your problem?   _____

17. Does walking down a sidewalk increase your problem?   _____

18. Is it difficult for you to concentrate because of your problem?   _____

19. Is it difficult for you to walk around your house in the dark because of your problem?   _____

20. Are you afraid to stay home alone because of your problem?   _____

21. Do you feel handicapped because of your problem?   _____

22. Has your problem placed stress on your relationship with friends or members of your family?   _____

23. Are you depressed because of your problem?   _____

24. Does your problem interfere with your job or household responsibilities? _____

25. Does bending over increase your problem?   _____

[a]From Jacobson & Newman 1990, with permission from American Medical Association.

The treatment program should be based on the functional deficits of the patient.

During the assessment of dizziness, it is important to determine if patients have fallen, how often they have fallen and whether they have had to seek medical intervention for a fall. Finding oneself suddenly and unexpectedly on a lower surface, usually the floor, is often defined as a 'fall'. Frequent falls (more than two within the past 6 months when no environmental hazards were present) are a reason for significant concern. These individuals should be treated more frequently in the clinic and be monitored closely at home by a family member. Patients who fall frequently might benefit from some type of alarm device to notify emergency personnel when a fall occurs.

Exercise

In an exercise program for a patient with vestibular dysfunction, the patient is asked to perform movements that increase symptoms. The objective is to let the patient feel dizzy in a safe environment. How quickly to advance a program is difficult to determine because if the exercises are progressed too rapidly, the patient may get worse, discontinue the exercises and not return for future therapy. It is often best to include a combination of easier and more difficult exercises so that the patient will be successful with at least a few of them. Keeping the number of exercises under five at each visit also helps with compliance.

When designing an exercise program, it is usually important to warn patients that they will initially and temporarily feel worse after the exercises. If the patient remains severely dizzy for as long as 20 min after the exercises have been completed, they were too difficult and must be modified in terms of intensity or number.

It is extremely important to get the patient to progress as quickly as possible while in a safe place so that confidence can be restored. Functional retraining, muscle strengthening, eye and head exercises and asking the patient to perform difficult tasks are components of an individualized exercise program for a patient with vestibular dysfunction (Box 60.2). Often a combination of balance and eye exercises

---

Box 60.2   Exercises for the patient with dizziness

1. Exercises for the patient who experiences dizziness with transitional movements
   - Head movements
     - Supine
     - Sitting
     - Standing
     - Walking
     - Walking and performing a functional activity
   - Functional activities
     - Pivots
     - Circle and figure-of-eight walking
     - Ball tossing
     - Obstacle course
2. Balance exercises
   - Consider the head, foot and arm positions and whether the eyes are open or closed
   - Use the Clinical Test of Sensory Organization to help plan treatment
   - Hip and ankle strategies
   - Weight shifting
   - Single-leg stance
   - Stepping forward and backward
   - Side stepping
   - Standing on foam
   - Kicking a ball
   - Walking backwards
   - Crossovers
   - Tandem walking
   - Romberg test
   - Step-ups
   - Moving objects to different surfaces
   - Tracing the alphabet
   - Heel raises
   - Racketball against the wall
   - Walking and carrying an object
   - Walking in a dark room
   - Catching a ball while sitting on a gym ball
   - Stepping on a compliant surface
   - Jump rope
   - Ankle 'proprioceptive' boards
   - Weight shifting with a weight around the waist
   - Elastic band exercises while standing on one leg
   - Heel walking
   - Single-leg stance while kicking a ball on a string
   - Bus step-ups
   - Standing on one leg and rotating the head
   - Functional movements for weight shift, e.g. golfing
   - Tilt boards
   - Toe walking
3. Eye movements (can be assessed with Frenzel glasses)
   - Examples of eye exercises
     - Head stable, eye tracking an object
     - Object stable with the head moving
     - Object and head both moving to track an object
   - Eye–head exercises
     - Focus on a card and move head to left and right
     - Track a moving object up and down
     - Focus on a card and move the head up and down
     - Move head and card in the same direction at arm's length
     - Look left and right quickly and focus on an object
     - Look up and at eye level at two cards, head still
     - Look up and at eye level at two cards, head moving
     - Move head and card up and down
     - Look right and left at the card while it is held ahead
     - Simon Says
     - Mall walking
     - Ping pong
     - Spin in a chair that rotates
     - Laser tag
     - Imaginary target exercise
     - X2 viewing
   - Otolith stimulation
     - Bouncing on a ball
     - Jump rope
   - Benign paroxysmal positional vertigo (BPPV) maneuvers
     - Epley maneuver
     - Semont maneuver
     - Brandt–Daroff exercises
     - Horizontal canalith repositioning maneuver (often called the Epley maneuver)

are provided simultaneously, with the older adult starting the exercises in 'safe' positions and progressing to situations in which balance is challenged, such as standing, walking or even reaching while standing.

Older adults most likely to benefit from a vestibular rehabilitation program include those with unilateral vestibular hypofunction (peripheral vestibular disorders) and those with bilateral peripheral vestibular disorders. Other patients who can be helped by physical therapy include those with head trauma, cerebellar atrophy or dysfunction, cerebellar stroke and multiple sclerosis. Patients who have been diagnosed with bilateral disorders may continue to improve with physical therapy for up to a year after the insult, although the functional result is not as successful as it is in patients with unilateral peripheral disorders. Patients with bilateral disorders often walk with a wide-based gait and may continue to require assistive devices after intervention (Telian et al 1991, Minor 1998, Herdman et al 2000, Brown et al 2001). It is much more difficult to treat individuals with central disorders, anxiety disorders and combined central/peripheral vestibular disorders than those who present with peripheral vestibular dysfunction (Whitney & Rossi 2000).

Older patients with dizziness can be helped by rehabilitation. At one time, it was thought that an improvement in the symptoms of such patients could not be made using a customized exercise program but this has been shown to be a false assumption (Whitney et al 2002).

One of the most important components of the exercise program is getting patients to comply with the prescribed exercise routine on a regular basis. When compliance is an issue, it may be necessary to treat these patients more frequently. Older adults may be fearful of performing exercises alone at home, even though a home exercise program always includes very specific instructions for performing the exercises safely.

The exercise most commonly recommended for older adults with dizziness is a walking program. Walking challenges the patient, especially outside the home, and exposes him or her to a wide variety of visual stimuli. However, in some older individuals, initiating a walking program may not be possible because they live alone and may be afraid of falling.

CONCLUSION

Dizziness is an elusive symptom that can be difficult to diagnose. Older adults present with many different causes of dizziness. These can be central, peripheral, psychiatric or based on various systemic diseases. Treatment is best initiated after a through medical workup to determine a medical diagnosis. If the cause of the dizziness is vestibular, individually tailored exercise is of great benefit in the recovery of functional skills.

References

Brown KE, Whitney SL, Wrisley DM, Furman JM 2001 Physical therapy outcomes for persons with bilateral vestibular loss. Laryngoscope 111:1812–1817

Cohen H, Ewell LR, Jenkins HA 1995 Disability in Meniere's disease. Arch Otolaryngol Head Neck Surg 121:29–33

De Vito F, Pagnini P, Vannuchi P 1987 Treatment of cupulolithiasis: critical observations on the Semont maneuver. Acta Otorhinolaryngol Ital 7:589–596

Epley JM 1980 New dimensions of benign paroxysmal positional vertigo. Otolaryngol Head Neck Surg 88:599–605

Furman JM, Cass S 1995 A practical work up for vertigo. Contemp Int Med 7:24–38

Furman JM, Cass SP 1999 Benign paroxysmal positional vertigo. N Engl J Med 341:1590–1596

Furman JM, Cass SP 2003 Vestibular Disorders: A Case Study Approach. Oxford University Press, New York

Gizzi M, Ayyagari S, Khattar V 1998 The familial incidence of benign paroxysmal positional vertigo. Acta Otolaryngol 118:774–777

Herdman SJ 2000 Vestibular Rehabilitation, 2nd edn. FA Davis, Philadelphia, PA

Herdman SJ, Blatt P, Schubert MC, Tusa RJ 2000 Falls in patients with vestibular deficits. Am J Otol 21:847–851

Jacob R, Furman J, Durrant JD, Turner SM 1996 Psychiatric aspects of vestibular disorders. In: Baloh RW, Halmagyi GM (eds) Disorders of the Vestibular System. Oxford University Press, New York, p 509–528

Jacobson GP, Newman CW 1990 The development of the Dizziness Handicap Inventory. Arch Otolaryngol Head Neck Surg 116:424–427

Katsarkas A 1999 Benign paroxysmal positional vertigo (BPPV): idiopathic versus post-traumatic. Acta Otolaryngol 119:745–749

Kroenke K, Lucas CA, Rosenberg ML et al. 1992 Causes of persistent dizziness – a prospective study of 100 patients in ambulatory care. Ann Int Med 117:898–904

Minor L 1998 Gentamicin-induced bilateral vestibular hypofunction. JAMA 279:541–544

Nunez RA, Cass SP, Furman JM 2000 Short- and long-term outcomes of canalith repositioning for benign paroxysmal positional vertigo. Otolaryngol Head Neck Surg 122:647–652

Peppard SB 1986 Effect of drug therapy on compensation from vestibular injury. Laryngoscope 96:878–898

Semont A, Freyss G, Vitte E 1988 Curing the BPPV with a liberatory maneuver. Adv Otorhinolaryngol 42:290–293

Sparto PJ, Whitney SL, Hodges LF et al 2004 Simulator sickness when performing gaze shifts within a wide field of view optic flow environment: preliminary evidence for using virtual reality in vestibular rehabilitation. J Neuroeng Rehabil 1:14

Telian SA, Shepard NT, Smith-Wheelock M, Hoberg M 1991 Bilateral vestibular paresis: diagnosis and treatment. Otolaryngol Head Neck Surg 104:67–71

Whitney SL, Rossi MM 2000 Efficacy of vestibular rehabilitation. Otolaryngol Clin North Am 33:659–672

Whitney SL, Wrisley DM, Marchetti GF, Furman JM 2002 The effect of age on vestibular rehabilitation outcomes. Laryngoscope 112:1785–1790

Whitney SL, Wrisley DM, Brown KE, Furman JM 2004 Is perception of handicap related to functional performance in persons with vestibular dysfunction? Otol Neurotol 25:139–143

Whitney SL, Marchetti GF, Morris LO 2005 Usefulness of the dizziness handicap inventory in the screening for benign paroxysmal positional vertigo. Otol Neurotol 26:1027–1033

Chapter 61

Balance testing and training

Diane M. Wrisley

CHAPTER CONTENTS

- Physiology of balance
- Balance assessment
- Treatment
- Evidence for the use of exercise to treat balance
- Conclusion

The medical and sociologic consequences of falls in the older adult are one of the largest public health issues. Thirty-five percent of adults over 65 years report falling more than once in the previous year, and this number increases to 50% in adults over 75 years (Campbell et al 1990, American Geriatrics Society et al 2001). Falls in the elderly are multifactorial and have been attributed to medication use, environmental challenges, cardiopulmonary compromise, cognitive changes, and sensory and motor deficits (Tinetti et al 1986). Once an older adult falls, changes occur (e.g. fear of falling, decreased mobility, speed, and fluency of movement) that increase their risk of falling. Therefore, it is essential that the geriatric specialist performs a thorough multifactorial balance evaluation and initiates treatment as early as possible. Definitions of key terms concerned with balance are included in Box 61.1.

Box 61.1   Definitions of key terms concerning balance (Nashner 1990, 1994, Allison 1995)

Balance: the ability to maintain the center of gravity over the base of support within a given sensoryenvironment
Static balance: the ability to hold a position
Dynamic balance: the ability to transition or move between positions
Automatic postural responses: operate to keep the center of gravity over the base of support in response to a stimulus or unexpected perturbation such as a slip or a jostle in a crowd
Anticipatory postural control: similar to automatic postural control but occurs prior to and in preparation for the perturbation
Volitional postural control: postural control under conscious control. Self-initiated perturbations that are strongly influenced by prior experience and instruction

Center of gravity: an imaginary point in space, calculated biomechanically from measured forces and moments, where the sum of all the forces equals zero. In a normal person standing quietly, it is located just forward of the spine at about the S2 level
Base of support: the body surfaces that experience pressure as the result of body weight and gravity. In standing, the base of support is the soles of the feet; in sitting, it is the thighs and buttocks. The narrower the base of support, the more difficult the balance task
Limits of stability: the limits to which a body can move in any direction without either falling (as the center of gravity exceeds the base of support) or establishing a new base of support by stepping or reaching (to relocate the base of support under the center of gravity)
Balance strategies: stereotypic sequences of muscle activity used to maintain upright. The most commonly suggested include the ankle, hip, and stepping strategies

PHYSIOLOGY OF BALANCE

Balance, the ability to maintain the center of gravity over the base of support within a given sensory environment, is composed of several subcomponents and influenced by several systems. Human balance is a complex neuromusculoskeletal process involving the sensory detection of body motions, integration of sensorimotor information within the central nervous system (CNS), and programming and execution of the appropriate neuromuscular responses. Figure 61.1 summarizes the organization of the human balance system. The brain uses visual, vestibular, and somatosensory systems to determine the body position and movement in space. Although there are age-related changes in these systems, older adults do not display increased postural sway compared with younger adults when standing or walking when they have all three senses available (Woollacott et al 1986). When older adults are first asked to balance on a posture platform under conditions of minimized somatosensory and visual input, half lose their balance (Woollacott et al 1986). With repeated exposure, however, they are able to learn to maintain their balance on the platform (Woollacott et al 1986). Interestingly, on further investigation, it was found that the falls correlated positively with subclinical pathologies in either the sensory or the motor systems (Woollacott et al

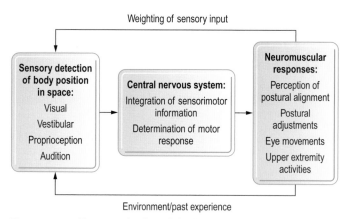

Figure 61.1   The organization of the human balance system.

1986). As sensory changes are common in older adults, the reader is referred to the previous chapters in this text on sensory changes in visual (see Chapter 53), somatosensory (see Chapter 51), and vestibular (see Chapters 54 and 60) systems for further evaluation and treatment techniques for these systems that will affect balance.

The information from the various sensory systems is relayed to the CNS and is integrated in several areas including the vestibular nuclei and the cerebellum prior to the generation of appropriate motor responses. Prioritization of use of sensory information for use by the CNS is most likely based on the availability of a particular sensory modality, the task at hand, and past experiences (Peterka 2002). The CNS then generates the appropriate motor responses to maintain upright body posture. Various balance strategies are thought to maintain balance depending on the speed of perturbation and the support surface. Slow, small perturbations on level surfaces result in muscle activity that is sequenced from distal to proximal (ankle strategy), while perturbations that are larger, faster, or on smaller surfaces result in muscle sequences from proximal to distal (hip strategy) (Nashner 1990). A stepping strategy is used when the perturbations take the center of gravity outside the base of support or limits of stability and is used to recover balance (Nashner 1990). Older adults frequently switch from an ankle strategy to a hip strategy during different conditions than younger adults such as walking on slippery surfaces or with smaller, slower perturbations (Horak et al 1989). Use of inappropriate balance strategies may contribute to falls in older adults.

There are many other factors that contribute to the ability to maintain an upright posture. First, musculoskeletal constraints must be met. Adequate range of motion must be available, especially in crucial joints such as the ankle and hip. Impaired range of motion of the neck or painful syndromes in the cervical muscles may lead to an altered representation of trunk and head movement and therefore cause imbalance. The proper generation of neuromuscular force is also essential to developing the appropriate balance strategies. The ability to sequence the muscles appropriately and the timing of the muscle activity are crucial and are sometimes the most difficult to retrain following injury (Horak & Shumway-Cook 1990). When automatic postural responses are examined, older adults demonstrate slowed onset and reversal in normal distal to proximal sequencing of muscle activation compared with younger adults (Woollacott 1990). Posture or alignment of bony segments can either assist with the production of the balance responses or make it more difficult to generate balance reactions. Maximizing a patient's postural alignment can assist in regaining their ability to generate balance responses (Horak & Shumway-Cook 1990). Although most of our balance reactions occur at a subconscious level, a patient's cognitive

status can influence their ability to generate the balance reactions necessary to maintain an upright posture. If a subject is easily distracted or has slow processing, he or she may not be able to react quickly enough to environmental changes to allow them to stay upright. This may be especially true if there is increased activity in the environment, if the patient is distracted by conversation, or if they are preoccupied (Shumway-Cook & Woollacott 2000). Many environmental factors can affect a patient's ability to maintain balance. Decreased or absent lighting, and soft, pliable surfaces decrease the sensory input available to the patient for spatial orientation. Small children or pets underfoot can cause sudden perturbations and make it difficult for a patient to maintain balance, especially if they already have an increased reaction time. Many classifications of medications, ranging from diuretics to CNS suppressants, can also impair a patient's ability to balance (Thapa et al 1995, Leipzig et al 1999).

BALANCE ASSESSMENT

The last two decades have seen a proliferation of tools for assessing balance. Some of these tools evaluate only one underlying impairment, and some are multidimensional. The tools run the range from highly technical and expensive to simple and portable. Table 61.1 provides an overview of various tools and the components of balance that they assess. Box 61.2 illustrates 'red flags' or signs and symptoms that indicate that the patient would benefit from further medical workup.

Box 61.2   Red flags – urgent referrals to physician for workup

Unexplained central nervous system signs – motor, sensory, or cognitive changes
Unexplained cranial nerve dysfunction
Unexplained sudden or unilateral hearing loss especially if accompanied by vertigo
Two or more falls in the previous 4 weeks
Inconsistencies in clinical examination

One of the most important areas that requires assess-ment when working with older adults is their risk of falling. Box 61.3 summarizes the risk factors that have been identified for falling in older adults. The reader is referred to the *Guidelines for the Prevention of Falls in Older Persons* (American Geriatrics Society et al 2001) that summarize the literature on the evaluation and treatment of fall risk in the older adult and provide recommendations.

Although self-report measures do not directly measure impairments, several self-report measures are available to allow the clinician to determine how stable the patient perceives that he or she is, and this will facilitate the clinician's ability to treat and assess for fall risk. Sometimes, patients will perceive that they are more stable than testing reveals. This indicates that they are either performing differently in the clinic or may be taking unnecessary risks at home and need some counseling regarding ways to decrease their fall risk. At other times, patients will perceive that they are less stable than tests reveal. These subjects may have a history of falling and have lost confidence in their balance abilities, causing them to decrease their activity (Lawrence et al 1998). Without intervention, this decrease in

Table 61.1   Evaluation tools for assessing balance

Self-perception scales	Falls Efficacy Scale (Tinetti et al 1990, 1994b)
	Modified Falls Efficacy Scale (Hill et al 1996)
	Activities-specific Balance Confidence Scale (Powell & Myers 1995)
Assessment of sensory components	Sensory Organization Test of Computerized Dynamic Posturography (Monsell et al 1997)
	Clinical Test of Sensory Interaction and Balance (Shumway-Cook & Horak 1986)
Assessment of motor components	Functional Reach Test (Duncan et al 1990)
	Multidirectional Reach Test (Newton 2001)
	Four Square Step Test (Dite & Temple 2002)
	Limits of Stability (El-Kashlan et al 1998)
	Motor Control Test (El-Kashlan et al 1998)
	Five times sit to stand (Csuka & McCarty 1985)
Multidimensional assessment	Performance Oriented Mobility Assessment (Tinetti 1986)
	Physical Performance Scale
	Berg Balance Scale (Berg et al 1992)
	Balance Evaluation Systems Test (BESTest) (Horak et al 2003)
Gait assessment	Timed 'Up & Go' (Podsiadlo & Richardson 1991)
	Dynamic Gait Index (Shumway-Cook & Woollacott 1995)
	Functional Gait Assessment (Wrisley et al 2004)
	Gait speed

Box 61.3   Risk factors for falls (American Geriatrics Society et al 2001)

Intrinsic
Lower extremity weakness
Poor grip strength
Balance disorders
Functional and cognitive impairments
Visual deficits
History of falls
Gait deficit
Visual deficit
Urinary incontinence
Extrinsic
Polypharmacy (four or more prescription medications)
Environmental
Poor lighting
Loose carpets

activity may lead to greater impairment and more balance problems (Lawrence et al 1998). Two of the most common self-report measures for balance function are the Falls Efficacy Scale (Tinetti et al 1990) and the Activities-specific Balance Confidence Scale (Powell & Myers 1995). Both the Falls Efficacy Scale [test–retest reliability Intraclass Correlation Coefficient, ICC, (2,1) = 0.91] (Tinetti et al 1990) and the Activities-specific Balance Confidence Scale have been shown to be reliable [test–retest reliability ICC (2,1) = 0.91] and valid. The Falls Efficacy Scale correlates with getting up from a fall and level of anxiety (Tinetti et al 1990). The modified Falls Efficacy Scale was developed to incorporate higher functional activities. It has high test–retest reliability (ICC = 0.93) and discriminates between older adults with and without a history of falling. Scores on the Activities-specific Balance Confidence Scale correlate with physical functioning and falls in community-living older adults (Myers et al 1998). Scores above 80% were strongly correlated with highly functioning community-dwelling older adults; scores between 50% and 80% were correlated with moderate physical functioning seen in older adults in retirement homes or with chronic disease; and scores below 50% were correlated with low physical functioning of older adults receiving home-care (Myers et al 1998).

Impairments in balance can be assessed using single-item balance tools such as the Romberg test, Functional Reach test (Duncan et al 1990), single limb stance (Bohannon et al 1984), or tandem stance (Fregly & Graybiel 1968). The greatest advantage of a single-item test is that it is easy to administer and generally provides a method for quick screening of balance function. The disadvantage of using a single-item test is that it only tests one aspect of balance. Without correlating findings with other tests, this may limit their usefulness in developing a treatment plan. These single-item tests have good reliability. The inability to maintain single limb stance for more than 5 seconds is correlated with increased risk of falls in older adults.

The ability to use sensory information for balance can be assessed using either high or low technology such as the Sensory Organization Testing (SOT) via the Equitest® or the Clinical Test of Sensory Interaction and Balance (CTSIB) or 'Foam and Dome' respectively (Shumway-Cook & Horak 1986). Each consists of six conditions designed to test whether the patient can utilize visual, vestibular, or somatosensory information for balance. Both the SOT and the CTSIB are reliable and valid (Monsell et al 1997, El-Kashlan et al 1998). The SOT provides an equilibrium score and additional information on motor strategies and the relative reliance on sensory information for balance. The CTSIB is a portable alternative that will provide similar information. Scores achieved on the CTSIB correlate moderately with scores achieved on SOT (Whitney & Wrisley 2004, Wrisley & Whitney 2004).

Several multidimensional balance assessments have been developed in order to take into account the many facets of balance in order to predict an individual's risk of falling. One of the primary benefits of multidimensional balance tests is that they assess several aspects of balance that are integrated into a single overall score. This makes them very useful for predicting one's risk of falling, but may make it more difficult to sort out which balance impairments should be addressed in treatment. Overall scores are used to determine fall risk (Tinetti 1986, Duncan et al 1990, Berg et al 1995, Shumway-Cook et al 1997a, 1997b, Newton 2001), a functional baseline before intervention, and to quantify the effectiveness of intervention (Rubenstein et al 2000). The therapist may need to look at the performance of individual test items or perform single-item assessments in order to identify the impairments that need to be treated. The inter- and intra-rater reliability of multidimensional tests is good to excellent (Tinetti 1986, Berg et al 1995, Newton 2001).

Walking is a complex balance task and a very functional means of both assessing and treating balance disorders. During ambulation, the center of gravity is moved outside the base of support, as in a fall. Then, there is recovery from the loss of balance by the base of support being reoriented with a step. Gait assessments allow us to measure a patient's ability to integrate balance and to measure balance during mobility. Assessments that appear to be particularly useful for gait are the Dynamic Gait Index (Shumway-Cook & Woollacott 1995, Shumway-Cook et al 1997a), the Functional Gait Assessment (Wrisley et al 2004), and the Timed 'Up and Go' (Podsiadlo & Richardson 1991). Functionally, patients need to be able to walk 1.22 m/sec to cross a street safely. Gait velocity can easily be calculated by timing a patient walking 6 m (20 ft) and dividing this distance by the number of seconds elapsed.

The assessment of an older adult's balance function may include self-perception measures, impairment-based or multidimensional tools, and will be directed by the purpose of the evaluation (e.g. fall risk assessment, diagnosis, or directing intervention). The assessment should include motor, sensory, musculoskeletal, and extrinsic factors underlying the balance dysfunction. A thorough balance assessment will guide treatment.

TREATMENT

Treatment of balance disorders is based on the specific impairments [e.g. range of motion (ROM), strength, decreased sensation, pain, use of sensory inputs, use of motor strategies, etc.] and functional limitations identified in the evaluation. Balance strategies and the ability to use sensory information for balance can be learned with the appropriate exercise and practice. For balance training, it is important to provide opportunities for patients to practice tasks that allow them to use the necessary balance strategies and, when at all possible, to incorporate the tasks into functional activities, as patients will be more likely to follow through with the exercise and to generalize the tasks they are learning. Safety is important for patients when working on balance. The exercises prescribed need to challenge the patient's balance and therefore are ones that may make them stumble or fall. Upper extremity support changes the sequence of muscle activation so that it originates in the upper extremities. This alteration in the sequence of muscle activity is not usually desirable if the goal of treatment is independent ambulation without an assistive device. For standing exercises, having the patient stand in a corner of the room with a chair in front of them provides a surface on all sides that can catch the patient, minimizing the chance of injury. It is unknown how frequently balance exercises need to be performed for maximum improvement. It is generally felt that patients need to practice

at least 4–5 days each week to see permanent change (American Geriatrics Society et al 2001).

Improving the use of balance strategies is best accomplished within functional activities, especially as balance strategies are rarely used alone. Table 61.2A provides a summary of exercises to improve balance strategies.

Age-related changes in sensory function and pathology of the different sensory systems may lead to patients having difficulty using sensory information for balance. Exercise can assist in training a patient to use a sense they are not using well or train them to compensate with an alternate sense. The general principle used when trying to maximize an individual's ability to use sensory inputs for balance is first to practice activities with all the sensory information available and then gradually to remove sensory information. Table 61.2B illustrates exercises that will stimulate the use of different sensory inputs.

Gait is the act of losing one's balance and then regaining it by taking a compensatory step. This makes it an excellent treatment tool for balance dysfunction experienced by the older adult. It is also very functional, as the majority of our patients have a primary goal of ambulation. There are many activities that can be introduced into gait to improve balance function. Ambulation with head turns in the yaw and pitch planes, at varying speeds, while negotiating objects, and on compliant surfaces or in varied lighting can all improve balance.

EVIDENCE FOR THE USE OF EXERCISE TO TREAT BALANCE

The majority of research on the effectiveness of exercise for balance has focused on older adults at risk of falling. Randomized clinical trials have demonstrated that exercise does improve balance in community-dwelling older adults (Tinetti et al 1994a, Lord et al 1995, Province & Rao 1995, Wolf et al 1996, Campbell et al 1999a, 1999b, McMurdo et al 2000, Rubenstein et al 2000, Steinberg et al 2000, Close et al 2005). For a thorough review of recent randomized clinical trials that have demonstrated that exercise does improve balance in community-dwelling older adults, the reader is referred to the review by Close et al (2005). However, several relevant points concerning exercise intervention can be deduced from these studies (American Geriatrics Society et al 2001): (i) the optimal type, duration, and intensity of exercise for fall prevention remain unclear; (ii) exercise intervention needs to be custom designed for each patient; (iii) exercise needs to be sustained; the successful programs lasted for more than 10 weeks; (iv) the only type of exercise that has been shown to decrease fall risk is T'ai Chi Ch'uan; and (v) exercise works best for fall prevention when combined with other forms of intervention such as home modification and education (American Geriatrics Society et al 2001).

CONCLUSION

Balance is a complex neuromusculoskeletal process involving sensory, skeletal, and motor components. Current research has shown that balance dysfunction is not a normal part of aging, but is often associated with a decline in the neuromuscular and sensory systems and should be taken seriously by healthcare practitioners working with this population. Functional balance presumes competence in a variety of areas. Healthcare practitioners need to address the

Table 61.2   Treatment strategies

A	Exercises to improve center of gravity control	Begin with slow weight shifts on a stable surface
		Add upper extremity activities, functional activities
		Progress the activity by:
		  Increasing the distance moved away from the midline
		  Alter the speed of movement
		  Add manual resistance
		  Narrow the base of support
		  Use an unstable surface, i.e. foam, rocker board, 2 × 4, half-roll
		  Add combined head and eye movement
		  Alter vision: dim lighting, close eyes, use opaque glasses

	Exercises that promote use of the ankle strategy	Small, slow perturbations on firm surface, either self- or externally generated Closed chain exercises such as stepping over a 2 × 4, walking Functional activities such as reaching to take objects off shelves, performing upper extremity activities in standing
	Exercises that promote use of the hip strategy	Moderate, rapid perturbations on narrow surfaces either self- or externally generated Tandem standing or walking Single limb support Functional activities such as reaching into the trunk of a car or laundry dryer, ascending and descending stairs
	Exercises that promote the use of the stepping strategy	Large, rapid perturbations either self- or externally generated that require the use of a step; progress from predictable to unpredictable Walking on uneven surfaces Stepping over obstacles

B	Exercises to stimulate the use of somatosensory inputs	Disadvantage vision while providing reliable somatosensory inputs on a stable surface:
		  Sit to and from stand with eyes closed
		  Ambulation with eye and head movements
		  Conflicting visual environments: crowds, striped curtains, moving visual surrounds, virtual reality

	Exercises to stimulate the use of visual inputs	Disadvantage somatosensory input while providing reliable visual cues (stable visual cues with landmarks):
		  Standing or sitting on a compliant surface or rocker board
		  Ambulate with foam boots
		  Instruct in visual fixation

	Exercises to stimulate the use of vestibular inputs	Disadvantage vision and somatosensation while providing reliable vestibular cues (detectable head position): Standing or ambulating on unstable or compliant surface with absent vision, destabilized vision, and inaccurate vision

sensory, motor, and integrative components of balance from both evaluative and training standpoints for the older adult. Balance in the older adult is not greatly different from balance in the younger adult, but the consequences of balance dysfunction may be greater, and their ability to adapt motor and sensory strategies may be slower. Therefore, one must recognize balance deficits early and implement successful intervention strategies proactively while not restricting the activity of older people.

References

Allison L 1995 Balance Disorders, 3rd edn. Mosby Year Book, St Louis, MO, p 802–837

American Geriatrics Society, British Geriatrics Society, American Academy of Orthopedic Surgeons Panel on Falls Prevention 2001 Guideline for the Prevention of Falls in Older Persons. J Am Geriatr Soc 49:664–672

Berg KO, Wood-Dauphinee SL, Williams JI et al 1992 Measuring balance in the elderly: validation of an instrument. Can J Public Health 83(suppl2):7–11

Berg KO, Wood-Dauphinee S, Williams JI 1995 The Balance Scale: reliability assessment with elderly residents and patients with an acute stroke. Scand J Rehabil Med 27(1):27–36

Bohannon RW, Larkin PA, Cook AC et al 1984 Decrease in timed balance test scores with aging. Phys Ther 64(7):1067–1070

Campbell AJ, Spears GF, Borrie MJ 1990 Examination by logistic regression modelling of the variables which increase the relative risk of elderly women falling compared to elderly men. J Clin Epidemiol 43(12):1415–1420

Campbell AJ, Robertson MC, Gardner MM et al 1999a Falls prevention over 2 years: a randomized controlled trial in women 80 years and older. Age Ageing 28(6):513–518

Campbell AJ, Robertson MC, Gardner MM et al 1999b Psychotropic medication withdrawal and a home-based exercise program to prevent falls: a randomized, controlled trial. J Am Geriatr Soc 47(7):850–853

Close JC, Lord SL, Menz HB et al 2005 What is the role of falls? Best Pract Res Clin Rheumatol 19(6):913–935

Csuka M, McCarty DJ 1985 Simple method for measurement of lower extremity muscle strength. Am J Med 78(1):77–81

Dite W, Temple VA 2002 A clinical test of stepping and change of direction to identify multiple falling older adults. Arch Phys Med Rehabil 83(11):1566–1571

Duncan PW, Weiner DK, Chandler J et al 1990 Functional reach: a new clinical measure of balance. J Gerontol 45(6):192–197

El-Kashlan HK, Shepard NT, Asher AM et al 1998 Evaluation of clinical measures of equilibrium. Laryngoscope 108(3):311–319

Fregly AR, Graybiel A 1968 An ataxia test not requiring rails. Aerospace Med 39:277–282

Hill KD, Schwarz JA, Kalogeropoulos AJ et al 1996 The modified falls efficacy scale. Arch Phys Med Rehabil 77:1025–1029

Horak FB, Shumway-Cook A 1990 Clinical Implications of Posture Control Research. APTA, Alexandria, VA, p 105–111

Horak FB, Shupert CL, Mirka A 1989 Components of postural dyscontrol in the elderly: a review. Neurobiol Aging 10(6):727–738

Horak FB, Frank JS, Meyer L et al 2003 The Balance Evaluations Systems Test: reliability, concurrent validity, and internal consistency. J Neurol Phys Ther 27(4):179

Lawrence RH, Tennstedt SL, Kasten LE et al 1998 Intensity and correlates of fear of falling and hurting oneself in the next year. J Aging Health 10:267–286

Leipzig RM, Cumming RG, Tinetti ME 1999 Drugs and falls in older people: a systematic review and meta-analysis: II. Cardiac and analgesic drugs. J Am Geriatr Soc 47(1):40–50

Lord SR, Ward JA, Williams P et al 1995 The effect of a 12-month exercise trial on balance, strength, and falls in older women: a randomized controlled trial. J Am Geriatr Soc 43(11):1198–1206

McMurdo ME, Millar AM, Daly F 2000 A randomized controlled trial of fall prevention strategies in old peoples' homes. Gerontology 46(2):83–87

Monsell EM, Furman JM, Herdman SJ et al 1997 Computerized dynamic platform posturography. Otolaryngol Head Neck Surg 117:394–398

Myers AM, Fletcher PC, Myers AH et al 1998 Discriminative and evaluative properties of the activities-specific balance confidence (ABC) scale. J Gerontol 53A(4):M287–M294

Nashner LM 1990 Sensory, Neuromuscular, and Biomechanical Contributions to Human Balance. APTA, Alexandria, VA, p 5–12

Nashner LM 1994 Evaluation of Postural Stability, Movement, and Control. Mosby, Philadelphia, PA

Newton RA 2001 Validity of the multi-directional reach test: a practical measure for limits of stability in older adults. J Gerontol A Biol Sci Med Sci 56(4):248–252

Peterka RJ 2002 Sensorimotor integration in human postural control. J Neurophysiol 88(3):1097–1118

Podsiadlo D, Richardson S 1991 The Timed 'Up & Go': a test of basic functional mobility for frail elderly persons. J Am Geriatr Soc 39(2):142–148

Powell LE, Myers AM 1995 The Activities-specific Balance Confidence (ABC) Scale. J Gerontol A Biol Sci Med Sci 50A(1):28–34

Province MA, Rao DC 1995 General purpose model and a computer program for combined segregation and path analysis (SEGPATH): automatically creating computer programs from symbolic language model specifications. Genet Epidemiol 12(2):203–219

Rubenstein LZ, Josephson KR, Trueblood PR et al 2000 Effects of a group exercise program on strength, mobility, and falls among fall-prone elderly men. J Gerontol A Biol Sci Med Sci 55(6):317–321

Shumway-Cook A, Horak FB 1986 Assessing the influence of sensory integration on balance: suggestions from the field. Phys Ther 66(10):1548–1549

Shumway-Cook A, Woollacott M 1995 Motor Control: Theory and Practical Applications. Williams and Wilkins, Baltimore, MD

Shumway-Cook A, Woollacott M 2000 Attentional demands and postural control: the effect of sensory context. J Gerontol A Biol Sci Med Sci 55(1):10–16

Shumway-Cook A, Baldwin M, Polissar NL et al 1997a Predicting the probability for falls in community-dwelling older adults. Phys Ther 77(8):812–819

Shumway-Cook A, Gruber W, Baldwin M et al 1997b The effect of multidimensional exercises on balance, mobility, and fall risk in community-dwelling older adults. Phys Ther 77(1):46–57

Steinberg M, Cartwright C, Peel N et al 2000 A sustainable programme to prevent falls and near falls in community dwelling older people: results of a randomised trial. J Epidemiol Community Health 54(3):227–232

Thapa PB, Gideon P, Fought RL et al 1995 Psychotropic drugs and risk of recurrent falls in ambulatory nursing home residents. Am J Epidemiol 142(2):202–211

Tinetti ME 1986 Performance-oriented assessment of mobility problems in elderly patients. J Am Geriatr Soc 34(2):119–126

Tinetti ME, Williams TF, Mayewski R 1986 Fall risk index for elderly patients based on number of chronic disabilities. Am J Med 80(3):429–434

Tinetti ME, Richman D, Powell L 1990 Falls efficacy as a measure of fear of falling. J Gerontol 45(6):239–243

Tinetti ME, Baker DI, McAvay G et al 1994a A multifactorial intervention to reduce the risk of falling among elderly people living in the community. N Engl J Med 331(13):821–827

Tinetti ME, Mendes de Leon CF, Doucette JT et al 1994b Fear of falling and fall-related efficacy in relationship to functioning among community-living elders. J Gerontol 49(3):140–147

Whitney SL, Wrisley DM 2004 The influence of footwear on timed balance scores of the modified clinical test of sensory interaction and balance. Arch Phys Med Rehabil 85(3):439–443

Wolf SL, Barnhart HX, Kutner NG et al 1996 Reducing frailty and falls in older persons: an investigation of Tai Chi and computerized balance training. Atlanta FICSIT Group. Frailty and Injuries: Cooperative Studies of Intervention Techniques. J Am Geriatr Soc 44(5):489–497

Woollacott M 1990 Postural Control Mechanisms in the Young and Old. APTA, Alexandria, VA, p 23–28

Woollacott MH, Shumway-Cook A, Nashner LM 1986 Aging and posture control: changes in sensory organization and muscular coordination. Int J Aging Hum Dev 23(2):97–114

Wrisley DM, Whitney SL 2004 The effect of foot position on the modified clinical test of sensory interaction and balance. Arch Phys Med Rehabil 85(2):335–338

Wrisley DM, Marchetti GF, Kuharsky DK et al 2004 Reliability, internal consistency, and validity of data obtained with the functional gait assessment. Phys Ther 84(10):906–918

Chapter 62

Fracture considerations

Timothy L. Kauffman, Carleen Lindsey and Rosanne Lewis

INTRODUCTION

The fracture of a bone has a profound impact on any member of the aging population, as the consequences may negatively impact on independence and can even lead to death (Cooper et al 1993). Fractures in aging individuals are usually associated with low bone mineral density and osteoporosis as defined by the World Health Organization in Box 62.1. It has been estimated that there are 75 million people in Europe, the USA, and Japan who have osteoporosis (European Foundation For Osteoporosis and Bone Disease & National Osteoporosis Foundation 1997).

Box 62.1   World Health Organization classification of skeletal status

- Normal: bone mineral density that is not more than one standard deviation below the young adult mean value
- Low bone mass or osteopenia: bone mineral density that lies between 1 and 2.5 standard deviations below the young adult mean value
- Osteoporosis: a value of bone mineral density that is more than 2.5 standard deviations below the young adult mean value
- Severe osteoporosis: a value of bone mineral density more than 2.5 standard deviations below the young adult mean value and the presence of one or more fragility fractures

---

Approximately one million Americans suffer fragility fractures each year at a cost of over 14 billion dollars (Kenny et al 2003). It has been estimated that costs related to osteoporosis will be equivalent to 2 million person–years of functional impairment and $45 billion in direct medical costs over the first decade of the twenty-first century (Chrisilles et al 1994).

In the United States, at least 90% of all hip and spine fractures among elderly white women and more than 70% of those among elderly white men may be attributed to osteoporosis (Melton et al 1997). The lifetime risk of fracture in women aged 50 years is approximately 16% for hip fractures, 15% for wrist fractures, and 32% for vertebral fractures (Cummings et al 1993). Based on 2000 US Census data, 44 million people with either osteoporosis or low bone mass represent 55% of the people aged 50 years or older in the United States. In 2002, it was estimated that over 10 million people already had osteoporosis, of whom approximately 80% were women. This figure will rise to almost 12 million by 2010, and to about 14 million by 2020 if additional efforts are not made to stem this disease, which may be largely prevented by lifestyle considerations and treatment when appropriate (National Osteoporosis Foundation 2002). Approximately 50% of all women will have osteoporosis by the age of 80 years. In contrast, a white man aged 50 years has approximately a 6% risk of hip fracture and a 16–25% risk of any osteoporotic fracture in his remaining life (Bilezikian et al 1999). Because of increasing life expectancy of the population, the number of people with osteoporosis will be augmented dramatically during the coming years, with huge health implications.

A bone fractures when a force or stress is placed upon it that is greater than the bone can withstand. Bone has a tensile strength of approximately 140 MPa (megapascals; one MPa equals 145 pounds per square inch) in the second decade of life, and it decreases to approximately 120 MPa by the eighth decade of life. The fracture threshold for the vertebrae and the epiphyseal areas of the femur is a bone density of less than $1 \, g/cm^3$ (Gerhart 1995). Even though the stiffness and strength of trabecular bone depends on bone density and the direction of loading, trabecular bone appears to fail at just under 1% strain no matter what the direction of loading (Chang et al 1999). The major physical difference between trabecular bone and cortical bone is the increased porosity exhibited by trabecular bone. This porosity is reflected by measurements of the apparent density (i.e. the mass of bone tissue divided by the bulk volume of the test specimen, including mineralized bone and marrow spaces). In the human skeleton, the apparent density of cortical bone is about $1.8 \, g/cm^3$, whereas the apparent density of trabecular bone ranges from approximately 0.1 to $1.0 \, g/cm^3$. A trabecular bone specimen with an apparent density of $0.2 \, cm^3$ has a porosity of about 90% (Hipp & Hayes 2003).

Fragility fractures are usually related to lower bone mineral density; however, recent evidence from the EPIDOS (Epidemiology of Osteoporosis) study, which was initiated in France in the early 1990s, indicated that over 50% of hip fractures in women over the age of 74 years were not associated with osteoporosis as determined by bone mineral density. Other factors found to be significant were decreased coordination and strength, and lower scores on mobility functional tests such as timed walking and chair rising (Robbins et al 2005).

NORMAL FRACTURE HEALING

Normal fracture healing can be divided into three overlapping phases. First, there is an immediate inflammatory phase in which there is bleeding resulting from the injury to the bone and surrounding soft tissue, and a hematoma forms (Fig. 62.1A). The bone cells at the fracture line die. The reparative, or proliferative, phase starts shortly after the injury, usually 24–48 hours if a good local blood supply to the fracture exists (Fig. 62.1B). Good reduction and immobilization of the fracture also help the bone during the reparative phase. Osteogenic cell proliferation lifts the fibrous layer of the periosteum from the bone and, somewhat more slowly, the osteogenic cells of the bone marrow cavity also proliferate (Fig. 62.1C). This proliferation gradually forms a collar, or callus, around the fracture line, which usually takes place in 2–4 weeks, but radiographic evidence of external callus formation may not appear until 3–6 weeks. A bone scan usually reveals increased metabolic activity shortly after the fracture and before the callus can be seen on a radiograph (McRae 1994).

The remodeling phase starts during proliferation as the osteogenic cells begin to differentiate into osteoblasts, which start to form bony trabeculae that bridge the living and dead bone across the fracture line (Fig. 62.1D). Some of the osteogenic cells differentiate into chrondrocytes and form cartilage in the fracture callus, which eventually calcifies, becoming bone. Osteoclasts gradually remove the necrotic bone at the fracture site. The callus, consisting mostly of cancellous bone that has now formed across the fracture site, is fusiform. The cancellous bone is slowly remodeled into compact bone and, finally, the original fracture line is no longer discernible (Koval & Zuckerman 1997).

FRACTURE REPAIR IN THE AGING INDIVIDUAL

The rate of fracture repair in the aging patient should always be considered to be similar to that of a younger person – that is, early callus formation in 2–4 weeks and bony bridging over the fracture in 6 weeks, as shown on radiographs. However, a host of factors may impede this normal progression. First, osteoporotic bone may not heal as well as bone with normal tissue density. The inflammatory response to the injury and the blood supply may be inadequate, and failure to immobilize the fracture site also delays the healing process. The role of morphogenetic proteins and growth factors in fracture healing in aging patients is unclear, but adequate nutrition is crucial. Overall health or frailty as well as cognition can delay the healing process as well.

In the case of open reduction and internal fixation of a fracture, there is greater risk of further bone injury, called a stress riser, due to the orthopedic hardware. The use of screws and plates may weaken or pull out from bone that is already osteopenic.

SPECIAL FRACTURES IN THE ELDERLY

Not all fractures in the elderly are considered to be complete fractures. Stress fractures, also referred to as insufficiency fractures, occur in areas of repeated trauma when bone remodeling is insufficient to repair the stresses of repetitive loading. Clinically, this is a particular concern when treating a patient who is at risk of increased bone fragility. Orthopedic internal fixation devices can become stress risers and cause increased loosening at the bone–appliance interface (Koval & Zuckerman 1997). People with spinal cord injury who have been fitted with a new orthotic device may develop stress fractures due to new movement abilities (Rafii et al 1982). The sedentary elderly are at risk when they start new, strenuous physical activities. Physically, these patients will present with pain, swelling, and warmth. Stress fractures or pseudofractures may arise in bone that has faulty mineralization, which results in the subsequent inadequate repair of microtraumas.

Microfractures of the bony trabeculae have been demonstrated. The proclivity of these microfractures to cause pain is unclear. However, they may progress and lead to the silent fractures that are recognized on radiograph but may be old fractures. Despite the radiograph evidence of fracture, a patient can be unaware of having experienced any frank trauma; hence the term 'silent fracture'. This may be one of the causes of the lumbar kyphosis that is seen in some individuals who spend excessive amounts of time sitting.

Occult fractures, also referred to as insufficiency fractures, are best diagnosed with a bone scan or magnetic resonance imaging (MRI). This type of fracture is usually intramedullary and undisplaced and frequently occurs as a result of some minor or major trauma, but radiograph examination is negative. Typically, occult fractures occur in the proximal femur or humerus after a fall, but they have also been reported in the sacrum, acetabulum, calcaneus, tibia and spine. Quickly, these patients present with moderate to severe pain and tenderness. There is a concomitant reduction in range of motion and strength and, if in the femur, there is a marked antalgic gait. In nursing and rehabilitation, this type of fracture should be treated seriously even if it has not been confirmed on initial radiograph. If pushed too aggressively, complete disruption of bone may occur. Protected ambulation with a walker is requisite while the femoral or pelvic occult fracture heals.

A pathological fracture results from primary or metastatic malignant tumors in bone. These types of fractures usually present as pain without any reported history of trauma; however, at times, metastatic bone disease is found in a patient who is being X-rayed because of trauma. Significantly, these patients complain of increased pain at night and of being awakened by the pain. The pain frequently increases with bedrest and the severity increases with time. Those presenting with primary tumors of the breast, prostate, thyroid, kidney, or other organ should be suspected of having metastatic disease if pain complaints fit these descriptions. Standard radiographs are helpful for specific bony sites; however, for diffuse bone metastasis, a nuclear medicine bone scan may be important for a total skeletal evaluation (see Chapter 14, Imaging).

FUTURE METHODS OF PROMOTING FRACTURE HEALING

As stated above, natural fracture repair in the elderly may not proceed in precisely the same pattern as repair proceeds in younger individuals. However, several medical and physical methods for enhancing bone repair are being investigated. A number of growth factors have been found that influence fracture repair, including

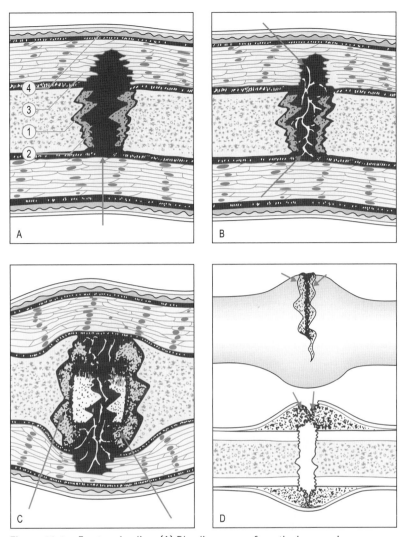

Figure 62.1   Fracture healing. (A) Bleeding occurs from the bone ends, marrow vessels, and damaged soft tissues, with the formation of a fracture hematoma that clots (closed fracture is illustrated). (1, periosteum; 2, haversian systems; 3, muscle; 4, skin). (B) The fracture hematoma is rapidly vascularized by the ingrowth of blood vessels from the surrounding tissues and, for some weeks, there is rapid cellular activity. Fibrovascular tissue replaces the clot, collagen fibers are laid down, and mineral salts are deposited. (C) New woven bone is formed beneath the periosteum at the ends of the bone. The cells responsible are derived from the periosteum, which becomes stretched over these collars of new bone. If the blood supply is poor, or if it is disturbed by excessive mobility at the fracture site, cartilage may be formed instead and remain until a better blood supply is established. (D) If the periosteum is incompletely torn, and there is no significant loss of bony apposition, the primary callus response may result in establishing external continuity of the fracture ('bridging external callus'). Cells lying in the outer layer of the periosteum itself proliferate to reconstitute the periosteum. (Reproduced with kind permission from McRae 1994.)

fibroblast growth factor, platelet-derived growth factor, transforming growth factor 13, and bone morphogenic protein. Insulin-like growth factor may stimulate fibroblast proliferation.

Ceramic composites of calcium phosphate have been used for bone grafts. Electrical stimulation and ultrasound at specific parameters are two physical modalities that are currently being used to promote fracture healing. Fracture treatment in the future is likely to involve active intervention to promote healing and thereby reduce morbidity.

THERAPEUTIC INTERVENTIONS

Osteoporosis-related fractures

Osteoporosis is caused by increased action of osteoclasts (cells that absorb bone) or decreased action of osteoblasts (cells that lay down bone). It affects cancellous (trabecular) bone more than cortical bone.

The areas of the human skeleton that are most likely to fracture as a result of osteoporosis are the neck of the femur, the vertebral bodies, and the wrist (Melton et al 1997). Compression fracture of a vertebral body is a common occurrence in an individual with osteoporosis, and it is often the first indication that a person has osteoporosis. Estrogen is protective of bone and prevents osteoporosis, whereas long-term steroid use has the effect of weakening the bone and increasing osteoporosis. Weight-bearing exercise has been shown to be protective of bone strength, and is associated with decreased bone resorption and increased osteogenesis (Nelson et al 1994, Ryan et al 1998, Kerr et al 2001). Postmenopausal women in Western culture are at the highest risk (see Chapter 19, Osteoporosis and Chapter 59, Hormone Replacement Therapy, for further discussion of this subject).

Treatment of someone with an osteoporosis-related fracture consists of promoting healing, preventing deformity, and facilitating the individual's return to full functioning. This type of fracture should not be viewed as an isolated event. It is usually the harbinger of future fractures. Thus, prevention of future fractures should be part of the treatment plan. In working with a patient who has had a compression fracture, the nurse or therapist should screen carefully for any signs of neurological compromise. By definition, compression fractures do not involve the posterior portion of the vertebral body and so do not involve a risk of protrusion of fractured bone into the spinal canal. If neurological signs are present, the client should be referred for studies to determine the presence of burst fracture or fracture dislocation.

Pharmacological interventions to promote healing

An individual with a compression fracture may be given medications that seek to restore bone strength. Current antiresorptive agents, chiefly bisphosphonates and selective estrogen receptor modulators, reduce fracture risk by 30–50% and teriparatide, a newly approved anabolic agent, reduces risk by 80+% (Heaney 2003). Alendronate and risedronate are bisphosphonates that inhibit bone resorption and probably do not impair bone formation. The nurse or therapist treating someone who is taking bisphosphonates may assist by ensuring that these medications are being taken correctly. They must be taken on an empty stomach with 8 ounces (236.6 mL) of water. The individual should be upright after ingestion and should wait 30 minutes before eating. The side effects of gastrointestinal upset may be worsened if these guidelines are not followed. Another medication that inhibits bone resorption is salmon calcitonin, which is either injected or used as a nasal spray. It can be given to those who cannot take any of the above medications. A postmenopausal woman may be given hormone replacement therapy; however, this practice has been dramatically limited since studies of combined estrogen plus progestin use for an average 5.2 years associated their use with an absolute excess risk of coronary heart disease events, strokes, pulmonary emboli, and invasive breast cancers (Writing Group for the Women's Health Initiative Investigators 2002).

Pain management

An individual with a spinal compression fracture is likely to have pain with movement and might need instruction in log-rolling (moving with no trunk rotation while rolling). The use of a neoprene lumbosacral corset with gel-foam lumbar support, clavicle strap, Spinomed or Jewett brace may prevent extraneous motion and thus minimize pain. In our experience, modalities such as gentle manual therapy, cold, heat and pulsed ultrasound with high-voltage galvanic electric stimulation are effective in reducing pain during the 6-week acute healing phase (see also Chapter 68, Conservative Interventions

for Pain Control). Caregivers also need to be instructed in safe transfers using the pelvis for contact guarding rather than putting any compression through the trunk. They also need to be made aware of bed and chair positioning with spinal alignment such that lumbar lordosis is supported and forward head with kyphosis posture minimized.

Prevention of further injury

Although the effects of a diet change on bone strength will take longer to be seen, the individual who has suffered a fracture may be amenable to changes in diet that will help to prevent future fractures. Referral to a registered dietician is indicated (see Table 62.1 for optimal calcium requirements, and further information about diet, calcium, and patient education can be found in Chapter 19, Osteoporosis).

All possible measures should be taken to prevent additional fractures and, above all, to avoid falling. A full balance evaluation and then interventions (see Chapter 61, Balance Testing and Training) based upon identified impairments need to be implemented as soon as the person is ambulatory. The environment should be inspected for and cleared of fall hazards. A gradual resumption of mobility is necessary to prevent other medical complications such as pneumonia. Indeed, the person should be encouraged to slowly increase his or her participation in the activities of daily living.

At that point, useful instruction must include a demonstration of how to perform activities without flexing the trunk. Sitting and forward flexion have been shown to increase intervertebral disk pressure, so these postures are to be avoided (Schultz et al 1982, Keaveny et al 1999). As the individual begins to tolerate sitting, the use of a lumbar support will help to achieve some measure of lordosis in the lumbar spine. A person with a spinal compression fracture may be given a walker to assist in ambulation, but a four-legged, or pick-up,

Table 62.1 Optimal calcium requirements

Group	Optimal daily intake (in mg of calcium)
Infants	
Birth–6 months	400
6 months–1 year	600
Children	
1–5 years	800
6–10 years	800–1200
Adolescents/young adults	
11–24 years	1200–1500
Men	
25–65 years	1000
Over 65 years	1500
Women	
25–50 years	1000
Pregnant and nursing	1200–1500
Over 50 years (postmenopausal)	
On estrogens	1000
Not on estrogens	1500
Over 65 years	1500

From Office of the Director 1994 NIH Consensus Statement. National Institutes of Health, Bethesda, MD, 12(4).

walker can place strain on the back because the individual must lean forward slightly to reach it, and then must lift it, which puts a great deal of pressure on the intervertebral disks and vertebral bodies. A walker with front wheels does not completely solve this problem, as the individual still has to lift the walker for turns and for backing up. In our experience, only a four-wheeled walker with hand-brakes and a folding seat provides the biomechanical protection necessary for the patient with a healing vertebral compression fracture.

Clinical experience shows that an individual with a history of compression fractures remains in a forward-flexed posture as a consequence of using a walker. The neurological system, particularly the vestibular system, learns that the 'normal' walking posture involves a forward-flexed trunk. Skeletal muscle lengths may change too, and contribute further to this new 'normal' posture. The person never experiences a truly upright posture and loses control of posterior sway, becoming fearful of standing up straight.

A

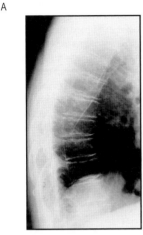
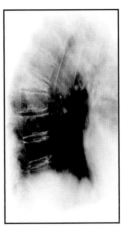

T7 vertebral height loss with initial fracture

T7 vertebral compression refracture

B

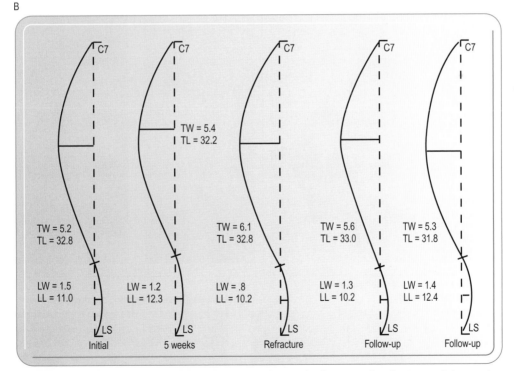

Figure 62.2   A 62-year-old woman with osteoporotic vertebral compression fracture, reinjury and recovery. (A) **Lateral spinal radiographs** for a 62-year-old woman with osteoporosis before and after her T7 vertebral refracture (right). (B) **Flexicurve kypholordosis** tracings during her rehabilitation at initiation, 5-week re-examination, immediately post refracture (coinciding with second radiograph), and at two more examinations throughout her rehabilitation. (TW = thoracic width (cm), TL = thoracic length, LW = lumbar width, LL = lumbar length.) Notice that her kyphosis increased noticeably after the second fracture, and diminished by the time of discharge.
(Printed with permission. Carleen Lindsey, PT, MS, GCS 2006.)

One means of preventing this problem is to have the individual work on exploring his or her limits of posterior stability (see Chapter 61, Balance Testing and Training) while standing in a place perceived as providing protection from a backwards fall.

The most useful exercise is 'wall arches', in which the person faces the wall and reaches upward, by sliding their hands up in from of themselves (Fig. 62.3). Wall slides, in which the person stands with his or her back to a wall, hands lightly on the walker, and moves up and down and side-to-side are also very useful. Progress can be made toward requiring less and less support from the wall and from the walker. When the person is ready to progress to trunk-strengthening activities, it is of paramount importance that the clinician understands the importance of maintaining spine neutral position for any abdominal exercises. A striking example of this was demonstrated in a prospective study in which subjects were divided according to the exercise regimen prescribed by their physician. Those who were prescribed extension exercises had a 16% incidence of new fractures, whereas those who were prescribed spinal flexion exercises (i.e. crunches) had an 89% incidence of new fractures. Some 53% of those who were prescribed combined flexion and extension exercises had new fractures, and 67% of those who were prescribed no exercise at all had new vertebral compression fractures (Sinaki & Mikkelsen 1984).

Prevention of further deformity

It is important for clinicians to carefully track the degree of spinal deformity when assessing progress and designing an effective exercise program both for individuals recovering from vertebral compression fractures and also for those with risk factors for further vertebral fractures.

Flexicurve ruler tracings, kyphometer measurement, and lateral radiographs have all been shown to be reliable methods for tracking kypholordosis alignment (Lundon et al 1998). Radiographs of a T7 vertebral compression fracture and subsequent refracture are shown in Figure 62.2A. Flexicurve tracings taken during rehabilitation of the same patient are shown in Figure 62.2B.

In our experience, this visual representation of spinal alignment can also serve as motivational feedback for patients during treatment.

During rehabilitation after a spinal compression fracture, it is vital to strengthen muscles that have become weak from disuse. Particular attention should be paid to exercises that encourage extension and upright posture. Of course, consideration must be given, during exercise programs, to restoring the length of tightened muscles and concurrently developing strength in them to provide the necessary stability. It is well documented that contracted muscles

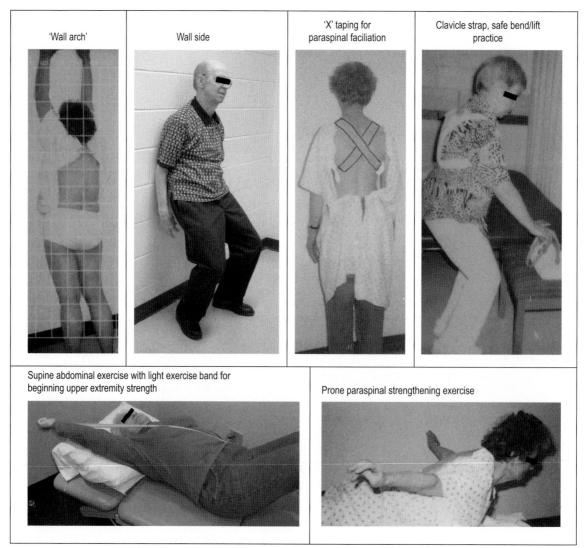

Figure 62.3   Exercises and postural protection for postvertebral compression fracture patients.
(Printed with permission. Carleen Lindsey, PT, MS, GCS 2006.)

require strengthening exercises after they have been stretched, or weakness and instability will prevail in that area.

Water exercises can be done, as the buoyancy of water provides a comfortable, gravity-free environment, but the client must eventually transition to a land-based program in order to develop strength and polish the skills necessary to live in a gravitational environment.

Various studies that have investigated methods of improving bone mineral density (BMD) have shown that weight-bearing exercises improve BMD in the lower extremities and the spine, and weight-training exercises, which include upper and lower extremity resisted exercises, improve BMD in the upper extremities as well as in the spine and lower extremities (Ayalon et al 1987, Dalsky et al 1988, Ryan et al 1998, Swezey et al 2000, Kerr et al 2001, Kelley et al 2002, Cussler et al 2003, Mitchell et al 2003, Waltman et al 2003). Many studies have also demonstrated that trunk extension exercise is a valuable tool not only for kyphotic deformity prevention but also for limiting spinal bone loss over time (Itoi & Sinaki 1994, Greendale et al 2002, Iki et al 2002, Sinaki et al 2002, Mitchell et al 2003, Gold et al

2004). Some abdominal and paraspinal strengthening exercises are included in Fig. 62.3.

Exercises should be instituted even with people who are not ambulatory because of the positive effects that exercise has on bones. For individuals who are attempting to regain mobility after an episode of bedrest necessitated by an osteoporotic fracture, balance exercises that address the individual's specific impairments and unique needs are necessary. Some generic exercises are included in Box 62.2. They are helpful as general exercises for middle-aged and older people, but it is important to remember the necessity of tailoring an exercise routine to the idiosyncrasies of the individual.

Vertebroplasty and kyphoplasty

While kyphoplasty and vertebroplasty have offered surgical hope for pain relief and, in many cases, vertebral height restoration following compression fracture (Lieberman et al 2001, Lane 2006), there are also

---

Box 62.2   Exercises for people 55 years old and older

These exercises are to be gradually increased. Work at your own pace and level of ability. Start with 5 or 10 repetitions and do fewer if you must or more if you can. Slowly increase by adding two to four or more repetitions every 5–10 days. Progress until you can do approximately 15–25 repetitions of each exercise. Do these exercises at least three times a week.

1 *High step*
Hold on to a chair for balance; stand up straight. Raise one foot off the floor so that your knee is as high as your hip. Reverse legs. Try not to lean on the chair too much. As you get stronger, you may be able to raise your leg higher, hold for a count of 5 (less if necessary), and decrease the amount of leaning on the chair.
Purpose: to increase hip and leg strength and balance

2 *Side step*
Hold on to a chair for balance; stand up straight. Move one leg out to your side and hold it in the air. Don't bend at the waist. Hold leg up for 5 seconds, or less if necessary. Reverse legs. At first, you may be unable to hold your leg in the air. If so, simply move your foot out to the side.
Purpose: to increase hip and leg strength and balance

3 *Stand up–sit down*
This is the key to being independent. Simply stand up, then sit down. To do this, you must get your feet under the front of the chair. Move your center of gravity forward and then up. If necessary, use the chair's arm rest. As you get stronger, decrease the amount of push that you need from your arms.
Purpose: to improve strength, balance, coordination, and joint motion

4 *Shoulder shrug*
Sit up or stand up straight. Shrug your shoulders up high and release. Pull your shoulders back. You should feel your shoulder blades pull together.
Purpose: to strengthen back, stretch chest muscles, and improve posture

5 *Cervical range of motion*
Sit up or stand up, head erect but not forward. Turn your chin to your left shoulder, then reverse to the right. Lean your ear to your left shoulder, then reverse to the right. Lightly place your finger on your chin and push your chin back. Do not roll your head back as if looking up at the ceiling.
Purpose: to improve posture, balance, and range of motion

6 *Walk, walk, walk*
Walk at whatever level of ability you have. If you can walk only 50 feet, start at that level and try to increase the distance and improve your gait speed. Avoid stops and starts. If you are walking longer distances, such as half a mile or longer in 5–10 minutes, do a little stretching before starting. When finishing your walk, cool down by simply walking slowly, stretching, and doing a few of these exercises or your favorite ones.
Purpose: to enhance overall health of muscles, bones, joints, circulation, heart, lungs, digestion, bowels, and mind

If you need help getting started or if you have any concerns about your health, show these exercises to your physician.

Reprinted with permission from Kauffman T 1987 Posture and age. Top Geriatr Rehabil 2:13–28. © Aspen Publishers Inc., New York

some very important precautions and limitations that need to be seriously considered. The available evidence suggests that these procedures can be effective and may be safe. However, existing studies evince significant risk of increased fracture risk for adjacent vertebrae, as well as a small but significant risk of cement leakage. The other problem is that the studies demonstrating minimal risks also have relatively short follow-up periods. Better clinical research is required to determine the true role of vertebroplasty and kyphoplasty among existing therapeutic options for vertebral compression fracture treatment (Grados et al 2000, Berlemann et al 2002, Donovan et al 2004, Bouza et al 2006). Physical therapy after surgery is also paramount for postural and strength training in order to minimize risks for further fracture.

CONCLUSION

Fractures are major problems for aging people and, in the great majority of cases, rehabilitation is a necessary follow-up. Understanding normal fracture healing and the possible factors that alter it will assist in the provision of optimal care. The special fractures such as the occult and insufficiency fractures and metastatic lesions are requisite considerations in geriatric rehabilitation. Proper therapeutic exercise, balance and gait training, pain control, and prevention of further injury facilitate rehabilitation and enable the patient to attain as high a quality of life as is possible.

References

Ayalon J, Simkin A, Leichter I et al 1987 Dynamic bone loading exercises for postmenopausal women: effect on the density of the distal radius. Arch Phys Med Rehabil 68:280–283

Berlemann U, Ferguson SJ, Nolte LP et al 2002 Adjacent vertebral failure after vertebroplasty. A biomechanical investigation. J Bone Joint Surg Br 84:748–752

Bilezikian JP, Kurland ES, Rosen CJ 1999 Male skeletal health and osteoporosis. Trends Endocrinol Metab 10:244–250

Bouza C, Lopez T, Magro A et al 2006 Efficacy and safety of balloon kyphoplasty in the treatment of vertebral compression fractures: a systematic review. Eur Spine J 15:1050–1067

Chang WC, Christensen TM, Pinilla TP et al 1999 Uniaxial yield strains for bovine trabecular bone are isotropic and asymmetric. J Orthop Res 17:582–585

Chrisilles E, Shireman T, Wallace R 1994 Costs and health effects of osteoporotic fractures. Bone 15:377–386

Cooper C, Atkinson EJ, Jacobsen SJ et al 1993 Population-based study of survival after osteoporotic fractures. Am J Epidemiol 137:1001–1005

Cummings SR, Black DM, Nevitt MC et al 1993 Bone density at various sites for prediction of hip fractures. The Study of Osteoporotic Fractures Research Group. Lancet 341:72–75

Cussler EC, Lohman TG, Going SB et al 2003 Weight lifted in strength training predicts bone change in postmenopausal women. Med Sci Sports Exerc 35:10–17

Dalsky GP, Stocke KS, Ehsani AA et al 1988 Weight-bearing exercise training and lumbar bone mineral content in postmenopausal women. Ann Intern Med 108:824–828

Donovan MA, Khandji AG, Siris E 2004 Multiple adjacent vertebral fractures after kyphoplasty in a patient with steroid-induced osteoporosis. J Bone Miner Res 19:712

European Foundation for Osteoporosis and Bone Disease (EFFO) & National Osteoporosis Foundation (NOF) 1997 Who are the candidates for prevention and treatment for osteoporosis? Osteoporos Int 7:1

Gerhart TN 1995 Fractures. In: Adams W, Beers M, Berkow R, Fletcher A (eds) Merck Manual of Geriatrics. Merck, Sharp and Dohme, West Point, PA, p 69–84

Gold DT, Shipp KM, Pieper CF et al 2004 Group treatment improves trunk strength and psychological status in older women with vertebral fractures: results of a randomized, clinical trial. J Am Geriatr Soc 52:1471–1478

Grados F, Depriester C, Cayrolle G et al 2000 Long-term observations of vertebral osteoporotic fractures treated by percutaneous vertebroplasty. Rheumatology (Oxford) 39:1410–1414

Greendale GA, McDivit A, Carpenter A et al 2002 Yoga for women with hyperkyphosis: results of a pilot study. Am J Public Health 92:1611–1614

Heaney RP 2003 Advances in therapy for osteoporosis. Clin Med Res 1:93–99

Hipp JA, Hayes WC 2003 Biomechanics of fractures. In: Browner B, Jupiter JB, Levine AM, Trafton PG (eds) Skeletal Trauma, Vol. 1. Saunders, Philadelphia, PA, p 90–119

Iki M, Saito Y, Dohi Y et al 2002 Greater trunk muscle torque reduces postmenopausal bone loss at the spine independently of age, body size, and vitamin D receptor genotype in Japanese women. Calcif Tissue Int 71:300–307

Itoi E, Sinaki M 1994 Effect of back-strengthening exercise on posture in healthy women 49 to 65 years of age. Mayo Clin Proc 69:1054–1059

Keaveny TM, Wachtel EF, Kopperdahl DL 1999 Mechanical behavior of human trabecular bone after overloading. J Orthop Res 17:346–353

Kelley GA, Kelley KS, Tran ZV et al 2002 Exercise and lumbar spine bone mineral density in postmenopausal women: a meta-analysis of individual patient data. J Gerontol A Biol Sci Med Sci 57:M599–M604

Kenny AM, Joseph C, Taxel P, Prestwood KM 2003 Osteoporosis in older men and women. Conn Med 67:481–486

Kerr D, Ackland T, Maslen B et al 2001 Resistance training over 2 years increases bone mass in calcium-replete postmenopausal women. J Bone Miner Res 16:175–181

Koval K, Zuckerman J 1997 Orthopaedic challenges in the aging population: trauma treatment and related clinical issues. Instructional course lectures (American Association of Orthopaedic Surgeons) 46:423–430

Lane NE 2006 Epidemiology, etiology, and diagnosis of osteoporosis. Am J Obstet Gynecol 194:S3–S11

Lieberman IH, Dudeney S, Reinhardt MK et al 2001 Initial outcome and efficacy of 'kyphoplasty' in the treatment of painful osteoporotic vertebral compression fractures. Spine 26:1631–1638

Lundon KM, Li AM, Bibershtein S 1998 Interrater and intrarater reliability in the measurement of kyphosis in postmenopausal women with osteoporosis. Spine 23:1978–1985

McRae R 1994 Practical Fracture Treatment, 3rd edn. Churchill Livingstone, New York, p 19

Melton LJ, Thamer M, Ray NF et al 1997 Fractures attributable to osteoporosis: Report from the National Osteoporosis Foundation. J Bone Miner Res 12:16–23

Mitchell MJ, Baz MA, Fulton MN et al 2003 Resistance training prevents vertebral osteoporosis in lung transplant recipients. Transplantation 76:557–562

National Osteoporosis Foundation 2002 America's Bone Health: The State of Osteoporosis and Low Bone Mass in Our Nation. National Osteoporosis Foundation, Washington, DC

Nelson ME, Fiatarone MA, Morganti CM et al 1994 Effects of high-intensity strength training on multiple risk factors for osteoporotic fractures: a randomized controlled trial. JAMA 272:1909–1914

Rafii M, Firooznia H, Golimbu C et al 1982 Bilateral acetabular stress fractures in a paraplegic patient. Arch Phys Med Rehabil 63(5):240–241

Robbins J, Schott, Garnero P et al 2005 Risk factors for hip fracture in women with high BMD: EPIDOS study. Osteoporos Int 16:149–154

Ryan AS, Treuth MS, Hunter GR et al 1998 Resistive training maintains bone mineral density in postmenopausal women. Calcif Tissue Int 62:295–299

Schultz AB, Andersson GBJ, Haderspeck K et al 1982 Analysis and measurement of lumbar trunk loads in tasks involving bends and twists. J Biomech 15:669–675

Sinaki M, Mikkelsen BA 1984 Postmenopausal spinal osteoporosis: flexion versus extension exercises. Arch Phys Med Rehabil 65:593–596

Sinaki M, Itoi E, Wahner HW et al 2002 Stronger back muscles reduce the incidence of vertebral fractures: a prospective 10 year follow-up of postmenopausal women. Bone 30:836–841

Swezey RL, Swezey A, Adams J 2000 Isometric progressive resistive exercise for osteoporosis. J Rheumatol 2:1260–1264

Waltman NL, Twiss JJ, Ott CD et al 2003 Testing an intervention for preventing osteoporosis in postmenopausal breast cancer survivors. J Nurs Scholarsh 35:333–338

Writing Group for the Women's Health Initiative Investigators 2002 Risks and benefits of estrogen plus progestin in healthy postmenopausal women: principal results from the Women's Health Initiative randomized controlled trial. JAMA 288:321–333

Chapter 63

Stiffness

Mark V. Lombardi and Lynn Phillippi

INTRODUCTION

Stiffness, or the loss of joint mobility, is a common complaint of the elderly. Stiffness limits numerous functional activities in the daily life of an elderly individual by interfering with the initiation and completion of movement patterns. Decreased activity increases the incidence of frailty (Wilson 2004). Frail individuals are at a significantly greater risk of poor outcomes and have also been reported to have higher levels of markers related to inflammation and clotting than nonfrail individuals. Frail individuals are clinically identified from those individuals having three of the five attributes of frailty: unintentional weight loss, muscle weakness, slow walking speed, exhaustion and low physical activity (Wilson 2004).

In the elderly, exudation of fibrinogen into extracellular tissue spaces increases, so more fibrin, an elastic filamentous protein, tends to be deposited in the tissue spaces of older people. Protein aggregation, while widely reported to be a common feature of physiological aging, is not clearly understood. If physical activity is not maintained, a complete breakdown of fibrin may not occur, and increased amounts of sticky fibrin may accumulate in the tissue spaces, producing the lesions that restrict movement between adjacent structures. Fibrinous adhesions also form in a localized area following damage to the tissues. These fibrinous adhesions, commonly referred to as 'cross-links', occur naturally during periods of immobilization or inactivity (Pickles 1983).

In many cases, restoration of normal physical activity is sufficient to cause the breakdown of fibrous adhesions. In some cases, when the mass has become consolidated, it may be necessary to intervene with massage, proprioceptive neuromuscular facilitation (PNF), stretching (using sustained, passive overpressure), graded mobilization techniques, or manipulation under anesthesia.

COMMON CAUSES OF STIFFNESS

Traditionally, the clinician has accepted stiffness to be a natural part of the aging process, perhaps without identifying the actual causes, some of which may be prevented and/or treated. Four common causes of stiffness are:

- biomechanical changes in connective tissue and related structures;
- hypokinesis;
- arthritis;
- trauma.

Biomechanical changes in connective tissue and related structures

Numerous characteristics of connective tissue and related structures cause stiffness in the elderly; a select few are highlighted here.

Myofibroblasts

Connective tissue cells that produce unusually large amounts of contractile proteins are termed myofibroblasts. When damage occurs in connective tissue, there are two stages of response: cell multiplication and increased cellular secretion. If hyperplasia creates excessive production of actomyosin, the resulting contractile force may be significant enough to prevent normal range of motion in the affected area.

In addition, numerous studies describe the natural loss of muscle mass in the aged. While loss of muscle mass has been identified as a natural occurrence in the aged, recent studies support strength training in the aged as a means of reversing or preventing declines associated with aging. It is important to note that studies estimate that the rate of muscle mass loss exceeds 3–5% per decade after age 60 years. Also, strength loss is estimated to reach 30% per decade after age 60 years (Watson 2000, Brennan 2002). Strength loss studies suggest that traditional aerobic and endurance training activities employed in rehabilitation, while effective in the reduction of coronary heart disease, may also contribute to positive changes in both muscle strength and bone density (Wallace & Cumming 2000, Kean et al 2004).

Collagen

Collagen is the main supportive protein in skin, tendon, bone, cartilage and connective tissue. A decrease in the elasticity of collagen and the volume of ground substance is associated with the aging process. Also, cross-linking between collagen fibers increases with age, inactivity, and trauma, thereby restricting the mobility of the connective tissue.

The decrease in ground substance creates a loss of critical inter-fiber distance, which restricts the ability of the fibers to move smoothly over each other. With intervertebral disk disease of the spine, decreased collagen mobility may compromise not only spinal mobility, but also spine length, which may also impair breathing patterns (Wilson 2004). Contractures, frequently the result of tight joint capsules, fibrotic or short muscles, or other scar tissues, are part fibrous adhesions and part collagenous shortening. Newly developed contractures have a greater portion of fibrinous adhesions, whereas chronic contractures are more collagenous. Normal activity may break down fibrinous adhesions, but collagenous shortening often requires heat, prolonged stretching, and possibly surgical intervention (see Chapter 17, Contractures).

Hyaluronic acid

Hyaluronic acid is secreted from the hyaline (articular) cartilage that covers the surface of synovial joints. Compression of the joint enhances this secretion, which entraps the synovial fluid among the hyaluronic acid molecules and lubricates the joint during movement. Secretion of hyaluronic acid decreases with age, thus causing a diminution in the effectiveness of joint lubrication (Pickles 1983). Another source of joint stiffness is said to occur as a result of 'articular gelling'. In healthy joints, surface-active phospholipids (SAPLs) inhibit the 'gelling' process (Hills & Thomas 1998). What triggers the 'deactivation' of SAPL in the joint is currently not known.

Cartilage

Cartilage, having no direct blood supply of its own, receives its nutrients from the blood flow in adjacent bones in the synovial fluid in the joint cavity. Chondroblasts secrete the glycoprotein chondroitin sulfate into the surrounding matrix and, through osmosis, attract water containing dissolved gases, inorganic salts, and other organic materials necessary for the normal cartilage cell metabolism. Dehydration occurs with increasing age because the secretion of chondroitin sulfate decreases (Pickles 1983). Normal loading and unloading of cartilage is necessary for movement of materials in and out of chondrocytes. Without compression, metabolites remain in the matrix and oxygen content is lowered, which causes a reduction in glycoprotein secretion and an increase in the collagen precursor, procollagen. This process may convert hyaline cartilage to fibrocartilage. After degeneration of the cartilage occurs, it is not reversible. However, further changes can be avoided through regular activities that promote alternating compression and relaxation of the joint.

Hypokinesis

Too little, or less than normal, movement is termed hypokinesis. Any joint or muscle that is put in its lengthened or shortened state for prolonged periods develops collagenous adhesions. To reduce the incidence of adhesions, physical activity several times during the day must be encouraged. One major problem confronting clinicians' successful treatment of their patients is compliance (Watson 2000, Brennan 2002). Clinicians are encouraged to individualize patient programs to increase compliance. Recommendations include identifying specific activities that interest the patient when developing treatment programs.

Arthritis

Osteoarthritis (the most common form of arthritis) as well as systemic and rheumatic arthralgias are common causes of decreased flexibility, or stiffness, in the elderly (Burbank et al 2002). Common areas identified usually involve the knees, hips, and distal interphalangeal joints of the hand. These complaints may be attributed to acute synovitis, minute fragments of articular cartilage in the synovial fluid, inability of the joints to glide smoothly, muscle spasms, osteophytes at the joint margins, stretching of the periosteum, or muscle weakness secondary to disuse.

Polymyalgia rheumatica, a systemic arthritis, is a syndrome that occurs in older individuals. It is characterized by pain, weakness, and stiffness in proximal muscle groups, along with swelling, fever, malaise, weight loss, and a very rapid increase in the erythrocyte sedimentation rate. The origin of the patient's complaint of pain is thought to be the result of stimulation of A delta mechanoreceptors and C polymodal nerve endings in the synovium and surrounding tissues (Kean et al 2004). The most commonly affected areas are the neck, back, pelvis, and shoulder girdle. Corticosteroid therapy is effective in the acute phase. However, following this phase, graded soft-tissue mobilization along with strengthening exercises can be helpful.

Trauma

Trauma caused by a significant external force, repetitive internal or external microtrauma, or surgery can produce long-standing soft-tissue changes and scarring. It is important to focus on how a particular trauma has affected the functional abilities of an elderly person. For example, have the biomechanics of an individual gait pattern been altered by trauma to the pelvic girdle? Decreased mobility of the pelvic girdle may limit the ability of the individual to propel the lower extremity during gait, to shift weight equally, to perform effective arm swing, and to maintain head, neck and trunk in alignment.

CONNECTIVE TISSUE AND STRETCHING TECHNIQUES

The unique qualities of deformation of connective tissues are referred to as viscoelastic ('viscous' refers to a permanent deformation characteristic and 'elastic' to a temporary deformation characteristic). The explanation of Cantu & Grodin (1992) is as follows.

The elastic component of connective issue represents the temporary change when subjected to stretch (spring portion of model). The elastic component has a poststretch recoil in which all the length or extensibility gained during stretch or mobilization is lost over a short period of time (Fig. 63.1); the elastic component is not well understood but it is believed to be the 'slack' taken out of connective tissue fibers.

The viscous (or plastic) component represents the permanent deformation characteristic of connective tissue. After stretch or mobilization, part of the length or extensibility gained remains even after a period of time (hyaluronic cylinder portion of the model). There is no postmobilization recoil or hysteresis in this component (Fig. 63.2).

If force is applied intermittently, as in progressive stretching, a progressive elongation may be achieved. In Fig. 63.3A, strain or percentage of elongation is plotted against time for the purposes of illustrating this phenomenon. If the stress is reapplied to the tissue, the curve looks identical, but starts from a new length (Fig. 63.3B).

Elastic model

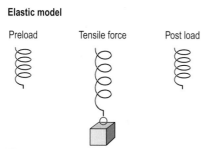

Figure 63.1   The viscoelastic model of elongation – an elastic component in which no permanent elongation occurs after application of tensile force.
(Reproduced with kind permission from Cantu & Grodin 1992.)

Plastic (viscous) model

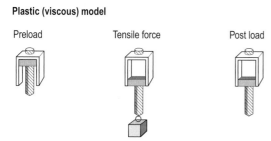

Figure 63.2   The viscoelastic model of elongation – a plastic component in which deformation remains after the application of tensile force.
(Reproduced with kind permission from Cantu & Grodin 1992.)

With each progressive stretch, the tissue has some gain in total length that is considered to be permanent.

In the clinical setting, the above description of elastic versus viscous deformation is evidenced by range of motion that is measured before intervention, immediately after intervention, and 1–2 days later when the patient returns for subsequent treatment. Although the patient may demonstrate an increase in the range of motion (the viscous portion) after intervention, part of that increased range may be lost from the elastic portion of the connective tissue by the time the patient returns for subsequent treatment. Repeated sessions along with an effective home exercise program should result in a overall increase in range of motion and improved function.

Connective tissue, like bone, responds to Wolff's law and adapts in the direction in which the stress is applied. Newly synthesized collagen will be laid down in the direction of the stress applied (Cantu & Grodin 1992). Therefore, it is critical to focus on effective home exercise programs that enhance optimal postural and movement retraining. An important factor to consider when stretching the connective tissue of the elderly is that the tissue responds optimally to slow and prolonged stretching. The elderly individual requires a longer time to loosen the connective tissue because of changes in biomechanical properties such as decreased ground substance and collagen flexibility. Heating modalities that produce tissue temperatures in the 42.5–45.0°C range in conjunction with prolonged stretching have been shown to produce a residual lengthening of tendons. Collagen fibers have to be heated to 42.5°C or above and have continuous force applied to them for at least 30 minutes. Ultrasound (at 1 MHz with an intensity of 1.0 W/cm^2 for 10 minutes) may be used to raise tissue temperature (Johnson 1994).

POSTURE, STIFFNESS AND MOBILITY

A common and often preventable postural change in the elderly is the forward-flexed posture. This posture exhibits varying degrees of forward-thrust head and shoulders, decreased chest and rib cage mobility, increased kyphosis, elevation of the first rib, decreased flexibility of hips and knees, and a shift in the center of gravity. Functionally, the individual has greater difficulty in performing sit-to-stand motions, walking on uneven services, turning, walking backwards, and performing abrupt starts and stops. As posture changes over time, collagenous adhesions increase, with resultant joint structural deformities. Table 63.1 highlights areas where the elderly commonly report stiffness and discomfort that limit functional activities and movements.

Pelvic mobility

Pelvic anterior/posterior tilts and diagonal motions should be assessed with the patient in side-lying, sitting, and standing positions. If restrictions exist, identify the tissues involved and perform soft-tissue mobilization and stretching techniques. Muscles commonly involved are the psoas major, the quadratus lumborum and the paraspinals. At the same time that the therapist is releasing the restriction, the patient can be performing an active movement such as the pelvic tilt, which may assist the release. As in all the following examples, it is important to educate the patient about how to improve functional movement patterns and to formulate an individualized home exercise program.

Trunk mobility

Assess the patient's trunk mobility in supine, side-lying, sitting and standing positions. Identify any restrictions in the abdominal muscles, such as the rectus abdominis or the lumbar extensors, and combine various trunk motions performed actively by the patient with soft-tissue release to the areas.

Hip mobility

Assess the patient in all the above positions with the patient performing the hip motions actively as much as possible. Pay particular attention to restrictions in the gluteal muscles, the rectus portion of the quadriceps, the hip adductors, the tensor fascia latae, and the iliotibial band.

Knee mobility

Assess the knee in the positions described above, focusing on the quadriceps, hamstring, and gastrocnemius muscles, as well as the mobility and tracking of the patellae. The hip, knee, and ankle should be assessed in isolation as well as in combination, including the trunk and pelvis, because areas of stiffness may involve muscles and connective tissues that cross over two joints.

Ankle mobility

In addition to assessing motions of the ankle, observe the position of the foot (pronation/supination) and restrictions in the talus/calcaneus and other bones of the foot, particularly in the standing position. Bressel & McNair (2002) reported that preliminary data from a study looking at ankle stiffness, in a small population of stroke

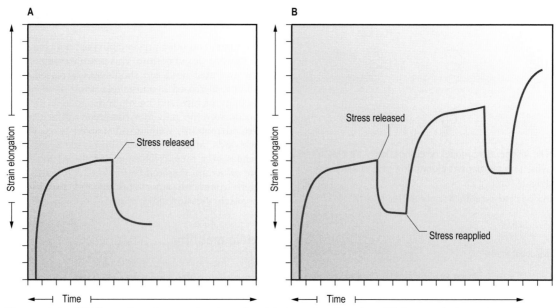

Figure 63.3 (A) Elongation of connective tissue (strain) plotted against time. (B) Repeated elongations of connective tissue (strain) plotted against time.
(Reproduced with kind permission from Cantu & Grodin 1992.)

Table 63.1 Areas of stiffness and discomfort and the muscles involved

Area of stiffness and discomfort	Key muscles involved
Pelvic girdle and trunk	Psoas, iliacus, quadratus lumborum
Hips	Rectus/hamstrings, internal/external rotators
Knees	Quadriceps, hamstrings
Ankles	Dorsi and plantar flexors, gastrocnemius, soleus, tibialis anterior, plantar fascia
Shoulders	Pectoralis major, pectoralis minor
Rib cage	Intercostals
Neck	Suboccipitals, scaleni

patients, showed that ankle stiffness decreases after both prolonged static and cyclic stretching.

Shoulder mobility

Assess the shoulder in all the positions described, noting restrictions in the pectoralis major and minor, the rotator cuff muscles, the long head of the triceps, and the latissimus dorsi. Scapular/humeral and scapular/thoracic motions should be evaluated along with motions in the rib cage, sternum and clavicles.

Head and neck mobility

Assess all motions and identify restrictions in the scaleni, upper trapezii, levator scapulae, sternocleidomastoids, and paraspinals of the cervical area. It is strongly recommended that the clinician should exercise caution when hyperextending the cervical spine to avoid potential compromise of the vertebral artery in those patients with cervical spondylosis.

Rib cage

Identify restrictions in the intercostal muscles, diaphragm and overall mobility of the rib cage. Stiffness or loss of flexibility of the thorax in the aging person can be partially reversed through soft-tissue mobilization and stretching techniques, movement re-education, and specifically designed home programs that focus on further resolving connective tissue restrictions. Great caution and individualized attention must be given to each patient because of a high risk of injury due to osteoarthritis, osteoporosis, and soft-tissue changes, especially skin atrophy. Improved posture facilitates other movements such as transfers, bed and mat mobility, ambulation and other functional activities.

CONCLUSION

Stiffness, a frequent symptom in geriatric patients, is caused by a variety of factors leading to functional declines in posture and mobility resulting in frailty. Some factors contributing to stiffness may be mitigated by proper assessment, appropriate heating modalities, therapeutic exercises and manual techniques. Regular slow, prolonged stretching is optimal to increase the length of connective tissues in aged people.

References

Brennan FH 2002 Exercise prescription for active seniors. Phys Sports Med 30(2):19–26

Bressel E, McNair PJ 2002 The effect of prolonged static and cyclic stretching on ankle joint stiffness, torque relaxation, and gait in people with stroke. Phys Ther 82(9):880–887

Burbank P, Reibe D, Padula CA et al 2002 Exercise and older adults: changing behavior with the transtheoretical model. Orthop Nurs 21(4):51–63

Cantu RI, Grodin AJ 1992 Histology and biomechanics of myofascia. In: Cantu RI, Grodin AJ (eds) Myofascial Manipulation: Theory and Clinical Application. Aspen Publishers, Gaithersburg, MD, p 25–46

Hills BA, Thomas K 1998 Joint stiffness and 'articular gelling': inhibition of the fusion of articular surfaces by surfactant. Br J Rheumatol 37(5):532–538

Johnson GS 1994 Soft-tissue mobilization. In: Donatelli RA, Wooden MJ (eds) Orthopedic Physical Therapy, 2nd edn. Churchill Livingstone, New York, p 697–756

Kean WF, Kean R, Buchanan WW 2004 Osteoarthritis: symptoms, signs and source of pain. Inflammopharmacology 12(1):3–31

Pickles B 1983 Biological aspects of aging. In: Jackson O (ed.) Physical Therapy of the Geriatric Patient. Churchill Livingstone, New York, p 27–63

Wallace BA, Cumming RG 2000 Systematic review of randomized trials of the effect of exercise on bone mass in pre- and postmenopausal women. Calcif Tissue Int 67(1):10–18

Watson C 2000 Aging and exercise: are they compatible in women? Clin Orthop Rel Res 372:151–158

Wilson JF 2004 Frailty – and its dangerous effects – might be preventable. Ann Intern Med 141(6):489–492

Chapter 64

Fatigue

Caroline O'Connell and Emma K. Stokes

Fatigue is hard to define. In the nineteenth century, Beard (1880) referred to fatigue as 'the Central Africa of medicine, an unexplored territory which few men enter'. Unfortunately, fatigue still remains a vague and difficult concept to define. Nevertheless, it is likely that most people will experience fatigue at one or more times in their lives. It can present in a multitude of ways, with a myriad of personal experiences and descriptions, such as mental exhaustion, lack of motivation, physical tiredness, and weariness.

FATIGUE – DEFINITIONS AND CONCEPTS

Fatigue is rarely a binary state, i.e. one has fatigue or one does not. At different times, everyone may experience levels of fatigue varying from mild to overwhelming. Within the concepts of fatigue, it is also important to consider a number of other descriptors of fatigue, namely normal, abnormal, peripheral, or central, in addition to the differing dimensions of fatigue. There is a clear distinction between *peripheral* and *central* fatigue. Peripheral fatigue is defined as a reduction in the maximal muscle force or motor output and is commonly due to overexertion, prolonged or strenuous physical activity. Central fatigue conversely refers to the general feeling often described as 'tiredness', 'weakness', 'languor', or 'sleepiness'. This may exist independently or may be due to some underlying psychological or pathological condition, as outlined in Table 64.1. It is accepted that 'normal' fatigue is a state of general tiredness that is the result of overexertion and can be ameliorated by rest. In contrast, 'abnormal' or 'pathologic' fatigue is a state characterized by weariness unrelated to previous exertion levels and is usually not ameliorated by rest. Both peripheral and central fatigue may exist in normal and abnormal states. This discussion focuses on this general tiredness and lack of motivation associated with central fatigue.

Ream & Richardson (1996), in a large-scale concept analysis review of fatigue literature, assimilated the pertinent information on fatigue in its various forms and proposed a clarified definition for the otherwise amorphous concept. The authors suggest 'fatigue is a subjective, unpleasant symptom which incorporates total body feelings ranging from tiredness to exhaustion creating an unrelenting overall condition which interferes with individual's ability to function to their normal capacity'.

Krupp (2003) suggests that the experience of fatigue reported by a patient may also be interpreted in different ways by different healthcare professionals – physiotherapists, oncologists, nurses, occupational therapists and neurologists. Nevertheless, she goes on to suggest that fatigue can be conceptualized in a number of different ways, included in Box 64.1. Fatigue is not one-dimensional; many authors report the importance of the various dimensions of fatigue. In designing an instrument to measure fatigue, Smets et al (1995) identified five discernible dimensions of fatigue, which are general fatigue, physical fatigue, reduction in activity, reduction in motivation and mental fatigue.

Table 64.1 Common conditions associated with fatigue

Infections	Lyme disease, HIV/AIDS, postpolio syndrome
Sequelae from neurological disorders	Head trauma, Parkinson's disease, stroke
Autoimmune disorders	Multiple sclerosis, systemic lupus erythematosus
Malignancy	Cancer-related anemia, chemotherapy
Endocrine disorders	Thyroid disorders
Hormonal imbalance	Pregnancy
Cardiac and pulmonary disorders	Obstructive sleep apnea, COPD, deconditioning
Postoperative states	
Fibromyalgia	
Rheumatoid arthritis	
Depression	

HIV, human immunodeficiency virus; AIDS, acquired immunodeficiency syndrome; COPD, chronic obstructive pulmonary disease.

Box 64.1   Concepts associated with fatigue (from Krupp 2003)

Decreased mental and physical endurance
Decreased motivation
Depletion of reserves
Fatigability
Inability to rise to the occasion
When healthy, performance that is less that one's
   expectations
Lassitude

Table 64.2   Instruments to measure fatigue

Name	Developed by	Populations validated
Brief Fatigue Inventory	Mendoza et al (1999)	Cancer patients, general population
Fatigue Assessment Instrument	Schwartz et al (1993)	General population, various medical conditions
Fatigue Descriptive Scale	Iriarte et al (1999)	Multiple sclerosis (MS)
Fatigue Impact Scale	Fisk et al (1994)	General population, MS, hypertension patients
Fatigue Scale	Chalder et al (1993)	General population
Fatigue Severity Scale	Krupp et al (1989)	General population, MS, systemic lupus erythematosus, chronic fatigue syndrome, depression
Fatigue Symptom Inventory	Hann et al (2000)	Cancer patients and general population
Iowa Fatigue Scale	Hartz et al (2003)	General population, range of different coexisting medical conditions
Multidimensional Fatigue Inventory	Smets et al (1995)	Radiotherapy patients, chronic fatigue syndrome, psychology and medical students, army recruits
Piper Fatigue Scale	Piper et al (1989)	Cancer, general population, postpolio syndrome
Visual Analog Fatigue Scale	Glaus (1993)	Cancer and gastrointestinal disease patients, general population

FATIGUE IN LATER LIFE

Are we more likely to be fatigued when we are older? Does the type of fatigue experienced throughout the course of life change? The findings are contradictory: Beutel et al (2004) observed, in a large sample of women, that all five dimensions of fatigue described above increased gradually over time. However, Watt et al (2000), investigating the levels of fatigue in people aged 20–79 years in a population-based study, found that most dimensions of fatigue decreased with age among healthy people, compared with an increase with age in the group with disease. Older people living in long-term care facilities may experience more fatigue symptoms (Liao & Ferrell 2000). Hence, all people, both ill and healthy alike, old and young, may experience fatigue. The likelihood of experiencing fatigue is increased in people suffering from a range of different medical conditions. These conditions are listed in Box 64.1, many of which can be more common in people over 65 years of age. It is probably more helpful to focus on what self-reported fatigue or tiredness is associated with, or a predictor of, in later life.

Avlund et al (1998) note that self-reported tiredness in functional mobility in people aged 70 years is strongly predictive of mortality during the following 10 years, even when disability at baseline is considered. Functional mobility in this study related to the performance of transfers, indoor and outdoor mobility in good and poor weather, and managing stairs. Avlund et al (2002) also noted a predictive association between people aged 75 years who report tiredness in four lower limb activities and onset of disability in the following 5 years. This association exists even when other variables associated with onset of disability are considered in the analysis. In this sample, Avlund et al (2001) also noted that men and women who self-reported tiredness in functional mobility at 75 years of age were twice as likely to be hospitalized in the year prior to follow-up, i.e. at 80 years, and were also more likely to use home help services.

It is important to take seriously reports of tiredness or fatigue by older people. Hence, measuring fatigue or tiredness in older people and exploring the reasons for its presence are significant because its report may be an early marker of coexisting disease or a decrease in functional reserve. If present, early intervention may prevent functional decline and/or highlight the need for more substantive evaluation.

MEASURING FATIGUE

Owing to the elusiveness of a precise definition of fatigue in the literature, an individual's reported perception of his or her fatigue has become the focus of fatigue measure-ment. These self-report scales have therefore become widely used. They also have the advantage of being easily understandable by the patient and requiring little prior training by the assessor. They are usually short and readily available. Self-report measures have different structures, from simple unidimensional measures such as the Visual Analog Fatigue Scale (Glaus 1993) to more complex measures encompassing the multidimensional nature of fatigue, such as the Multidimensional Fatigue Inventory (Smets et al 1995). Table 64.2 contains some of the commonly used self-report scales, along with the populations in which they have been validated. One particular measure of value for use with older people is the Multidimensional Fatigue Inventory (MFI-20) (Smets et al 1995). The Multidimensional Fatigue Inventory is a 20-item self-report instrument that acknowledges the comprehensive nature of fatigue. It divides fatigue into the following dimensions: general fatigue, physical fatigue, mental fatigue, reduced motivation and reduced activity. It has been validated in both healthy older people and those with a range of common conditions. The creators found the instrument to have good internal consistency and construct validity (Smets et al 1995). The MFI-20 is copyrighted on the

Form 64.1 The Multidimensional Fatigue Inventory (MFI-20)

Instructions

By means of the following statements we would like to get an idea of how you have been feeling lately. There is, for example, the statement:

'I FEEL RELAXED'

If you think that this is entirely true, that indeed you have been feeling relaxed lately, please place an X in the extreme left box; like this:

yes, that is true [| | |] no, that is not true

The more you disagree with the statement, the more you can place an X in the direction of 'no, that is not true'. Please do not miss out a statement and place one X next to each statement.

1.	I feel fit	yes, that is true	[			]	no, that is not true
2.	Physically I feel only able to do a little	yes, that is true	[			]	no, that is not true
3.	I feel very active	yes, that is true	[			]	no, that is not true
4.	I feel like doing all sorts of nice things	yes, that is true	[			]	no, that is not true
5.	I feel tired	yes, that is true	[			]	no, that is not true
6.	I think I do a lot in a day	yes, that is true	[			]	no, that is not true
7.	When I am doing something, I can keep my thoughts on it	yes, that is true	[			]	no, that is not true
8.	Physically I can take on a lot	yes, that is true	[			]	no, that is not true
9.	I dread having to do things	yes, that is true	[			]	no, that is not true
10.	I think I do very little in a day	yes, that is true	[			]	no, that is not true
11.	I can concentrate well	yes, that is true	[			]	no, that is not true
12.	I am rested	yes, that is true	[			]	no, that is not true
13.	It takes a lot of effort to concentrate on things	yes, that is true	[			]	no, that is not true
14.	Physically I feel I am in a bad condition	yes, that is true	[			]	no, that is not true
15.	I have a lot of plans	yes, that is true	[			]	no, that is not true
16.	I tire easily	yes, that is true	[			]	no, that is not true
17.	I get little done	yes, that is true	[			]	no, that is not true
18.	I don't feel like doing anything	yes, that is true	[			]	no, that is not true
19.	My thoughts easily wander	yes, that is true	[			]	no, that is not true
20.	Physically I feel I am in an excellent condition	yes, that is true	[			]	no, that is not true

Thank you very much for your cooperation.

©E. Smets, B. Garssen, B. Bonke. Reprinted with permission.

names of the authors and is reproduced here with permission (Form 64.1). The scoring system and conditions of use are available from Dr E.M.A. Smets, Medical Psychology Academic Medical Center, University of Amsterdam, PO Box 22660, 1100 DD, Amsterdam, The Netherlands, e-mail: e.m.smets@amc.uva.nl.

INTERVENTIONS FOR FATIGUE

To date, there exists no standardized intervention for fatigue. The treatment approaches taken depend largely on the suspected underlying pathology resulting in the fatigue. For example, people with anemia may notice an improvement in fatigue levels following iron supplementation, while it may be appropriate to prescribe medications and support for sleep apnea in other cases. Other pharmacologic interventions suggested for fatigue are insulin to control blood sugar and thyroxine to regulate thyroid function. The link between fatigue and depression may indicate that antidepressive treatment will ameliorate the effects of fatigue. Advice on nutritional support and correct dietary supplements has been demonstrated to reduce self-reported fatigue levels. Increasingly, exercise has been recommended for its role in increasing general fitness levels and thus reducing fatigue.

References

Avlund K, Schultz-Larsen K, Davidsen M 1998 Tiredness in daily activities at age 70 as a predictor of mortality during the next 10 years. J Clin Epidemiol 51(4):323–333

Avlund K, Damsgaard MT, Schroll M 2001 Tiredness as a determinant of subsequent use of health and social services among nondisabled elderly people. J Aging Health 13(2):276–286

Avlund K, Damsgaard MT, Sakari-Rantala RI 2002 Tiredness in daily activities among nondisabled old people as a determinant of onset of disability. As a predictor of mortality during the next 10 years. J Clin Epidemiol 55:965–973

Beard G 1880 A Practical Treatise on Nervous Exhaustion (Neurasthenia): its Symptoms, Nature, Sequences, Treatments. William Wood, New York

Beutel ME, Weidner K, Schwarz E et al 2004 Age-related complaints in women and their determinants based on a representative community study. Eur J Obstet Gynecol Reprod Biol 117:204–212

Chalder T, Berelowitz G, Pawlikowska J et al 1993 Development of a fatigue scale. J Psychosom Res 37:147–153

Fisk JD, Pontefract A, Ritvo PG et al 1994 The impact of fatigue on patients with multiple sclerosis. Can J Neurol Sci 21(1):9–14

Glaus A 1993 Assessment of fatigue in cancer and non-cancer patients and in healthy individuals. Support Care Cancer 1(6):305–315

Hann DM, Jacobsen PB, Axxarello LM et al 1998 Measurement of fatigue in cancer patients: development and validation of the fatigue symptom inventory. Qual Life Res 7:301–310

Hartz A, Bentler S, Watson D 2003 Measuring fatigue severity in primary care patients. J Psychosom Res 54:515–521

Iriarte J, Katsamakis G, De Castro P 1999 The fatigue descriptive scale (FDS): a useful tool to evaluate fatigue in multiple sclerosis. Multiple Sclerosis 5(1):10–16

Krupp LB 2003 Fatigue, 1st edn. Elsevier Science, Philadelphia, PA

Krupp LB, LaRocca NG, Muir–Nash J, Steinberg AD 1989 The fatigue severity scale: application to patients with multiple sclerosis and systemic lupus erythematosus. Arch Neurol 46:1121–1123

Liao S, Ferrell BA 2000 Fatigue in an older population. J Am Geriatr Soc 48(4):426–430

Mendoza TR, Wang XS, Cleeland CS et al 1999 The rapid assessment of fatigue severity in cancer patients: use of the Brief Fatigue Inventory. Cancer 85(5):1186–96.

Piper BF, Lindsey AM, Dodd MJ et al 1989 The development of an instrument to measure the subjective dimension of fatigue. In: Funk SG, Tornquist EM, Champagne MT, Copp LA, Wiese RA (eds). Key aspects of comfort: Management of pain, fatigue, and nausea. Springer, New York, pp 199–208

Ream E, Richardson A 1996 Fatigue: a concept analysis. Int J Nurs Stud 33(5):519–529

Smets EM, Garssen B, Bonke B, De Haes JC 1995 The multi-dimensional fatigue inventory (MFI): psychometric qualities of an instrument to assess fatigue. J Psychos Res 39:315–325

Schwartz JE, Jandorf L, Krupp LB 1993 The measurement of fatigue: a new instrument. J Psychosom Res 37:753–762

Watt T, Groenvold M, Bjorner JB et al 2000 Fatigue in the Danish general population. Influence of sociodemographic factors and disease. J Epidemiol Commun Health 54:827–833

Chapter 65

The function of the aging hand

Eli Carmeli and Dario G. Liebermann

INTRODUCTION

The hand is the most active and important part of the upper extremity. The function of the hand and its quality of performance are based on many components such as psychological, musculoskeletal, sensory and social. Hand function declines with age and, therefore, for clinicians working with elderly people it is crucial to understand the possible functional deterioration in order to be able to offer primary and secondary prevention programs.

The anatomy and biomechanics of the hand are complex. As we age, several intrinsic and extrinsic factors may be involved in the age-related functional decline; thus, the hands undergo changes even without evidence of trauma or disease. Many of the obvious changes are not a consequence of aging so much as a consequence of inactivity.

This chapter aims to provide an overview of the effect of the aging process on hand anatomy and function.

HAND AGING: A PREDICTABLE PROCESS

Hand function is crucial for maintaining independence during daily life activities. It has been demonstrated that a reduction in hand-grip strength can predict the risk of future disability in aged people (Carmeli et al 2003). Natural and expected aging changes are genetically and environmentally determined and contribute to the normal decline. However, metabolic disorders such as rheumatoid arthritis, osteoporosis, diabetes mellitus, sarcopenia along with accumulative trauma disorders (i.e., due to repetitive movements), comorbidity, and behavioral factors (i.e. declining physical activity, lack of motivation) have a direct effect on the normal prehension patterns (grasping wrapping and pinching). Additionally, they are important factors that determine the age-related functional impairment of the hand.

As people get older, errors in the performance of manual skills are accompanied by a progressive decline in perceptual–motor abilities. Longer reaction times, deterioration of sensory capacity and a decrease in muscle power contribute to the functional deterioration in hand dexterity in the elderly. The outcome is an overall change in hand coordination that cannot be viewed in isolation from the parallel changes in sensorimotor capabilities, particularly the deterioration of vision. It seems suitable for the present discussion to refer to the decrease in hand function with age as a problem of hand–eye coordination. In the following sections, the link between vision and hand movements will be discussed within a developmental perspective.

HAND EVALUATION IN PRACTICE

A first assessment of hand function is carried out at an early stage using a clinical examination. It can provide the alert observer with a wealth of information about the patient's habits, personality and physical health.

Hand structure and function are very complex issues to investigate because of their multifactorial nature, particularly within the continuum of a natural aging process. As an integrated functional unit, the human hand performs a wide variety of tasks that require comprehensive examination. Although it is difficult to isolate any single prehension pattern as being the most relevant to assess function, tests of hand grip strength, using a digital grip myometer, are usually used to evaluate possible functional limitations and to anticipate future clinical needs.

The first components of the hand–eye system that need to be evaluated in order to assess the hand–eye function are:

1. *hand anatomy*: muscles and tendons, intrinsic bones and joints, fingernails;
2. *hand neurology*: cutaneous and motor nerves;
3. *hand metabolism and physiology*: skin dexterity and vascularization;
4. *hand motor behavior*: prehension patterns, hand and finger functional movements, control and sensorimotor integration during task-oriented reaching and grasping performances.

THE FINGERNAILS

In the healthy individual, the fingernails grow continuously at a rate of 0.5–1.0 mm per week. However, such a growth rate may slow during severe illness, and such slowing may produce a 'coronary groove' in the nail plate. This groove moves distally when normal nail growth resumes. After the age of 80 years, the rate of female nail growth is greater than that in males. The normal nail has a hard area near its root but, under pathological conditions such as a deficit of albumin, cirrhosis, or renal insufficiency, the whole nail plate is solid and white. Lymphatic disorders might cause thickened and yellow nails. Metal mineral deficiency (of iron or zinc) may result in a 'spoon-shaped' nail. The 'club-shaped' or 'drumstick' nail appears following respiratory, heart or intestinal diseases. Hypertrophic nails are commonly associated with connective tissue disorders such as dermatomyositis. However, age-related nail changes are less specific and involve discoloration, changes in contour and roughness of the nail plate. The most common disorder of aging fingernails is fungal infection, which is only a source of 'cosmetic distress'.

THE SKIN

There are many characteristic changes in the skin of the hand that result from poor dermatological conditions underlying disease and metabolic disorders. The clinician should be specifically aware of the following: chronic and pernicious anemia, liver disease, Raynaud's phenomenon, lupus erythematosus, diabetes mellitus, thyroid disease, and other unspecified skin alterations such as pigmentation, cutaneous infarcts and vasculitis.

The aging skin of the dorsal side of the hand is often fragile, dry, inelastic and wrinkled, and heals slowly after injuries such as cuts, abrasion or burns.

A reduction in tactile sensation is also notable, accompanied by fewer mechanosensory receptors at the fingers. These changes in sensory perception might affect the basic functions of the hand and fingers such as touch, force, grip and slow response time.

INTRINSIC MUSCLES, BONES, AND JOINT

The hand's diminished muscle mass and strength are not as prominent changes in elderly people as they are in other skeletal muscles. The decline in hand-grip strength has been shown to enable predicting the risk of future dysfunction. The decrease in grip strength may be a result of disuse and physical inactivity of the upper limb musculature, and/or eventually due to biochemical changes in the aging tendon tissue. The latter is particularly important for an effective transmission of forces from the extrinsic forearm muscles to the hand, and for the performance of fast and precise finger motion. Hand-grip strength deteriorates more extensively in patients diagnosed with rheumatoid arthritis and osteoarthritis, and is secondary to various conditions such as Dupuytren's contracture, Marfan's syndrome, Raynaud's disease, myotonia and hypocalcemia.

NERVE CHANGES

Loss of normal hand motor function is seen as a result of trauma or disease of the peripheral motor and/or sensory neurons. For example, a demyelinization of the neuronal axons, a diminished axon diameter, a decline in active motor units (mainly in the thenar group), axonal transportation interferences, and nerve compression (the cervical–thoracic zone or more distally as in carpal tunnel syndrome) can be expressed in the form of hand malfunction. Effects of morphological and chemical changes in the central nervous system (CNS) are widely reported (Kandel et al 2000) in the literature with regard to hand motor control. Many movement disorders of central origin may primarily manifest in the inability to move one or both hands. The fine tremor signs in conditions of thyrotoxicosis and the resting tremor of Parkinson's disease or multiple sclerosis are just a few examples of a central impairment that is expressed in aberrant hand movements. Possible explanations for the link between central pathologies and the hand are explained next.

HAND MOTOR CONTROL

The 'reaching-to-grasp' movement is a skill that humans develop early in life and may be representative of aging processes. The reaching-related muscles are centrally represented in a neural circuitry that is rather differentiated from that of other systems (Kuypers 1973). The neural substrates responsible for the orientation of the hand, the preshaping of the finger aperture, and the actual prehension of an object, for example, are different from those responsible for achieving the posture of the arm and trunk during the manipulation of objects (Humphrey 1979).

Based on the findings of Kuypers (1973), common models of arm motor control have regarded the 'transport' of the hand and the 'grasp' of an object as one functional unit. This view is supported by experimental observations showing that these two kinematically defined aspects (reaching for an object and grasping the object) are independently planned even though they are executed in parallel (Jeannerod 1988). A clinical implication of such a functional linkage is that reaching, grasping or both may be affected by the site of the injury regardless of age.

Hand and arm timing behavior has been described by Jeannerod (1988) who showed that the transport of the hand to a target and the timing of the finger opening–closure to grasp an object are finely tuned. Such timing is extremely important for daily life activities as well as for communicating our thoughts. The functional importance of hand actions is such that finger, hand, and forearm musculatures are extensively represented in the motor brain within large somatotopic neural maps (Kandel et al 2000). Such a widespread central representation of arms, hands and fingers is, perhaps, an evolutionary expression of its functional importance but, paradoxically, this increases the likelihood of damage to the associated neural nets as a result of local malady or trauma. Such extensive internal representation of the hand in the brain explains why many CNS pathologies become manifested in the form of negative or positive hand-related motor signs.

'Plasticity' is a fundamental characteristic of the CNS tissue but, at different ages, people differ in their ability to adapt. After injury or disease, elderly subjects often witness changes in the ability to move the hands. Age does not facilitate adaptation, thus, training is crucial for future functioning. Massive practice should be used to enhance the plastic processes in the brain. In the condition known as webbed-finger syndrome (syndactyly), which is characterized by fusion of the fingers at birth, the lack of individual finger movement is accompanied by lack of representation in the brain in the corresponding somatotopic area. As evidence of the plastic brain adaptability, within a few weeks after surgical intervention and therapeutic training, it is possible to observe a reorganization of the motor maps. Single neuronal activity of each digit within the hand area may be recorded from the brain upon movement of fingers that never moved before (Kandel et al 1995).

During movements of the hand, the brain must also regulate the transformation between the actual hand–arm positions relative to external objects. This requires the use of information from visual and proprioceptive sources. That is, hand movements cannot be studied in isolation with no regard for other systems. People learn to reach for fragile objects differently than toward other objects and make the required adjustments based on vision. The appropriate posture of the hand and the parallel finger aperture and prehension of an object all depend on the visual perception of that object.

Jeannerod (1988) suggested different visuomotor channels for the transport of the hand to an object and for its grasp. The first channel is related to external object coordinates in space and, thus, large axial muscles are activated to bring the upper arm into an appropriate posture and transport the hand close to the object. This part of the skill is less affected by object characteristics. Thus vision is restricted to defining the object spatial coordinates and movement. Hand orientation and grasping actions, on the other hand, are influenced by previous forearm–hand movements and require visual perception of the object characteristics to make preparatory adjustments in finger aperture and closure. The latter depends on visual feedback and involves more 'complex' perceptual processes.

VISION

The differences between the dependence of the transport and grasp components on vision have been associated with peripheral and central vision respectively. Vision deteriorates with age, although we become highly dependent on it. The link between the aging hand and the aging visual system is relevant here. Central vision (CV) and peripheral vision (PV) differ in many anatomical and functional respects. CV is restricted to the central receptor area of the retina (the fovea), where 'cone' cells are highly concentrated and project directly into 'column' arrangements in the visual brain (occipital brain areas 17 and 18). Cells in the fovea capture light (in daylight conditions) within the frequency spectrum that allows perception of color. Because of the high spatial resolution (high acuity), the fovea is adapted for conveying information that allows for the recognition of objects and the perception of subtle object features such as line orientation, junctions, diagonal lines at different angles (Hubel & Wiesel 1977).

Some eye-movement types (e.g. saccades) are intended to bring the fovea 'on target'. Once the gaze is locked, the lens of the eye focuses on the object, and a recognition process starts before the object is grasped. Central vision facilitates visual perception of objects in three dimensions by adding, depth via stereopsis (two eyes at a fixed distance seeing the same object from a different perspective).

During PV, the remaining area of the retina (outside the fovea) is used. In the periphery, cells called 'rods' have adapted for sensing light in dark conditions (black–white changes or shadows). Rods gradually decrease in density outwards. Such cells arrangement enables PV to be sensitive to movement because changes in object position projected on two separated and contiguous cells on the retina will result in time derivatives (velocity sensing) that increase when the space between cells increases (lower spatial resolution). As the spatial resolution decreases toward the periphery. People tend to look for moving objects using peripheral vision. The retina may be regarded as an 'outgrowth' of the brain, and also the functional organization of cells in the retina is an expression of evolution. In the above discussion, it is postulated that hand transport toward an object is associated with the more primitive PV, while the grasp is associated with CV because finger aperture and closure are related to the visual object characteristics (Humphrey 1979).

Kuthz-Buschbeck and colleagues (1998) reported interesting findings in the development of functional hand characteristics in children. Infants appear to show a mature stereotypic pattern of moving the arm, and couple it to the fingers opening as early as 24 months after birth. Purposeful reaching and a fine timing of arm and hand movements start as early as 3–4 months of age (Konczak & Dichgans 1997). This process is parallel to the development of vision and plays a fundamental role in the timing of the arm transport and hand grasp actions. At about 12 years old, children develop age-appropriate patterns of motion (Kuthz-Buschbeck et al 1998). At this age, the occlusion of central vision (preventing children from seeing the object with the fovea) causes excessive finger aperture during the transport, when attempting to grasp the object (Kuthz-Buschbeck et al 1998). With experience throughout early infancy, adulthood, and old age, subtle control strategies are adopted. Over time, they may become embedded within the neural system. As aging is accompanied by a loss of visual functions, e.g. a decrease in visual acuity, a slowing down of the saccadic eye movements, and a decrease in the ability to focus on targets, eye muscles weaken as do the eye lens muscles, and thus vision becomes blurred. Eventually, such a deterioration in vision results in poor hand–eye coordination. Elderly people are able to recalibrate the sensorimotor processes for using the hands. Nevertheless, they appear to fail in implementing already structured hand control strategies that they develop through life (Bock 2005). In conclusion, an aging hand is the result of combined cognitive, visual and motor factors.

ERGONOMIC DEVICES

Everyday tools are not initially designed for elderly people. Mobile phone use, nail scissors, microwave, keyboard and even withdrawing money from an automated teller machine (ATM), etc. are beyond the manual capabilities of the large majority of elderly people. These advanced technological devices are usually designed with small and too close punched buttons, and with instrumental active daily living apparatus (IADLs) that are not 'user-friendly' or ergonomically suited for grabbing, holding, switching or tuning.

An example of this problem is the transcutaneous electrical nerve stimulation (TENS) unit. Although an effective non-narcotic pain control device, TENS units, because of their poor design, are usually too difficult for use by aging people.

CLINICAL ASSESSMENTS

In order to clinically assess hand functions, in the context of clinical neuropsychology tasks, several tests have often been used by physical and occupational therapists such as the grooved pegboard test, Crawford small parts dexterity test, Box and Blocks test, finger tapping test, tracing test, Jebsen Taylor hand function, and other tests. Each test has its merits and should be applied according to the needs.

THERAPEUTIC TRAINING

A routine training program is indispensable for improving hand functions. Such exercise training should be designed: (i) to recover impairments such as muscle weakness and decrease in range of motion; and (ii) to expand psychomotor functions and fine motor coordination necessary for ADLs and IADLs using tools and apparatus for the elderly people.

CONCLUSION

Hand functioning mirrors the brain's normal functioning by means of an extensive net of connections. Hands as well as eyes may be viewed as extensions of the brain toward the periphery. Humans at all ages use their hands to communicate and adapt to the demands imposed by the surroundings. In order to meet such demands, the arm, hand and fingers act as one functional unit in close cooperation with vision. Elderly people often lose hand ability and become restricted, not only in the motor sense, but also in other regards such as in their perception of the environment. As far as motor control is concerned, an 'aging hand' cannot be addressed without acknowledging an aging visual system and, most importantly, an aging brain.

References

Bock O 2005 Components of sensorimotor adaptation in young and elderly subjects. Exp Brain Res 160:259–263

Carmeli E, Patish H, Coleman R 2003 The aging hand. J Gerontol A Biol Sci Med Sci 58(2):146–152

Hubel DH, Wiesel TN 1977 Functional architecture of macaque monkey visual cortex. Proc Royal Soc London B 198:1–59

Humphrey DR 1979 On the organization of visually directed reaching: contributions by nonprecentral motor areas. In: Talbott RE, Humphrey DR (eds) Posture and Movement. Raven Press, New York, p 51–112

Jeannerod M 1988 The Neural and Behavioral Organization of Goal-directed Movements. Oxford University Press, Oxford

Kandel ER, Schwartz JH, Jessel TM 1995 Essentials of Neural Science and Behavior. McGraw-Hill, New York

Kandel ER, Schwartz JH, Jessel TM 2000 Principles of Neural Science, 4th edn. McGraw-Hill, New York

Konczak J, Dichgans J 1997 The development toward stereotypic kinematics during reaching in the first 3 years of life. Exp Brain Res 117:346–354

Kuthz-Buschbeck JP, Stolze H, Jöhnk K et al 1998 Development of prehension movements in children: a kinematic study. Exp Brain Res 122:424–432

Kuypers HGJM 1973 The anatomical organization of the descending pathways and their contributions to motor control especially in primates. In: Desmedt JE (ed) New Developments in Electromyography and Clinical Neurophysiology, Vol. 3. Karger, Basel, p 38–68

Chapter **66**

Overweight and obesity

Richard W. Bohannon

INTRODUCTION

The National Institutes of Health (NIH) classifies body weight (Table 66.1) on the basis of body mass index [BMI; weight (kg)/height (m^2)]. The agency defines overweight and obesity as a BMI of 25.0–29.9 kg/m^2 and $\geq$30.0 kg/m^2 respectively (National Institutes of Health 1998). The combined prevalence of overweight and obesity is high among elders. In the United States, between 1999 and 2002, the prevalence of overweight and obesity combined was 39.4% for 60- to 69-year-olds and 25.3% for individuals at least 70 years old (Silventoinen et al 2004). Both mean BMI and the prevalence of overweight are increasing in all western European countries, Australia, the United States and China (Silventoinen et al 2004).

Numerous untoward consequences are associated with increased body weight. Among elders in the United States, obesity is associated with an estimated 111 909 excess deaths (Flegal et al 2005). Overweight and obesity are accompanied by numerous comorbidities. The relationship between weight and type 2 diabetes is particularly

strong, with Colditz et al (1995) showing that women experience a 25% increase in the relative risk of diabetes for each added unit of BMI over 22.0 kg/m^2. Other comorbidities accompanying increased body weight include hypertension, coronary artery disease, stroke, respiratory problems (including sleep apnea), osteoarthritis, and some forms of cancer among elders who are overweight or obese (National Institutes of Health 1998).

As concerned as rehabilitation professionals should be about these comorbidities, it is the functional limitations accompanying increased body weight that are particularly relevant to their practice. The combination of increased body fat and decreased strength (which typically occurs with aging) can render demanding activities such as standing from a chair or climbing stairs painful, difficult, or impossible (Sarkisian et al 2000, Larrieu et al 2004, Bohannon et al 2005). Consequently, it is essential that rehabilitation professionals address the body composition of their patients. Hereafter, some fundamentals of the examination and interventions for overweight and obesity are covered.

EXAMINATION

Based on its practicality, BMI is recommended by the US Preventive Services Task Force for screening adults for obesity (McTigue et al 2003). Indeed, the measurement of weight and height, on which the BMI is based, is possible for most adults. When height and weight cannot be measured directly, they can be obtained by self-report. However, the accuracy of BMI may be compromised by the tendency of individuals to underreport weight and to overstate height (Niederhammer et al 2000). Regardless of the source of the height and weight information used in its calculation, the BMI has limitations. These include the propensity of elders (particularly women with osteoporosis) to lose stature with age and the failure of BMI to differentiate between lean body mass and fat mass.

Alternatives to the BMI exist. Underwater weighing and X-ray absorptiometry provide more specific information about adiposity but are generally impracticable in rehabilitation settings. Bioelectrical impedance is applicable in some settings, but is influenced by hydration and by other variables used with its predictive algorithms. Skinfold measurements are relatively easy to obtain, and measurements from a single site (e.g. subscapular) may be sufficient (Garn et al 1971). The relationship of central adiposity to cardiovascular disease renders waist circumference a useful supplement to BMI (National Institutes of Health 1998). Waist circumference should be measured just above the pelvic crest, parallel to the floor, while individuals stand. A man is considered to be at high risk of weight-related

Table 66.1 Classification of body weight according to the National Institutes of Health

Classification	Body mass index (kg/m^2)
Underweight	<18.5
Normal weight	18.5–24.9
Overweight	25.0–29.9
Obese (class I)	30.0–34.9
Obese (class II)	35.0–39.9
Obese (class III)	$\geq$40

comorbidities if his waist circumference exceeds 102 cm (40 in); for women, the criterion is 88 cm (35 in).

INTERVENTIONS

For elders who are overweight or obese, even small losses of weight have been shown to be highly advantageous. Larsson & Mattsson (2003), for example, found that obese women who achieved a 10% weight loss realized significant improvements in walking speed, oxygen consumption, pain and perceived exertion. Felson et al (1992) discovered that individuals who achieved a weight loss of 2 or more BMI units (about 5.1 kg) over a 10-year period reduced their likelihood of developing knee osteoarthritis by more than 50%. Given such findings, health professionals should not be shy about engaging patients about their weight. Patients are generally desirous of advice about diet, assistance with setting weight goals, and recommendations regarding exercise (Potter et al 2001). These desires are within the realm of five basic strategies that can be used alone or in combination in an effort to promote weight loss. They are diet, physical activity, behavior therapy, pharmacotherapy and bariatric surgery (National Institutes of Health 1998).

Dietary therapy focuses on reduced caloric intake. Low-calorie diets (800–1500 kcal/day) can reduce total weight by a mean 8% over a period of 6 months. Unfortunately, weight loss thus achieved is usually not sustained (National Institutes of Health 1998).

Physical activity is often reduced in overweight and obese elders. As walking activity decreases, percentage overweight increases (Tryon et al 1992). As sitting time increases, BMI increases (Brown et al 2003). Aerobic exercise regimens, which serve to increase activity over baseline, are able to produce modest weight losses (3.0 kg for men and 1.4 kg for women) (Garrow & Summerbell 1995). Such exercise can take many forms, but research indicates that elders prefer walking as a mode of exercise (McPhillips et al 1989). For elders tolerant of progressive walking, pedometry can be used to monitor and reinforce activity. For individuals unable to tolerate sufficient walking to achieve a therapeutic benefit, alternatives not entailing the full load of body weight may be indicated. These include recumbent cycling or aquatic activities. Resistance exercise should be considered as it may enable elders to better handle their weight and to increase their muscle mass and energy expenditure. In lieu of, or in addition to, formal exercise interventions, elders can expend a considerable amount of energy by walking rather than driving short distances, taking stairs instead of elevators, and resisting the unnecessary use of 'labor-saving devices' (Lanningham-Foster et al 2003). Such activities warrant fostering.

Behavior therapy is multifaceted, but much of it is directed at changing dietary and exercise behavior. Key components include, but are not limited to: training in self-monitoring, self-control, exercise and diet information, stimulus control strategies, reinforcement, problem solving and goal setting, behavior modification, family support, stages of change, cognitive restructuring, peer relations and maintenance strategies. Behavioral therapy has been described as offering benefits that are supplemental to those provide by other approaches (National Institutes of Health 1998).

When more conservative approaches prove insufficient, drugs or surgery may be appropriate. Several drugs, including sibutramine and orlistat, can be prescribed. As part of a comprehensive program, they can contribute to weight loss 'when used for 6 months to 1 year' (National Institutes of Health 1998). For patients with severe obesity, bariatric surgery (either open or laparoscopic) is immensely successful in causing weight loss. Weight loss is greatest in the first year or two after surgery and ranges from about 20% to 40%. In the Swedish Obese Subjects Study, patients' weight losses were still 16.3% after 8 years and 16.1% after 10 years (Sjöström et al 2004). Bariatric surgery has a powerful effect on some of the comorbidities that tend to accompany obesity. During the first years after surgery, diabetes, hypertension and sleep apnea are resolved or improved in the vast majority of cases.

CONCLUSION

Rehabilitation professionals are well positioned to serve elders who are overweight and obese. Such service first requires the objective documentation of weight status. Thereafter, interventions can be initiated. Although some interventions (e.g. drugs or surgery) may not be (per se) within the scope of rehabilitation practice, aspects of diet, exercise, and behavioral therapy can be incorporated with modest effect. As patients are open to such interventions, they should not be neglected.

References

Bohannon RW, Brennan P, Pescatello L et al 2005 Relationship among perceived limitations in stair climbing and lower limb strength, body mass index, and self-reported stair climbing activity. Top Geriatr Rehab 21: 350–355

Brown WJ, Miller YD, Miller R 2003 Sitting time and work patterns as indicators of overweight and obesity in Australian adults. Int J Obes 27:1340–1346

Colditz GA, Willett WC, Rotnitzky A, Manson JE 1995 Weight gain as a risk factor for clinical diabetes mellitus in women. Ann Intern Med 122:481–486

Felson DT, Zhang Y, Anthony JM et al 1992 Weight loss reduces the risk for symptomatic knee osteoarthritis in women. The Framingham Study. Ann Intern Med 116:535–539

Flegal KM, Graubard BI, Williamson DF, Gail MH 2005 Excess deaths associated with underweight, overweight, and obesity. JAMA 293:1861–1867

Garn SM, Rosen NN, McCann MB 1971 Relative values of different fat folds in a nutritional survey. Am J Clin Nutr 24:1380–1381

Garrow JS, Summerbell CD 1995 Meta-analysis: effect of exercise, with or without dieting, on body composition of overweight subjects. Eur J Clin Nutr 49:1–10

Lanningham-Foster L, Nysse LJ, Levine JA 2003 Labor saved, calories lost: the energetic impact of domestic labor-saving devices. Obes Res 11:1178–1181

Larrieu S, Pérès K, Letenneur L et al 2004 Relationship between body mass index and different domains in older persons: the 3C study. Int J Obes 28:1555–1560

Larsson UE, Mattsson E 2003 Influence of weight loss programmes on walking speed and relative oxygen cost (%$\dot{V}O_2$ Max) in obese women during walking. J Rehabil Med 35:91–97

McPhillips JB, Pelletera KM, Barreto-Connor E et al 1989 Exercise patterns in a population of older adults. Am J Prev Med 2:65–72

McTigue K, Harris R, Hemphil B et al 2003 Screening and Interventions for Obesity in Adults. Summary of the Evidence. Originally published in Ann Intern Med 139(11):933–949. Agency for

Healthcare Research and Quality, Rockville, MD http://www.ahrq.gov/clinic/3rduspstf/obesity/obessum.htm

National Institutes of Health 1998 Clinical Guidelines on the Identification, Evaluation, and Treatment of Overweight and Obesity in Adults. The Evidence Report. NIH Publication No. 98-4083. NIH, Bethesda, MD

Niederhammer I, Bugel I, Bonenfant S et al 2000 Validity of self-reported weight and height in French GAZEL cohort. Int J Obes 24:1111–1118

Potter MB, Vu JD, Croughan-Minihane M 2001 Weight management: what patients want from their primary care physicians. J Fam Pract 50:513–518

Sarkisian CA, Liu H, Gutierrez PR et al 2000 Modifiable risk factors predict functional decline among older women: a prospectively validated clinical prediction tool. J Am Geriatr Soc 48:170–178

Silventoinen K, Sans S, Tolonen H et al for the WHO MONICA Project 2004 Trends in obesity and energy supply in the WHO MONICA project. Int J Obes 28:710–718

Sjöström L, Lindroos A-K, Peltonen M et al 2004 Lifestyle, diabetes, and cardiovascular risk factors 10 years after bariatric surgery. N Engl J Med 351:2683–2693

Tryon WW, Goldberg JL, Morrison DF 1992 Activity decreases as percentage overweight increases. Int J Obes 16:591–595

Chapter 67

Evaluation of pain in older individuals

John O. Barr

INTRODUCTION

Pain is the symptom that most commonly prompts individuals to seek healthcare. Over 80% of older adults have at least one chronic condition that results in some type of discomfort, including pain (Burke & Jerret 1989). While arthritis is the most common cause of pain, other conditions that result in chronic pain for the elderly include cancer, compression fracture, degenerative disk disease, diabetic peripheral neuropathy, hip fracture repair, postherpetic or trigeminal neuralgia and stroke. Although the incidence of pain increases with age, reports of pain tend to decrease slightly among the oldest individuals (Ferrell & Ferrell 1996). Older people frequently believe that pain is an inevitable consequence of aging that must simply be endured. Upon being questioned, they may deny being in pain out of fear of medical procedures and related expenses, loss of autonomy and possible institutionalization. Unfortunately, across the continuum from acute postoperative to chronic persistent pain, older people experience less than optimal pain management. Inadequate assessment and undertreatment of pain remain two primary problems for older individuals (Taylor et al 2005).

The atypical presentation of pain in the elderly complicates its clinical evaluation. The cardinal signs of inflammation, including pain, redness, elevated temperature and swelling, are less pronounced in older individuals. For example, acute myocardial infarction can occur without significant pain, while conditions such as appendicitis, bowel gangrene, peptic ulcers and pneumonia may result in only mild discomfort. Instead of producing pain, these conditions may contribute to other behavioral signs such as confusion and fatigue. Conversely, pain that is less common in the elderly, such as headache, can signal serious medical problems such as cerebrovascular accident and temporal arteritis (Tierney et al 2003). The interdependence of chronic pain and depression has been thought to be even greater for older people. However, younger individuals with rheumatoid arthritis have been found to be more likely to report depressive symptoms and to have higher levels of daily stress and higher levels of pain than older people (Wright et al 1998).

EVALUATION OF PAIN

Key professional organizations (e.g. the American Geriatrics Society Panel on Persistent Pain in Older Persons 2000) and regulatory agencies (e.g. Joint Commission on Accreditation of Healthcare Organizations 1999) have advocated improved assessment and treatment of pain experienced by older people. Appropriate evaluation of pain involves the synthesis of information derived from the patient's history, subjective interview, objective physical examination and special tests (e.g. laboratory, imaging, electroneuromyography, etc.). The evaluation should clarify the underlying basis for pain and guide therapeutic interventions or result in referral for other specialized healthcare services. Importantly, this evaluation provides baseline information needed to determine the effectiveness of treatment. Periodic re-evaluation allows assessment of the response to treatment, including adverse reactions. The evaluation of pain is unfortunately complicated by its very personal and subjective character. The manner in which an individual reports pain is related to a range of factors that include age, cognitive status, gender, personality, ethnic/cultural background, behavioral needs and past pain experiences.

The patient/client history should include information about current medical conditions and medications that are prescribed: over-the-counter and natural or home remedies. Past interventions that have been both successful and unsuccessful in controlling pain should also be noted. It may be possible to determine patient expectations for or biases against certain interventions, and also to gain further insight as to why a prior treatment was a success or a failure. For example, a previous lack of patient education may have contributed to poor adherence to a prior pain management strategy.

The individual should be given the opportunity to freely verbalize complaints of pain and related symptoms (e.g. aching, burning, fatigue, joint locking, joint warmth, paresthesia, stiffness, etc.). The clinician should then direct specific questions concerning the onset, occurrence (e.g. at rest vs. activity), intensity (current vs. greatest and least during a specific time period), quality, distribution and duration of pain. Situations that aggravate and relieve pain should be identified (e.g. types of movement, postures, rest, etc.). The patient can mark a body diagram to document the location(s) and quality of their pain (Fig. 67.1). Assessment of behavioral indicators of pain is especially useful for documenting the presence of pain in individuals with limited verbal or impaired cognitive abilities (Box 67.1).

Box 67.1 Behaviors that are recommended to be described when assessing pain in older individuals who are nonverbal or cognitively impaired

Change in behavior
- Change in socialization, mood, or psychosocial function
- Change in activities of daily living or function
- Change in appetite
- Restlessness
- Agitation or aggressiveness
- Change in sleep pattern
- Change in ambulation

Change in body language
- Facial expression, grinding teeth or grimacing
- Change in body movement (includes stillness, decreased movement, guarding, holding body part, change in posture, limited range of motion, limping or increased muscle tension or tone)
- Unspecified

Vocalization
- Moaning or groaning
- Crying or calling out
- Sighing or grunting
- Unspecified

Reproduced with kind permission from Molony et al 2005.

The objective examination should focus on physical signs or impairments thought to be associated with a given pain problem (e.g. edema, gait parameters, joint tenderness, muscle strength and endurance, posture, pulmonary functions, range of motion, skin temperature, tissue healing, tolerance to palpation, etc.). Typically, there are reduced levels of activity and functional independence, so it is important to evaluate physical function including activities of daily living (ADL) and physical performance related to occupational and recreational pursuits. It should be recognized that some ADL assessment tools (e.g. the Katz Index of ADL or the Barthel Index) do not represent an adequate range of functional activities for community-active older people, while other tools require too high a level of functioning for some institutionalized cognitively impaired elderly individuals (e.g. the Physical Performance Test). Weiner et al (1996) found that observational analysis of simulated ADL performance was sensitive and valid in assessing pain behavior in older people with chronic low back pain. Importantly, functional limitations should be translated into treatment plan outcome goals.

PAIN ASSESSMENT TOOLS

A number of pain assessment tools have been developed in an attempt to document clinical pain more objectively. The most basic tool for the assessment of pain intensity is the Verbal Descriptor Scale (VDS; also called the 'Verbal Rating Scale'). Patients are instructed to rate their pain intensity as being 'none', 'mild', 'moderate', 'severe', or 'unbearable'. This scale is preferred by individuals who find it easy to understand, resulting in low failure rates for their scoring. Lack of sensitivity in detecting changes based on the limited number of rating categories is the primary limitation of this type of scale. The Iowa Pain Thermometer (IPT) combines an expanded VDS and a pain thermometer (PT) (Taylor et al 2005).

The Numeric Rating Scale (NRS; also call the Pain Estimate or PE) requires patients to rate the severity of their pain on a scale of 0 to 10, or 0 to 100 ('0' indicating no pain, and endpoints of '10' or '100' representing the worst possible pain that could ever be imagined). Understanding the definitions related to these endpoints is critical. If a patient mistakenly believes that a rating of '100' is to indicate 'the worst pain I've ever had', pain that is even more severe the next day could not be properly rated. The primary advantages of this approach are that it is easy to understand and that ratings can be done verbally.

The Visual Analogue Pain Scale (VAPS) employs a horizontal 10-cm line with 'no pain' at the left and 'pain as bad as it could be' at the right (Fig. 67.2). Patients mark one location on the line corresponding to the intensity of their pain. This scale may also be vertically oriented. An alternative format requires the rating of pain relief, employing scale anchors of 'complete pain relief' and 'no pain relief'. A major limitation of visual analogue scales is that they rely on vision and motor control, which may be limited in some older patients. While it has been suggested that elderly individuals may

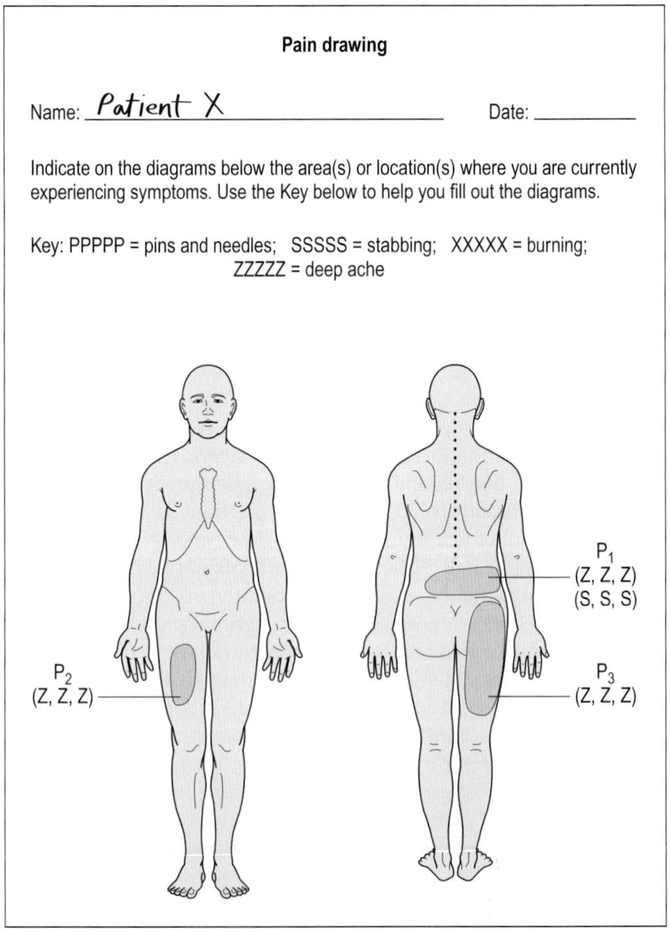
Pain drawing
Name: Patient X
Date:
Indicate on the diagrams below the area(s) or location(s) where you are currently experiencing symptoms. Use the Key below to help you fill out the diagrams.
Key: PPPPP = pins and needles; SSSSS = stabbing; XXXXX = burning; ZZZZZ = deep ache
P1 (Z, Z, Z) (S, S, S)
P2 (Z, Z, Z)
P3 (Z, Z, Z)

Figure 67.1 Body diagram completed by a patient to indicate location and quality of pain.
(Pattern resulting from right L4–5 lumbar foraminal stenosis with neurogenic claudication. Provided courtesy of Mark J. Levsen, Assistant Professor, Physical Therapy Department, St Ambrose University, Davenport, IA, USA.)

have difficulty with the abstract thought processes required to use visual analogue scales, these scales been found to be useful and reliable with older patients (Herr & Mobily 1993).

The Graphic Rating Scale (GRS) combines a visual analogue pain rating scale with word descriptors (e.g. mild, moderate, severe). It is important that the word descriptors be placed without spacing along the line between endpoint anchors in order to improve the distribution of patient responses.

Herr and colleagues have provided support for the use of the Faces Pain Scale (FPS) with both cognitively intact and cognitively impaired older individuals (Herr et al 1998, Taylor et al 2005). This scale consists of seven cartoon facial depictions arranged in order from least to most distressed (Fig. 67.3).The patient points to the face that best represents the intensity of their pain. An ordinal pain intensity value ranging from 0 (face at left) to 6 (face at right) is then assigned by the clinician. In order to improve visualization by some older patients, it has been suggested that the height of the faces be increased to 4 cm, and facial markings be darkened and slightly separated.

The McGill Pain Questionnaire (MPQ) is the most widely recognized multidimensional tool for assessing pain in the general population. It includes a body diagram for locating sites of pain. Sensory, affective and evaluative qualities of pain are assessed using a pain rating index that is based on word descriptors. Pain intensity is measured with a five-category present pain intensity scale. A short form of the MPQ has reduced tool administration time from 15 minutes to 5 minutes or less (Melzack 1987). Although this short form may be less fatiguing, complex word descriptors may present difficulty to some individuals based on their educational level, verbal intelligence and cognitive impairments.

Most of these pain rating scales have been criticized for focusing on the intensity of pain while excluding other important qualitative pain characteristics. It has been recommended that a comprehensive evaluation of pain should include both unidimensional (e.g. VDS, VAPS) and multidimensional (i.e. MPQ) measures as each assesses an important part of the overall pain experience (Gagliese & Melzack 1997). Alternatively, the 24-item Geriatric Pain Measure questionnaire assess pain intensity, patient disengagement, and pain during ambulation, strenuous activities, and other activities (Ferrell et al 2000).

To date, only a small number of studies have critically assessed methods of rating pain used exclusively by older individuals. Goode & Barr (1993) found that a majority of community-active older people felt that the PE (i.e. NRS) was both easier to use and better described their recollected pain than the VAPS. Utilizing the FPS, NRS, VAPS and VDS with cognitively intact older individuals, almost half of whom were African Americans, Stuppy (1998) concluded that a majority preferred the FPS, which was also valid and reliable. Herr & Mobily (1993) determined that community-based elderly people preferred and found the VDS easier to use than the VAPS, the NRS or the PT. Using ambulatory geriatric clinic patients, Ferrell et al (2000) reported that the GPM was both valid and reliable. Wynne et al (2000) found that more than half of their cognitively impaired long-term care residents could utilize the FPS, VAS and VRS, but not the McGill word scale; lower cognitive function made completion of these scales more difficult. Examining cognitively impaired community elderly (mean Mini Mental State Exam score = 15.7), Krulewitch et al (2000) determined that over 40% could complete the VAS, FPS and the Philadelphia Pain Intensity Scale. For those able to complete one or two scales, the greatest number completed the Philadelphia Scale. This six-item scale requires patients to assess pain at four points in time (i.e. over past few weeks, right now, at its worst and at its least) and to determine how much pain has interfered with daily activities [using integer ratings from '1' (not at all) to '5' (extremely)], and to note how many days a week that pain gets really bad. Further research is needed to determine the intertester reliability and validity of this scale (Parmelee 1994). Most recently, Taylor et al (2005) reported that both cognitively intact and cognitively impaired older assisted living residents preferred the VDS and IPT over the NRS and FPS. Concurrent validity was support for all assessment tools, except for the FPS when used by the cognitively impaired group. Test–retest reliability was acceptable for the cognitively intact subjects using all these assessment tools, but was unacceptable for the cognitively impaired group for all tools except the VDS.

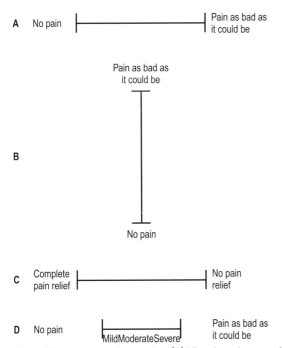

Figure 67.2 Simple pain rating scales. (A) Visual analogue pain rating scale (horizontal). (B) Visual analogue pain rating scale (vertical). (C) Visual analogue pain relief rating scale. (D) Graphic rating scale.
(Reproduced with permission from Barr 2000.)

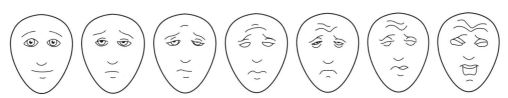

Figure 67.3   The faces pain scale.
(Reproduced with permission from Bieri et al 1990.)

A number of practical suggestions for assessing pain experienced by older people have appeared in the literature (Herr & Mobily 1991, Taylor et al 2005). The health status of the patient/client, severity of pain and ability to cooperate should guide the number and complexity of evaluation sessions needed for adequate pain assessment. It is crucial to establish good rapport and to avoid being rushed during evaluation sessions, both increasingly difficult tasks in today's healthcare system. Impairments in vision, hearing, speech, and mental processes should be taken into account and accommodated as these will have a direct impact on the use of specific pain assessment tools. Lighting should be adequate and larger print on evaluation tools may be needed. The patient must be able to successfully use a pain measurement tool, with supervision and even coaching if necessary. In the presence of cognitive impairment, time must be provided for patients to assimilate questions and to formulate their responses. A daily pain log or diary can be used by patients and caregivers to document pain intensity, medications, response to treatment, and functional activities. Family members, friends, and other healthcare workers can provide useful information about changes in behavior or functioning related to pain. Observational assessment, with inferences drawn from facial expression, body language, and other nonverbal behaviors, can be used to identify pain in severely demented older people (Box 67.1).

CONCLUSION

Appropriate evaluation of pain is critical to effective pain management for older people. Clinicians should utilize an individualized approach when evaluating pain, taking into account an array of age-related factors and patient/client preferences in the selection of a pain assessment tool. Specific diagnoses associated with aging (e.g. dementias, including Alzheimer's disease) will require the development, validation and reliability testing of new pain assessment tools.

References

American Geriatrics Society Panel on Persistent Pain in Older Persons 2000 Clinical practice guidelines: the management of persistent pain in older persons. J Am Geriatr Soc 50:S205–S224

Barr JO 2000 Conservative pain management for the older patient. In: Guccione AA (ed.) Geriatric Physical Therapy, 2nd edn. Mosby, St Louis, MO

Bieri D, Reeve RA, Champion GD et al 1990 The Faces Pain Scale for the self-assessment of the severity of pain experienced by children: development, initial validation, and preliminary investigation for ratio scale properties. Pain 41:139–150

Burke SO, Jerret M 1989 Pain management across age groups. West J Nurs Res 11:164–178

Ferrell BA, Stein WM, Beck JC 2000 The Geriatric Pain Measure: validity, reliability and factor analysis. J Am Geriatr Soc 48(12):1669–1673

Ferrell BR, Ferrell BA (eds) 1996 Pain in the Elderly. IASP Press, Seattle, WA

Gagliese L, Melzack R 1997 Chronic pain in elderly people. Pain 70:3–14

Goode J, Barr JO 1993 Comparison of two methods of pain assessment by the elderly: pain estimate (PE) vs. visual analogue scale (VAS). Phys Ther 73:6S

Herr KA, Mobily PR 1991 Complexities of pain assessment in the elderly: clinical considerations. J Gerontol Nurs 17:12–19

Herr KA, Mobily PR 1993 Comparison of selected pain assessment tools for use with the elderly. Appl Nurs Res 6:39–46

Herr KA, Mobily PR, Kohout FJ et al 1998 Evaluation of the faces pain scale for use with elderly. Clin J Pain 14:29–38

Joint Commission on Accreditation of Healthcare Organizations 1999 Pain Management Standards. Available: http://www.jcaho.org. Accessed 27 July 2005

Krulewitch H, London MR, Skakel V et al 2000 Assessment of pain in cognitively impaired older adults: a comparison of pain assessment tools and their use by nonprofessional caregivers. J Am Geriatr Soc 48:1607–1611

Melzack R 1987 The short-form McGill Pain Questionnaire. Pain 30:191–197

Molony SL, Kobayashi M, Holleran EA, Mezey M 2005 Assessing pain as a fifth vital sign in long-term care facilities: recommendations from the field. J Gerontol Nurs 31(3):16–24

Parmelee PA 1994 Assessment of pain in the elderly. In: Lawton MP, Teresi J (eds) Annual Review of Gerontology and Geriatrics. Springer, New York

Stuppy D 1998 The Faces Pain Scale: reliability and validity with mature adults. Appl Nurs Res 11(2):84–89

Taylor JT, Harris J, Epps CD et al 2005 Psychometric evaluation of selected pain intensity scales for use with cognitively impaired and cognitively intact older adults. Rehabil Nurs 30(2):55–61

Tierney LM, McPhee SJ, Papadakis MA (eds) 2003 Current Medical Diagnosis and Treatment, 42nd edn. Lange Medical Books/McGraw-Hill, New York

Weiner D, Pieper C, McConnell E et al 1996 Pain measurement in elders with chronic low back pain: traditional and alternative approaches. Pain 67:461–467

Wright GE, Parker JC, Smarr KL et al 1998 Age, depressive symptoms, and rheumatoid arthritis. Arthritis Rheumatol 41:298–305

Wynne CF, Ling SM, Remsburg R 2000 Comparison of pain assessment instruments in cognitively intact and cognitively impaired nursing home residents. Geriatr Nurs 21(1):20–23

UNIT **9**

Special physical therapeutic intervention techniques

Chapter **68**

Conservative interventions for pain control

John O. Barr

INTRODUCTION

Successful physical rehabilitation of older people requires that pain be eliminated or minimized to a level that allows the improvement of related impairments [e.g. weakness, low endurance, loss of joint range of motion (ROM), etc.], the removal of functional limitations (e.g. inability to ambulate independently, ability to sit for only brief periods, etc.) and the prevention of disability (e.g. inability to work at community food bank or to travel to visit grandchildren, etc.). Analgesic medications are the most common treatment used for pain management in older adults. However, hazards associated with some popular medications used for pain control by the elderly are becoming increasingly well known. Factors related to proper pharmacological management of pain are discussed in Chapter 12. Although Clinical Practice Guidelines established by the American Geriatrics Society emphasize pharmacologic interventions for persistent pain, nonpharmacologic approaches alone or in combination with medications should be an integral part of care (American Geriatrics Society Panel on Persistent Pain in Older Persons 2002). Proper use of conservative interventions for pain control can lessen the need for medications and may allow postponement of elective surgery for some painful conditions that are common in older adults. Unfortunately, conservative nonpharmacologic interventions are still often not used in the management of some diagnoses associated with pain in older individuals (Shrier et al 2006), and some interventions commonly recommended for pain control may not be frequently employed (Leseberg & Schunk 1990). Importantly, patients aged 55 years and older benefit as much as, if not more than, younger patients who participate in multidisciplinary chronic pain rehabilitation (Middaugh et al 1988).

This chapter reviews evidence regarding the effectiveness of conservative interventions commonly used to control pain experienced by older people (i.e. individuals aged 55 years and more). Interventions discussed include assistive devices and orthotics, massage, electrical stimulation, thermal agents, and exercise. Information from systematic reviews focused on diagnoses common for older people, and randomized control trials (RCTs) limited to older individuals are emphasized. The former include reviews conducted by the Philadelphia Panel (2001) and the Cochrane Collaboration (2006). Theoretical mechanisms of action for these interventions in controlling pain are outlined in Box 68.1 (Barr 2000).

ASSISTIVE AND ORTHOTIC DEVICES

Properly selected and fitted assistive or orthotic devices act to limit mechanical forces that would otherwise stimulate pain at a site of pathology, inflammation or trauma (see Box 68.1). Canes and walkers are among the most common assistive devices used by older individuals with pain. Hip joint contact forces can be reduced by over 30% using a cane held in the hand opposite to the involved hip. Raised seats on toilets and chairs act to limit joint forces at the hips and knees during push-off from a seated position.

Impact-absorbing shoes may help to relieve foot, ankle, knee and hip pain from osteoarthritis (OA). Hodge et al (1999) assessed foot orthotics (prefabricated, standard custom molded, custom with metatarsal bar, custom with metatarsal dome) for older patients with rheumatoid arthritis (RA). Pressure at the first and second metatarsal heads was significantly reduced by all orthoses tested. The standard custom molded and dome orthoses significantly decreased walking pain. However, only the dome orthosis significantly decreased pain during standing, and it was preferred by a majority of patients. A pilot study by Seligman & Dawson (2003) demonstrated that a combination of customized heel pads and soft orthotic inserts produced a significant decrease in heel pain from plantar fasciitis.

Knee pain from medial compartment OA may be decreased by the use of lateral heel wedges in shoes. These wedges shift more of the joint loading to the lateral side of the knee. With medial femorotibial osteoarthritis, Maillefert et al (2001) found that, when compared with neutral insoles, laterally wedged insoles were associated with significantly decreased nonsteroidal anti-inflammatory drug (NSAID) consumption at 6 months. However, scores on Western Ontario & McMaster Universities Osteoarthritis (WOMAC) index subscales for pain, joint stiffness and physical function did not differ significantly for the two types of insoles. In a 2-year follow-up, Pham et al (2004) found essentially the same outcomes, plus no significant difference in the rates of joint space narrowing. Interestingly, using lateral wedges in combination with subtalar straps for 6 months, Toda &

Box 68.1 Primary theoretical mechanisms of action for conservative interventions used to manage pain (adapted from Barr 2000)

Decrease activity of nociceptors or their sensory neurons

Limit mechanical stresses through:
- Use of assistive gait device (e.g. cane or walker) or orthotic (e.g. shoe insert, splint or brace)
- Minimizing effects of gravity via hydrotherapy or swimming
- Preventing acute edema formation with ice, compression and elevation
- Resorption of chronic edema via mild heat, massage, elevation, compression or electrical stimulation
- Elongation of connective tissue using vigorous heat (diathermy or ultrasound) and prolonged stretch
- Restoration of normal joint arthrokinematics via joint mobilization, stretching or strengthening exercise
- Application of ergonomic principles

Limit effects of depolarizing and sensitizing agents through:
- Enhanced local circulation with mild to moderate heat, massage, exercise or electrical stimulation
- Decreased local metabolic activity with cryotherapy (e.g. cold pack or ice massage)
- Decreased muscle spasm via heat, cold, massage, TENS or exercise

Create local anesthetic or anti-inflammatory effects through:
- Iontophoresis (e.g. with lidocaine (lignocaine) or dexamethasone)
- Phonophoresis (e.g. with hydrocortisone)
- Cryotherapy (e.g. cold pack or ice massage)
- TENS

Increase activity of mechanoreceptors or their sensory neurons

Stimulate mechanoreceptors through:
- Passive and active joint range of motion (ROM) exercise
- Joint mobilization
- Comfortable massage (e.g. effleurage and petrissage)
- Voluntary (e.g. walking, swimming, bicycling) or electrically stimulated exercise

Directly stimulate large-diameter neurons from mechanoreceptors through:
- Comfortable low- to moderate-intensity TENS (e.g. conventional, pulse-burst or modulated TENS)

Increase descending or spinal level inhibition within the central nervous system

Use of uncomfortable 'counterirritants' such as:
- Intense massage (e.g. vigorous kneading, strong friction, acupressure, connective tissue massage)
- Uncomfortable but tolerated TENS (e.g. strong low-rate, brief-intense or hyperstimulation TENS)
- Uncomfortable brief ice massage

TENS, transcutaneous electrical nerve stimulation.

Tsukimura (2004) demonstrated significant decreases in both the femorotibial angle and pain but no significant changes with traditional insoles. Knee braces incorporating a varus unloader increase femorotibial separation during walking and can be used for unicompartmental knee pain, but these have not been found to be effective for obese patients with knee OA (Buckwalter et al 2001). Systematically reviewing brace and orthotic effectiveness in the treatment of knee OA, Brouwer et al (2005) concluded that laterally wedged insoles decrease pain medications and may decrease pain, and a knee brace is better than a neoprene sleeve in improving pain, stiffness and function; however, a 13% incidence of low back, foot sole and posterior knee pain is associated with strapped insoles.

Spinal orthoses can provide varying degrees of immobilization, plus important tactile cues, for patients with neck and back pain. While a soft cervical collar does little to immobilize, tactile cueing can help a patient with mild spondylosis to limit motion or improve alignment of the cervical spine. For a patient with RA and atlantoaxial subluxation, a rigid Philadelphia collar or a sternal–occipitoandibular immobilizer (SOMI) may be required.

Kyphosis related to spinal osteoporosis often causes chronic upper and middle back pain in older women. A cruciform anterior spinal hyperextension (CASH) orthosis or Jewett hyperextension orthosis can be used to limit spinal flexion. In contrast, an orthosis that limits extension, such as a Williams flexion orthosis, can be used to control pain from spinal stenosis. Compression fractures from spinal osteoporosis

may call for a thoracic lumbosacral orthosis (TLSO). Pfeifer et al (2004) evaluated the 'Spinomed', a lightweight perispinal metal orthosis, with an abdominal pad and shoulder straps. It was worn a mere 2 hours per day by women with osteoporotic vertebral fractures. At the end of 6 months, orthosis wearers demonstrated: a 38% decrease in 'average' pain; a 27% decrease in limits of daily living; an 11% decrease in kyphotic angle; a 25% decrease in sway; and an increase of 73% in back extension and 58% in abdominal flexor strength.

Special considerations

When using assistive devices to limit forces on the lower extremities or spine, the clinician should be careful not to overload the patient's upper extremities. Adverse effects of orthotic use include skin breakdown due to pressure from orthotic components, psychological dependency, and weakening of muscles whose action has been limited by the orthosis. Proper evaluation, selection, fit and short-term use of assistive devices and orthotics can help to prevent these problems.

MASSAGE

Massage is defined as the intentional and systematic manipulation of soft body tissues to enhance health and healing (Benjamin &

Table 68.1 Common modes of transcutaneous electrical nerve stimulation (TENS) for pain (adapted from Barr 2000)

Mode classification	TENS unit output characteristics	Electrode site options	Desired perceptual–motor experience
'Conventional'	Frequency: 10–100 Hz Intensity: low to medium	At perimeter of painful area; over nerve to region; or at segmentally related area	Comfortable paresthesia superimposed on painful area, or in segmentally related area
'Strong low-rate' (or 'acupuncture-like')	Frequency: <10 Hz Intensity: high	Over nerve related to muscle in or remote from painful area	Uncomfortable rhythmic muscle contractions at patient tolerance
'Brief-intense'	Frequency: 60–150 Hz Intensity: high	Over nerve related to muscle in or remote from painful area	Uncomfortable tetanic muscle contraction that fatigues, at patient tolerance
'Pulse-burst'	Frequency: high (60–100 Hz) modulated by low (0.5–4 Hz) Intensity: low to high	Over nerve related to muscle in or remote from painful area	Weak to strong intermittent tetanic muscle contraction and paresthesia
'Modulated'	Frequency, pulse duration, or amplitude modulated separately or together Intensity: low to high	Any of these listed sites	Weak to strong sensation, with or without muscle contraction; may minimize perceptual accommodation
'Hyperstimulation'	Frequency: 1–100 Hz Intensity: high, based on current density	Acupuncture points	Sharp burning sensation at tolerance; no muscle contraction

Tappan 2005). There are many varieties of massage, ranging from the comfortable and gentle superficial stroking of effleurage, to the invigorating kneading of petrissage, to uncomfortable forms of deep friction massage. Potential mechanisms underlying pain relief with these various forms of massage are noted in Box 68.1.

Although the Philadelphia Panel (2001) concluded that there were insufficient data for the general population to reach a conclusion about the effect of massage for low back pain, neck pain, and shoulder pain, a systematic review by Furlan et al (2002) determined that massage can provide some relief for subacute and chronic back pain, especially in combination with stretching exercises and patient education.

A limited number of studies on massage have been conducted exclusively with older individuals. While slow stroke back massage used with older nursing home and hospice homecare patients significantly decreased heart rate and blood pressure and significantly increased skin temperature after the intervention, pain was not assessed in these studies (Fakouri and Jones 1987, Meek 1993). Sansone & Schmitt (2000) had trained certified nursing assistants (CNAs) to provide 'tender touch' massage to older nursing home residents suffering from chronic pain and dementia over a period of 12 weeks. Patients experienced decreased pain and anxiety scores, and the CNAs reported improved ability to communicate with the residents. Mok & Woo (2004) determined that 10 minutes of nightly slow stroke back massage given to hospitalized patients with shoulder pain after cerebrovascular accident was associated with significantly decreased pain and anxiety that lasted for up to 3 days when compared with a control group.

Special considerations

Massage is a safe intervention with a low risk of adverse effects. General contraindications for massage include skin infections, active inflammation, and deep vein thrombosis. Specific contraindications for massage can be related to both the underlying pathology and the amount of force provided by a specific massage procedure.

Contraindications would include, for example: superficial stroking over open wounds and areas of acute inflammation or infection; kneading massage to limbs at risk of deep vein thrombosis, with a nonconsolidated fracture, active cancer tumor, thrombophlebitis, or during anticoagulant therapy; and friction massage over a recently healed burn wound.

Vigorous massage strokes, such as deep effleurage or petrissage, should not be applied to fragile skin that is prone to tearing, as is encountered with many frail elderly individuals. Because of massage's influence in lowering heart rate and blood pressure, the clinician must be aware of other medical conditions (e.g. postural hypotension) that could be aggravated. Older individuals may require special positioning to receive massage based on underlying medical conditions (e.g. severe chronic obstructive pulmonary disease, preventing the use of a recumbent position) or deformity (e.g. severe kyphosis, limiting positioning in prone lying) (Benjamin & Tappan 2005).

ELECTRICAL STIMULATION

Clinical electrical stimulation as done by nonphysician rehabilitation professionals (e.g. physical therapists, occupational therapists, nurses and their assistants) is done using electrodes placed on the surface of the skin to stimulate nerves transcutaneously. More specifically, transcutaneous electrical nerve stimulation (TENS) involves the stimulation of cutaneous and peripheral nerves to control pain. At least six types, or 'modes', of TENS have been described in the literature: conventional (or 'high frequency'), strong low-rate (or 'acupuncture-like'), brief intense, pulse-burst, modulated and hyperstimulation (Barr 2000). Box 68.1 outlines the potential mechanisms of action for these common TENS modes.

Each mode of TENS involves specific electrical stimulator output characteristics that produce different perceptual-motor experiences related to the relief of pain (see Table 68.1). Placement of electrodes varies with the TENS mode used and can include positioning of a pair of electrodes: at the perimeter of the painful area (i.e. 'bracketing' the area); over a cutaneous or peripheral nerve proximal to the painful area; over a peripheral nerve to a muscle in the painful area; with one electrode over the site of pain and the other paraspinally over the related segmental nerve root; or at related acupuncture points.

The Cochrane Collaboration has published systematic reviews concerned with electrical stimulation for pain control, which have included older patients among their subjects. Osiri et al (2000) assessed the effectiveness of TENS in treating knee OA. Pain relief from TENS and acupuncture-like TENS delivered over at least 4 weeks was significantly better than placebo treatment; knee stiffness was also significantly improved by TENS. Different TENS modes (high-rate and strong-burst) had significant benefit in pain relief over placebo. The Philadelphia Panel (2001) also found clinically important benefit for pain and patient global assessment, and noted good evidence to include TENS as an intervention for pain associated with knee OA. However, electrical stimulation/TENS was determined either to be of no benefit or to have insufficient data relative to low back pain, knee pain after surgery or associated with tendonitis, chronic neck pain, and for non-specific shoulder pain or shoulder pain from calcific tendonitis.

Two other applications of electrical stimulation have been systematically reviewed. Brosseau et al (2003) evaluated the effectiveness of TENS for the treatment of RA of the hand. Acupuncture-like TENS was determined to be beneficial in reducing resting pain (but not grip pain) and joint tenderness, and in improving muscle power compared with placebo. Conventional TENS had no clinical benefit for pain compared with placebo. Oddly, more patients receiving conventional TENS than acupuncture-like TENS were reported to have assessed their RA disease activity as decreasing. Price & Pandyan (2000) assessed the efficacy of common forms of surface electrical stimulation for preventing and treating poststroke shoulder pain. Evidence from the RCTs reviewed was not seen to either confirm or refute that electrical stimulation (including TENS) to the shoulder after stroke influenced reports of pain; however, passive lateral rotation of the shoulder appeared to benefit. No adverse effects were documented.

To date, only a small number of studies have been found that examined the effect of TENS exclusively with older adults. Grant et al (1999) compared acupuncture with TENS for chronic back pain. Both interventions significantly improved pain scores and decreased analgesic intake after 4 weeks of treatment and for up to 3 months after treatment. Barr and associates (2004) applied conventional TENS, high-intensity pulse-burst TENS, and sham TENS to assisted-living residents with chronic musculoskeletal pain. Pain was decreased significantly for both conventional and pulse-burst TENS, averaging 23% and 32% respectively. Not surprisingly, low-intensity conventional TENS was found to be more comfortable than high-intensity pulse-burst TENS. Most recently, Defrin et al (2005) treated patients with knee OA with either innocuous or noxious (hyperstimulation) intensities of interferential current (IFC) electrical stimulation. IFC to the knee produced significant decreases in chronic pain and morning stiffness, and significant increases in ROM and pain threshold. ICF was deemed to be very effective (with hyperstimulation being most effective in decreasing the intensity of knee pain).

Special considerations

The most common problem associated with TENS for a small number of patients at any age is dermatitis at the electrode sites. Dry skin associated with aging and the use of alcohol-based skin care products can increase skin resistance to the flow of electrical current, which then requires higher intensity stimulation. This may cause discomfort and irritation to the skin. The use of additional electrode gel, slight moistening of an electrode's synthetic surface, and hydration of the skin with a nonalcohol-based cream can lower skin impedance and increase comfort for these patients. Regular use of alternate electrode sites can prevent the breakdown of fragile skin due to the cumulative effects of allergic, chemical, electrical and mechanical irritation. To prevent tearing of the skin during electrode removal, electrodes should be peeled off gently and slowly while holding down the underlying skin.

The primary contraindication for TENS in older adults is use near areas with implanted electrical devices, such as older demand-type (synchronous) cardiac pacemakers that may be affected by the field generated by the stimulator. All patients with cardiac pacemakers should be electrically monitored during initial trials and extended use of TENS. If interference is noted, it may be possible to have the cardiologist reprogram the pacemaker to a lower level of sensitivity (Chen et al 1990).

In order to facilitate appropriate use and adherence, rehabilitation professionals should be familiar with the options available for TENS units and their components. TENS units that require no adjustment of complex controls may be best suited for a patient with cognitive limitations who needs to use TENS as part of a home program. Self-adhering electrodes or electrodes that are incorporated into a band with a Velcro closure may be the best option for an older adult with limited mobility or impaired hand dexterity.

THERMAL AGENTS

The thermal agents used in pain control include a variety of therapeutic cooling and heating modalities that have both direct and reflex effects. Thermal agents can target body tissues at various depths, ranging from the skin to the muscle/bone interface. The effective depths of penetration for common thermal agents are depicted in Table 68.2.

Superficial heating agents (e.g. hot packs, warm hydrotherapy, paraffin, fluidotherapy and infrared) or deep heating agents (e.g. short-wave and microwave diathermy, and ultrasound) can be used to increase blood flow, membrane permeability, tissue extensibility and joint ROM in ways that can contribute to decreasing pain. Heat and cold alter both peripheral and central nervous system excitability, and can thus serves as a means of modulating pain. Brief uncomfortable application of cold (e.g. brief ice massage) can be used as a 'counterirritant' to decrease pain (see Box 68.1 for the theoretical mechanisms of action).

The Philadelphia Panel (2001) determined in the general population that thermal agents were either of no benefit or lacked evidence to either include or exclude them as a therapeutic intervention for chronic low back pain, neck pain, shoulder pain and knee pain from OA or after surgery. However, ultrasound was found to have a clinically important benefit in managing pain associated with shoulder calcific tendonitis.

Only a couple of additional systematic reviews have been conducted for thermal agents. Robinson et al (2002) evaluated thermotherapy used for RA. While no significant effects on pain were determined for hot or ice packs, positive results on pain were seen with paraffin wax baths and nonresisted exercise after four consecutive weeks of treatment. Assessing thermotherapy for treatment of OA, Brosseau et al (2004) determined that, while ice massage had significant beneficial effect on knee ROM, strength and function, and cold packs decreased swelling, neither had a significant impact on pain.

Over the past 50 years, a large number of studies have attempted to establish either the efficacy or the effectiveness of thermal agents

Table 68.2 Depth of effective penetration into the body by common thermal agents (reproduced with permission from Barr 2000)

Thermal agent	Depth into soft tissues
Cold pack	2 mm–4 cm
Hot pack	2–5 mm
Hydrotherapy (warm)	2–5 mm
Paraffin	2–5 mm
Fluidotherapy	2–5 mm
Infrared	
Nonluminous	2–5 mm
Luminous	5 mm–1 cm
Short-wave diathermy (27.12 MHz; subcutaneous fat <2 cm thick)	1–3 cm
Microwave diathermy (2450 MHz; nondirect contact applicator; subcutaneous fat <0.5 cm thick)	1–5 cm
Ultrasound	
3 MHz	1–2 cm
1 MHz	1–5 cm

in controlling pain and related clinical problems. Unfortunately, only a few studies have specifically focused on older patients. In some instances, opposing thermal agents (i.e. cold vs. heat) have been shown to have equivalent effects on pain for some clinical pain problems. Hamer & Kirk (1976) compared cryotherapy (i.e. towels dipped in crushed ice and water) with ultrasound in the treatment of chronic shoulders that included active and passive exercise. While both agents were associated with improved pain, there were no significant differences between treatments relative to pain grade improvement, number of treatments, or shoulder rotation. Williams et al (1986) compared cold and hot packs, both combined with exercise, in treating RA affecting the shoulder. Although both groups demonstrated improvement, there were no significant between-group differences for changes in pain or shoulder ROM (flexion or abduction). These findings may reflect separate but equally potent mechanisms of pain relief, which, when combined with exercise, act to further control pain and enhance function. Assessing the effects of short-wave diathermy (SWD) vs. a placebo control treatment on knee OA, Wright (1964) determined better, but not significantly greater, long-term improvements for SWD. Also evaluating effects for knee OA, Clarke et al (1974) found that ice bags applied above and below the knee produced short-term significant improvements in knee pain and stiffness in comparison with both actual and sham SWD.

The proposed theoretical mechanisms of action may not be supported (Box 68.1), however. For example, Klemp et al (1982) determined that ultrasound treatment of chronic fibromyotic upper trapezius muscles actually resulted in a significant *decrease* in muscle blood flow during treatment. Interventions that can afford pain relief for older people need not be technically complex. Robinson & Benton (2002) determined that the use of warm blankets for elderly hospitalized patients produced reduced levels of discomfort (e.g. pain, being cold or feeling anxious).

Special considerations

A range of precautions for thermal agents used with older adults have been discussed by Kauffman (1987). Contributing to an increased risk of thermal injury are factors such as: decreased hypothalamic thermoregulatory system reactivity; decreased autonomic and vasomotor responses; impairments in the circulatory system; loss of sweat glands; atrophy of skin and related reduction in circulation; decreased sensation of thirst; and decreased perception of thermal gradients. Medications can impair thermoregulatory control. For example, vasodilation of the skin may be hampered by diuretics which limit volume expansion. Anticholinergic drugs, dermatologic conditions and spinal cord lesions can impair sweating. Long-term use of steroids produces fragile capillaries easily damaged by thermal agents. Skin vasodilation from the heating of large body surface areas can produce hazardous demands on cardiac output. Cold agents may produce short-term increases in systolic and diastolic blood pressures, posing a risk for hypertensive patients. Cold agents may be associated with increases in mechanical stiffness of joints and cold intolerance for some patients.

Considerations for older patients when using thermal agents include (Barr 2000):

1. Selecting an appropriate thermal agent for a given clinical condition. Deep heating of joints involved with pathologies such as OA should be avoided because it may contribute to temperature-sensitive enzymatic lysis of joint cartilage. Superficial moist heating for less than 20 minutes has actually been shown to produce lowering of joint temperature. However, with arthritic knees, intra-articular temperature 3 hours after treatment is increased by superficial heat and decreased by superficial cold agents (Oosterveld & Rasker 1994).

2. Lowering temperatures for heating agents and increasing temperatures for cooling agents. Hot and cold packs will need to be better insulated by using a greater thickness of toweling. If the patient can only be positioned comfortably by resting on top of these packs, additional layers of toweling must be used because of compression of the insulating layers.

3. Producing a slower rate of temperature change, particularly for ultrasound, which provides rapid deep temperature elevation. This can be accomplished by using a lower intensity, faster sound head movement and less overlap of sound head strokes.

4. Shortening treatment time. The traditional 30 minutes for superficial heating agents may need to be limited to no longer than 20 minutes. More conservative treatment durations for deep heating agents may be appropriate. For example, it may be necessary to perform ultrasound for 5 minutes for each 150 cm^2, as opposed to 5 minutes for an area two to three times the sound head area (20–30 cm^2).

Although the above modifications may improve the safety of thermal agents used with older patients, further research is needed to determine whether the resultant treatment effects are increased or diminished.

EXERCISE

Exercise programs can range from low intensity (e.g. walking) to high intensity (e.g. strengthening or endurance exercises) and may include specific types of exercises, such as trunk flexion, extension or 'core' strengthening programs. Various forms of exercise may be employed to modulate pain either directly or indirectly, as depicted in Box 68.1.

A direct effect on pain may be achieved by increasing input from joint mechanoreceptors through passive or active exercise. Indirect effects of exercise on pain may be related to: increased blood flow that disperses chemical depolarizing/sensitizing agents; decreased edema; inhibition or fatigue of muscle spasm; enhanced ROM, flexibility, strength or endurance, which may improve biomechanical factors; and relaxation and reduction in anxiety. Additionally, exercise is an important adjunct to other interventions (e.g. thermal agents, patient education, etc.) in attaining significant relief from chronic pain (Allegrante 1996).

In the general population, the Philadelphia Panel (2001) determined that therapeutic exercise has clinically important benefit for: low back pain (i.e. postsurgical, subacute, and chronic, but not for acute); knee pain (i.e. associated with OA; but not when done preoperatively for postsurgical pain); and chronic neck pain. Insufficient evidence was found relative to shoulder pain due to calcific tendonitis or non-specific shoulder pain. A systematic review by van Baar et al (1999) determined that there was evidence of beneficial effects of exercise for OA of the knee or hip. However, a more recent systematic review by Fransen et al (2001) using more extensive databases found that, although land-based exercise reduced pain and improved physical function for patients with knee OA, studies were insufficient to determine the value of exercise for hip OA.

A few specific RCTs warrant specific mention. Minor et al (1989) compared 12 weeks of aerobic walking, aerobic aquatics, nonaerobic active ROM, and relaxation exercises for chronic RA and OA. Both the aerobic and the nonaerobic exercises demonstrated significant improvements in pain, and there was no significant difference between these groups. Ferrell et al (1997) assigned older adults with chronic musculoskeletal pain to 6 weeks of a supervised program of walking, a pain education program (i.e. demonstrations on heat, cold, massage, relaxation and distraction), or 'usual care' (i.e. continuation of already prescribed treatments, printed information about pain management, and weekly phone calls from a nurse educator). Pain improved significantly for patients in both intervention programs but not for those receiving usual care. Baker et al (2001) assessed the effectiveness of a 4-month progressive high-intensity home exercise program (HEP) on knee OA for community-dwelling elderly people (vs. nutrition education as a control group). Outcomes included significantly greater improvements for the HEP (vs. the control group) relative to pain, strength, and improved function. Evaluating the impact of a 12-week Sun-style T'ai Chi exercise program for women with knee OA, Song et al (2003) found that T'ai Chi was associated with significantly less joint pain and stiffness, fewer difficulties in physical function, improved balance, and increased abdominal muscle strength in comparison with a nonexercise control group. Most recently, Lin et al (2004) evaluated the effectiveness of a 12-month community-based water exercise program for sedentary community-dwelling elderly individuals (vs. monthly education combined with quarterly phone calls). Exercise participants had significantly better improvements in pain, physical function, ability to ascend/descend stairs, and both hip and knee ROM; however, differences were not significant for quadriceps strength and for ratings of psychological well-being.

While all the above-noted studies support the effectiveness of exercise in helping to control pain experience by older people, the effects of a specific period of training do have their limits. Reassessing patients with OA of the knee and hip who had participated in 12 weeks of exercise administered by a physical therapist, van Baar et al (2001) found that a small to moderate effect on pain persisted at 6 months, but not at 9 months, post intervention. Rather than viewing exercise as a one-time rehabilitative intervention, appropriate exercises should be a regular component of a fitness program to ensure healthy aging and to compress morbidity.

Special precautions

Appropriate precautions should be followed when using exercise for pain management with older adults. During strenuous resistive exercise, a hypertensive patient who performs a Valsalva's maneuver risks a dangerous elevation in blood pressure. Severe osteoporosis and degeneration of the alar ligaments in the cervical spine in patients with RA may pose limitations for even gentle ROM exercises. Vigorous eccentric exercise in both young and old subjects induces muscle soreness 24–48 hours later. Although tissue repair rates are similar to those for younger subjects, older individuals show significantly greater muscle shortening following eccentric exercise. This may predispose the older individual to a greater risk of injury with additional exercise.

CONCLUSION

A range of conservative interventions can be successfully employed for pain control with older people. Based on studies conducted to date, the best support exists for the use of therapeutic exercise.

Practitioners who lack formal training in the use of these interventions, or do not have these interventions within their scope of practice, will need to refer patients to other members of the rehabilitation team. Historically, physical therapists have been educated in how to evaluate patients for and treat with the interventions discussed in this chapter. Increasingly, nurses and occupational therapists are being trained to use some of these interventions (e.g. heat/cold, massage, and TENS). Healthcare professionals must be knowledgeable about the strength of evidence supporting the use of conservative interventions for pain control.

Based on the limited research available (especially related to assistive devices, orthotics, and thermal agents), it is often difficult to either accept or exclude selected interventions for use in pain management with older individuals. Improved research methodologies will need to be employed in order to better examine the effectiveness and efficacy of conservative interventions, both singly and in combination, to manage a wider range of painful conditions commonly experienced by older people.

REFERENCES

Allegrante JP 1996 The role of adjunctive therapy in the management of chronic nonmalignant pain. Am J Med 101 (suppl1A):33S–39S

American Geriatrics Society Panel on Persistent Pain in Older Persons 2002 Clinical practice guidelines: the management of persistent pain in older persons. J Am Geriatr Soc 50:S205–S224

Baker KR, Nelson ME, Felson DT et al 2001 The efficacy of home based progressive strength training in older adults with knee osteoarthritis: a randomized controlled trial. J Rheumatol 28(7):1655–1665

Barr JO 2000 Conservative pain management for the older patient. In: Guccione AA (ed) Geriatric Physical Therapy, 2nd edn. Mosby, St Louis, MO, p 351–375

Barr JO, Weissenbuehler SA, Cleary CK 2004 Effectiveness and comfort of transcutaneous electrical nerve stimulation for older persons with chronic pain. J Geriatr Phys Ther 27(3):93–99

Benjamin PJ, Tappan FM 2005 Tappan's Handbook of Healing Massage Techniques – Classic, Holistic, and Emerging Methods. Pearson Prentice Hall, Upper Saddle River, NJ

Brosseau L, Judd MG, Marchand S et al 2003 Transcutaneous electrical nerve stimulation (TENS) for the treatment of rheumatoid arthritis in the hand. Cochrane Database Syst Rev Issue 2:CD004377. DOI: 10.1002/14651858.CD004377

Brosseau L, Judd MG, Marchand S et al 2004 Thermotherapy for treatment of osteoarthritis. Cochrane Database Syst Rev Issue 4:CD004522. DOI: 10.1002/14651858.CD004522

Brouwer RW, Jakma TSC, Verhagen AP et al 2005 Braces and orthoses for treating osteoarthritis of the knee. Cochrane Database Syst Rev Issue 1:CD004020. DOI: 10.1002/14651858.CD004020.pub2

Buckwalter J, Stanish W, Rosier R et al 2001 The increasing need for nonoperative treatment of patients with osteoarthritis. Clin Orthop Rel Res 385:35–45

Chen D, Philip M, Philip P et al 1990 Cardiac pacemaker inhibition by transcutaneous electrical nerve stimulation. Arch Phys Med Rehabil 71:27–30

Clarke GR, Willis LA, Stenners L et al 1974 Evaluation of physiotherapy in the treatment of osteoarthrosis of the knee. Rheumatol Rehabil 13:190–197

Cochrane Collaboration 2006 Online. Available: http://www.cochrane.org/index0.htm. Accessed 17 April 2006

Defrin R, Ariel E, Peretz C 2005 Segmental noxious versus innocuous electrical stimulation for chronic pain relief and the effect of fading sensation during treatment. Pain 115(1–2):152–160

Fakouri C, Jones P 1987 Relaxation Rx: slow stroke back rub. J Gerontol Nurs 13(2):32–35

Ferrell B, Josephson K, Pollan A et al 1997 A randomized trial of walking versus physical methods for chronic pain management. Aging 9:99–105

Fransen M, McConnell S, Bell M 2001 Exercise for osteoarthritis of the hip or knee. Cochrane Database Syst Rev Issue 2:CD004376. DOI: 10.1002/14651858.CD004376

Furlan AD, Brosseau L, Imamura M et al 2002 Massage for low-back pain. Cochrane Database Syst Rev Issue 2:CD001929. DOI: 10.1002/14651858.CD001929

Grant D, Bishop-Miller J, Winchester D et al 1999 A randomized comparative trial of acupuncture versus transcutaneous electrical nerve stimulation for chronic back pain in the elderly. Pain 82:9–13

Hamer J, Kirk JA 1976 Physiotherapy and the frozen shoulder: a comparative trial of ice and ultrasonic therapy. NZ Med J 83:191–192

Hodge M, Bach T, Carter G 1999 Orthotic management of plantar pressure and pain in rheumatoid arthritis. Clin Biomech 14:567–575

Kauffman T 1987 Thermoregulation and use of heat and cold. In: Jackson OL (ed) Therapeutic Considerations for the Elderly. Churchill Livingstone, New York

Klemp P, Staberg B, Korsgard J et al 1982 Reduced blood flow in fibromyotic muscles during ultrasound therapy. Scand J Rehabil Med 15:21–23

Leseberg KA, Schunk C 1990 TENS and geriatrics. Clin Manage Phys Ther 10(6):23–25

Lin SY, Davey RC, Cochrane T 2004 Community rehabilitation for older adults with osteoarthritis of the lower limb: a controlled clinical trial. Clin Rehabil 18(1):92–101

Maillefert J, Hudry C, Baron G et al 2001 Laterally elevated wedged insoles in the treatment of medial knee osteoarthritis: a prospective randomized controlled study. Osteoarthritis Cartilage 9:738–745

Meek SS 1993 Effects of slow stroke back massage on relaxation in hospice clients. Image J Nurs Sch 25(1):17–21

Middaugh S, Levin R, Kee W et al 1988 Chronic pain: Its treatment in geriatric and younger patients. Arch Phys Med Rehabil 69:1021–1026

Minor MA, Hewitt JE, Webel RR et al 1989 Efficacy of physical conditioning exercise in patients with rheumatoid arthritis and osteoarthritis. Arthritis Rheumatol 32:1396–1405

Mok K, Woo CP 2004 The effects of slow-stroke back massage on anxiety and shoulder pain in elderly stroke patients. Compl Ther Nurs Midwifery 10(4):209–216

Oosterveld FG, Rasker JJ 1994 Effects of local heat and cold treatment on surface and articular temperature of arthritic knees. Arthritis Rheumatol 37(11):1578–1582

Osiri M, Brosseau L, McGowan J et al 2000 Transcutaneous electrical nerve stimulation for knee osteoarthritis. Cochrane Database Syst Rev Issue 4:CD002823. DOI: 10.1002/14651858. CD002823

Pfeifer M, Begerow B, Minne HW 2004 Effects of a new spinal orthosis on posture, trunk strength, and quality of life in women with postmenopausal osteoporosis. Am J Phys Med Rehabil 83:177–186

Pham T, Maillefert JF, Hudry C et al 2004 Laterally elevated wedged insoles in the treatment of medial knee osteo-arthritis. A two-year prospective randomized controlled study. Osteoarthritis Cartilage 12(1):46–55

Philadelphia Panel 2001 Philadelphia Panel evidence-based clinical practice guidelines on selected rehabilitation interventions. Phys Ther 81:1629–1730

Price CIM, Pandyan AD 2000 Electrical stimulation for preventing and treating post stroke shoulder pain. Cochrane Database Syst Rev Issue 4:CD001698. DOI: 10.1002/14651858.CD001698

Robinson S, Benton G 2002 Warmed blankets: an intervention to promote comfort for elderly hospitalized patients. Geriatr Nurs 23(6):320–323

Robinson VA, Brosseau L, Casimiro L et al 2002 Thermotherapy for treating rheumatoid arthritis. Cochrane Database Syst Rev Issue 2:CD002826. DOI: 10.1002/14651858.CD002826

Sansone P, Schmitt L 2000 Providing tender touch massage to elderly nursing home residents: a demonstration project. Geriatric Nurs 21(6):303–308.

Seligman DA, Dawson DR 2003 Customized heel pads and soft orthotics to treat heel pain and plantar fasciitis. Arch Phys Med Rehabil 84(10):1564–1567.

Shrier I, Feldman DE, Gaudet MC et al 2006 Conservative non-pharmacological treatment options are not frequently used in the management of hip osteoarthritis. J Sci Med Sports May 9(1–2):81–86

Song R, Lee EO, Lam P et al 2003 Effects of tai chi exercise on pain, balance, muscle strength, and perceived difficulties in physical functioning in older women with osteoarthritis: a randomized clinical trial. J Rheumatol 30(9):2039–2044

Toda Y, Tsukimura N 2004 A six-month follow-up of a randomized trial comparing the efficacy of a lateral-wedge insole with subtalar strapping and an in-shoe lateral-wedge insole in patients with varus deformity osteoarthritis of the knee. Arthritis Rheumatol 50(10):3129–3136

van Baar M, Assendelft WJ, Dekker J 1999 Effectiveness of exercise therapy in patients with osteoarthritis of the hip or knee. Arthritis Rheumatol 12:1361–1369

Williams J, Harvey J, Tannebaum H 1986 Use of superficial heat vs. ice for the rheumatoid arthritic shoulder: a pilot study. Physiother Canada 38:8–13

Wright V 1964 Treatment of osteoarthritis of the knees. Ann Rheum Dis 23:389–391

Chapter 69

Gait training

Patricia A. Hageman

CHAPTER CONTENTS

- Defining the problem
- Gait assessment
- Gait training
- Conclusion

DEFINING THE PROBLEM

Gait training is one of the most frequently prescribed rehabilitation techniques for the older adult because gait is the most common of all human movements and, as such, any pathology that affects it requires immediate attention. Normal gait includes a complex sequence of limb motions that propel the body in an energy-conserving, stable and shock-absorbing manner. Rehabilitation therapists must be aware that a healthy geriatric gait includes a wide variety of 'normal', yet disruptions in the sequence of actions are easily identified (see Table 69.1).

Gait changes due to aging, disease or disability become problematic when the individual suffers pain, has difficulty maintaining balance, lacks sufficient endurance or has insufficient ability to ambulate to meet his/her activities of daily living (ADL). Gait disorders are associated with falls in older adults. This is clinically relevant because falling is one of the leading causes of injury-related deaths among elderly people (Runyan et al 2005). For many older adults, the inability to ambulate safely results in loss of independence and frequently results in the need for institutional assistance (Guralnik et al 1994, Quadri et al 2005).

GAIT ASSESSMENT

Gait analysis must be conducted in order to determine what gait deviations and/or problems are present. There are many valid and reliable gait assessment tools that are appropriate for use with the older client. Observational gait analysis is routinely performed by clinicians and refers to the use of qualitative methods to assess gait deviations (McGinley et al 2003, Ranchos Los Amigos National Rehabilitation Center 2001). Other gait assessment methods utilize measures of distance, stability and time (see Table 69.2). Assessment of gait speed is important as it has been shown to be the single best predictor of disability and frailty among older adults (Guralnik et al 2000).

When assessing gait, the healthcare provider must consider that many specific pathologies (orthopedic, neurological, biomechanical, cardiopulmonary) may contribute to gait deviations, and that the typical elderly client usually presents with multiple problems. Individual pathologies (i.e. stroke, Parkinson's disease, etc.) may result in a typical pattern of gait deviation, but many elderly adults have one or more common gait deviations.

The *International Classification of Diseases*, 9th edition (ICD-9) recognizes the existence of gait abnormalities that have causes that cannot be clearly determined but that produce symptoms that represent important problems in medical care. The ICD-9 codes include code 781.2 Abnormality of Gait, which describes ataxic, paralytic, spastic or staggering gait patterns. The code 719.7 Difficulty in Walking is appropriate to use for individuals who demonstrate a limp or related problems during gait that are due to unspecified disorders of the pelvic region, thigh, lower leg, ankle and foot. Both codes may be appropriate to describe the gait conditions for which many elderly people require training.

GAIT TRAINING

Findings from the results of gait analysis are used to design appropriate interventions. Gait difficulties may be attributed to impaired motor control, abnormal joint range of motion, impaired sensation and/or pain. The challenge for the healthcare provider is to determine the relationship between impairments and deviations (Ranchos Los Amigos National Rehabilitation Center 2001). A single impairment can result in multiple deviations. For example, decreased plantar flexor muscle function may result in excess knee flexion, excess dorsiflexion and lack of heel off during single limb support. A single deviation may also be caused by multiple impairments. For example, excess plantar flexion may be caused by either a plantar flexion contracture or plantar flexion spasticity. Some suggested intervention strategies for common gait deviations of the elderly are included in Table 69.3.

Gait training may involve any combination of: (i) mobility and transfer activities; (ii) pregait mat and standing activities; (iii) static and dynamic balance activities; (iv) interventions during gait; and (v) adaptation of assistive devices or environment in order to reduce gait deviations.

Mobility and transfer activities include rising-to-standing and returning-to-sit. Compared with young adults, healthy older adults show similar patterns of rising from sitting, although they tend to minimize the forward body displacement during returning-to-sit. Frail elderly people frequently demonstrate difficulty in initiating

Table 69.1 Normal vs. pathological gait in the elderly

Parameter	Normal aging gait	Pathological gait
Speed	Decreased self-selected and fast speed, although ability remains to voluntarily increase speed from self-selected to fast speed	Significant decrease in free velocity (<0.85 m/s) with loss of ability to voluntarily increase speed from self-selected gait speed
Step/stride lengths	Smaller step and stride lengths but symmetrical	Significant decrease in step and stride length and/or nonsymmetrical steps
Step width	Averages 1–4 in	Step width is >4 in or less than 1 in; or too much or too little step width variability
Toe clearance	Small toe clearance	Either large toe clearance or tripping or both
Ankle–foot	Mild decrease in force at push-off and/or slight decreases in plantar flexion and dorsiflexion range of motion	Large toe clearance or tripping or both; forefoot or foot-flat contact during initial contact; excess plantar flexion or dorsiflexion
Knee	Range of motion from 5° flexion during weight acceptance to 60° of flexion during swing limb advancement	Limited or excessive flexion, wobbling; extension thrust
Hip	15–20° of flexion during weight acceptance and 15–20° of apparent hyperextension at terminal stance	Limited flexion or extension; 'past retract' meaning a visible forward and then backward movement of the thigh during terminal swing; excessive abduction or adduction; excessive or limited internal or external rotation
Pelvis	5° of forward rotation during weight acceptance; and 5° of backward rotation at terminal stance and preswing; iliac crest on reference limb is higher or equal to the iliac crest on the opposite side during midstance	Limited or excess rotation forward or backward; pelvic drop; pelvic hiking
Trunk	Erect	Forward, backward or sideways lean

Table 69.2 Gait assessment and outcome measures

Measure	Description	Findings
Dynamic Gait Index (Shumway- Cook et al 1997)	Eight elements are assessed on 0–3 scale where 3 = normal, 2 = mild impairment, 1 = moderate impairment, 0 = severely impaired. Items include: (i) 20-ft gait on level surface (pattern, speed, assistive device, balance) (ii) Change in gait speed from comfortable to fast (iii) Gait with horizontal head turns (iv) Gait with vertical head turns (v) Gait and pivot turn (vi) Step over obstacle (shoe box) (vii) Step around obstacles (cones at 6-ft intervals) (viii) Steps (using rail if necessary)	Scores of ≤19 are predictive of falls in older community-living adults
Gait Abnormality Rating Scale (GARS) (Wolfson et al 1990)	Gait is rated according to 16 elements on a four-point scale ranging from 0 to 3 where 0 is normal. Items include: (i) Variability of stepping and arm movements (ii) Guardedness in stepping and arm swing (iii) Weaving (iv) Waddling (v) Staggering	A higher GARS score indicates a more impaired gait. GARS score >18 indicates patients who are at the greatest risk of falls

(Continued)

Table 69.2   (*Continued*)

Measure	Description	Findings
	(vi) Lower extremity % time in swing (vii) Lower extremity heel contact at heel strike (viii) Lower extremity hip ROM (ix) Lower extremity knee ROM (x) Elbow extension (ROM) (xi) Shoulder extension (ROM) (xii) Shoulder abduction (pathological increase) (xiii) Arm–heel strike synchrony (xiv) Head position (check for head held forward) (xv) Shoulder position (check for elevation) (xvi) Trunk position (check for trunk flexion forward)	
Gait Abnormality Rating Scale – Modified (GARS-M) (VanSwearingen et al 1996)	Gait is rated according to seven elements on a four-point scale ranging from 0 to 3 where 0 is normal. GARS-M includes items i, ii, v, vii, viii, xi and xiii from GARS (listed above)	A higher GARS-M score indicates a more impaired gait. GARS-M scores >8 indicates those who are at the greatest risk of falls
Gait Speed (Guralnik et al 2000; Steffen et al 2002)	Instructions are 'to walk at your normal comfortable walking speed' and 'to walk as fast as you comfortably can' over an established distance (typical distances are 6 or 10 m). Note whether the distance measured included acceleration and deceleration. If preferred, measure the time to complete three consecutive stride lengths within a 9-m distance	Gait speed that is <0.8 m/s indicates a high risk of falls and/or disability
Performance Oriented Mobility Test (Tinettti 1986)	Nine elements on the Balance test (maximum score = 16) plus 10 elements on the Gait test (maximum score = 12) are assessed on either a 0, 1 or 0, 1, 2 scale with higher scores associated with better performance. Balance test items include: (i) Sitting balance (0, 1) (ii) Arise from chair (0, 1, 2) (iii) Attempts to arise from chair (0, 1, 2) (iv) Immediate standing balance upon arising (0, 1, 2) (v) Standing balance, feet close together (0, 1, 2) (vi) Standing balance with nudge to subject's sternum (0, 1, 2) (vii) Standing balance, feet close together, eyes closed (0, 1) (viii) Standing turn 360° continuity of steps (0, 1) and steadiness (0, 1) (ix) Sitting down from standing (0, 1, 2) Gait test items include: (i) Examine hesitancy at initiation of gait (0, 1) (ii) Right swing foot step length (0, 1) (iii) Right swing foot clearance (0, 1) (iv) Left swing foot step length (0, 1) (v) Left swing foot clearance (0, 1) (vi) Step symmetry (0, 1) (vii) Step continuity (0, 1) (viii) Path deviation, if any, over 10-ft course (0, 1, 2) (ix) Trunk sway or walking aid, if any (0, 1, 2) (x) Walking stance – stride width (0, 1)	Scores <19 indicate a high risk of falling, scores of 19–24 indicate moderate risk of falling, scores of 25–28 indicate a low risk of falling

(*Continued*)

Table 69.2 (*Continued*)

Measure	Description	Findings
Timed 'Up & Go' test (Podsiadlo & Richardson 1991)	Using stopwatch, start timing at 'go'. Start position is fully seated in the back of chair. Use chair with armrests. Time the period to rise from seated chair, walk 3 m, turn around, walk back to chair and sit. Document whether performed with or without use of arms (arms to be crossed over chest upon rising from chair) and whether assistive device was used	Young adults generally score <10 seconds; Older adults who take ≥13.5 seconds to perform the TUG are at greater risk of falls. Scores >30 seconds identifies individuals who will have significant difficulties in ADLs
Walk Tests (2 or 6 or 12 min) (Butland et al 1982, Enright & Sherrill 1998, Eng et al 2002)	These tests estimate maximum oxygen consumption. Using standardized instructions, the patient is instructed to walk as far as possible in the time permitted. Prediction equations of the total distance walked during the first time 6-min walk for healthy adults (40–80 years): For men: distance (m) = [7.57 × height (cm)–(5.02 × age)– 1.76 × weight (kg)]–309 m. For women: Distance (m) = [2.11 × height (cm)– 2.29 × weight (kg)]–(5.78 × age) + 667 m	Mean (SD) distances for healthy individuals aged 61± 12 years: 2-min test: 149± 35 m 6-min test; 413± 107 m 12-min test: 774± 229 m Mean (SD) distances for individuals with a diagnosis of stroke: 2-min test: 62.5± 8.5 m 6-min test: 267.7± 89.7 m 12-min test: 530.5± 184.9 m

Table 69.3   Potential intervention strategies for common gait deviations

Observed deviation	Strategy
Difficulty rising from sitting	Scoot forward in chair, lean forward to rise Push from chair; strengthen triceps/latissimus dorsi Adapt chair height/firmness
Trunk forward lean (flexed posture)	Reduce hip flexor or other contractures, if present Strengthen hip extensors and ankle plantar flexors Provide feedback for normal posture Raise height of walker or cane, if needed
Trunk backward lean	Provide feedback for normal posture Strengthen hip flexors Practice disassociation of trunk muscles from pelvic motion
Trunk sideways lean	Strengthen hip abductors Correct leg length discrepancy
Trunk and pelvis decreased rotation	Practice trunk rotation exercise on mat, in sitting and standing Attempt four-point gait drills Use PNF facilitation during gait Facilitate trunk rotation on upper body ergometer
Foot clearance	Strengthen and facilitate dorsiflexors Reduce lower extremity contractures, if any Assess appropriateness of ankle–foot orthosis (AFO)
Decreased push-off at terminal stance	Strengthen plantar flexors Facilitate awareness of ankle push-off during gait
Decreased endurance	Adapt gait with appropriate assistive device to pattern that requires less energy (e.g. convert four-point gait to swing-to pattern, use wheeled walker vs. standard walker, etc.) Progress distances traveled and speed
Decreased balance	Assess need for assistive device Provide postural control training Assess and modify footwear Modify environment for safety (e.g. increase lighting, clear pathways, etc.)

rising-to-standing and tend to perform a rapid descent when returning-to-sit. Activities to facilitate safe chair rising and sitting should include using the upper extremities for assistance and facilitating awareness of body position relative to the chair. Floor-to-stand transfers are recommended for individuals who are tolerant of these high-level activities.

Pregait exercises are designed primarily to improve trunk and extremity strength and control. Strength training should be directed toward improving lower extremity strength, particularly of ankle plantar flexors and dorsiflexors, quadriceps, hip abductors, and hip extensors at an intensity sufficient to result in improvement (70–80% of the one-repetition maximum). Upper extremity strengthening should be conducted to improve strength of the latissimus dorsi and triceps. Appropriate mat exercises include pelvic tilt movements, hip raising (bridging), trunk twisting, sitting push-ups (latissimus dorsi dips), and quadriped activities including rocking and arm and leg reaching. Pregait standing activities include weight shifting, arm raising, chair push-ups, toe raising, hip hiking and leg swinging, and a progression of drills from four-point to swing-to to swing-through. Advanced standing activities include sideways and backwards

ambulation. These pregait standing activities may be progressed from using the parallel bars to using an assistive device to freestanding movement. Normal postural alignment should be encouraged in all activities.

Static and dynamic balance activities for gait training may be performed in sitting and standing positions. Sitting activities include controlled reaching and leaning within the base of support, with movement side-to-side, forward and backward. Sitting postural control may be challenged by using external disturbances such as a gentle push. Standing balance may be enhanced with the use of weight-shifting activities in which the patient is asked to move as far in all directions as he or she is comfortably able without needing to bend at the hips or take a step. Controlled reaching, lifting and weight-shifting activities assist in training for standing balance. The level of difficulty may be increased by performing reaching, lifting, and weight-shifting activities while standing on high-density foam. Sophisticated computerized force platform systems offer monitoring for various weight-shifting and response activities, which might include responding to a moving floor in some cases. Evidence suggests that the older adult may demonstrate better balance during gait

Table 69.4 Considerations for prescribing assistive devices for gait

Device	Objective	Considerations for prescription
Cane –single point –broad based –small based –rolling quad	Enhances stability through weight redistribution; compensates for losses in vision and proprioception	Appropriate for individuals who need balance and stability assistance with minimal weight-bearing shift (up to 25%) Coordination needed to use effectively; may not be appropriate for elderly people with impairments in cognition or coordination Single point offers the least weight-bearing shift and broad base offers the most weight-bearing shift Rolling quad is effective for use in individuals with limited upper extremity strength or coordination
Crutches –axillary –Loftstrand	Permits significant weight-bearing shift from legs to arms	Permits more weight-bearing shift (50% or greater) than a cane (up to complete nonweight-bearing on one leg) Less stable than a walker Requires good balance and upper body strength Inappropriate use of axillary crutches may result in brachial plexus injuries Loftstrand crutches permit hand use and reaching
Walkers –standard –rolling –hemi –platform –rollators	Offers greater stability and significant weight-bearing shift from legs to arms	Provides more weight-bearing shift (50% or greater) than a cane but with more stability than crutches; difficult to maneuver on stairs Standard offers the greatest stability but may be difficult for older adults to maneuver; requires more attentional demand and has greater destabilizing effects compared with the rolling walker Rolling walker is less stable than standard but is easier to propel for those with upper body weakness; reduces energy costs by 5% compared with standard walkers Rollators have the advantages of a rolling walker with brakes and a seat Hemi walker allows a large base of support for individuals with one functional arm Platform walkers are heavy and increase energy cost but permit weight-bearing shift through the humerus

when wearing either a laced firm thin-soled walking or athletic shoe as opposed to walking barefoot or in high-heel shoes (Arnadottir & Mercer 2000, Koepsell et al 2004).

Interventions during gait should focus on reducing deviations, improving gait efficiency and safety, and increasing endurance. Interventions during gait include assessment for assistive devices (a cane, crutches, a walker, orthoses), feedback for movement control (manual, electrical stimulation, biofeedback, visual), practice of dynamic balance, and progression from performing the standing activities listed above within the parallel bars to performing them outside the bars. Treatment progression may advance from even surfaces to uneven surfaces, ramps and stairs. Forward gait training may be progressed to side-stepping, turning, backward stepping, reaching and carrying objects. Practice in stepping over obstacles and climbing stairs is relevant to improving the functional mobility of the client. Because attentional demands may affect the gait of an older client, training for gait safety during challenging or distracting situations may be appropriate (de Hoon et al 2003, Jaffe et al 2004).

The prescription of an appropriate assistive device may help the client to improve balance and mobility without loss of stability as well as reducing lower limb loading (Bateni & Maki 2005). Advantages and disadvantages of various assistive devices for geriatric gait training are included in Table 69.4.

Most gait training programs focus on achieving mobility with stability prior to emphasizing increases in gait velocity. It is clinically relevant that self-selected gait speed is related to maximum oxygen consumption. With healthy aging, individuals have progressively smaller aerobic reserves. Gait disorders, as well as the use of assistive devices, add to the energy demands of walking. For these reasons, it is highly recommended that therapists monitor the vital signs of older adults during gait training. Endurance training has been shown to improve gait and balance in older adults (Sauvage et al 1992, Buchner et al 1997).

Environmental concerns include assessment of the distances and velocities that have to be covered, the surfaces traveled, the safety of paths, and transfers at home and in the community. Where possible, environmental modifications should be made to increase safety and reduce the risk of falling.

Technology is increasingly being used for gait training. Walking on a treadmill, with some body weight supported via a harness connected to an overhead support system, is a method of treating walking impairments post stroke. Preliminary results using this body weight support treadmill training have shown improvement in gait speed and endurance (Mosely et al 2003). Another high-technology option for gait training includes the use of robotic gait orthoses, which guide the patient's legs according to a preprogrammed physiological gait pattern. Both technologies are thought to enhance motor learning for locomotion by optimizing task-specific training (Malouin et al 1992, Mosely et al 2003); however, both are costly in terms of equipment and human resources.

CONCLUSION

Declining mobility is a common complaint among aging people, and it is likely to lead to diminutions in the performance of daily living activities and the quality of life. Gait training interventions include corrections of deviations during ambulation, as well as activities to improve the strength, mobility, balance and endurance needed for gait. Various pathologies may contribute to declining mobility and pathological gait in an elderly person, but significant improvements may be documented by using appropriate assessment tools and interventions.

References

Arnadottir SA, Mercer VS 2000 Effects of footwear on measurements of balance and gait in women between the ages of 65 and 93 years. Phys Ther 80:17–27

Bateni H, Maki BE 2005 Assistive devices for balance and mobility: benefits, demands and adverse consequences. Arch Phys Med Rehabil 86:134–145

Buchner DM, Cress ME, de Lateur BJ et al 1997 A comparison of the effects of three types of endurance training on balance and other fall risk factors in older adults. Aging (Milan, Italy) 9:112–119

Butland RJ, Pang J, Gross ER et al 1982 Two-, six-, and 12-minute walking tests in respiratory disease. Br Med J 284:1607–1608

de Hoon EW, Allum JH, Carpenter MG et al 2003 Quantitative assessment of the stops walking while talking test in the elderly. Arch Phys Med Rehabil 6:838–842

Eng JJ, Chu KS, Dawson AS et al 2002 Functional walk tests in individuals with stroke: relation to perceived exertion and myocardial exertion. Stroke 33:756–761

Enright PL, Sherrill DL 1998 Reference equations for the six-minute walk in healthy adults. Am J Respir Crit Care Med 158:1384–1387

Guralnik JM, Simonsick EM, Ferrucci L et al 1994 A short physical performance battery assessing lower extremity function: Association with self-reported disability and prediction of mortality and nursing home admission. J Gerontol 49:M85–M94

Guralnik JM, Ferrucci L, Pieper CF et al 2000 Lower extremity function and subsequent disability: consistency across studies, predictive models, and the value of gait speed alone compared to the short physical performance battery. J Gerontol 55:M221–M231

Jaffe DL, Brown DA, Pierson-Carey CD et al 2004 Stepping over obstacles to improve walking in individuals with poststroke hemiplegia. J Rehabil Res Dev 41:283–292

Koepsell TD, Wolf ME, Buchner DM et al 2004 Footwear style and risk of falls in older adults. J Am Geriatr Soc 52:1495–1501

McGinley JL, Goldie PA, Greenwood KM et al 2003 Accuracy and reliability of observational gait analysis data: judgments of push-off in gait after stroke. Phys Ther 83:146–160

Malouin F, Potvin M, Prevost J et al 1992 Use of an intensive task-oriented gait training program in a series of patients with acute cardiovascular accidents. Phys Ther 72:781–793

Moseley AM, Stark A, Cameron ID et al 2003 Treadmill training and body weight support during walking after stroke. Cochrane Database Syst Rev Issue 3:CD002840

Podsiadlo D, Richardson S 1991 The timed 'Up & Go': a test of basic functional mobility for frail elderly persons. J Am Geriatr Soc 39:142–148

Quadri P, Tettamanti M, Bernasconi S et al 2005 Lower limb function as predictor of falls and loss of mobility with social repercussions one year after discharge among elderly inpatients. Aging Clin Exp Res 17:82–89

Ranchos Los Amigos National Rehabilitation Center 2001 Observational Gait Analysis Handbook. Los Amigos Research and Education Institute: Downey, CA

Runyan CW, Casteel C, Perkis D et al 2005 Unintentional injuries in the home in the United States Part I: Mortality. Am J Prev Med 28:73–79

Sauvage LR, Myklebust BM, Crow-Pan J et al 1992 A clinical trial of strengthening and aerobic exercise to improve gait and balance in elderly male nursing home residents. Am J Phys Med Rehabil 71:333–342

Shumway-Cook A, Baldwin M, Polissar NL et al 1997 Predicting the probability for falls in community-dwelling older adults. Phys Ther 77:812–819

Steffen TM, Hacker TA, Mollinger L 2002 Age- and gender-related test performance in community-dwelling elderly people: Six-Minute Walk Test, Berg Balance Scale, Timed Up & Go Test, and gait speeds. Phys Ther 82:128–137

Tinetti ME 1986 Performance-oriented assessment of mobility problems in elderly patients. J Am Geriatr Soc 34:119–126

VanSwearingen JM, Paschal KA, Bonino P et al 1996 The modified Gait Abnormality Rating Scale for recognizing the risk of recurrent falls in community-dwelling elderly adults. Phys Ther 76:994–1002

Wolfson L, Whipple R, Amerman P et al 1990 Gait assessment in the elderly: a gait abnormality rating scale and its relations to falls. J Gerontol 45:M12–M19

Chapter 70

Orthotics

David Patrick

CHAPTER CONTENTS

INTRODUCTION

An orthosis is a mechanical device applied to the body in order to support a body segment, correct anatomical alignment, protect a body part or assist motion to improve body function (Bunch 1985). In accomplishing these objectives, orthotic devices assist in promoting ambulation, reducing pain, preventing deformity and allowing greater activity. Orthotic devices are often indicated as a component of the rehabilitation process for a variety of diseases and conditions that affect the geriatric population. Successful orthotic intervention when working with aging individuals demands a practical balance between the objectives that are ideally desired and what the elderly individual will reasonably tolerate.

Orthotic devices accomplish their objectives by applying forces to the involved body segments. As a rule, the more aggressive the orthotic intervention, the greater the force generated (Edelstein 1995). In general, elderly individuals are less tolerant of the resultant discomfort of aggressive orthotic intervention, and their skin and subcutaneous tissue are less tolerant of the external forces generated. This frequently results in the need to compromise between an ideal and an acceptable orthotic outcome and to choose more 'forgiving' orthoses in terms of comfort and tolerance, that is less rigid orthotic devices. This discussion focuses on the lower extremity and spinal orthotic interventions, which are commonly associated with the geriatricpopulation.

LOWER EXTREMITY ORTHOTIC SYSTEMS

Shoes

Proper distribution of forces in order to maintain the integrity of the skin of the foot is of primary importance. The shoe should fit properly, and the volume of the shoe should appropriately accommodate the foot and any additions such as a foot orthotic or plastic ankle–foot orthosis (AFO). Generally, a sneaker with a removable inlay or an extra-depth shoe with a removable inlay is recommended. The inlay can be removed to accommodate fluctuating edema or the addition of an orthosis. In unilateral involvement, the inlay can remain in the shoe on the uninvolved side, maintaining the fit on that side and balancing the patient in terms of height. It is recommended that the shoe should have a soft upper (the portion of the shoe covering the dorsum of the foot) to reduce pressure in the presence of minor foot deformities such as bunions or hammer toes. Severe foot deformities may require a custom shoe made from a cast of the individual's foot.

Foot orthotics

In general, flexible accommodative orthotics for the purpose of distributing forces to protect the skin and promote comfort are indicated. The bones of the foot of the geriatric patient are often functionally adapted, and the joints may be restricted in terms of range of motion (ROM). Thus, attempting biomechanical correction may be inappropriate, and may thereby contraindicate the use of rigid orthotic devices and necessitate careful consideration of the application of even semirigid devices.

Ankle–foot orthotics (AFO)

AFOs are frequently utilized with the elderly to improve ambulation status and gait quality. AFOs are capable of controlling the foot and ankle directly and the knee indirectly. For example, by positioning the ankle in dorsiflexion, a knee flexion moment can be produced to control genu recurvatum. Also, positioning the ankle in plantar flexion can produce a knee extension movement to assist in stabilizing the knee. Neuromuscular conditions, such as hemiparesis, resulting from a cerebral vascular accident as well as musculoskeletal pathologies such as arthritis commonly result in foot and ankle dysfunctions in the geriatric population that can be managed in part with AFOs.

A common challenge is deciding whether to use a plastic or a metal AFO system. The metal AFO has little skin contact except for the calf band and shoe, which are the reaction points of the orthosis. This quality is a distinct advantage of the metal system for patients with fluctuating edema or poor skin integrity. In comparison, the total contact nature of the plastic AFO results in a greater ability to control the foot and ankle. Additionally, the plastic AFO is lighter in weight, more cosmetically acceptable, and has the practical advantage of easy interchange among shoes. Plastic AFOs would appear to be the orthosis of choice for geriatric patients whenever possible. One strategy to determine whether a metal AFO system is indicated for a particular patient is to consider the sensory status and volume stability (i.e. the presence or absence of fluctuating edema) of the patient and the reliability of the patient or support person to monitor the skin integrity of the involved lower extremity. Negative findings in two of these categories would indicate consideration of a metal AFO instead of a plastic orthosis.

A soft AFO such as a neoprene ankle sleeve may be appropriate for controlling minor discomfort from arthritis or to encourage ankle stability when a more rigid system cannot be tolerated. Such orthoses accomplish their goals remarkably well in some cases by retaining heat and providing proprioceptive and kinesthetic sensory input.

Knee–ankle–foot orthoses (KAFOs)

Although AFOs are tolerated well by the geriatric population, the addition of a knee joint and a thigh cuff to form a KAFO system results in a much less acceptable orthotic intervention. A KAFO has the advantage of controlling the knee as well as the foot and ankle directly, and indirectly influences the hip joint. A KAFO is the orthosis of choice in the presence of severe genu recurvatum, or knee buckling, which cannot be managed with an AFO.

Historically, a knee that buckled during weight-bearing required the use of a locking-type knee joint. This satisfied the need to stabilize the knee during the stance phase of gait. However, it prevented knee flexion at swing phase, resulting in a less than desirable gait pattern that was energy consuming. As an alternative, stance control knee joints are now available. These joints lock the knee during the stance phase of gait but allow knee flexion during the swing phase. Some offer a limited degree of resisted knee flexion before locking, which helps to normalize the gait pattern at initial stance.

Additionally, significant coronal plane instabilities at the knee (genu varum or valgum) are effectively managed by a KAFO. Less severe knee problems may be managed using a knee orthosis (KO), but the shortened lever arm (the shorter length of the orthosis) results in greater skin pressures, and the softer nature of the elderly patient's lower extremity (LE) musculature can create suspension problems as the KO tends to slide distally during use. One advantage of the KAFO is that the footplate serves to maintain the orthosis in its proper position.

Hip–knee–ankle–foot orthoses (HKAFOs)

The addition of a hip joint and pelvic band to a KAFO results in an orthosis that is difficult to don and doff, less comfortable than shorter ones, and more cumbersome to wear. For the geriatric population, the hip joint and pelvic band are most commonly added when rotation control of the LE is required.

Hip orthoses

A hip orthosis is commonly used with the elderly to limit the extent of hip joint adduction and flexion following the dislocation of a hip arthroplasty (hip rotation is controlled to a lesser degree). Premanufactured systems are available that allow the limits of hip ROM to be adjusted as required to protect the hip adequately and simultaneously allow the patient to perform the activities of daily living.

Knee orthoses

A postoperative knee orthosis is commonly used after a knee arthroplasty. The knee orthosis is usually designed to allow ROM adjustment in graduating increments, as desired. A soft knee orthosis is commonly used to address arthritis-related pain and promote knee stability through a greater kinesthetic awareness. A knee orthosis with wraparound closure design is recommended for the elderly patient to facilitate donning and doffing. Some orthopedists order knee immobilizers postoperatively for their patients who have had total hip replacements. The rationale is that by preventing knee flexion, the operative hip flexion will be reduced, thereby mitigating the risk of dislocation. This technique should be considered for individual patients only in the early postoperative period as it does impede mobility and may cause knee stiffness and hip pain because of the long lever arm.

Fracture orthoses

Fracture orthoses are utilized with the geriatric population when surgical repair is contraindicated, or to reduce the amount of time the joints surrounding a fracture have to be immobilized in a cast. This reduces the potential negative effects of immobilization such as contractures and phlebitis. Additionally, LE fracture orthoses may reduce the period of recumbency, thereby minimizing the risk of potentially life-threatening complications such as pneumonia. Fracture orthoses are tightened circumferentially around the involved area and, using the hydraulic effect of soft tissues (the noncompressibility of fluids) and gravity, they transmit forces that realign and support the fracture site while allowing motion in the surrounding joints (Bunch et al 1985). Fracture orthoses must be worn snugly; they are commonly used for the management of nondisplaced or minimally displaced fractures, especially those of the humerus, tibia, radius and ulna.

SPINAL ORTHOTIC SYSTEMS

Spinal orthotic intervention is particularly challenging when dealing with the elderly population. Older patients commonly present with a variety of pathologies involving the spine and soft tissues of the trunk that could well be treated by the application of a spinal orthosis. Tolerance to wearing such a device, however, is limited, particularly in the cases of the more rigid systems and those that cover an extensive body area.

Spinal orthoses accomplish their objectives through one or more of the following biomechanical principles:

1. three-point pressure control;
2. indirect transfer of load by increasing intra-abdominal pressure;
3. correction of spinal alignment;
4. sensory feedback (kinesthetic reminder) (Edelstein 1995).

Three-point pressure control (the design of the orthosis) determines which spinal motions are limited. The magnitude of control (the degree of limitation) is directly related to the rigidity of the orthosis and the degree of tightness with which it is worn. A rigid orthosis is capable of applying greater forces to the body to restrict motion than is a more flexible system. However, the geriatric patient is less tolerant of the resulting discomfort and potential breathing restriction, and the skin of the older patient is less capable of withstanding the forces generated without its integrity being compromised. The decision to use a rigid rather than a more flexible system should therefore be based on the degree to which spinal motion restriction is required. For example, a geriatric patient with an unstable fracture of the spine requires a rigid orthotic system to restrict motion in the involved spinal segment, whereas management of a stable compression fracture offers greater latitude to use a more flexible and lightweight device without compromising the patient's safety. It should be noted that a more rigid device is often preferred in terms of protecting the involved spinal segment, but the decision to use a more flexible system is based on the practical issue of orthotic tolerance and thus compliance with wearing the orthosis. The ideal orthosis serves no purpose at all if it is not worn and, particularly with the geriatric population, it is sometimes necessary to make practical decisions that involve relinquishing orthotic control to gain patient acceptance.

Soft and rigid spinal systems applied to the trunk typically incorporate a means of applying abdominal pressure, thereby increasing intra-abdominal pressure, which has been shown to reduce the load on the vertebrae and intervertebral disks. Some literature (Kulkarni & Ho 2005) suggests that this may be the primary effect of the corsets and soft binders that are frequently used in geriatric applications.

The principle of correcting spinal alignment is seldom applied to the geriatric population because of restriction of spinal flexibility and poor tolerance of the required forces.

Flexible spinal orthoses serve to limit motion by acting as kinesthetic reminders to volitionally restrict movement as opposed to exerting three-point pressure control. Motion restriction accomplished through a flexible orthosis would obviously be better tolerated by the elderly.

Cervical orthoses (COs)

Among cervical orthoses (COs), soft cervical collars are well tolerated and provide reasonable control of cervical flexion and extension. The Philadelphia collar offers greater control than the soft cervical collar and is also reasonably well tolerated.

Cervical–thoracic orthoses (CTOs)

When more definitive control of the cervical spine and upper thoracic region is required, a cervical orthosis with a thoracic extension is indicated. Rigid four-poster and sternal–occipital–mandibular immobilizer (SOMI) systems are difficult for the elderly to tolerate. The Minerva CTO tends to be better tolerated without sacrificing spinal control.

Thoracolumbosacral orthoses (TLSOs)

TLSOs are utilized to address spinal pathologies from approximately the T6 to the L3–4 region. An overshoulder overlap may allow control of the T4–5 levels, and a cervical extension addition to the TLSO is recommended for more definitive control above the T6 level. TLSOs most effectively control the T12–L1 region and offer diminishing control of spinal segments further away from this region. Rigid immobilization is typically accomplished using a 'body jacket' made of plastic with a soft foam interface (lining). Soft, high-density body jackets can incorporate high-density outer foam instead of plastic. Plastic stays (permanent or removable) or a plastic frame can be incorporated into the foam for additional restriction of motion if desired. These systems, when custom fabricated, offer excellent alternatives to the rigid body jacket. They tend to be much better tolerated by the elderly patient and offer moderately effective restriction of spinal motion (Lusardi & Nielsen 2000).

The TLSO corset (semiflexible) is often used for patients whose acceptance of a more rigid spinal orthosis is questionable or for patients who require minimal restriction of spinal motion. Compression fractures are very common in the geriatric population, and frequently an attempt is made to manage them with a corset. Rigid systems such as the Taylor and Knight–Taylor are less frequently used for the elderly because they are difficult to tolerate.

Lumbosacral orthoses (LSOs)

Utilized to address spinal pathologies from approximately L1 to L4–5, the LSO most effectively controls the L3–4 spinal level. As with the TLSO, a rigid system is used in the presence of spinal instability, whereas more flexible systems are preferred and better tolerated by the geriatric population, and should be used whenever possible. Corsets are commonly used to manage soft-tissue injuries that result in back pain. The custom-made, soft, high-density LSO is an excellent alternative to the rigid body jacket or corset, offering a balance between comfort and control. It should be noted that successful orthotic outcomes with the soft, high-density system appear to be more readily accomplished in patients with average to thin body types. Again, rigid LSO systems such as the Chairback and Knight are poorly tolerated by geriatric patients.

CONCLUSION

The use of orthotics to support a body segment, correct anatomical alignment, protect a body area or assist body movement is an important therapeutic consideration in geriatric rehabilitation. It is crucial to involve the patient in the choice of orthotic design whenever possible in order to attain a balance between objective ideals and patient adherence. Attention must be given to possible harmful effects of the orthotic device on the skin and the subcutaneous connective tissues of older people.

REFERENCES

Bunch W 1985 Atlas of Orthotics: Biomechanical Principles and Application. Mosby, St Louis, MO
Edelstein JE 1995 Orthoses. In: Myers RS (ed) Saunders Manual of Physical Therapy Practice. WB Saunders, Philadelphia

Kulkarni SS & Ho S 2005 Spinal orthotics. Available: http://www.emedicine.com/pmr/topic173.htm. Accessed February 20 2006
Lusardi M & Nielsen CC 2000 Orthotics and Prosthetics in Rehabilitation. Butterworth-Heinemann, Boston

Chapter 71

Prosthetics

David Patrick

INTRODUCTION

The elderly make up the largest group of patients requiring lower extremity (LE) amputations; peripheral vascular disease (PVD) and complications of diabetes are the leading causes (in May 2002). Progress in the fields of rehabilitation and prosthetics has resulted in a large number of geriatric amputees being successfully fitted with prostheses and subsequently requiring rehabilitation.

EVALUATING THE PATIENT

The physical therapy program starts with a comprehensive evaluation of the patient. This is particularly important with the elderly amputee who commonly presents with a number of comorbid conditions that can affect his or her functional outcome. A format for the evaluation of the LE amputee is provided in Form 71.1. The following elements represent important considerations in the evaluation and treatment of the geriatric amputee.

Age

Consider overall wellness and conditioning, functional abilities, and motivation as being more important than chronological age.

Secondary diagnosis

Investigate the presence of comorbid conditions. Elderly vascular amputees can demonstrate multiple secondary conditions in addition to the amputation. The presence of cardiac disease is common, as the same factors that increase the incident of PVD in diabetics also increase the incidence of atherosclerotic coronary artery disease. This leads to an increased death rate (there is an estimated 25–50% 3-year survival for a person with diabetes, with a major amputation)

(Sanders 1986) and an increase in the symptoms of angina, congestive heart failure (CHF) and arrhythmias.

Cognitive status

Determine the patient's ability to understand and remember instructions. Provide instructions in writing that clearly state the wearing schedule of the shrinker, socks and prosthesis. Review the instructions with the patient frequently. Direct the patient to maintain a written diary of sock-ply use and color code the various sock plies to assist the patient in maintaining proper socket fit.

Wheelchair

Recommend the availability of a lightweight, easily transportable wheelchair for long-distance transportation, limited ambulation endurance, discontinued prosthetic use (because of skin breakdown) and prosthetic breakdown. Bilateral LE geriatric amputees commonly depend on wheelchairs or powered mobility as an option to walking with prostheses, particularly for long distances.

Transfers and mobility

Train patients to change position slowly to avoid episodes of syncope that could result in loss of balance. Reduced proprioceptive feedback through the prosthetic extremity, and the predisposition of the elderly for postural hypotension, increase the risk of balance loss when changing position.

Ambulation

Prioritize the maintenance of skin integrity, the prevention of falls and the control of energy expenditure. Assess the patient's ability to ambulate with an assistive device without a prosthesis.

Skin integrity

The loss of elements of the connective tissue, the thinning of the dermis, and alterations in the content of elastin and collagen represent characteristic skin changes that occur with aging and predispose the amputee to skin breakdown during prosthetic use (see Chapter 52, Skin Disorders). Particularly with the transtibial (below-knee) amputee, use a conservative, methodical progression of weight-bearing and ambulation distance and continue to monitor the skin of the residual limb (in the past, it was referred to as the stump) on a

Form 71.1 Sample lower extremity amputee evaluation form

Date therapy initiated _____

Name _____ Age _____ Room # _____

Diagnosis (date/cause of amputation) _____
_____

Secondary diagnosis _____

Precautions _____

Past medical history _____
_____

Social history _____
_____

Orientation and ability to follow directions _____

Functional level

  1. Wheelchair _____

  2. Transfers _____

  3. Bed mobility _____

  4. Sitting balance _____

  5. Standing balance _____

  6. Ambulation – level surface without prosthesis _____

     – level surface with prosthesis _____

     – elevations without prosthesis _____

     – gait deviations _____

  7. Floor transfer _____

  8. Donning/doffing prosthesis _____

  9. Residual limb wrapping _____

10. Endurance _____

Residual limb length: below knee – left or right

    a. _____ cm from MTP to end of bone

    b. _____ cm from MTP to end of flesh

Residual limb length: above knee – left or right

    a. _____ cm from perineum to end of bone

    b. _____ cm from perineum to end of flesh

Girth measurements: reference point

Date					
Proximal					
Distal					

	(R) – ROM – (L)	(R) – Muscle strength – (L)
Hip flexion		
Hip extension		
Hip abduction		
Hip external rot		
Hip internal rot		
Knee flexion		
Knee extension		
Ankle P/F		
Ankle D/F		

Knee A-P stability (L) _____ (R) _____

Knee M-L stability (L) _____ (R) _____

(Continued)

Residual limb condition:

Shape _____

Scar _____

Skin _____

Bones _____

Musculature _____

Sensation _____

Pulses _____

Phantom sensation/pain _____

Description of prosthetic appliance: _____

_____

Condition of remaining LE:

Skin condition _____

Pulses _____

Sensation _____

Ulcerations _____

Upper extremities:

ROM (L) WNL except for _____

(R) WNL except for _____

Strength: (L) WNL except for _____

(R) WNL except for _____

Back _____

Abdominals _____

Additional comments: _____

_____

Goals: Treatment plan:

_____   _____

Date   Therapist

---

frequent basis. Consider shear force-absorbing socket interfaces and prosthetic components to reduce forces on the residual limb.

Fall prevention

Conservative advancement of assistive devices is recommended, prioritizing safety over progression. In the author's experience, the transfemoral (above-knee) geriatric amputee is less prone to skin breakdown than the transtibial amputee, but the transfemoral amputee is at greater risk of falls.

Energy expenditure

The geriatric amputee should not be encouraged to walk at a 'normal' walking speed. Allowing the patient to self-select ambulation velocity results in a more normal rate of metabolic energy expenditure, decreasing perceived exertion and potential cardiac difficulties. A slower self-selected walking velocity should be expected at higher amputation levels (Bowker & Michael 1992).

Prosthetic donning and doffing

Difficulty in donning and doffing the prosthesis may result from limitations in manual dexterity as well as visual dysfunction. Self-suspending systems, Velcro closures vs. buckles, and oversized extensions on belts and socket inserts should be considered.

Range of motion (ROM)

Adequate ROM is required for successful prosthetic outcome. Degenerative joint disease predisposes elderly amputees to contractures. Common areas of LE contractures include:

- the partial foot level: plantar flexors (due primarily to muscle imbalance);
- the transtibial level: knee flexors and hip flexors; and
- the transfemoral level: hip flexors, hip abductors, hip external rotators.

Strength and endurance

Deconditioning is common with aging and may limit the ability to participate in the rehabilitation program. Initiate a strengthening and endurance program as soon after surgery as possible.

Volume containment

Controlling the volume of the residual limb is an important aspect of preparing it for definitive prosthetic fitting, reducing pain in the limb that is related to edema and facilitating healing after the amputation surgery. Comorbid conditions such as renal failure and dialysis or CHF predispose the geriatric amputee to significant girth fluctuations. Shrinker socks are recommended instead of Ace wraps because of the relative ease of donning and the greater consistency of fit (they require less frequent reapplication and adjustment). A rigid dressing should be considered when protection of the residual limb is a priority. Regular girth measurements of the residual limb are recommended to monitor the effectiveness of the volume containment program.

Sensation

Sensory examination is important for accurate prediction of the amputee's ability to detect abnormal forces during prosthetic use and to detect soft-tissue trauma in the remaining limb. Vascular insufficiency, and particularly diabetes, may result in polyneuropathy involving the sensory nerve fibers, predisposing the elderly amputee to skin problems.

Condition of the remaining lower extremity

It is essential to examine the remaining LE for evidence of vascular insufficiency or sensory deficits that could lead to further amputation. Unilateral amputees with diabetes have more than a 40% risk over 4 years of having an amputation of the remaining LE (Sanders 1986). Polyneuropathy associated with diabetes may involve sensory, motor and autonomic nerve fibers. Motor deficits may cause atrophy of the foot intrinsics and muscle imbalances in the foot, resulting in foot deformity and skin injury caused by fitting problems with shoes. Sensory deficits result in the lack of an appropriate avoidance response to abnormal forces. Autonomic involvement may result in dry skin, which creates greater susceptibility to breakdown and infection. The importance of this evaluation cannot be overemphasized, as a peripheral neuropathy has been identified as the primary underlying cause of amputation in the elderly with diabetes. Patient education that emphasizes proper footwear and skin management is an essential component of the amputation prevention program.

PROSTHETIC PRESCRIPTION

Advances in the technology of prosthetic components have improved the possibility of successfully fitting the geriatric amputee with a prosthesis. Innovations in socket designs, lightweight components, improved suspensions and stable knee design options all contribute to improved prosthetic tolerance and better functional outcomes for elderly amputees. The application of advanced prosthetic components also results in increased expense, so judgments must be made about the relative costs and benefits of these components to each patient. The Lower Limb Prosthetics Medical Review Policy (LLPMRP) developed by Medicare structures financial sponsorship of the various prosthetic ankle, foot and knee components based on the patient's anticipated functional outcome (Box 71.1). The LLPMRP should be considered by the prosthetics team in the process of prescribing prostheses for the many geriatric amputees with Medicare coverage.

Box 71.1   Medicare's Lower Limb Prosthetics Medical Review Policy (LLPMRP)[a]

A determination of the medical necessity for certain components/additions to the prosthesis is based on the patient's potential functional abilities. Potential functional ability is based on the reasonable expectations of the prosthetist and ordering physician, considering factors including, but not limited to:

a. the patient's past history (including prior prosthetic use, if applicable)
b. the patient's current condition, including the status of the residual limb and the nature of other medical problems, and
c. the patient's desire to ambulate

Clinical assessments of patient rehabilitation potential should be based on the following classification levels:

Level 0:   Does not have the ability or potential to ambulate or transfer safely with or without assistance and a prosthesis does not enhance the patient's quality of life or mobility

Level 1:   Has the ability or potential to use a prosthesis for transfers or ambulation on level surfaces at fixed cadence. Typical of the limited and unlimited household ambulator

Level 2:   Has the ability or potential for ambulation with the ability to traverse low-level environmental barriers such as curbs, stairs or uneven surfaces. Typical of the limited community ambulator

Level 3:   Has the ability or potential for ambulation with variable cadence. Typical of the community ambulator who has the ability to traverse most environmental barriers and may have vocational, therapeutic, or exercise activity that demands prosthetic utilization beyond simple locomotion

Level 4:   Has the ability or potential for prosthetic ambulation that exceeds basic ambulation skills, exhibiting high-impact stress or energy levels. Typical of the prosthetic demands of the child, active adult or athlete

In the following sections, the determination of coverage for selected prostheses and components with respect to potential functional levels represents the usual case. Exceptions will be considered in an individual case if additional documentation is included that justifies the medical necessity. Prostheses will be denied as not medically necessary if the patient's potential functional level is '0'

(continued)

Feet

A determination of the type of foot for the prosthesis will be made by the prescribing physician and/or the prosthetist based upon the functional needs of the patient. Basic lower extremity prostheses include a SACH foot. Prosthetic feet are considered for coverage based upon the functional classification:

External keel, SACH foot, or single-axis ankle/foot are covered for patients with a functional level 1 or above

Flexible keel foot and multiaxial ankle/foot candidates are expected to demonstrate a functional level 2 or greater functional need.

Flex-foot system, energy-storing foot, multiaxial ankle/foot dynamic response, or flex-walk system or equal are covered for patients with a functional level 3 or above

Knees

Basic lower extremity prostheses include a single-axis, constant-friction knee. Prosthetic knees are considered for coverage based upon functional classification:

Fluid and pneumatic knees are covered for patients with a functional level 3 or above

Other knee–shin systems are covered for patients with a functional level 1 or above

Ankles

Axial rotation units are covered for patients with a functional level 2 or above

Sockets

No more than two of the same socket inserts are allowed per individual prosthesis at the same time.

Socket replacements are considered medically necessary if there is adequate documentation of functional and/or physiological need. There are situations where the explanation includes but is not limited to: changes in the residual limb; functional need changes; or irreparable damage or wear/tear due to excessive patient weight or prosthetic demands of very active amputees

[a]From US Department of Health and Human Services.

Preparatory vs. definitive prosthesis

A preparatory prosthesis is strongly recommended over a definitive prosthesis as the first prosthetic device for a geriatric amputee. The preparatory prosthesis includes basic components that are easily adjusted but is not finished cosmetically. The preparatory prosthesis allows earlier prosthetic fitting by avoiding the need to wait until shrinkage of the residual limb is complete (Edelstein 1992). This may help to prevent secondary complications resulting from immobility that are potentially life-threatening to the elderly patient. The definitive prosthesis is the finished product, with all the appropriate components and cosmetic touches. The definitive prosthesis is fitted when the residual limb size stabilizes.

Endoskeletal vs. exoskeletal design

The exoskeleton design has a hard, laminated plastic shell that provides the weight-bearing support. In contrast, the endoskeletal design consists of a tubular structure that constitutes the internal support to which the foot, ankle and knee assemblies are attached. The endoskeleton is covered with a pliable surface that is shaped and colored to match the opposite limb.

Endoskeletal prosthetic design is usually recommended for geriatric amputees because of the ease with which adjustments can be made and components interchanged, the reduced weight and the cosmetic benefits in transfemoral applications. Weight restrictions have been identified by the manufacturers of some endoskeletal components (Bowker & Michael 1992).

Prosthetic sockets

At the level of the transtibial amputation, the patellar tendon-bearing (PTB) socket with a soft insert is commonly utilized. A patient with fragile skin or sensitivity in the residual limb may benefit from soft insert materials such as silicone that are designed to dissipate shock and shear forces. A flexible inner socket supported in a rigid outer frame may result in greater comfort for the elderly amputee by providing relief to pressure-sensitive structures. The flexible inner socket also facilitates necessary socket adjustments (American Academy of Orthotists and Prosthetists 2004).

After a transfemoral amputation, a geriatric patient can be successfully fitted with either a quadrilateral or an ischial containment socket. A patient with a short residual limb, poor residual limb muscle tone, obesity, or a high activity level would be expected to achieve the greatest benefit from the ischial containment socket design (Patrick 1995). The elderly amputee may experience more comfort when sitting if he or she has chosen a flexible socket design that is capable of accommodating its shape to the supporting surface.

Prosthetic suspensions

The following prosthetic suspensions are recommended for transtibial-level amputation:

- supracondylar cuff with Velcro closure on strap;
- supracondylar wedge self-suspension with tab extensions attached to medial and lateral insert wings;
- sleeve suspension (determine if the patient has the hand dexterity to manage the sleeve);
- silicone suction suspension (consider the patient's ability to manage the sleeve and the patient's skin's tolerance to silicone);
- joint and corset (which may be necessary because of hypersensitivity, skin problems, or knee joint pathology that prohibits full weight-bearing through the residual limb).

For transfemoral-level amputation, the following prosthetic suspensions are suggested:

- Neoprene belt with Velcro closure;
- hip joint and pelvic band with Velcro closure (indicated when hip stability or rotational control is required);
- silicone suction.

Prosthetic feet

The weight of the foot and function of the foot's keel in relation to the patient's activity level are the two primary considerations for the geriatric amputee (Patrick 1993). The keel provides the inner rigidity of structure to control the function of the prosthetic foot.

SACH feet

The solid ankle, cushion heel (SACH) feet are low cost and dependable. Geriatric lightweight versions are available. The rigid keel can interfere with the ability of the amputee to roll over the forefoot during the terminal stance phase.

Single-axis feet

These feet more readily plantar flex from heel strike to foot flat during the early loading phase of gait. Single-axis feet are recommended for the geriatric transfemoral amputee using an unlocked knee when greater knee stability during the early stance phase of gait is desired.

Multiple-axis feet

Accommodating to uneven surfaces, multiple-axis feet are recommended for geriatric patients with sensitive skin, who may benefit from the reduction in shear forces transmitted to the prosthetic socket–skin interface. Typically, this is a heavier prosthetic foot.

Elastic keel feet

The flexible nature of the elastic keel foot facilitates ambulation by allowing easier rollover at the terminal stance phase of gait. Lightweight designs are available. This prosthesis is appropriate for the moderately active individual.

Dynamic response feet

Typically more expensive, dynamic response feet are appropriate for an individual with a high activity level. They incorporate foot keels that bend in response to the patient's weight during rollover, then 'spring back', providing propulsion during the push-off phase of gait.

Prosthetic knees

Insuring knee stability during stance is the highest priority for the geriatric transfemoral-level amputee. Lightweight versions of the various designs of prosthetic knees are available and are recommended for consideration for the elderly amputee (Patrick 1993).

Manual-locking knees

Maximum knee stability during gait is important, and manual-locking knees provide it, but the resulting gait is the least cosmetic because the knee remains in extension during the swing phase. Manual-locking knees are appropriate when it is necessary to prevent knee buckling during weight-bearing.

Weight-activated friction knees (safety knees)

Frequently used with geriatric patients, weight-activated friction knees provide inherent knee stability during the stance phase by locking in response to the patient's weight-bearing, then unlocking, allowing the knee to bend during the swing phase, which provides a more natural gait appearance.

Polycentric knees

Inherent alignment stability is provided by polycentric knees, but they are not commonly used by geriatric patients because of their greater weight and complexity.

Hydraulic or pneumatic swing-phase controls

A very active individual might consider hydraulic or pneumatic swing-phase controls.

The Otto Bock C-leg

This is a prosthetic knee option that provides an electronically controlled swing and stance phase. It features swing-phase and stance-phase movements that are controlled by software algorithms in an onboard microprocessor. This results in a knee with a large degree of adjustability to different walking speeds and variations in terrains (www.ottobockus.com).

CONCLUSION

Amputations occur with increasing incidence as age increases. The conditions that most commonly necessitate amputation are peripheral vascular disease and complications of diabetes. Because of the high frequency of comorbid conditions in the elderly patient, comprehensive examination and evaluation are requisite. A preparatory prosthesis is strongly recommended for the geriatric patient because it allows early fitting and thus discourages the secondary complications of immobility. The various types of prosthetic components should be studied, and then chosen to meet the individual patient's needs. The patient's date of birth is less important when considering a prosthesis than overall wellness, fitness, functional ability and motivation.

References

American Academy of Orthotists and Prosthetists 2004 Post-operative management of the lower extremity amputee. J Prosthet Orthot 16(suppl3): S1–S26

Bowker JH, Michael JW 1992. Atlas of Limb Prosthetics: Surgical, Prosthetic, and Rehabilitation Principles. Mosby-Year Book, St Louis, MO

Edelstein JE 1992 Lower limb prosthetics. Topics Geriatr Rehabil 8:1

May BJ 2002 Amputations and Prosthetics: A Case Study Approach, 2nd edn. FA Davis, Philadelphia, PA

Otto Bock healthcare products. Available: http://www.ottobockus.com/products/lower_limb_prosthetics/c-leg_benefits.pdf. Accessed February 21 2006

Patrick DG 1993 Prosthetics and geriatric patients. Phys Ther Today 16:4

Patrick D 1995 Prosthetics. In: Myers R (ed.) Saunders Manual of Physical Therapy Practice. WB Saunders, Philadelphia, PA

Sanders GT 1986 Lower Limb Amputations: a Guide to Rehabilitation. FA Davis, Philadelphia, PA

Chapter 72

Complementary therapies for the aging patient

Carol M. Davis

CHAPTER CONTENTS

INTRODUCTION

Alternative and complementary therapies, or holistic therapies, are becoming more common in the healthcare of older individuals in the United States. First, let us define the terms we often read with this topic. 'Holistic' therapies are those therapies that emphasize the mind and the body working together to bring about the desired affect. For example, in T'ai Chi, patients are told to bring their attention to a spot just below the umbilicus and drop their minds into their bodies like sand in an hourglass, and then lead their movement from that place. Mind and body working together, with the breath coordinated in a specific way, is the mark of a 'holistic' therapy.

When the term 'alternative' is used, it often refers to a therapy that is not known to be part of allopathic medicine, nor is it listed as a therapeutic measure in traditional 'gold standards' of care. The therapy is an *alternative* to standard care. An example would be when a patient turns to acupuncture for pain relief rather than taking acetaminophen (paracetamol). When the term 'complementary' is used, it often refers to a therapy that, again, is not part of standard allopathic regimens, but is used 'in addition to' standard care rather than replacing the care, so it 'complements' the care. This happens, for example, when physical therapists utilize Barnes' method (bioenergetic) of myofascial release as a way of preparing a person's soft tissue for traditional exercise programs. 'Integrative' therapy is a term used when traditional and holistic therapies are closely interwoven in care, *integrated* to the point that nontraditional and traditional methods flow together. As more holistic therapies become validated by the traditional gold standard randomized controlled trial, they are being integrated more smoothly into comprehensive care programs. Many hospitals have begun including wellness and prevention programs that integrate T'ai Chi, yoga, and Pilates as part of their outpatient clinics' group exercise programs.

Whether alternative, complementary or integrative is used, there is another, more profound, definition of holistic therapies that has to do with a theory about how they work. This author most commonly uses the term 'complementary' therapies when referring to those therapies that, granted, are not listed as standard for allopathic care, that integrate the mind and the body together in their action, thus are 'holistic', and, here is the difference – that have as their basic goal to unblock body energy (chi) that is not flowing freely, for whatever reason, and therefore the body/mind is hindered from healing itself, or self-regulating. Fundamental to this viewpoint is the belief that the body and mind cannot be separated, and that all the cells of the body vibrate naturally for their own healing. This natural vibration is facilitated by the flow of a vital energy, or chi, and this natural state of healing flow can be interrupted by injury, toxins, imbalances, etc., which causes the body energy or chi to become blocked, to not flow smoothly. When this happens, the body/mind becomes vulnerable to bacterial and viral invasion, endocrine imbalance (diabetes, depression), and loss of self-regulation that insures proper pH, body temperature, pituitary function, etc. With this in mind, the goal then becomes to restore the flow of chi so the body can once again heal itself, or self-regulate.

WHY COMPLEMENTARY THERAPIES LACK UNIVERSAL ACCEPTANCE

Controversy over the use of holistic therapies relates to the resistance of some to using any therapy that has not been proven efficacious by traditional randomized controlled trial (Harris 2001). However, many alternative and complementary therapies arise from an eastern philosophy in contrast to western Cartesian and Newtonian thought. Traditional or mechanistic therapies, based on the physics of Isaac Newton, aim to 'fix what is broken'. The reliability and validity of traditional therapies is proven by randomized trials that can replicate the efficacy of an approach when the same outcome is observed within a variety of patients using the same process over and over.

As complementary therapies are those therapies that aim to restore balance or homeostasis by removing blocks to the flow of bioelectric body energy, or chi, they do not lend themselves readily to validation by research methods that count on replication of the exact process. A subject's energy pattern and flow will change as it is impacted by the energy of the examiner. Thus, for example, a therapist placing her hands under the cranium of a patient to feel the craniosacral rhythm will impact that rhythm with her own energy that is emitted from her hands in the process. A second therapist attempting to validate the flow of the craniosacral rhythm at the feet will also be observing the flow of the patient and his energy flow. To then try to attempt inter-rater reliability between the two therapists with the patient's energy as that which is constant becomes an impossibility, as was shown by Rogers et al (1998).

THE SCIENCE OF MECHANISTIC VS. HOLISTIC THERAPIES

Traditional mechanistic science or reductionism has its roots in the early seventeenth century. The philosopher René Descartes claimed that the best way to elevate and organize the search for truth would be to eliminate that which could not be observed with the five senses. All that could not be seen was to be ignored, and only that which could be measured and experienced was suitable in the scientific search for cause and effect. Later, Sir Isaac Newton developed the theory of gravity, outlined mathematical rules of physics and described the theories upon which contemporary science is based. It is from this foundation that the randomized controlled trial has its base as a way of insuring that the experimental variable is, indeed, causing the outcome, and not chance, or 'placebo' (Davis 2004).

In the early 1900s, Einstein suggested another way of viewing reality based on his understanding of the behavior of subatomic particles. Subsequently, quantum physics and systems theory (from biology) formed the basis for the theoretical foundation of holism, a concept that attempts to describe the outcomes of alternative and complementary therapies (Davis 2000). Holism as a concept is based on current knowledge of molecules, atoms and electron behavior, and states that it is no longer useful to regard humans solely as machines that can be fully understood simply by reducing the whole and analyzing the parts. The uniqueness and challenge of the human organism lies in how it is organized and how the parts interact and exchange information. Atoms and their electrons and other subatomic particles provide the basis of wave theory, bioelectromagnetism, energy and thus the flow of chi (Davis 2000, Oschman 2000).

Holism focuses on balance and integration of all the interacting elements of the system. Information inherent in the organization of a system gets lost in the separation of the parts (Schwartz & Russek 1997). The whole is more than simply the sum of the parts. For example, no matter how thoroughly one studies hydrogen and oxygen, one cannot understand water from that study. When two hydrogen atoms and one oxygen atom come together to form water, their electrons not only share orbits, but also they share information that results in the formation of the new system, the new substance. Information sharing is the key to electron flow. All systems 'work' by way of electrons sharing information.

COMPLEMENTARY THERAPIES IN THE CARE OF AGING PATIENTS

A variety of complementary therapies have been found to be useful for all people, and particularly useful in caring for older people. Generally, each of these therapies aims to increase the flow of healthy bioelectric energy and, as a result, restore balance or homeostasis in the mind/body and restore information flow that facilitates the body's natural state of wholeness and healing (Davis 2000, 2004).

The manual therapies

These include myofascial release (Barnes method), craniosacral therapy, Rosen method, rolfing, hellerwork, soma, neuromuscular therapy, osteopathic and chiropractic medicine. The manual therapies involve the use of hands directly on the body/mind surface, thereby stimulating bioelectromagnetic force. Research by Hunt (1989), Zimmerman (1990), Seto et al (1992), and Rubik (1995) documents the measure of energy flow from the body and suggests that both mechanical and energy forces stimulate responses from the tissues.

Mind/body interventions

These include psychotherapies, support groups, meditation, and imagery, hypnosis, dance and music therapy, art therapy, prayer, validation therapy, neurolinguistic psychology (Masin 2006), biofeedback (Bottomley 2004a), yoga (Taylor 2004) and T'ai Chi (Bottomley 2004b). These mind/body interventions demonstrate how movement and verbal and nonverbal communication with the mind/body seem to open up new pathways for thought and, therefore, unblock energy flow or chi. A growing body of literature examines the effects of T'ai Chi on the ability to prevent falls in elderly people and on quality of life (Wolf et al 1997).

Movement awareness techniques

These include the Feldenkrais method (Stephens & Miller 2004), the Alexander technique (Zuck 2004), and the Trager approach (Stone 1997). It is postulated that these movement awareness techniques help people recognize the way they move habitually. By practicing new ways of moving and identifying habitual postural holding patterns, energy trapped in tissue while maintaining habitual postures is freed.

Traditional Chinese medicine

These methods include acupuncture (LaRiccia & Galantino 2004), acupressure, polarity (Sharp 1997), reflexology (Sharp 1997), Touch for Health (Sharp 1997), Jin Shin Do (Mik 1997) and Qi Gong (Bottomley 2004c). These approaches within the system of traditional Chinese medicine focus on enhancing the flow of chi along body pathways or meridians.

Bioelectromagnetics

Thermal applications of nonionizing radiation, such as radiofrequency hyperthermia lasers, low-energy laser (Reddy 2004), radiofrequency surgery, radiofrequency diathermy and nonthermal applications of nonionizing radiation, are used for bone repair and wound healing. Biomicroelectromagnetics is the term applied to the energy that seems to emanate from the hands of people who have proven to be healers (Rubik 1995). Credible research exists on the effects of electromagnetic energy for wound healing and bone repair (Midura et al 2005).

Influence of the mind on the body

Mind/body medicine links traditional research methods with holistic healthcare practices. The influence of the mind on the body was first introduced by Herbert Benson's research on Tibetan monks who could control their autonomic nervous system. These monks could lower their body temperature and respiration rates, and enter a wakeful hypometabolic physiological state at will (Wallace et al 1971). Ader & Cohen (1991) coined the term *psychoneuroimmunology*, wherein the mind affects the immune system via the autonomic nervous system and the 'fluid' nervous system, another name given to the neurotransmitters and neuropeptides. Pert (2002) articulated the physiological functioning of the fluid nervous system, which manifests through the effects of thought on neurotransmitters, neuropeptides and steroids in the body. This biochemistry differs from the flow of chi, but both concepts reinforce the theory that the mind and the body are inseparable, and that the mind communicates with every cell in the body.

Complementary therapies are energy-based therapies that require belief in the phenomenon of vital flow of energy in the body. We can observe energy at work in the body in many ways: electrocardiograms, electroencephalograms and electromyograms all measure the energy output from various organs. The piezoelectric effect enables osteoblastic activity that keeps our bones structurally intact. Biomicroelectropotentials, or the exchange of subtle energies in electromagnetic fields that emanate from the hands of healers, are being researched (Seto et al 1992, Rubik 1995).

Traditional therapies applied from a holistic approach

In working with older people, massage, exercise and relaxation can be approached by practitioners in a conventional way, where the intention is a mechanical effect on a part (e.g. pushing fluid out of an edematous extremity), or it can be approached in a holistic way, where the intention is to influence the flow of vital energy and bring about homeostasis (e.g. manual lymph drainage that 'energetically' opens up lymph passages in the opposite side of the body from the edematous extremity so it can receive the fluid that is pushed out) (Funk 2004).

Researchers confirm the importance of hope and faith in one's physician and practitioners. How this facilitates healing still remains unclear, but to ignore the positive effect of therapeutic presence is to neglect a powerful intervention (Greer 1999). How practitioners are with their patients, not just what they do, is important. The exchange of energy with the intention to serve and facilitate healing is critical.

Myofascial release – Barnes method

This bioenergetic technique developed by Barnes (1990) is an effective manual therapy for older patients with diminished hydration of tissue, myofascial shortening and cross-linked collagen restrictions in their bodies. Other therapeutic approaches that use the term 'myofascial release' refer to a mechanistic impact on tissue by way of stretching and mechanically pressing on trigger points to try to influence the circulation to the area and the length of tissue mechanically, rather than energetically. In contrast, with Barnes' method of myofascial release, the practitioner places his or her hands directly on the skin of the patient, and with slight pressure, separates the hands, eliminating the flexibility of the skin between the hands so that the tissue is taught, and then gently waits with this traction until the tissue responds energetically under the surface of the practitioner's hand. Within 90–120 seconds, the tissue begins to move in a flowing manner. The practitioner follows the flow of the tissue with his or her hands in order to increase the length of the tissue as the myofascia 'softens' underneath the hands. The cause of this softening of tissue, experienced by practitioners and patients alike, is unknown. It is believed to be the effect of mechanical stress in gravity along with the therapist's energy – the piezoelectric effect – on the polyglycoid layer of the collagen of the myofascia, which increases tissue length and results in a release of trapped energy. It has been hypothesized that mechanical force may be transformed into a chemical response within the collagen of the myofascia, causing a flow of the polyglycoid layer of the collagen by way of the piezoelectric effect. The result is that the tissue under the therapist's hands seems to be 'melting' as it releases. Recent research by Wang et al (2005) revealed

that human cells send biochemical messages to each other as a result of tiny mechanical jabs. Actin filaments and microtubules in the fascia function as conduits for the spread of biochemical signals.

The patient then has more freedom to move, gains better posture and a relief of the pain caused by myofascial restriction (Barnes 1990). Fascial restrictions released in this way over time result in improved balance and strength and help to eliminate pain and poor posture. Multiple outcome case studies on myofascial release demonstrate improvements in the quality of life of older people and the prevention of chronic musculoskeletal problems (Barnes 1990).

It is believed that complementary therapies have an effect on patients by way of the energy that emanates from the healer's hands (Hunt 1989, Zimmerman 1990, Seto et al 1992). As we move into the next century, many researchers and practitioners in healthcare are seriously exploring new ways of viewing reality. What we know about quantum physics and systems theory, the inadequacies of conventional medicine in overcoming chronic illness and autoimmune disease, and the growing tendency of patients and clients to seek out complementary therapies, positions healthcare practitioners and medical researchers on the verge of a revolution in the linear and materialistic view of reality.

BENEFITS OF COMPLEMENTARY THERAPIES WITH OLDER PATIENTS

Alternative and complementary therapies are increasingly being used by older patients and physical therapists treating older patients because of their proven success in relieving pain and improving quality of life. As more research is done, we will be able to explain better how this takes place.

Most of our elderly patients have many chronic problems. Treating one problem with traditional healthcare may negatively impact other comorbid conditions. Traditional healthcare emphasizes the use of medications which often interact with one another. Complementary therapies aim to impact the whole of the patient to restore the flow of natural body energy, or chi.

Most older patients are dehydrated and experience postural problems that exacerbate pain and pathology. Complementary therapies, along with proper hydration and exercise, can restore balance and improve posture. T'ai chi has been shown to help reduce the tendency to fall, common in older patients (Wolf et al 1997, Bottomley 2004b). Holistic therapies stress empathic communication between therapist and patient, and involve the patient in goal setting and problem solving. Older patients appreciate being treated in humanistic and caring ways that are emphasized in holistic therapies. Finally, many of the complementary therapies are pleasurable. Older people enjoy the socialization of T'ai chi and yoga classes, for example.

CONCLUSION

Complementary, alternative, integrative therapies are holistic approaches to healthcare, many of which have been used successfully for centuries around the world in other cultures. A growing body of research evidence suggests that holistic therapies have much to offer for older patients in rehabilitation, and as approaches that help to prevent the usual changes with aging and promote wellness. As more healthcare professionals use and research these therapies, two major advantages will emerge: patients will be better served for their chronic problems that are not well treated allopathically, and we will come to better understand the quantum physics at work in human biophysiological functioning.

References

Ader R, Cohen N 1991 The influence of conditioning on immune responses. In: Ader R, Felten DL, Cohen N (eds) Psychoneuro-immunology, 2nd edn. Academic Press, San Diego, CA, p 611–646

Barnes JF 1990 Myofascial Release/the Search for Excellence. Rehabilitation Services, Paoli, PA

Bottomley J 2004a Biofeedback: connecting the body and mind. In: Davis CM (ed.) Complementary Therapies in Rehabilitation – Evidence for Efficacy in Therapy, Prevention and Wellness, 2nd edn. Slack, Thorofare, NJ, p 131–156

Bottomley J 2004b T'ai chi: choreography of body and mind. In: Davis CM (ed.) Complementary Therapies in Rehabilitation – Evidence for Efficacy in Therapy, Prevention and Wellness, 2nd edn. Slack, Thorofare, NJ, p 109–130

Bottomley J 2004c Qi Gong for health and healing. In: Davis CM (ed.) Complementary Therapies in Rehabilitation – Evidence for Efficacy in Therapy, Prevention and Wellness, 2nd edn. Slack, Thorofare, NJ, p 253–282

Davis CM 2000 The science behind complementary and alternative therapies or holistic approaches to healing. Orthoped Phys Ther Clin North Am 9(3):291–302

Davis CM 2004 Quantum physics and systems theory – the science behind complementary and alternative therapies. In: Davis CM (ed.) Complementary Therapies in Rehabilitation – Evidence for Efficacy in Therapy, Prevention and Wellness, 2nd edn. Slack, Thorofare, NJ, p 15–24

Funk B 2004 Complete decongestive therapy. In: Davis CM (ed.) Complementary Therapies in Rehabilitation – Evidence for Efficacy in Therapy, Prevention and Wellness, 2nd edn. Slack, Thorofare, NJ, p 83–98

Greer S 1999 Mind–body research in psychooncology. Adv Mind–Body Med 15:236–281

Harris S 2001 Challenging myths in physical therapy. Phys Ther 81:1181–1182

Hunt VV 1989 Infinite Mind – the Science of the Human Vibrations of Consciousness. Malibu Publishing, Malibu, CA

LaRiccia PJ, Galantino ML 2004 Acupuncture theory and acupuncture-like therapeutics in physical therapy. In: Davis CM (ed.) Complementary Therapies in Rehabilitation – Evidence for Efficacy in Therapy, Prevention and Wellness, 2nd edn. Slack, Thorofare, NJ, p 307–320

Masin H 2006 Communicating to establish rapport and reduce negativity using neurolinguistic psychology. In: Davis CM (ed.) Patient Practitioner Interaction – An Experiential Manual for Developing the Art of Health Care, 4th edn. Slack, Thorofare, NJ, pp 149–166

Midura RJ, Ibiwoye MO, Powell KA et al 2005 Pulsed electromagnetic field treatments enhance the healing of fibular osteotomies. J Orthop Res 23(5):1035–1046

Mik GH 1997 Jin shin do. In: Davis CM (ed.) Complementary Therapies in Rehabilitation – Holistic Approaches for Prevention and Wellness, 1st edn. Slack, Thorofare, NJ, p 257–266

Oschman J 2000 Energy Medicine – The Scientific Basis. Churchill-Livingstone, Edinburgh

Pert C 2002 The wisdom of the receptors: neuropeptides, the emotions and body–mind. Adv Mind–Body Med 18(1):30–35

Reddy GK 2004 Biomedical applications of low-energy lasers. In: Davis CM (ed.) Complementary Therapies in Rehabilitation – Evidence for Efficacy in Therapy, Prevention and Wellness, 2nd edn. Slack, Thorofare, NJ, p 357–374

Rogers JS, Witt PL, Gross MT, Hacke JD 1998 Simultaneous palpation of the craniosacral rate at the head and feet: intrarater and interrater reliability. Phys Ther 78:1175–1185

Rubik B 1995 Energy medicine and the unifying concept of information. Altern Ther Health Med 1:34–39

Schwartz GE, Russek LG 1997 Dynamical energy systems and modern physics: fostering the science and spirit of complementary and alternative medicine. Altern Ther Health Med 3(3):46–56

Seto A, Kusaka C, Nakazato S et al 1992 Detection of extraordinary large bio-magnetic field strength from human hand. Acupuncture Electro-Therapeut Res Int J 17:75–94

Sharp M 1997 Polarity, reflexology and touch for health. In: Davis CM (ed.) Complementary Therapies in Rehabilitation – Holistic Approaches for Prevention and Wellness, 1st edn. Slack, Thorofare, NJ, p 235–256

Stephens J, Miller TM 2004 Feldenkrais method in rehabilitation. Using functional integration and awareness through movement to explore new possibilities. In: Davis CM (ed.) Complementary Therapies in Rehabilitation – Evidence for Efficacy in Therapy, Prevention and Wellness, 2nd edn. Slack, Thorofare, NJ, p 201–218

Stone A 1997 The Trager approach. In: Davis CM (ed.) Complementary Therapies in Rehabilitation – Holistic Approaches for Prevention and Wellness, 1st edn. Slack, Thorofare, NJ, p 199–212

Taylor MF 2004 Yoga therapeutics: an ancient practice in a 21st century setting. In: Davis CM (ed) Complementary Therapies in Rehabilitation – Evidence for Efficacy in Therapy, Prevention and Wellness, 2nd edn. Slack, Thorofare, NJ, p 157–178

Wallace RK, Benson H, Wilson AF 1971 A wakeful hypometabolic physiologic state. Am J Physiol 221(3):795–799

Wang Y, Botvinick E, Zhao U et al 2005 Visualizing the mechanical activation of Src. Nature 434:1040–1045

Wolf SL, Coogler C, Tingsen X 1997 Exploring the basis of Tai Chi Chuan as a therapeutic exercise approach. Arch Phys Med Rehabil 78:886–892

Zimmerman J 1990 Laying-on-of-hands healing and therapeutic touch: a testable theory. BEMI Currents, J Bio-Electro-Magnetics Inst 2:8–17

Zuck D 2004 The Alexander technique. In: Davis CM (ed) Complementary Therapies in Rehabilitation – Evidence for Efficacy in Therapy, Prevention and Wellness, 2nd edn. Slack, Thorofare, NJ, p 179–200

Chapter 73

Aquatic therapy

Beth E. Kauffman and Benjamin W. Kauffman

INTRODUCTION

Aquatic physical therapy may be one of the most dynamic modalities used in the treatment of the older adult. For many reasons, it is underutilized in today's healthcare settings. Throughout history, aquatic therapy has been used for healing, strengthening and relaxation. The Native Americans used hot springs for healing purposes. The Greeks and Romans used the 'baths' for relaxation. Franklin Delano Roosevelt along with many others with polio and postpolio syndrome used and acknowledged the benefits of water. The aquatic setting for physical therapy can be utilized in many different ways including gait training, improved cardiovascular efficiency, strengthening, balance, improved neuromuscular coordination, reduction of muscle spasms or tightness in joints, and edema control and wound care in specialized hydrotherapy settings.

PROPERTIES OF WATER

Part of the reason why therapy in water is so advantageous is because of the density of water. Hydrostatic pressure is an important concept in aquatic therapy; it is the static force of the water pressing against a person or object. Also, this force creates the upward thrust that we experience known as buoyancy. It is important to note that buoyancy has a direct effect on therapeutic exercise. For example, as the patient performs standing hip abduction, the limb is assisted by buoyancy. During the limb's return to neutral, increased hip adductor force is required to overcome buoyancy. Therefore, buoyancy can be assistive and resistive at the same time (Atkinson 2005). A person's body mass index (BMI), adipose tissue vs. muscle mass, is the primary determining factor in the degree to which a person sinks or floats. Muscle mass has a greater density than water, causing it to sink. Adipose tissue is less dense, causing it to float. Each individual's unique level of buoyancy requires appropriate flotation devices or weights, depending upon the desired effects of treatment. Buoyancy allows the body to be unloaded. The greater the depth of submersion, the less the effect of gravity on body weight. A basic breakdown of buoyancy and the unloading of gravity on a patient goes as follows: waist deep 50%; chest deep 75%; neck deep 90% of body weight (Atkinson 2005). The exact percentage of unloading may vary by gender and mass (Thein & Brody 1998). Hydrostatic pressure increases the efficiency of the heart by helping in venous return. It also applies compression to joints, muscles and soft tissue, facilitating reduction of swelling and adding lymphatic drainage (Jamison 2005).

Hydrodynamics, another important concept in aquatic therapy, is the force created when moving through water, causing resistance in front of the object. By changing the shape or surface area of an object, one can increase or decrease the hydrodynamic resistance (Thein & Brody 1998). By increasing the speed of movement, the resistance of the water becomes greater. In other words, the harder you push, the harder water pushes back. Water itself will not create a greater force of resistance than that which the individual is able to perform. This concept makes exercise in water a safe alternative to resistance training on land. Equipment, such as webbed gloves or water paddles, can be added to increase resistance. In some aquatic pools, the use of jets can add an increased level of resistance, or could be used for massage post exercise. It should be noted that an increase in water turbulence, even by a small amount, can significantly increase resistance depending on the activity (Atkinson 2005). This is important to remember when performing a group aquatic session.

A therapist or group leader should be cognizant that light refraction occurs when light passes from air to water, causing a perception of bending. This is caused by the reduction in the speed at which light is traveling upon entering the water. This bending may cause a visual disturbance to the patient's balance mechanism (Atkinson 2005).

SPECIAL CONSIDERATIONS IN THE AGING ADULT

The aquatic therapy setting may be more beneficial to people who have a history of being comfortable in the water. They do not need to be swimmers; however, that is advantageous with advanced activities. It is possible for people with a fear of water or who have previously had a bad experience to benefit from aquatic therapy. Patience and encouragement are important with every individual, but for those with a fear of water, it is imperative. Flotation devices may need to be used by the patient to increase their confidence.

A complete initial examination and evaluation by a physical therapist is essential for assessing each individual's needs, which must be performed prior to entering the water. This requisite is to screen individuals who may not be candidates for aquatic therapy and to establish goals of care (Geigle & Norton 2005). It is important to note that some patients may need assistance changing into their bathing suits, or entering and exiting the water. Some may require full assistance throughout the entire treatment session with the clinician in the water assisting. Being in the water with the patient is advantageous but not always necessary, depending on the activity or performance level. Some aging adults may not have been in a bathing suit for many years and may feel uncomfortable or self-conscious. It is recommended that, prior to entering the pool for the first time, the patient understands what is going to happen during the session.

Ideal water temperature for a therapeutic pool should be between 88°F and 93°F or 31–34°C. Depending on the patient, the diagnosis, and indications, the ideal water temperature may differ. A temperature less than 85°F (29°C) is too cool for many older patients. Their speed of movement will typically be slower, and they will not be generating as much additional body heat. Sustained exercise at temperatures greater than 95°F is too hot with respect to cardiovascular and thermoregulatory systems. Greater than 100°F is dangerous for persons with heart conditions and is considered unsafe for exercise.

The amount of work being performed by the patient is deceiving, on account of the buoyancy and resistance of the water. Thus, it is important to monitor the patient during exercise to determine exertion and fatigue levels. On land, it is common to use heart rate and oxygen saturation for monitoring a person's level of fitness or stress on the body. However, in water, these are not the most accurate or good determiners of exertion. When comparing the cardiac response of deep water running (up to the neck) with shallow water running (up to the xiphoid process), heart rate is 10 beats per minute slower in the deeper water (Robertson et al 2001). This is due to the hydrostatic pressure adding in venous return and other possible hemodynamic changes. It is suggested that one use a Perceived Exertion Scale, physical observation, as well as a Talk Test: shortness of breath while trying to talk will provide clues about the patient's exertion level. Skin coloration changes may include paleness, redness, blotchiness and/or excessive sweating. These are warning signs of overexertion or overheating. When submerged in water, it is difficult for the body to thermoregulate due to the radiant and conduction temperature gain or loss in water. Simply communicating with the patient about their general feeling may provide clues as to how the patient is tolerating the level of exercise, temperature and overall intervention.

Dehydration is an important concern with the older adult. Hydration should be included in a comprehensive aquatic therapy program. Patients should be encouraged to drink 8 oz (240 mL) of water at least 1 hour before entering the pool. They should be reminded that drinking or eating large amounts prior to entering the water might cause cramping. Patients exercising in the water do sweat, and they may not realize it. Water should be available before, during or after each session. It is important to encourage patients to void prior to aquatic sessions. The hydrostatic pressure on the abdomen stimulates the internal organs and facilitates kidney function and lymph return, which may increase the need to void (Atkinson 2005).

It is important to asses skin integrity prior to entering the water. An open wound is contraindicated for the aquatic setting, except when it is specifically being used as a wound care modality. A person's skin may be sensitive to pool chemicals; thus, chlorine or bromine as well as pH levels need to be observed and maintained. Usually, smaller indoor pools use bromine; larger or outdoor pools typically use chlorine as the sanitizing agent. Chlorine is harder on the skin; it tends to dry it out more rapidlly. Ideally, pool pH should be 7.4–7.6: higher or lower may cause skin irritation. Having the patient shower prior to and after aquatic sessions assists with the maintenance of chemical levels as well as protecting the patient's skin. Aqua shoes may also be worn to protect feet and maintain skin integrity, especially in people with diabetes. Shoes aid in traction, increasing confidence and avoidance of falls secondary to slipping.

There are many considerations to remember when deciding if aquatic therapy is appropriate for a particular patient (Morris 2005). In addition to medical screening and the above-mentioned concerns, there are contraindications (Hayes 1983) for aquatic therapy including:

1. active bleeding or open wounds;
2. significant bowel or bladder incontinence;
3. acute inflammatory conditions, i.e. fracture or neurological trauma;
4. significant cardiac or respiratory instability;
5. any unstable medical condition;
6. fever or infection.

EFFECTIVENESS OF WATER THERAPY

Exercise, rehabilitation and training in water is effective for elite athletes and people in mid- to late life with a variety of diagnoses (Thein & Brody 1998, Binkley et al 2002, Pechter et al 2003). After 12 weeks of low-intensity aquatic exercise by people with mild to moderate renal failure, Pechter et al (2003) reported beneficial effects in all cardiopulmonary functional measurements and significant changes in resting blood pressure, proteinuria, lipid peroxidation and serum glutathione. Similarly, oxygen uptake was significantly improved in hypertensive elderly inner city females after 10 weeks of a water exercise program. Also, heart rate response to submaximal walking in the water declined significantly as did systolic blood pressure (Binkley et al 2002). Significant gains in peak torque measurements have been reported after 12 weeks of graded aquatic exercise (Kendrick et al 2002). After 5–6 weeks of water exercise by individuals in the eighth and ninth decades of life, significant improvements have been shown on balance measurements in the Functional Reach Test (Simmons & Hansen 1996) and on the Berg Balance Scale (Douris et al 2003). A series of papers from France reported that 3 weeks of spa therapy including water exercise for people in their early fifties to middle sixties with chronic low back pain or osteoarthritis of the spine, hips, or knees had beneficial effects on pain, drug use, functional impairment, Waddell index, and quality of life. Follow-ups at 3–9 months showed continued benefits (Guillemin et al 1994, Nguyen et al 1997, Constant et al 1998).

CONCLUSION

Clinician expertise may be a limiting factor in choosing the patient population able to benefit from aquatic therapy. It is important for clinicians working in the realm of aquatic therapy to attend continuing education courses, and to learn proper techniques that will most benefit their patients. Care should always be aimed at meeting mutually agreed upon needs and goals. Aquatic therapy adds an excellent modality to meet goals as well as to enhance health and well-being.

References

Atkinson K 2005 Hydrotherapy in orthopaedics. In: Atkinson K, Coutts F, Hassenkamp AM (eds) Physiotherapy in Orthopaedics. Elsevier, Oxford p 312–351

Binkley H, Kendrick ZV, Doerr E et al 2002 Effects of water exercise on cardiovascular responses of hypertension elderly inner-city women. J Aquatic Phys Ther 10(1):28–33

Constant F, Guillemin F, Colin JF et al 1998 Use of spa therapy to improve the quality of life of chronic low back pain patients. Med Care 39:1309–1314

Douris P, Southard V, Varga C et al 2003 The effect of land and aquatic exercise on balance scores in older adults. J Geriatr Phys Ther 26(1):3–6

Geigle P, Norton C 2005 Medical screening for aquatic physical therapy. J Aquatic Phys Ther 13(2):6–10

Guillemin F, Constant F, Colin JF et al 1994 Short and long term effect of spa therapy in chronic low back pain. Br J Rheumatol 33:148–151

Hayes K 1983 Manual for Physical Agents, 4th edn. Appleton and Lange, Norwalk CT, p 17–21

Jamison L 2005 Aquatic therapy for the patient with lymphedema. J Aquatic Phys Ther 13(1):9–12

Kendrick ZV, Binkley H, McGettigan J et al 2002 Effects of water exercise on improving muscular strength and endurance in suburban and inner-city older adults. J Aquatic Phys Ther 10(1):21–28

Morris DM 2005 The 'go' or 'no go' decision in aquatic physical therapy. J Aquatic Phys Ther 13(2):4

Nyugen M, Revel M, Dougados M 1997 Prolonged effects of 3 week therapy in a spa resort on lumbar spine, knee and hip osteoarthritis: follow-up after 6 months. A randomized controlled trial. Br J Rheumatol 36:77–81

Pechter U, Ots M, Mesikepp S et al 2003 Beneficial effects of water-based exercise in patients with chronic kidney disease. Int J Rehabil Res 26(2):153–156

Robertson JM, Brewster EA, Factora KI 2001 Comparison of heart rates during water running in deep and shallow water at the same rating of perceived exertion. J Aquatic Phys Ther 9(1):21–26

Simmons V, Hansen P 1996 Effectiveness of water exercise on postural mobility in the well elderly: an experimental study on balance enhancement. J Gerontol Med Sci 51:M233–M238

Thein JM, Brody LT 1998 Aquatic-based rehabilitation and training the elite athlete. J Orthop Sports Phys Ther 27(1):32–41

UNIT **10**

Social and government implications, ethics and dying

Chapter 74

Legal considerations

Ron Scott and Timothy L. Kauffman

INTRODUCTION

Rehabilitation professionals and support personnel who treat geriatric patients face potential malpractice liability exposure for their conduct, just as healthcare professionals do in any other care delivery setting. The majority of the reported physical therapy healthcare malpractice cases published in the legal literature involve geriatric clientele as plaintiffs, or parties bringing legal action against their healthcare providers.

The United States is a highly litigious society. In 1992, approximately 19 million new civil lawsuits between private parties were initiated nationwide. Although only a small proportion of these legal cases involved healthcare malpractice, the risk of liability exposure in healthcare practice generally, and in geriatric rehabilitation practice in particular, is significant. Geriatric rehabilitation professionals must strike a careful balance between providing optimal quality patient care (a prospect made more difficult in the current cost containment-focused managed care environment) and minimizing their own healthcare malpractice liability risk exposure incident to practice (Scott 1997).

In a recent study of 1452 closed malpractice claims, Studdert et al (2006) found that 3% of the claims had no verifiable medical injuries and 37% were not associated with errors in care. However, payment for 28% of claims not involving errors averaged $313 205, which was significantly lower than the average payment of $521 560 in claims in which errors were involved.

Medical malpractice has attracted a great deal of attention because of rising insurance and healthcare costs.

The average payment for malpractice claims for physicians and other licensed providers was about $300 000 for all settlements and $500 000 for trial verdicts (General Accounting Office 2003). This drove up the cost of malpractice insurance for a general surgeon in Philadelphia, PA, by 43% from the year 2000 to 2003 (from $33 684 to $72 518).

As a result, 93% of surveyed specialist physicians reported practicing defensive medicine (Studdert et al 2005).

In geriatric rehabilitation, professional practice in compliance with legal standards also includes knowledge by caregivers of, and compliance with, the Patient Self-Determination Act and state statutory reporting requirements for suspected elder abuse, among a myriad of other relevant laws. Because nearly one-third of the population over age 55 years is employed, healthcare professionals should also be cognizant of laws protective of the employment rights of their geriatric clients, including the Age Discrimination in Employment Act, the Americans with Disabilities Act, and the Family and Medical Leave Act (Scott 1998a, 1998b).

HEALTHCARE MALPRACTICE

Negligence

Healthcare malpractice is defined as physical and/or mental injury incurred by a patient in the course of healthcare examination or intervention, coupled with a legal basis for imposing civil liability on a healthcare provider for the harm suffered by the patient. Traditionally, the only basis for imposing healthcare malpractice liability was professional negligence, or substandard care.

In a professional negligence lawsuit brought by a patient against a healthcare professional, the patient must normally prove four core elements by a preponderance, or greater weight, of evidence. These four elements are:

- that the defendant healthcare professional owed a special duty of care to the plaintiff-patient;
- that, in the course of healthcare delivery, the healthcare professional breached, or violated, the duty owed, by failing to meet at least minimally acceptable care standards;
- that the breach of duty by the healthcare provider caused injury to the patient; and
- that the patient sustained injuries of the type for which a judge or jury may legally order compensation in the form of a money damages judgment, designed to make the patient 'whole' again.

In addition to being legally responsible for his or her own conduct, a healthcare professional providing geriatric rehabilitation is also normally vicariously, or indirectly, responsible for the conduct of supportive personnel acting under the supervision of the licensed or certified professional. Healthcare professionals must clearly communicate orders to support personnel to whom care tasks are delegated, and establish competency standards and actually assess the competency of supportive personnel on an ongoing basis.

Additional legal bases for malpractice

Other legal bases for imposing healthcare malpractice liability, in addition to professional negligence, include:

- intentional misconduct, including battery (injurious or otherwise offensive physical contact with a patient) and sexual battery (physical contact intended to gratify a healthcare provider's illicit sexual desires);
- strict product liability, for patient injury by dangerously defective treatment-related equipment, such as durable medical equipment supplied to a geriatric client; and
- breach of contract liability, for failure to fulfill a therapeutic promise made to a patient.

Geriatric rehabilitation professionals and clinic and agency managers are advised to develop, educate staff about, and enforce formal risk management policies and procedures designed to minimize healthcare malpractice liability exposure of professional employees and organizations. Legal counsel should be consulted proactively for advice on developing and implementing such initiatives (Scott 1997, 1998a, 1998b).

Consider the following hypothetical example:

A home health physical therapist is charged by a geriatric patient with sexual battery. In this case, involving myofascial release, there was, in fact, no therapist misconduct; the patient was simply confused about the nature of the therapeutic touch and honestly believed it to be improperly applied by the therapist to her torso. What risk management measures should the physical therapist and agency have undertaken to prevent this kind of allegation?

The agency and its professional and support staff should have developed and practiced under a professional–patient relations policy that requires:

1. patient understanding of and informed consent for intensive hands-on therapy, such as myofascial release and massage;
2. notification by the treating healthcare provider to the patient of the right to have a same-gender chaperone present during treatment (such a policy obligates the employer to make available a chaperone upon the patient's request); and
3. respect by providers for patient autonomy and modesty, including appropriate patient draping procedures prior to and during treatment.

In this scenario, the physical therapist faces primary liability exposure for his or her conduct, and the employing agency possible vicarious liability for the physical therapist/employee's conduct within the scope of employment.

PATIENT INFORMED CONSENT

In any healthcare delivery setting, adult patients with full mental capacity have the right to give informed consent before evaluation or intervention. The duty to make relevant information disclosure and obtain patient informed consent to treatment is premised on respect for patient autonomy, or self-determination. Although the exact disclosure requirements for patient informed consent vary from state to state, the following elements are commonly included:

- disclosure of the patient's diagnosis and relevant information about a proposed intervention;
- disclosure of serious risks of possible harm or complication associated with a proposed intervention that would be material to the patient's decision about whether to accept or refuse the intervention;
- discussion about the expected benefits, or goals, associated with the proposed intervention; and
- disclosure of reasonable alternatives to a proposed intervention, and their material risks and benefits,
- after the above disclosure elements are discussed with the patient, the provider is additionally obligated to solicit and satisfactorily answer the patient's questions and formally ask for patient consent to proceed before doing so.

It may not be necessary to individually document in patients' records each patient's informed consent for routine care. An agency, institution, or group may elect instead to memorialize an informed consent policy in a policy and procedures document; orient providers upon employment of their informed consent obligations; monitor informed consent processes on an ongoing basis; and reinforce the duty to obtain patients' informed consent with providers on a regularly recurring basis during in-service education.

Managed care 'gag clause' employment provisions requiring providers to refrain from discussing with patients care options that are not offered by patients' insurance plans derogate from respect for patient autonomy and the informed consent requirement for disclosure of reasonable alternatives to proposed care options, and are therefore unethical and, in many jurisdictions, illegal (Scott 1997).

REPORTING SUSPECTED ELDER ABUSE

Geriatric rehabilitation professionals have a legal duty to act reasonably to identify elder abuse in their clients and to take appropriate action to prevent further abuse. This may include reporting suspected elder abuse to social service departments or agencies or to law enforcement agencies, as appropriate (Joshi & Flaherty 2005).

Elder abuse may be less often recognized and reported by healthcare professionals than 'domestic' or child abuse. Most state laws on reporting abuse provide for qualified immunity from defamation or other bases of liability for persons making good faith reports of suspected abuse.

Signs and symptoms of possible elder abuse may be present in a geriatric client and in the client's abuser, who may be present with the client during examination or treatment. Signs and symptoms in the geriatric client may include, among others: unexplained or untreated injuries; reticence; poor hygiene; malnutrition and dehydration; and dirty or inappropriate dress for conditions. Indices of elder abuse in abusers, who may be caregivers or family members, include, among others: aggression toward or verbal abuse of the geriatric patient; speaking for the client during an examination or treatment; and indifference to instructions or suggestions offered by the provider (Scott 1997).

Consider the following case:

Mr Doe is an 83-year-old patient who is status post-right cerebrovascular accident, with mild left upper limb hemiparesis. He has just been referred as an outpatient to ABC Rehab, Inc. His examining physical therapist notices the following about Mr Doe:

1. He is accompanied by his 51-year-old daughter, Sue, who does most of the talking for the patient.
2. He has scratches and petechiae on the dorsal forearms.
3. He is dressed in a Navy pea-coat, long-sleeved shirt, and wool trousers, despite it being June and 78°F.

How should the physical therapist proceed, based on the above information?

Based on the presentation above, Mr Doe may be a victim of elder abuse. The physical therapist should annotate pertinent objective examination findings in Mr Doe's health record and should consult with a supervisor or professional colleague about this patient. The therapist may also, as an exercise of professional judgment, report his or her suspicion to the facility's social service department for follow-up. Whether or not a report to social service department is made at this time, the physical therapist should closely monitor Mr Doe for any further indicators of possible abuse.

PATIENT SELF-DETERMINATION ACT

The Patient Self-Determination Act (PSDA) of 1990 is a federal statute that memorializes a patient's right to control routine and extraordinary treatment-related decisions. The PSDA, like the law of patient informed consent, is premised on respect for patient autonomy.

The PSDA does not create any new substantive patient rights; it simply requires healthcare facilities – including hospitals and long-term care facilities – to ask patients about any advance directives that they might have in effect and to honor the provisions of those advance directives.

Advance directives are legal instruments that memorialize patients' desires regarding care options in the event of such patients' incapacitation. They are of two basic types: living wills, which spell out patients' wishes concerning the scope of permissible healthcare interventions in the event of patient incapacity; and durable powers of attorney for healthcare decisions, which empower third parties to act on behalf of incapacitated patients. Patient health records should include information about existing patient advance directives.

Health Insurance Portability and Accountability Act of 1996

The Health Insurance Portability and Accountability Act (HIPAA) became effective in 2003. The intention of the law is to make health insurance more portable, especially as people change jobs, and to prevent healthcare fraud and abuse. It requires all healthcare practitioners, healthcare plans, and healthcare clearinghouses (electronic billing services) to protect patient health information including demographic data as well as any other information that may potentially identify an individual. HIPAA regulations do not supersede existing federal or state laws. The confidentiality protection in HIPAA has caused problems for families and adult protective services working with elder abuse (Dyer et al 2005).

Direct access to physical therapy

The World Confederation of Physical Therapy (WCPT) consists of 92 member countries that represent more than 250 000 physical therapists. Most member countries have laws that require physical therapists to have a physician referral; however, an evolution is occurring toward direct access to physical therapy services by the patient/consumer. As reflected in a WCPT report, the outcomes of educational programs for physical therapists in South Africa, Australia, Norway, Jamaica, Canada and Brazil are intended for graduates to work autonomously and/or in primary care (Takahashi et al 2003).

In the United States, 42 states have laws permitting direct access to physical therapy services. Also, in military settings, direct access has been in effect in various forms since 1972. In a recent large study involving direct access in Army, Navy and Air Force healthcare sites, 50 799 patients were evaluated without any documented adverse events as a result of the physical therapy diagnosis or management. Also, there were no disciplinary actions, litigations, license or credential problems for the physical therapists involved in this direct access care (Moorer et al 2005).

EMPLOYMENT PROTECTION FOR OLDER WORKERS

There are three federal statutes that serve primarily to protect the employment interests of older workers. These are the Age Discrimination in Employment Act, the Americans with Disabilities Act, and the Family and Medical Leave Act (Scott 1997, 1998a, 1998b).

The Age Discrimination in Employment Act (ADEA) of 1967 prohibits employer discrimination against workers aged 40 years or older. The broad prohibition of discrimination against older workers encompasses nearly all aspects of the employment relationship, from recruitment and selection to training and promotion to employee benefits. Under case law developed after implementation of the ADEA, employers may discharge older workers from employment if such workers contractually waive their ADEA rights in exchange for monetary compensation.

The Americans with Disabilities Act (ADA) of 1990 offers significant protection from discrimination to older workers and patients. Under Title I of the ADA, business organizations having 12 or more workers are prohibited from discriminating against physically or mentally disabled employees, and must provide reasonable accommodation for employees' disabilities that affect their ability to carry out essential functions of their jobs. Title III of the ADA protects the rights of disabled consumers to equal access to public accommodation, including privately owned healthcare facilities.

The Family and Medical Leave Act (FLMA) of 1993 requires employers having 20 or more full-time employees to allow employees to take up to 12 weeks per year of unpaid, job-protected leave for personal or family illness or for adoption or childbirth. Unlike the ADEA and the ADA, which are enforced by the federal Equal Employment Opportunity Commission, the FLMA is administered by the federal Department of Labor.

Consider the following scenario:

A 68-year-old rehabilitation client informs a physical therapist during the patient history interview of circumstances that might constitute employment discrimination (age-related discharge) related to the client's disability. What should the therapist do?

Even though the therapist is generally familiar with employment laws, the therapist should not attempt to advise the client about possible legal options. Instead, the therapist should inform the client of the right to seek legal advice with an attorney of choice or through the public service county bar association's legal referral service, which is available in every county and parish in the United States at no cost or for a low charge for 'initial' legal advice.

CONCLUSION

Geriatric rehabilitation professionals must be cognizant of key laws and legal requirements affecting their practice and their clients' civil rights. Under managed care, the rehabilitation milieu has become extremely business-like and impersonal, making malpractice avoidance more difficult. Clinicians and managers must simultaneously strive for optimal quality patient care and effective clinical risk management in order to survive and thrive.

Knowledge of laws respecting patient autonomy, including the PSDA concerning patients' advance directives, and of employment protection benefiting elderly clients, enables geriatric rehabilitation professionals to better serve their clients. Legal advice, however, should be given to clients only by attorneys.

The information presented in this chapter is intended as legal information only and not as specific legal advice for any health professional. Individual legal advice can be given only by a person's personal or institutional attorney, based on the distinct laws of the particular jurisdiction (state or federal law, as applicable).

Acknowledgment

The kind reviews and suggestions of Michael A. Roman Esq. and Russell W. Stabler Esq. are acknowledged.

References

Dyer C, Heisler C, Hill C et al 2005 Community approaches to elder abuse. Clin Geriatr Med 21:429–447

General Accounting Office (GAO) 2003 Medical Malpractice Implications of Rising Premiums on Access to Health Care. GAO-03-836. Available: www.gao.gov/cgi_bin/getrpt? GAO-03-836. Accessed November 5 2006

Joshi S, Flaherty J 2005 Elder abuse and neglect in long term care. Clin Geriatr Med 21:333–354

Moorer J, McMillian D, Rosenthal M et al 2005 Risk determination for patients with direct access to physical therapy in military health care facilities. J Orthopaed Sports Phys Ther 35:674–678

Scott RW 1997 Promoting Legal Awareness in Physical and Occupational Therapy. Mosby-Year Book, St Louis, MO

Scott RW 1998a Health Care Malpractice: A Primer on Legal Issues for Professionals, 2nd edn. McGraw-Hill, New York

Scott RW 1998b Professional Ethics: A Guide for Rehabilitation Professionals. Mosby-Year Book, St Louis, MO

Studdert D, Mello M, Sage W et al 2005 Defensive medicine among high-risk specialist physicians in a volatile malpractice environment. JAMA 293:2609–2617

Studdert D, Mello M, Gawande A et al 2006 Claims, errors, and compensation payments in medical malpractice litigation. N Engl J Med 354:2024–2033

Takahashi S, Killette D, Eftekari T 2003 Exploring Issues related to the Qualifications Recognition of Physical Therapists. World Confederation for Physical Therapy, London

Chapter 75

Ethics

Mary Ann Wharton

INTRODUCTION

Decisions regarding moral choices, what is right vs. what is wrong, are difficult, and they frequently complicate treatment interventions and service delivery in geriatric rehabilitation. These moral decisions are often made more limited by factors such as ageism, societal attitudes and available reimbursement for healthcare services. This is especially true in the current healthcare delivery system, which intermingles patient care with technology, a reimbursement-driven environment and a societal mandate to conserve healthcare dollars. An understanding of the concept of professionalism and of ethical principles and theory can provide a framework for analyzing the values involved in moral decision-making in geriatrics.

PROFESSIONALISM, ETHICS AND GERIATRIC PHYSICAL THERAPY PRACTICE

It has been said that every clinical decision involving a patient has a moral or ethical dimension. The physical therapist's response to this ethical circumstance requires that the therapist possesses the moral courage to formulate a reply to the ethical situation and implement a decision that will benefit the patient. This ability to act ethically on behalf of a patient's needs is inherent in the notion of professionalism.

In our society, a professional is regarded as possessing more than a body of knowledge and technical expertise. A true professional is expected to perform a valuable service to society. In exchange for autonomy to make decisions on behalf of vulnerable patients and on behalf of society, a professional is expected to abide by high ethical standards. In essence, they are expected to exercise professional expertise responsibly, and to make accountable decisions that are in the patient's and societies' best interests (Swisher 2005). The American Physical Therapy Association (APTA), recognizing the intimate relationship between professionalism and ethics, has adopted a consensus document that identifies the core values of professionalism in physical therapy practice. These core values can be viewed as guiding principles for the ethical treatment of patients, especially those older individuals who are entrusted to our care. The core values are account-ability, altruism, compassion and caring, excellence, integrity, professional duty and social responsibility (APTA 2003).

ETHICS AND MORALITY

Morality is defined by Churchill as 'behavior according to custom' (Henderson & McConnell 1997). It is further defined by Purtilo as guidelines that are designed to preserve the fabric of society (Purtilo 2005). Ethics, on the other hand, can be viewed as 'a systematic reflection on and analysis of morality' (Purtilo 2005). As such, ethics is based on principles that provide a conceptual framework within which it is possible to place perceptions of ethical cases and problems. These principles allow the imposition of some sense of artificial order on a story, and they affect peoples' response to it. Ethical concepts are tied to society's customs, manners, traditions and institutions. In essence, these concepts define how members of a society deal with the world (Elliott 1992).

Professional ethics that arise in the context of healthcare provide guidelines that are ultimately no different from those that arise from religious, philosophical, cultural and other societal sources (Purtilo 2005). Ethical situations in geriatrics are no different from the ethical situations in other aspects of healthcare. Similar reasoning processes should be observed to answer questions of morality when dealing with older individuals.

ETHICAL PRINCIPLES

Ethical principles serve as one tool for solving complex ethical problems. Ethical theories provide a sense of order. They can help to simplify a complicated case for initial problem-solving, and that simplification in itself can be useful in ordering and focusing a wide range of disparate intuitions (Elliott 1992).

The foundational principles of biomedical ethics that govern geriatric rehabilitation professionals include the following ethical duties and rights:

- beneficence – the duty to do the best possible;
- nonmaleficence – the minimal duty to do no harm;
- justice – the allocation of time and resources; and
- autonomy – the ethical right of self-determination.

Autonomy

Respect for patient autonomy is an ethical principle that requires further understanding and definition. According to the ethical principle of autonomy, the patient has the right to actively negotiate his or her own healthcare decisions. In geriatrics, issues of autonomy may revolve around questions of individual capacity and competency to make decisions. Healthcare providers must recognize that questions of patient competency are determined legally and are not to be presumed by the professional or by family members or caregivers.

In general, the decision-making capacities of older individuals with cognitive deficits must be respected as long as possible. For patients with dementia, determination of capacity and competency is especially problematic. However, the respect for autonomy must be balanced with the notion of protection of that individual from potential harm. The tension between autonomy and protection may direct caregivers to make decisions that are in conflict with patient wishes. Ethically, the rights of the individual to express a choice regarding his or her care should be made in light of several observations, including the severity of the dementia, the presence or absence of actual mental illness, the physical and functional state of the individual and the availability of family and community resources (Brindle & Holmes 2005).

A concern specific to the autonomy of the older patient may be the reliance of the professional on family members or caregivers to make decisions for that individual even when the older patient is legally competent to make the decision himself or herself. In these situations, in which the older client is legally competent, the moral and legal appropriateness of consulting such individuals must be determined by the patient. This is an especially difficult issue for caregivers when the patient is ill, recovering from surgery or pathological insult, or taking certain medications, all of which can negatively affect the patient's judgment.

One factor that may influence the ability of older individuals to make autonomous healthcare choices is their own beliefs or expectations regarding healthcare. Specific factors to consider might include whether they view healthcare as a right or a privilege. They must also analyze whether they believe that they are a passive recipient of healthcare vs. the more current concept that stresses an individual's responsibility to actively participate in the rehabilitation process.

Informed consent, which provides the legal basis for autonomy, requires patient education according to the 'reasonable man standard'. Specifically, this standard obliges the healthcare professional to provide information in terms understandable to a reasonable individual of like circumstances. Informed consent is recognized as one way to achieve patient adherence.

Scott (1997), in his work on legal awareness, notes that the legal disclosure requirements vary from state to state, but commonly include the following:

- the patient's diagnosis and pertinent evaluative findings;
- the nature of a proposed or ordered intervention;

- any material risks for harm or complication associated with the proposed intervention;
- reasonable alternatives, if any, to the proposed intervention; and
- the goals of the intervention.

Scott (1997) goes on to state that the goals of rehabilitation intervention must be jointly developed and implemented by the patient and the rehabilitation professional. Both parties to the rehabilitation 'contract' then feel that they have a stake in achieving an optimal patient outcome.

An additional factor to consider with respect to ethics and patient autonomy is the issue of paternalism. Paternalism may be defined as coercion, or interference with another person's freedom of action. The healthcare professional justifies paternalism by reasons related to the welfare and happiness of the individual being coerced. In the ethics of healthcare, paternalism stems from the principle that the practitioner should act to bring about the maximum benefit for the patient, even at the expense of the patient's autonomy. It is rooted in the healthcare provider's knowledge and professional understanding coupled with the duty of beneficence and the healthcare provider's desire to bring about the best outcome. In its extreme, paternalism can result in a violation of autonomy, which is not considered acceptable in this society. On the other hand, contemporary health-care may accept gentle paternalism, which combines with informed consent to achieve patient adherence. In geriatrics, questions of competency frequently complicate this issue (Weiss 1985).

The issues of patient autonomy and paternalism may also be complicated by Medicare and other insurance regulations that require specified treatment times and frequencies. Thus, the ill or depressed patient may be coerced into going to rehabilitation in order to protect Medicare payment benefits, which may be suspended if the patient fails to attend the regulated number of daily hours or treatment days per week, depending upon the treatment setting – rehabilitation unit or skilled nursing facility respectively. Some medical providers maintain the attitude that the patient may not refuse the required care, which is paternalistic.

FIDELITY, VERACITY, CONFIDENTIALITY

Secondary ethical duties inherent in healthcare include the following:

- Faithfulness, or the fidelity/fiduciary relationship: entails meeting a patient's reasonable expectations.

- Truth-telling, or veracity and honesty: obligates a healthcare provider not only to the patient but also to other sources such as the reimbursement source (this is a frequent source of conflict).

- Confidentiality, or the patient's expectation that the healthcare provider will honor personal information as private: requires that a healthcare provider only shares sensitive information with those who have a legitimate right to know. The legal basis for confidentiality exists in the constitutional concept of the right to privacy.

VIRTUE ETHICS AND THE ETHICS OF CARE

Traditional bioethical principles may have limited value in guiding ethical decisions that must be made daily when caring for geriatric patients in today's complex healthcare environment. Virtue ethics is another theory that may provide the physical therapist with insight into ethical care. Virtue ethicists look at character, rather than rules, for moral guidance in patient care decisions. Therefore, virtue ethics is considered as a theory of being that focuses on the character of the moral agent rather than on the acts of that agent. For example, a virtue ethicist would look at the patience of the therapist treating the older individual, rather than judge the lack of productivity that resulted from the therapist taking additional time to address the complex concerns of an older patient. A virtue is defined as a good habit that balances excesses and deficiencies. As agents, physical therapy practitioners may apply virtue ethics to geriatric care by developing trusting relationships with patients, being compassionate, and developing a deep awareness of the lives and wishes of the patient. Compassion is considered a cardinal virtue of physical therapists treating geriatric patients, and moral and ethical actions are guided by that compassion (Nalette 2001).

Regardless of the ethical theory, when physical therapists deliberate an ethical concern or attempt to determine a solution to an ethical situation, the goal should be to provide a caring response. In spite of competing loyalties, the primary loyalty must be to the patient, and the caring response must lead to a conclusion with purposeful action. Purtilo states that care means 'seeking the deepest understanding of what that other person really needs. Care is what you pay attention to. And that's important within the health professional–patient relationship. . .' (Ries 2003). Ethically, it means going beyond evidence-based practice that simply looks at the results of research studies and, instead, incorporates the essence of true evidence-based practice, which includes client-centered goals in patient care (Wong et al 2000). This may involve helping the patient to understand how your knowledge and expertise may benefit them, and empowering older patients to make decisions that are in their best interests. It means listening to the older individual's story, and respecting their ideas, concerns, and perspectives as you jointly develop a meaningful plan of care (Ries 2003).

CODES OF ETHICS

One hallmark of a profession is its adoption and enforcement of a code of ethics. An underlying assumption is that a code of ethics articulates the values of that profession and holds members of the discipline accountable for adhering to ethical standards. The purpose of a code is to make positive statements of ethical values and to educate professionals about the ethical dimensions of practice. Perhaps more importantly, a code of ethics is meant to educate the public through statements of what can be expected from members of that profession. As such, a code of ethics is an official statement by the profession that is intended to promote public trust. It serves as a guide for professionals to solve moral problems. However, it is not a substitute for good moral judgment or personal commitment.

The World Confederation of Physical Therapy (WCPT) has adopted ethical principles that are recognized as prototypes for member organizations to develop their own code of ethics or code of conduct (see Box 75.1). The ethical principles articulated by WCPT can offer ethical guidance for physical therapists providing care for geriatric patients. Specifically, Principle 1 states that physical therapists respect the rights and dignity of all individuals. This principle directs practitioners to respect patients regardless of age, culture or disability. It implies the right to privacy and confidentiality. It requires respect for patient autonomy. It states that physical therapists have the absolute responsibility to act professionally when involved with patient care. Principle 2 requires that physical therapists comply with laws and regulations that govern the practice of physical therapy in the country in which they work. In addition to licensing laws, this principle implies that therapists in the United States who treat older individuals have knowledge of the legal implications of informed consent. It also implies that therapists

| Box 75.1 | WCPT ethical principles/declarations of principle |

Physical therapists:

1. Respect the rights and dignity of all individuals
2. Comply with the laws and regulations governing the practice of physical therapy in the country in which they work
3. Accept responsibility for the exercise of sound judgment
4. Provide an honest, competent, and accountable professional service
5. Are committed to providing quality services according to quality policies and objectives defined by their national physical therapy association
6. Are entitled to a just and fair level of remuneration for their services
7. Provide accurate information to clients, to other agencies and the community about physical therapy and the services physical therapists provide
8. Contribute to the planning and development of services that address the health needs of the community

Reproduced with kind permission from the WCPT (http://www.wcpt.org/policies/principles/ethicalprinciples.php).

understand the regulations related to Medicare reimbursement. Principle 3 states that physical therapists accept responsibility for the exercise of sound judgment. Inherent in this principle is the notion of professional independence and autonomy and the idea that a therapist is qualified to make judgments regarding the physical therapy plan of care. Implied is that the therapist is working within the scope of the profession, is competent based on knowledge and skill, has made an appropriate assessment and determined a diagnosis, and will implement the plan of care based on the assessment and diagnosis. Principle 4 directs physical therapists to provide honest, competent, and accountable professional service. This principle directs therapists to understand the nature of the services they provide, including the costs associated with that service. It also instructs therapists to maintain competency through professional development and participation in ongoing continuing education. It directs therapists to keep adequate client records and to disclose those records only to individuals who have a legitimate right to access the information contained in the documentation. Included in this principle is the notion that ethical practice takes precedence over business practices in the provision of physical therapy services. Principle 5 states that physical therapists must be committed to providing quality services according to the policies and objectives defined by their national physical therapy association. As stated, this principle requires physical therapists to be aware of current standards of practice, and to participate in ongoing education to update knowledge and skills consistent with current evidence and research. Principle 6 identifies the physical therapist's entitlement to just and fair remuneration for services rendered. Principle 7 directs therapists to provide accurate information to clients and the public regarding physical therapy services. Principle 8 requires therapists to contribute to the planning and development of services that address the health needs of the community. This principle obliges therapists to work toward achieving justice in the provision of healthcare for all people, and may be particularly applicable in view of the needs and access to care provided for geriatric clients under the current constraints imposed by healthcare regulations and financing in the United States healthcare delivery system (WCPT 2006).

The APTA's code of ethics, 2000 revision, is markedly similar to the principles adopted by the WCPT. This code of ethics contains 11 principles that direct physical therapists to respect the rights and dignity of all individuals; provide compassionate and trustworthy care; comply with laws and regulations that govern physical therapy practice; exercise sound professional judgment; achieve and maintain professional competency; maintain high standards for practice, education, and research; seek deserved and reasonable remuneration for services; provide accurate information to patients and consumers; protect the public from unethical, incompetent, and illegal acts; address the health needs of society; and respect the rights, knowledge, and skills of colleagues and other healthcare professionals (APTA 2006a). Similarly, APTA adopted seven standards of ethical conduct for the physical therapist assistant. These standards direct physical therapist assistants to respect the rights and dignity of all individuals, provide compassionate and trustworthy care, provide only selected physical therapy interventions under the supervision and direction of a physical therapist; comply with laws and regulations governing physical therapy; achieve and maintain competence; make judgments commensurate with educational and legal qualifications; and protect the public from unethical, incompetent and illegal acts (APTA 2006b). Physical therapists and physical therapist assistants who provide care for older individuals are responsible for maintaining the standards of ethical conduct when providing patient care, regardless of association membership.

WCPT's ethical principles and the code of ethics and standards of ethical conduct for the physical therapist assistant adopted by the APTA can provide valuable guidance for physical therapists and physical therapist assistants who provide care to geriatric patients. In addition to the ethical theories and principles, they articulate principles that direct responsible, ethical and caring practice.

SOURCES OF CONFLICTS IN GERIATRIC REHABILITATION

Several broad sources of ethical conflicts in geriatric rehabilitation have been outlined by Guccione & Shefrin (1993). They can be listed as follows:

Personal vs. professional beliefs

In dealing with older patients, a healthcare professional must recognize that occasionally a conflict exists between personal feelings about a patient or situation and professional duties. The professional must know how to weigh personal values against professional obligations and responsibilities.

An interdisciplinary team's perception and conflicts

Expectations of team members involved in the care of geriatric patients may differ or not be clearly understood. Conflicts may develop regarding the role and responsibility of each professional. It is important that each individual in the team clarifies the promises implicit in the commitment to work in an interdisciplinary team.

Organizational and societal conflicts

Current healthcare reflects rapid changes in delivery and service models, especially as managed care principles have come to predominate in organizations. Conflict often exists between the healthcare professional's obligation to the patient and obligations to the organization. Our society expresses a wide variety of opinions about the attitude that should be taken toward elders. Recent dilemmas involve the allocation of healthcare resources, especially the financing of care and reimbursement for services. Therapists must look at each case on an individual basis and at the same time consider that case in the context of societal issues.

ETHICAL DECISION-MAKING

Purtilo (2005) has identified the following six-step process as a tool that can be used to address ethical problems:

1. gather relevant information;
2. identify the type of ethical problems;
3. use ethics theories or approaches to analyze the problem;
4. explore the practical alternatives;
5. complete the action; and
6. evaluate the process and outcome.

SPECIAL TECHNIQUES TO PROMOTE ETHICAL DECISION-MAKING IN GERIATRIC CARE

A variety of techniques can be used to promote ethical decision-making in geriatric care. Included in these techniques are value histories, use of ethics committees and team conferences, and recognition of legal remedies, including guardianship and power of attorney (Henderson & McConnell 1997).

Value history

A value history is a summary of a patient's values and beliefs. The information is obtained prior to the onset of a cognitive impairment that impedes the exercise of autonomous judgment. It can be constructed with the help of family members or significant others. This tool helps to preserve respect for the individual patient and his or her autonomy.

Ethics committees

Groups of individuals in an institution may be identified as an ethics committee. Such committees have the authority to facilitate the resolution of ethical dilemmas in healthcare. They can develop policy and guidelines, provide consultation and case review, offer theological reflection, and educate others in the institution regarding matters of morality. Membership varies and is often determined by the purpose of the committee. Generally, membership includes attorneys, clergy, ethicists, medical practitioners and community representatives. Specific limits of authority vary, depending on the policy developed by the institution. One model specifies optional consultation with the committee, leaving compliance with their recommendations to the discretion of the professionals involved in the case. Another model specifies mandatory review of certain decisions, for example those regarding life support measures, but continues to allow professionals to retain their authority in the final decision. A third model dictates mandatory review by the ethics committee and mandatory compliance with its conclusions.

Team conferences

The interdisciplinary team may be used for additional input when ethical issues about patients must be addressed. In order to effectively consider issues of morality and value as they affect geriatric patient care, both patients and appropriate family members and caregivers should be included in the team.

Legal remedies

In situations where an older individual is unable to make competent determinations regarding care, the right to make decisions may be delegated to other caregivers or surrogates through legal mechanisms such as guardianship or power of attorney.

- *Guardianship*: a mechanism that allows a surrogate or surrogates to exercise rights for an older person who is no longer mentally competent.

- *Power of attorney*: a form of voluntary guardianship in which a competent individual freely appoints a surrogate decision-maker. The decision may be invalidated automatically in some states if the individual becomes incompetent, but some states recognize a durable power of attorney, which does not expire if an individual becomes mentally incompetent. The authority of a durable power of attorney can include the ability to make healthcare decisions.

The relationship between ethical and legal obligations

Scott (1997) summarized the relationship between ethical and legal obligations. In geriatric rehabilitation, discipline-specific professional codes of ethics govern the official conduct of members of that discipline if they are members of the professional association that promulgates and enforces the ethics rules. Rule of law, on the other hand, governs the conduct of all members of society. Currently, in healthcare, the ethical duties and the law have become blended to the point where they are often interchangeable. For example, it is a violation of civil and criminal law and of health professional ethical mandates to commit sexual battery upon a patient. Similar parallels exist in the commission of healthcare fraud, professional practice without the requisite license or certification, and other activities of clinical practice (Scott 1997).

SPECIAL AREAS OF ETHICAL CONCERN IN GERIATRIC REHABILITATION

Discharge planning

Complex ethical concerns can be identified with respect to discharge planning in geriatric rehabilitation. Typically, discharge involves transition from a hospital to a site of continuing care. It can also be viewed as a transition from illness to rehabilitation and health. Ethical conflicts can be identified in relation to patient autonomy and involvement in the decision-making process. Additionally, ethical concerns may be identified with respect to discharge plans as they impact on the interests of multiple parties, including the patient, the family, the healthcare providers, the institutions, the reimbursement sources, the referral sources and society itself. Specific concerns arise in the context of the current United States healthcare delivery systems. The system typically accessed by employed, middle-income Americans is based on prospective payment systems with defined lengths of stay and managed care principles designed to control the expenditure of healthcare dollars. Healthcare providers caring for patients funded through this system may experience pressure to advocate discharge plans that put financial considerations ahead of decisions that are in the patient's best interest

and safety. As the healthcare delivery systems designed for the unemployed, uninsured, and largely minority Americans, the military medical care system, and the veterans administration healthcare system adopt managed care principles in an effort to conserve healthcare dollars, healthcare practi-tioners working in these delivery systems may experience similar pressures (Torrens 2002).

One variable in discharge planning may be that the healthcare providers' prescription for long-term care may not show sufficient respect for individual autonomy. Typically, an individual's ability to participate in any decision-making process is determined, at least in part, by performance on mental status examinations. These examinations, although considered to be reliable in judging mental capacity, are of limited value in judging capacity to make complex decisions related to discharge. Of primary importance is that such examinations fail to account for an elderly individual's ability to function in the community, based on social ability and the strength of support networks, in spite of the fact that both these factors are strong predictors of success in community living. An ethical decision related to discharge that truly accounts for patient autonomy should include some prediction of the individual's ability to address the challenges of independent living (Dubler 1988).

If the individual with dementia wishes to be discharged to their own home, that option should be considered in view of the individual's age, physical dependency, cognitive impairment, and competency to perform physical, mental and functional tasks. An attempt must be made to determine whether the individual who wishes to return home has adequate insight into his or her level of dependency in order to address safety issues. In order to facilitate successful discharge home, an assessment must be made of whether that individual's needs could be met through a holistic flexible care plan that utilizes community teams and ongoing assessment and observation (Brindle & Holmes 2005).

Another factor that complicates the ethics of discharge plans is that every decision affects the rights of many people and must account for competing obligations. It is widely recognized that the elderly individual has the moral and legal right to decide autonomously what is appropriate. However, the impact of that decision on the rights, duties, and obligations of family members must also be considered. Specifically, the patient's goal must be accommodated to the family's ability and willingness to help, if such support is part of the proposed discharge plan. Bioethics has historically largely ignored the rights of families. Although families are traditionally obliged to care for each other in ways not expected from friends, neighbors and strangers, the burden of care associated with prolonged life of individuals with chronic and debilitating injuries is an important factor for consideration. Therefore, the obligation to care for family members must be balanced against the obligation of the family member to care for their own physical and emotional needs (Haddad 2000). While the rights of family members must be factored into discharge plans, they must not have more influence on the plan than the rights of the older patient. One current temptation is to consult and address the needs of family members while virtually ignoring the decision-making right and ability of the older individual, even when that individual is capable of involvement in the process.

From an administrative standpoint, discharge involves balancing the good of the patient against other goods, including the needs of the hospital and of society. Conflicts may arise between the financial interests of the institutions and society and the welfare of the patients. These are especially evident when financial considerations are viewed in light of the mission of the institution and its administrative obligations to the staff and the community. The code of ethics of the American College of Hospital Administrators specifically addresses such conflicts of interest by stating that the welfare of the individual must prevail. The code, however, is silent on issues of conflicts in administrative obligations. Therefore, an underlying motivation in effecting the discharge or transfer of a patient from an institution may be the administrative obligation to insure that the institution remains viable. This obligation may be seen to supersede the obligations of the institution to the community, the medical staff, and even the patient. As a result, the needs of individual patients may play a relatively minor role in ethical frameworks espoused by some administrators. Rather, in this context, a patient's needs are balanced against the needs and interests of others. This may pose an ethical dilemma for those caregivers directly involved in effecting an appropriate discharge plan for an individual patient (Spielman 1988).

Discharge plans that involve placement in long-term care are often among the most difficult. The health delivery system provides the older individual with little opportunity to choose either the site of care or its details. Such decisions are often made by discharge planners or social workers who have little opportunity to consult with the individual patient. Frequently, the discharge plan is determined without discussing the circumstances with the patient, family or caregiver, and is based on the physician's judgment that the older patient 'needs 24-hour care'. Additionally, the patient is rarely informed that the primary purpose of the discharge planner is to facilitate prompt discharge while automatically following rules for referral to postacute care settings. The older individual is expected to make a critical life decision with inadequate time and information and may be being advised by professionals who have not fully disclosed the constraints imposed on them by their jobs. Furthermore, little consideration is given to the individual's right to make an informed, autonomous decision to return home when that decision is considered risky or hazardous by the physician or healthcare team. This is often the result not only of the healthcare professionals' desire to do what they know is best for the patient, but also of the fear of litigation resulting from the adverse outcome of a risky discharge decision (Kane 1994).

Recurrent ethical conflicts may revolve around discharge orders that violate the conscience of those caring for the patient but do not necessarily violate the law. An example of a recurring theme seen in geriatric care would be situations in which discharge is planned for patients who are medically ready, but a discharge location that meets the patient's and family's need is not available. In these situations, the therapist and discharge planner recognize that the geriatric patient's needs may be in conflict with the discharge order. In this case, it may be argued that hospitals are held to a higher standard than a patient's medical status alone. Discharge must not be effected until there is adequate care and support in the home or an appropriate healthcare facility. The institution must not discharge a patient under adverse conditions, whether of medical status or social support. On the other hand, patients have no right to prolong their stay simply because they are comfortable or the desired discharge destination is not available. Patient autonomy is not absolute in this example, and questions of distributive justice must be considered, and patient's rights must be balanced against institutional policies. The institution might argue that the patient is entitled to be discharged to a facility as long as it meets minimally acceptable criteria, and has no right to demand discharge to the best possible facility. Such a discharge would serve the principle of justice as this same standard would apply to all patients. On the other hand, consistency offers only a minimal standard of justice. It does not take into consideration the impersonality of the institution in enforcing its own regulations. In attempting to do the right thing in these cases, the therapist and discharge planner are continually presented with a hopeless choice and an unfair set of circumstances. There are no easy answers at the individual case level. In these types of situations, practitioners may look to preventive ethics, which focuses on the overall problem rather than the individual case. The right thing to do, then, becomes the mandate to change conditions so that a more equitable, ethical solution may be effected for future cases (Moody 2004).

Ethics and long-term care

Long-term care, in current health services delivery, refers to a broad range of services that are available to assist an individual who has functional impairments. These services can include personal care, social support and health-related services. Settings for the provision of long-term care include an individual's home as well as a variety of institutional setting. The same ethical issues described above arise in the care of any older person receiving long-term care.

As noted previously, a primary ethical concern in decisions about long-term care involves the admission process itself. Frequently, decisions are made with little respect for patient autonomy. An individual may be denied the right to choose what is perceived as a risk-laden choice (to remain at home), and that may be a violation of his or her autonomy. In order to preserve autonomy and allow a patient to return home, he or she must understand the risks and consequences and must also understand that the decision should not have an adverse impact on the rights of others.

Another consideration in long-term care is the issue of privacy and dignity. Providers of geriatric rehabilitation services must be cognizant of individual dignity when assisting with personal care services such as bathing and toileting. In institutional settings, sensitivity to issues of privacy and dignity must be heightened, as the environment, by its nature, is not conducive to either. Examples of situations that may lead to violation of these rights include multiple occupancy rooms, responsiveness to call buttons, and the use of first names without permission from the patient.

Rehabilitation in long-term care may evoke ethical dilemmas unique to that setting. By definition, rehabilitation implies fostering maximum patient independence in functional tasks. Geriatric patients seek long-term care precisely because they are dependent to some degree. An ethical challenge exists between respecting a patient's autonomy and complying with his or her request for help and encouraging independence. In a broader sense, a similar challenge may exist in decisions related to protecting a patient from risky situations such as falls or adverse health events. Healthcare providers must determine when a person needing care should be allowed to consciously choose a course that professionals consider risky in order to maximize values vs. allowing a patient to be unattended and potentially unsafe.

The lack of patient autonomy in long-term care living environments may be the result of the caregivers' and administrators' roles, their job descriptions, the physical environment, and the regulations that govern these institutions. Administrators and staff may be trained to be task oriented, which provides little opportunity to consider autonomy or even clients' involvement in daily decisions about their own care. The physical environment is often one of little space for storage of clothing and personal possessions, minimal security for personal items, and limited privacy. Care plans and routines dominate the timing and the content of daily activities. Regulations, although designed to protect the welfare and safety of residents, frequently discourage residents' participation in decision-making and often allow for little freedom of choice. Examples include restrictions on what residents can keep in their rooms, requirements about supervision and the charting of patient activity, and safety requirements. Conversely, some regulations may enhance patient autonomy, such as those that mandate the availability of consumer information, enforce privacy regulations, and place limits on the use of restraints (Kane 1994).

The Center for Advocacy for the Rights and Interests of the Elderly (CARIE) developed a curriculum for guiding and improving ethical decision-making in long-term care. The program is based on the premise that long-term care involves the overall well-being of the resident, including the emotional, spiritual, psychological and social well-being, as well as the physical health of the resident. It takes into account the relationships that exist with family members, friends, and staff that may be supported and strengthened by including them in the resident's care. The program recognizes that long-term care residents have physical dependencies and often suffer from dementing illnesses, and recognizes that the experience of dependency is magnified by the variety of ways in which a resident relies upon facility staff. The Center's model recognizes that traditional bioethics is inadequate to address the ethical issues confronting staff and residents in long-term care. The resulting curriculum, '*Promises to Keep: Creating an Ethical Culture in Long-Term Care*', represents an ethics education curriculum that proposes commitment to the resident as the ethical basis of the long-term care admission. The program identified five themes: health, safety, pain and suffering, respect for personhood, and life story. These themes are coupled to commitments to preserve and promote the resident's health, protect the resident's safety, palliate the pain and suffering, practice respect and care for the attributes of personhood, and provide opportunity and support for the continuation and completion of the resident's life story. In this model, health is concerned with maximizing functional ability rather than curing disease, and safety addresses the resident's interaction with the external environment. Spiritual and emotional pain is deemed to be as important as physical pain. Life story is viewed as a continuation of that person's being, and involves honoring, encouraging and supporting in the resident the qualities that are associated with personhood including self-awareness, intentionality, decision-making, agency, emotions, relationships and creativity. CARIE developed a five-step process called IDEAS, which provides a framework for working through care dilemmas to reach ethical solutions. The steps are: (i) identify the ultimate issues, stakeholders, and other decision points; (ii) develop a resident narrative; (iii) explore all conceivable responses to the issue; (iv) assess each response in light of the provider's commitments to the residents; and (v) select a course of action and create an implementation plan. This program contributes to care providers' ability to identify ethical dilemmas and provides a process for examining and sensitively resolving problems that are unique to long-term care (Mathes et al 2004).

Restraints

The use of restraints in the care of the elderly poses several ethical and legal questions that must be addressed by healthcare providers. A restraint is defined as any device that restricts freedom of movement. The rationale for restraint use with the elderly is frequently cited as prevention of injury to self or others, but often the underlying motivation is fear of institutional liability.

When considering the use of restraints to control a patient for safety or because of behavior, the rehabilitation professional must be cognizant of the fact that the literature reports little scientific basis to support the efficacy of restraints in safeguarding patients from harm (Hieleman 1991, Moss & LaPuma 1991). In fact, adverse effects cited in relation to restraint use include such consequences as reduced functional capacity secondary to immobilization, as well as physiological changes including contractures, decreased muscle mass and strength, loss of bone integrity, decubitus ulcers, and adverse psychological response to stress. It should also be noted that, with respect to geriatric rehabilitation, the use of restraints is inconsistent with and frequently in conflict with the goals of rehabilitation (Hieleman 1991).

Hieleman (1991) identifies several issues that must be addressed when weighing the option of using restraints:

- informed consent;
- risk vs. benefit analysis;
- determination of competency;
- the resident's rights and empowerment; and
- risk reduction.

It should be noted that the use of restraints without the patient's informed consent may be legally restricted. The Omnibus Budget Reconciliation Act (OBRA) of 1987 strongly implies that nursing facilities must obtain informed consent for whatever approach is taken to effect resident safety. Also, the Fourteenth Amendment to the US Constitution guarantees freedom from harm and unnecessary restraints (Moss & LaPuma 1991).

It may be ethically permissible to override the refusal of a competent patient to apply a mechanical restraint if that individual is jeopardizing the safety and welfare of others. In such cases, the ethical principle of preventing harm to others supersedes the patient's right to refuse, and the negative rights of an individual to be free from interference ends as the autonomy of others is violated. In this case, the professional must balance professional responsibility to an individual patient with societal and legal obligations to protect public health (Moss & LaPuma 1991).

If restraints are used as a punitive measure, there is no ethical justification for their application. Such a practice would be defined as abusive.

When the use of restraints is consistent with treatment goals, their application may be ethically indicated. One example is when a restraint such as wrist cuffs is applied to prevent interference with a life-sustaining treatment such as a nasogastric tube. In such cases, it should be emphasized, the treatment goal is to restore the patient to health (Moss & LaPuma 1991).

Managed care

Part of the tradition of health professionals' service toward society's common good is based on the notion of altruism, or selfless concern for the welfare of the patient. Patients are viewed not as customers, but as individuals who are vulnerable and require the intervention of the healthcare provider. In turn, physical therapists promise to meet the health needs of the patient under the ethical principles of do no harm and provide benefit, while fostering autonomy and justice. In essence, the healthcare professional is a trustee who works for the good of the client and knows the limits of his or her expertise. However, in the current healthcare delivery system that embraces managed care principles, this concept may be challenged, especially when treating older patients who come to us with complex medical and social problems that require our professional expertise and interventions (Nalette 2001). As such, managed healthcare poses special challenges in geriatric rehabilitation and ethics. One consideration is the managed care organization, structure and function itself. In the managed care structure, there are multiple actors with incompatible interests. For example, the rehabilitation provider has a fiduciary responsibility to patients, but may also be an employee of or contractor with the organization. The organization itself may have legal and financial obligations to shareholders to maintain low cost, yet an ethical obligation to patients to provide quality care.

Another current source of ethical conflict is the morality of market-driven healthcare, which has the potential to threaten professionalism. The introduction of market-driven practices into healthcare may divide professional loyalties between providing the best treatments in order to improve the patient's quality of life and keeping expenses to a min-imum by limiting services, increasing efficiency, and lesse-ning the amount of time spent with each patient. The result may be that the professional must choose between the best interests of the patient and economic survival. Frequently, reimbursement drives the care.

The integrity of the patient–provider relationship may also be threatened in the current healthcare delivery climate. Focus on the patient is the primary concern of healthcare. Managed care, however, may threaten this relationship through policies that deny access to care, restrict the professional's ability to perform tests, and withhold or limit treatment. Such policies create conflicting loyalties and undermine the trust between provider and patient. The provider may be in the dual and potentially conflicting positions of being guardian of society's resources and being a primary advocate for the individual patient (AMA 1995, Kassirer 1995, Rodwin 1995). With respect to geriatric patients, it can be stated that, ethically, the profession may not be able to afford to rehabilitate someone who is about to die, in which case rehabilitation would not be effective anyway. On the other hand, it is imperative that the professional never withholds treatment just because a person is old. The difficulty lies in determining who is ready to die and who may benefit, and how much, from rehabilitation efforts.

Managed care may impact on the ethical principle of patient autonomy, and it potentially threatens the patient's freedom of choice. When healthcare coverage is provided as an employee or retirement benefit, the employee's choice may be even more restricted. In order to take advantage of healthcare coverage as a benefit, the employee or retiree is often forced to accept a plan that limits service access and does not meet healthcare needs. A person has the responsibility of understanding the terms of his or her own healthcare plan (AMA 1995, Emmanuel & Dubler 1995).

One more factor related to patient autonomy is the perceived right to have all treatment choices funded. It is paramount to acknowledge that autonomy does not guarantee funding. Rather, some balance must be achieved between conserving society's healthcare dollars and paying for ind-ividual healthcare needs. Providers and elderly patients must recognize that autonomy also entails responsibility. It obliges individuals to use resources wisely, to assist in conserving resources, and to live a healthy lifestyle.

In 2000 and 2001, the American College of Physicians, with the Harvard Pilgrim Health Care Ethics Program, convened a group of patients, physicians, managed care representatives and medical ethicists. The purpose of the meeting was to develop a statement of ethics for managed care. The statement that they developed offers guidance on preserving the patient–client relationship, patient rights and responsibilities, confidentiality and privacy, resource allocation and stewardship, the obligation of health plans to foster an ethical environment for the delivery of care, and the clinician's responsibility to individual patients, the community and public health. The statement identifies four ethical principles to address the ethical challenges posed by limitations realized in association with managed care and that recognize that healthcare resources should be distributed justly. Principle I addresses the relationships that are critical in the delivery of health services. It states that health plans, purchasers, clinicians and patients should be characterized by respect, truthfulness, consistency, fairness and compassion. Principle II states that health plans, purchasers, clinicians and the public share responsibility for the appropriate stewardship of healthcare resources. One tenet of this principle is that a clinician's first and primary duty is to promote the good of the patient while honoring the responsibility to practice effective and efficient healthcare that utilizes healthcare resources responsibly. It also states that health plans should engage purchasers in discussions about the health coverage that can reasonably be met, and that health plans should work with purchasers to insure that benefit packages are consistent with the healthcare needs and cultural norms of the purchasers' constituents. Contracts must not only contain costs, but should enhance efforts to improve quality care. Principle III states that all parties should foster an ethical environment for the delivery of effective and efficient quality healthcare. Financial incentives should enhance the provision of quality care and support professional ethical obligations. Principle IV states that patients should be well informed about care and treatment options and the financial and benefit issues that affect the provision of care (Povar et al 2004).

Elder abuse

Abuse of the elderly may take many forms, from causing actual physical harm or mental anguish to denial of needed medical and social services to financial exploitation. Abusive behavior toward the elderly may come from family members, caregivers or healthcare providers themselves. Often, the abuse may not be overt or intentional, but may stem from personal and professional values, including the desire to protect the elderly patient at the expense of his or her right to make autonomous choices.

One ethical consideration that must be acknowledged when healthcare providers become aware of actual abuse is the need to maintain a balance between sensitivity to patient trust and the need to abide by regulatory statutes that mandate reporting. This is especially important if knowledge of the abusive situation was gained through confidential disclosure of information (Guccione & Shefrin 1993).

As recognized previously, components of elder abuse must be acknowledged in discharge planning, use of restraints and denial of services enforced through regulations and managed care.

CONCLUSION

Ethical concerns and sources of conflict abound in regard to the rehabilitation of the geriatric patient. It is imperative that the healthcare practitioner who works with elders should be sensitive to these issues, understand the underlying ethical principles, acknowledge the legal basis of these principles and incorporate moral values into the decision-making process.

References

American Medical Association (AMA) 1995 Council on Ethical and Judicial Affairs, Ethical issues in managed care. JAMA 273:338–339

American Physical Therapy Association (APTA) 2003, Professionalism in Physical Therapy. Available: http://www.apta.org/AM/Template.cfm?Section=Professionalism/&TEMPLATE=/CM/ContentDisplay.cfm&CONTENTID=21299. Accessed April 6, 2006

American Physical Therapy Association (APTA) 2006a, APTA Code of Ethics. Available: http://www.apta.org/AM/Template.cfm?Section=Ethics_and_Legal_Issues1&CONTENTID=21760&TEMPLATE=/CM/ContentDisplay.cfm. Accessed April 30, 2006

American Physical Therapy Association (APTA) 2006b, APTA Standards of Ethical Conduct for the Physical Therapist Assistant

Available: http://www.apta.org/AM/Template.cfm?Section=Ethics_and_Legal_Issues1&CONTENTID=23729&TEPLATE=/CMM/ContentDisplay.cfm. Accessed April 6, 2006

Brindle N, Holmes J 2005 Capacity and coercion: dilemmas in the discharge of older people with dementia from general hospital settings. Age Ageing 34:16–20

Dubler NN 1988 Improving the discharge planning process: distinguishing between coercion and choice. Gerontologist 28:76–81

Elliott C 1992 Where ethics comes from and what to do about it. Hastings Cent Rep 22:28–35

Emmanuel EJ, Dubler NN 1995 Preserving the physician–patient relationship in the era of managed care. JAMA 273:338–339

Guccione AA, Shefrin DH 1993 Ethical and legal issues in geriatric physical therapy. In: Guccione AA (ed.) Geriatric Physical Therapy. Mosby-Year Book, St Louis, MO

Haddad A 2000 Acute care decisions. Ethics in action. RN 63:21–22, 24

Henderson ML, McConnell ES 1997 Ethical considerations. In: Matteson MA, McConnell ES, Linton AD (eds) Gerontological Nursing Concepts and Practice, 2nd edn. WB Saunders, Philadelphia, PA

Hieleman F 1991 Restraint reduction in nursing facilities: the issues involved in decision-making. Geri-topics 14:26–27

Kane RA 1994 Ethics and long-term care. Clin Geriatr Med 10:489–499

Kassirer JP 1995 Managed care and the morality of the marketplace. N Engl J Med 33:50–52

Mathes M, Reifsnyder J, Gibney M 2004 Commitment, relationship, voice: cornerstones for an ethics of long-term care. Ethics, Law, Aging Rev 10:3–24

Moody HR 2004 Hospital discharge planning: carrying out orders? J Gerontol Social Work 43:107–118

Moss RJ, LaPuma J 1991 The ethics of mechanical restraints. Hastings Cent Rep 21:22–25

Nalette E 2001 Physical therapy: ethics and the geriatric patient. J Geriatr Phys Ther 24(3):3–7

Povar GJ, Blumen H, Daniel J et al 2004 Academia and clinic. Ethics in practice: managed care and the changing health care environment: Medicine as a Profession Managed Care Ethics Working Group Statement. Ann Intern Med 141:131–136

Purtilo R 2005 Ethical Dimensions in the Health Professions, 4th edn. Elsevier Saunders, Philadelphia, PA

Ries E 2003 The art and architecture of caring. PT Mag 11(4):36–43

Rodwin MA 1995 Conflicts in managed care. N Engl J Med 332:604–607

Scott RW 1997 Informed consent. In: Scott RW (ed.) Promoting Legal Awareness in Physical and Occupational Therapy. Mosby, St Louis, MO

Spielman BJ 1988 Financially motivated transfers and discharges: administrators' ethics and public expectations. J Med Humanities Bioeth 9:32–43

Swisher LL 2005 Ethics in geriatric physical therapy. An independent home study course for individual continuing education. Section on Geriatrics, APTA

Torrens PR 2002 Overview of the organization of health services in the United States. In: Williams SJ, Torrens PR (eds) Introduction to Health Services, 6th edn. Delmar Publishers, Albany, NY

WCPT 2006 World Confederation for Physical Therapy. Declarations of Principle, Appendix to WCPT Ethical Principles. Available: http://www.wcpt.org/policies/principles/appendixethical.php. Accessed April 6, 2006

Weiss GB 1985 Paternalism modernized. J Med Ethics 11:184–187

Wong RA, Barr JO, Farina N et al 2000 Evidence-based practice: a resource for physical therapists. Issues Aging 23(3):19–26

Chapter 76

Physical therapy and the generational conflict

Timothy L. Kauffman and Megan Laughlin

INTRODUCTION

The conflict between the older generation and the younger generation is an age-old problem. The issue is particularly poignant in societies and nations that do not venerate their seniors. Physical therapy care in an aging world population was the subject of an editorial 19 years ago in which T. F. Williams, former Director of the National Institute of Aging in the United States, was quoted as saying, 'Of all human beings who have ever lived on the earth and have reached age 65 years, the majority are alive today' (Williams 1987). 'This statement holds significant implications for the society in general and especially for healthcare providers and their aged patients' (Kauffman 1988). By now, everyone has heard the demographic litany about the increasingly aging population and the rising costs of caring for the elderly. The problem that we, as a civilization, face is how to handle this growing dilemma, both fiscally and ethically.

PARTISAN POLITICS

A member of the US House of Representatives addressed a group of physical therapists at the 1996 Combined Sections Meeting of the American Physical Therapy Association. He presented a scenario in which a family had a choice between healthcare for a terminally ill mother or more money for the discretionary use of the younger family members through tax savings derived from reduced healthcare benefits for Medicare patients and pensioners. The Congressman insisted that we must cut the healthcare benefits, even though it is cold-hearted, because we must offer hope and a future (which is being 'warm-hearted') to our children and grandchildren. This simplistic either/or verbiage is the source of an increasingly intense generational conflict that pits one generation against another.

A similar perspective was promoted by a World Bank economist concerning the aging population in the former Soviet bloc countries of Eastern Europe. 'I tell people in Eastern Europe that pensions policy is impoverishing their children. The demands of pensioners are taking food out of the mouths of working people's children' (Kohli 1996).

Dollars, euros, yen, and the other monetary units drive this conflict, aided by partisan politics, abuse of elders by the media (Cohen 1994) and in health delivery (Commission for Healthcare Audit and Inspection, CHAI, 2006) and sensationalism. Political concerns about healthcare costs are heard around the world, especially in countries with aging populations.

The generational conflict can also be seen in the workforce as middle-aged and older people hold the highest paid and most authoritative jobs. Because those positions are occupied, younger people cannot move up the business ladder as easily. In the US, there are approximately 77 million people who were born between 1945 and 1963, the 'baby boomers'. Beneath them in age is 'generation X, born between 1964 and 1983, which is about 48 million strong (Karp & Sirias 2001). This is part of the demographic that is manipulated in the conflict of 'us against them', especially because older people use more healthcare and social security/pensioner dollars/euros (Vladeck 2005).

DEMOGRAPHICS

According to World Health Organization data, in 2000 there were 600 million people living in the world who were aged 60 years and older. It is projected that there will be 1.2 billion people over this age by 2025 and 2 billion by the year 2050. This is a worldwide phenomenon. By 2025, 75% of the aging persons will be living in the developing world. The fastest growing cohort in the developed world is that group of old-old people over the age of 80 years (WHO 2006).

Europe was the first region in the world in which the demographic transformation resulting from increased life expectancy was manifested. It has the highest proportion of old people in the world. Of 11 European countries, Italy has the highest population of people aged 65 years and older (18.6%), followed by Sweden (17%) and Germany (16.6%) (Carpenter 2005). Italy, with a low birth rate and rapidly aging society, now has the oldest population of all the European countries. They have relatively underdeveloped community care services, and many are supported at home by extended families with minimal formal care (Carpenter 2005). Despite the various languages, cultural heritages and political histories, Europe is considered a homogeneous society. Nevertheless, European countries have diverse healthcare and social care structures, and this has created a unique opportunity to study different models of care (Carpenter 2005).

The European Observatory on Health Care Systems recently studied health delivery systems in eight different countries, all of which provide some type of universal healthcare financed through public funding (Dixon & Mossialos 2002). It is interesting to note that Australians have bipartisan support for improving access and equity for its Medicare system, which is a more comprehensive program than it is in the US. However, the impact of the aging population and how to provide care were acknowledged challenges for health systems in New Zealand and the European Union, especially Denmark, France and Sweden.

The European Union recently funded the Aged in Home Care project, which included the development of the inter *Resident Assessment Instrument* (interRAI), which assesses the needs of older people. It is now in use in over 30 countries and has the potential to improve the understanding and measurement of effectiveness, efficiency and quality of care of healthcare services provided to people of various ages in different settings (Carpenter 2005).

Living Well in Later Life, A review of progress against the National Framework for Older People (Commission for Healthcare Audit and Inspection, CHAI, 2006) was an effort to look at social and health services for the elderly in the UK. In its framework, data are presented that can be interpreted from generational differences. People 65 years old and older account for 16% of the population in the UK, but they use almost two-thirds of general and acute hospital beds. In 2003/4, 43% or £16 billion, of the National Health Service's (NHS) budget was consumed by the same age group. Similarly, 44% or £7 billion of the social services budget was spent for this same age group. This official government report was met with criticism because of the '. . . "patronising and thoughtless" manner in which NHS hospitals and care institutions treat older patients'. It was noted that the ruling Labour party featured better care for the elderly and that may not be happening (Laurance 2006).

The need to grapple with these demographic and financial issues is very real. Across the European Union, 80% of social protection expenditures are for old-age pensioners (Watson 1995).

A similar trend is occurring in the US, where the over-85 age group is growing the fastest. Currently, in the US, there are 36 million people aged 65 years and over, and 4.5 million over 85 years. By the year 2050, both these populations will have increased significantly with 80 million people aged 65 years and older and 20 million people over the age of 85 (Louria 2005). Researchers in Europe have found that, in industrialized countries, the population of centenarians has doubled each decade since 1950 (Kinsella 2005). Adding to the Medicare problem is the looming postwar baby boom cohort, which reaches retirement age beginning in 2010. Someone retiring today can anticipate spending 25–29% of their adult life in retirement but, with increasing longevity to 95 years, this percentage increases to 40% (Louria 2005), Compounding the problem further is the fact that the US birth rate reached unprecedented lows in the mid-1970s (Ycas 1994), which means that the taxpaying workforce will be smaller when the mandated social costs are likely to be the highest ever. If current retirement trends continue, there will be a shortage of workers by 2025 (Vladeck 2005).

POLITICAL DECISIONS

The zenith of the generational conflict in the US occurred in November 1995. That was when the American people suffered through the debacle of the closing down of the US government. The closure occurred because it was announced by some that Medicare, the American old-age healthcare system, would be bankrupt by the year 2000 or shortly thereafter. The impasse resulted because of partisan political maneuvering by a Congress that wanted to cut costs and to eliminate the US federal debt in order to save something for future generations. Blocking this move was President Clinton, who wanted to protect the healthcare benefits for the elderly.

In November 2005, the administrator of the Centers for Medicare and Medicaid Services (CMS) released an updated physician fee schedule, indicating that payment rates per service for physicians' services will be reduced by 4.4% for 2006. 'The existing law calls for a decrease in payment rates for physicians in response to continued rapid increases in use of services and spending growth, and Medicare does not have the authority to change this', said CMS Administrator Mark B. McClellan. Similar changes in fee schedules have also affected rehabilitation services, with reimbursement for physical therapy services decreasing. This presents a challenge to healthcare providers who are dedicated to providing the best quality of care, but with diminishing financial resources (CMS 2005).

In the UK, the demographic reality has also had an impact on access to universal healthcare. Shortages of primary care providers are a factor (Dixon & Mossialos 2002). Young (1996) indicated that the pressure for shorter lengths of stay has reduced rehabilitation services for the elderly. A projected deficit of nearly £800 million has worsened the care especially for the elderly (Laurance 2006).

It is a profound truth that democratic governments built on consensus and compromise must painfully allocate limited resources to numerous mandated, needy and exigent programs and projects.

FORMER SOVIET BLOC

The difficulty of developing workable and ethical solutions to problems of healthcare and aging may be greater in the countries of the former Soviet bloc. The paternalistic system of government provided many social supports for retirees, including free healthcare and medications, which improved life expectancy in the 1980s. However, many societal changes took place after the fall of the Communist system. In Russia, life expectancy for males dropped to 57.6 years during the 7 years between 1987 and 1994. This was attributed to a variety of reasons including environmental degradation, accidents, excessive alcohol use, poor diet and deterioration in health services (Kinsella 2005). In the present period of transition, the rehabilitation possibilities in Hungary, for example, are limited by few resources and few healthcare specialists, which may account for the extensive use of medication there (Blasszauer 1994). In Georgia (in the former Soviet Union), only 0.59% of the gross domestic product (GDP) was spent on healthcare in 1999, and only 22% of healthcare expenses were covered by state or municipal budgets or insurance.

PARADIGM SHIFT

The drawing here (Fig. 76.1), by the German artist Bernd Stolz, illustrates the problem by depicting the weight (or burden) of the young and the old resting upon the shoulders of healthy, young, working adults. The question to be answered is, must the generational difference be viewed as an either/or situation? The answer is no. What if the headlines in the newspapers reported that nearly 100% of education costs go to persons under the age of 19 years? Should pensioners in the UK stop paying community charges and other taxes that benefit younger persons? Public education in the US is funded largely by real estate taxes on property owners. Some fixed-income Medicare retirees must sell their homes because they can no longer afford their real estate taxes.

In the US, the federal government spends about 40% of its budget on services that go mostly to older people for the benefits of social

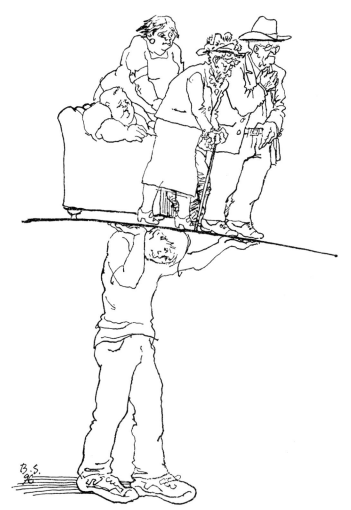

Figure 76.1   Bernd Stolz, 1996.

return to work out of financial necessity, many may return as healthy, involved, active and productive members of society, thereby helping to counteract the shrinking workforce and the financial burden on this workforce (Louria 2005).

Lubitz et al (1995) took a sample of actual 1990 Medicare costs and simulated lifetime costs for people who became Medicare beneficiaries in that year and for people who will enter the system in 2020. These writers suggested that the effect of increased longevity on Medicare cost per individual may be minimal, even though the overall costs will, of course, increase because of the greater number of enrollees. Physical therapy, both rehabilitative and preventive, is integral to the compression of morbidity and, thus, to the control of costs.

The trend toward home healthcare (Dall 1994), which should clearly involve rehabilitation care, may help to reduce costs to the system and possibly to preserve individual dignity and family integrity (Allert et al 1994). However, the trend is not without problems. It shifts the costs to families, which already provide the majority of care for the elderly (Topinková 1994), and it may increase stress on the caregivers. Over the past 20 years, the population of people aged 75 years and older has increased by two-thirds, but the use of nursing homes has only increased minimally. This can be attributed to the increase in community-based alternatives to long-term care as well as the improved health of old people. Despite the current trend toward less frequent and later child-bearing, growing longevity is leading toward families with three and four surviving generations. As baby boomers age, there is now a large population of older people with surviving adult children. Baby boomers are moving quickly between childcare responsibilities and caring for aging parents. What will happen as the baby boom generation, who outnumber their children, continues to age (Vladeck 2005)? Recognizing these increased burdens on families, a plan was designed in Germany to help families to offset these additional costs, but the demand exceeded what the system could manage (Karcher 1995). Also, family structures are changing as more women enter the workforce, and social and international mobility is increasing (McCormick & Rubenstein 1995). Better screening of individuals through the use of a geriatric intermediate-care facility may help to predict those who are likely to be discharged home and, thus, to prevent institutionalization. However, this study conducted in Japan did not deal with the changing structure of the family and workforce (Ishizaki et al 1995).

security, Medicare, Medicaid and veterans. In contrast, state and local governments spend about 37% of their budgets on benefits to the younger population in the form of education at all levels and criminal justice (Vladeck 2005). When the debate about the costs for healthcare and social care for the elderly are couched in terms of generational conflict, these data on spending levels are not included.

Harbingers of doom aside, not all the information is catastrophic. First, although the population of the world is aging, the morbidity of the aging population is being compressed into a shorter time period (Mor 2005). Of persons in the US over the age of 85 years, 80% are not living in nursing homes, and half of the over-85-year-old patients in nursing homes are there because of chronic conditions that have definable and modifiable antecedent risk factors (Lubitz et al 1995). Although studies in the nineteenth century demonstrated that the death rate increased exponentially with age, more recent studies have found a decline in mortality at age 80 years and older, and the age of mortality deceleration is rising. This creates a society of older people with healthy attributes (Kinsella 2005). This means that people are living longer and healthier lives. This, it is hoped, will reduce the per capita cost. That is, adding years to life does not automatically mean adding excessive cost to the system. This presents a promising scenario for counteracting the costs of an aging society for future decades and centuries. Although old and very old people may

THE ROLE OF HEALTHCARE PROVIDERS

Healthcare providers are very much involved in the entire process. We are involved as caregivers with our patients and our families. We are involved as researchers hoping to find better ways of providing the best possible care within the social structures and financial constraints of each country, and we share that information through this text and many others. We are involved as citizens, hoping that our governments will listen to our needs and the needs of our patients. We, as healthcare providers, are the future elderly ourselves. We can look forward to living longer and healthier lives than past generations. For these reasons, it is crucial that we voice our concerns, needs, and ideas for our future. We are seeking the wisdom and ability to amalgamate our personal interests with our professional interests and the interests of our societies. However, Binstock (1986), past president of the Gerontological Society of America, reminds us of an enduring and universal truth: 'Politics, not research, will resolve value conflicts regarding the nature and extent of hardship and what actions, if any, governments should undertake to alleviate hardships'. Maybe we need to remind our politicians that 'When, due to financial restrictions, resources are allocated in a hard and pitiless manner, society's response to its vulnerable old and ill members becomes an even greater sign of its humaneness' (Allert et al 1994).

NO EASY ANSWERS

The determination to remain independent despite the travails of age-related pathology and the fear of becoming a burden on family and society is an attitude that correlates with the compression of morbidity. This phenomenon of aging has forced society to consider issues such as advance directives or living wills and do-not-resuscitate orders. Hesse (1995) reported that, in persons 85 years old and older, during terminal hospitalizations, there have been significant declines in high-intensity medical interventions such as cardiopulmonary resuscitation, invasive tests and minor surgery. Requiring consent to treatment may reduce undesired and costly medical and surgical interventions. Palliative care must be maintained out of human decency, and this requires physical therapy for comfort and for pain control. At this time, there is very little support for the highly emotional subjects of euthanasia, (deliberate acts that lead directly to death) or assisted suicide (the provision to a knowing patient of medical means to cause self-death). Civilization must continue to wrestle with these issues, especially as we enter this age of aging.

CONCLUSION

The issues of generational conflict are not new, and they need not be magnified. The biblical story of Abraham and Isaac serves as a concluding comment. Abraham, a centenarian, was tempted by God to sacrifice his only son, Isaac, who was then only a lad. Abraham instructed his servants to wait for him and Isaac and stated, 'We will return.' Seeing the wood, fire and knife, Isaac asked, 'Where is the lamb?' Abraham answered, 'God will provide himself a lamb' [Genesis 22:1–13, Authorized (King James) version]. The important message is that Abraham never lost sight of what he needed to do, which was to obey God and sacrifice his son, the next generation. In this story, a desirable solution to Abraham's dilemma was reached. As this world ages, the solution will be found by young people and old people working together for the common good. We, as healthcare providers, must be participants in that solution.

References

Allert G, Sponholz C, Baitsch H 1994 Chronic disease and the meaning of old age. Hastings Cent Rep 24:11–13

Binstock R 1986 Perspectives on measuring hardship: concepts, dimensions, and implications. Gerontologist 26:60

Blasszauer B 1994 Institutional care of the elderly. Hastings Cent Rep 24:14–17

Carpenter G 2005 Aging in the United Kingdom and Europe – a snapshot of the future? J Am Geriatr Soc 53:310–313

Centers for Medicare and Medicaid Services (CMS) 2005 CMS announces payment update and policy changes for Medicare physician fee schedule. Available: http://www.cms.hhs.gov/apps/media/press/release.asp?Counter +1709. Accessed November 3, 2005

Commission for Healthcare Audit and Inspection (CHAI), 2006 Living Well in Later Life, London. Available: http://www.healthcarecommission.org.uk/assetRoot/04/02/46/42/04024642.pdf. Accessed 18 April, 2006

Cohen GD 1994 Journalistic elder abuse: it's time to get rid of fictions, get down to facts. Gerontologist 34:399–401

Dall J 1994 The greying of Europe. Br Med J 309:1282–1285

Dixon A, Mossialos E 2002 Health Care Systems in Eight Countries: Trends and Challenges. The London School of Economics & Political Science, London, p 1–129

Hesse KA 1995 Changes in the way we die. Arch Intern Med 155:1513–1518

Ishizaki T, Kai I, Hisata T et al 1995 Factors influencing users' return home on discharge from a geriatric intermediate care facility in Japan. J Am Geriatr Soc 43:623–626

Karcher H 1995 Germany's home care scheme faces problems. Br Med J 310:1025

Karp HB, Sirias D 2001 Generational conflict – a new paradigm for teams of the 21st century. Gestalt Rev 5(2):71–87

Kauffman T 1988 Physiotherapy as the world ages. Physio Theory Pract 4:61–62

Kinsella K 2005 Future longevity – demographic concerns and consequences. J Am Geriatr Soc 53:299–303

Kohli M 1996 The problem of generations: family, economy, politics. Public Lectures No. 14, delivered at Collegium Budapest

Laurance J 2006 The great betrayal: how the NHS fails the elderly. Available: http://news.independent.co.uk/uk/health_medical/article353861.ece. Accessed March 27, 2006

Louria D 2005 Extraordinary longevity: individual and societal issues. J Am Geriatr Soc 53:317–319

Lubitz J, Beebe J, Baker C 1995 Longevity and Medicare expenditures. N Engl J Med 332:999–1003

McCormick WC, Rubenstein LZ 1995 International common denominators in geriatric rehabilitation and long-term care. J Am Geriatr Soc 43:714–715

Mor V 2005 The compression of morbidity hypothesis: a review of research and prospects for the future. J Am Geriatr Soc 53:308–309

Topinková E 1994 Care for elders with chronic disease and disability. Hastings Cent Rep 24:18–20

Vladeck B 2005 Economic and policy implications of improving longevity. J Am Geriatr Soc 53:304–307

Watson R 1995 Making the most of ageing populations. Br Med J 310:554

World Health Organization (WHO) 2006 The world is fast ageing – have we noticed? Available: www.who.int/ageing/en/. Accessed 16 February, 2006

Williams TF 1987 The future of aging. Arch Phys Med Rehabil 68:335–338

Ycas MA 1994 The challenge of the 21st century: innovating and adapting social security systems to economic, social, and demographic changes in the English-speaking Americas. Soc Secur Bull 57:3–9

Young J 1996 Caring for older people: rehabilitation and older people. Br Med J 313:677–681

Chapter 77

Medicare

Timothy L. Kauffman

INTRODUCTION

In the United States, the rehabilitation of geriatric patients takes place largely within the Medicare and Medicaid systems. As the population ages, the systems have become an increasingly partisan political battleground with a moderate to high level of distrust, frustration and confusion among the various players on the field, including the beneficiaries and their advocates, lobbyists and families; the care providers, both individuals and institutions; the insurance companies; and the politicians and regulatory bureaucrats.

There is some justification for this sociopolitical quagmire because the Medicare and Medicaid systems are large, changing and expensive. Over 42 million people are covered by the Medicare system, and Medicaid enrollees amount to over 44 million beneficiaries, of whom almost half are children (Centers for Medicare & Medicaid Services (CMS) 2005). Medicare accounts for about one-third of all payments to hospitals and one-fifth of payments to physicians. In 1999, over $387 billion were spent on personal healthcare by people aged 65 years and older (Keehan et al 2004). The Medicare system paid 46% and Medicaid 15% of these costs. Including all healthcare programs directed by the CMS, the cost in 2004 to the federal government was $449.9 billion or 19.6% of the federal budget (CMS 2005).

The alarm about Medicare costs and expenditures has been ringing for almost two decades because of the looming demographic shift of the initial wave of postwar baby boomers reaching Medicare age in the year 2011. The good news is that the average rise in Medicare costs started to decline in 1996 (Keehan et al 2004) and continued to decline through 2004 (CMS News 2006). This may be due to changes in the health insurance system (Keehan et al 2004) or possibly improved lifestyle habits which compress morbidity (Hubert et al 2002).

The bad news is that the system is mired in a political debate about the future based on demographics. At this time, the population of Americans who are 65 years old or older is just under 13% of the total. The percentage is projected to increase to 15.7% by 2019 and to 21.3% by 2049 (Keehan et al 2004). Unfortunately, the political rhetoric offers solutions of cutting costs, stopping fraud, more choices/options and reducing (rationing) services. Because there will be more Medicare beneficiaries, this does not mean there will be more services. This debate and failure to solve this demographic imperative have been ongoing for decades (see Binstock & Post 1991).

HISTORY

The bill that initiated the Medicare program was signed into law by President Lyndon Johnson on July 3 1965. Symbolically, he signed the bill at the Truman Library in Independence, Missouri, because President Harry Truman had publicly endorsed and fought for government health insurance in the 1940s and 1950s. Interestingly, at that time, then Senator Lyndon Johnson was only one of several southern Democratic senators who supported President Truman's legislative effort. Truman's ideas were not new, as they were based on European hospital insurance models that were shaped at the turn of the century. Truman's proposals were defeated by Congress in 1951, but the tenets were debated and reworked during the Eisenhower administrations, which offered scaled-down alternatives under the name 'medicare'.

As President, John Kennedy determined that hospital healthcare for the aged was 'must have' legislation. Introduced by Representative Cecil King (Democrat, California) and Senator Clinton Anderson (Democrat, New Mexico), the bill was blocked by opponents, including Senator Wilbur Mills (Democrat, Arizona). Kennedy's death and Johnson's landslide victory in 1964 led to a new makeup of Congress. By then, Mills not only supported the Anderson–King Bill (hospital insurance, now known as Medicare Part A), he also expanded it to outpatient services (now known as Medicare Part B). Thus, Title XVIII of the Social Security Act became the law of the land, and the Medicare system went into effect 11 months later on 1 July 1966.

The Medicaid legislation was also enacted in 1965 as Title XIX to provide for a combined federal and state program for poor families. Medicaid covers children and some long-term care service, but it varies with the state (Moon 1995, Poen 1996).

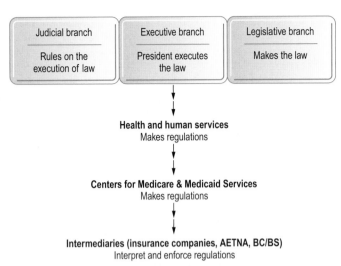

Figure 77.1 The key players in the Medicare system are in all three branches of the federal government.

THE KEY PLAYERS

The American government is based on a system of checks and balances, so it should be no surprise that this comes into play within the Medicare system too. The key players are in all three branches of the government, as shown in Fig. 77.1. First of all, Congress enacted the legislation that authorized the Medicare system. Congress can and does alter the system by passing new laws; indeed, the Balanced Budget Act (BBA) of 1997 has had a strong impact on geriatric rehabilitation. Prior to passage of the BBA, there were almost 11 000 home health agencies and, by 2004, the number was reduced to 7519 (Keehan et al 2004). Likewise, the Medicare Modernization Act of 2003 expanded the Medicare program to a new option called Medicare Part D for drug coverage. This also carries a premium projected to be an average of $32.20, per month depending upon the choice of coverage. This new elective program is administered by the Supplemental Medical Insurance Trust (Hoffman et al 2005).

A second and equal player is the Chief Executive, or President, who signs the legislative bills into law. The President is responsible for executing the law. This is done by asking the appropriate executive branch department to implement the wishes of Congress. In 1965, it was John Gardner, the Secretary of Health, Education and Welfare, who was responsible for promulgating the regulations to implement the grand idea of providing healthcare to elderly Americans. In 1980, during the Jimmy Carter administration, the Department of Health, Education and Welfare was dismantled, and the new Health and Human Services Department emerged. Thus, the law comes from the Congress and the regulations come from the Department of Health and Human Services (HHS). Most changes in the Medicare system now take place through the regulatory process.

Shortly after the inception of the Medicare system, the Department of Health, Education and Welfare recognized that it did not have expertise in administering the financial aspect of federally mandated healthcare programs. Thus, the Health Care Financing Administration (HCFA) became a new federal agency, and it oversaw all the financial aspects of the Medicare and Medicaid systems and the regulatory process. In 2001, HHS Secretary Tommy Thompson reorganized the system and changed the name to Centers for Medicare & Medicaid Services (CMS). In today's healthcare arena, it appears at times that CMS's purpose is to control costs, not to assist in the delivery of care.

CMS is not designed as an insurance company, so it contracts with private insurance companies to administer the Medicare regulations and to handle the reimbursement and healthcare delivery processes. These fiscal intermediaries, or insurance companies, also reinterpret and implement the Medicare regulations that come from the Department of Health and Human Services and from CSM. The intermediaries will, at times, release guidelines for implementing the regulations.

There is no single fiscal intermediary for the entire Medicare system. Thus, the interpretation of the regulations is not uniform. This causes some confusion among care providers and patients, especially as they move from one location to another in the United States. Further confounding the situation is the tendency toward larger and larger business organizations for healthcare delivery; thus, one may be providing rehabilitation services in Massachusetts when the Medicare intermediary is located in Tennessee. Also, the healthcare provider companies may further refine and make declarations in writing concerning what is coverable or allowable according to their interpretations of the intermediary guidelines or CMS regulations.

Several other government agencies are involved in overseeing the implementation of the Medicare system too. They are the US General Accounting Office (GAO), which is occasionally funded to review the system to determine its appropriateness. For example, the GAO released a report (GAOI HRD-87-91) in July 1987 that has had a profound effect upon geriatric rehabilitation. It said that rehabilitation services were being paid for by the Medicare system without receipt of adequate information. This was the major justification for the tightening of requirements for documentation. Another very important report (GAOI PEMD-93-97) was released by the GAO in August 1993; it found that the methods being used by four Medicare carriers to pay claims under the supplemental medical insurance program, or Medicare Part B, were not effective in determining whether the medical care was appropriate or not. Thus, since this report, greater emphasis has been placed on establishing medical necessity.

Also, the Office of the Inspector General of the Department of Health and Human Services is at times called upon to review the implementation of the Medicare system. Additionally, the Office of Management and Budget and the Congressional Budget Office are involved in auditing the Medicare programs and forecasting future expenses.

A third equal player in the Medicare system is the judiciary branch, as lawsuits are brought by Medicare beneficiaries or plaintiffs against the Medicare system. A major case was the *Fox* v. *Bowen* decision in 1986, which had a profound impact upon outpatient geriatric rehabilitation by implementing screens or edits that delimited the length and number of treatments allowable according to diagnosis.

SOCIAL SECURITY TRUST FUNDS

As mentioned above, during the historic debate over the Medicare legislation, the initial thrust was to provide hospital insurance, with acute care benefits in mind. This is administered under the Hospital Insurance Trust Fund (HI) and is best recognized as Medicare Part A. Currently, Medicare beneficiaries are required to pay $952 (up from $764 in 1998) as a deductible for the first day in the hospital. After 61 days, a co-payment is implemented at $238 (up from $191.00 in 1998) until day 90, after which the co-payment increases to $476 (up from $382 in 1998). HI, or Medicare Part A, also pays for 'inpatient' care and services provided in a patient's home if there is reasonable rehabilitation potential and the patient is currently housebound. This will be discussed in further detail later. Hospice care is usually Part A as well.

As mentioned above, in its historic context, the Medicare Part B system, or Supplemental Medical Insurance (SMI), was added to the legislative effort late in the process. It provided for outpatient services. In addition to these two social security trust funds, there are the Old Age and Survivors Insurance (OASI) and Disability Insurance. The most well-recognized social security payment system falls under the OASI program. This is the program to which employers and employees contribute and, upon retirement or if the worker dies, payment is made to the employee or to his or her survivors respectively. At the present time, one can retire at age 65 years and receive full social security benefits; the age will rise to 67 years by the year 2027. The OASI, or social security fund, currently brings in more money through payroll deduction taxes than it spends. This payroll deduction tax is 6.2%, which is deducted from employees' wages, plus an additional 6.2%, which is contributed by employers. This amounts to a payroll deduction tax of 12.4% to support the OASI. Further, the Medicare Hospital Insurance Trust Fund is supported by an additional payroll deduction tax amounting to 2.9%, which is split evenly between the employee and the employer, coming to a contribution of 1.45% from each. At this time, the Hospital Insurance Trust Fund for Medicare Part A is also solvent but is the focus of major political and public discussion.

The Medicare Part B system, or SMI trust fund, is supported by the payment of premiums by beneficiaries. Typically, when an individual turns 65 years of age, he or she is able to receive retirement benefits under the OASI system. At that time, the Medicare retiree receives the Hospital Insurance Part A protection without any further financial outlay. However, the Medicare Part B system is financed by a deduction from the social security retirement amount as a premium payment for the SMI or Part B insurance. In 1966, this SMI premium amounted to $3.00 per month and, by 1996, this premium amount had increased to $42.50. In 1997/8, the amount rose to $43.80 and is now $88.50 in 2006. The increased monthly Part B premiums are projected to bring improved outpatient care, especially for mammograms, pap smears, prostate and colorectal cancer screening, some bone mass measurements and diabetes self-management. There is a great deal of discussion about this changing amount and possibly attaching it to a means test or allowing people to opt out of the system. At the present time, Medicare Part B pays for 80% of allowable expenses and carries a $124 annual deductible.

CRITERIA FOR MEDICARE REIMBURSEMENT

Geriatric rehabilitation services are covered by the Medicare system when there is an expectation of restoring the patient's level of function if it has been compromised by an injury or illness. Repetitive care to maintain a level of function is not eligible for reimbursement. It is crucial to have an appropriate diagnosis, with specific treatment goals, both short term and long term. The frequency of treatment should be enumerated and, for Part A, there is a minimum of 5 days per week. In most rehabilitation units, treatment takes place twice daily for a minimum of 4 hours at least 5 days a week, sometimes 7 days a week. For Medicare Part B, rehabilitation services are supposed to take place at least three times per week; however, this regulatory perspective has become very difficult to achieve in the outpatient setting as Congress and HHS have established a cap or limit on Part B services of $1740 starting in 2006. Obviously, both these guidelines may have to be modified in order to meet the individual patient's illnesses, schedules, and other confounding factors in the delivery of healthcare. These confounding situations should be recorded in the patient's chart.

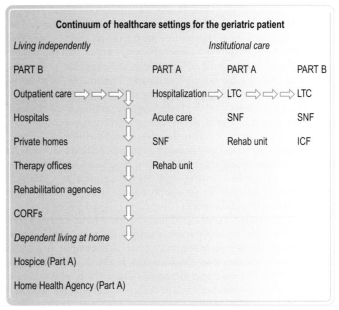

Figure 77.2 The delineation between Part A and Part B of Medicare should not be based on the skilled nature of the services, but should be based on sociomedical decisions that determine the place of care. SNF, skilled nursing facility; LTC, long-term care; ICF, intermediate care facility.

MEDICARE PARTS A AND B: THE CONFUSION

As stated above, Medicare Part A is a hospital insurance; however, services under the HI trust fund may be rendered in a hospital, rehabilitation unit, hospice system, skilled nursing facility or home healthcare situation. In contrast, coverage under Medicare Part B may take place in an outpatient setting in the hospital, a patient's home, an extended care facility, rehabilitation agency, comprehensive outpatient rehabilitation facility (CORF) or other outpatient treatment center. Additionally, it may be rendered to an individual who is living in a skilled nursing facility in a long-term care setting. Thus, the strict nomenclature of inpatient vs. outpatient care is not fully appropriate. This continuum of healthcare under the Medicare system is shown in Fig. 77.2. From the rehabilitation perspective, there should be no difference in the sophistication of the level of care rendered to a patient, whether it falls under Part A or Part B. The differentiation arises only from the sociomedical factors that necessitate inpatient rather than outpatient care.

HOME HEALTH SERVICES

Geriatric rehabilitation taking place in the home is largely a result of legislative and regulatory decisions made in the 1980s. At that time, the prospective payment system (PPS) with diagnosis-related groups (DRGs) was enacted, which encouraged hospitals to discharge people as quickly as possible. The concept behind this PPS was that the efficient hospitals would benefit and the inefficient hospitals would suffer financial demise. However, as the late Senator John Heinz reported, the DRG system encouraged patients to leave hospitals 'sicker and quicker'.

As a result, the home healthcare industry grew so rapidly that, by the late 1990s, it had become a major concern for budget watchers because of the increase in home healthcare costs. Home health services are usually covered under Medicare Part A, provided certain criteria are met. As stated above, the patient must have an appropriate diagnosis, and there should be a reasonable expectation that the patient will recover from the condition. Obviously, in the geriatric setting, the functional declines are not always clearly attributable to an acute episode, and this creates some ambiguity about medical necessity.

A person who requires skilled rehabilitative services must be determined to be confined to home in order to receive home healthcare. Also, the physician must certify that the patient is confined to home. If the patient is able to leave home, it should be achievable only with considerable and taxing effort. The patient may leave home for short durations to obtain medical care such as outpatient dialysis, chemotherapy, radiation or for an occasional trip to a barber or a walk or drive around the block.

Further, the patient is considered housebound if he or she has a condition or illness that restricts the ability to leave home except with assistance from another person or requires special transportation, or leaving home is contraindicated. Any condition such as a stroke that may cause the loss of the use of the upper extremities so that the patient is unable to open doors or use handrails will fit the criteria of being housebound. Posthospital care with resultant asthenia or weakness, pain or other medical conditions that restrict activities also qualify the patient for home healthcare. For example, a person with atherosclerotic cardiovascular disease may have cardiac risk with physical activity and should not be leaving home. Additionally, a psychiatric problem in which a patient refuses to leave home or a circumstance in which it is unsafe to leave a person unattended may qualify the person as housebound.

The patient is not confined to home if he or she has the ability to obtain healthcare in an outpatient setting. The aged person who does not often travel from home because of feebleness and insecurity brought on by advanced age would not be considered to be housebound for the purposes of receiving home health services unless he or she meets one of the above conditions.

THE MEDICAID SYSTEM

The Medicaid system is a federally mandated program under Title XIX, which is administered by the individual states, so there is discrepancy concerning who and what is covered by the program. Basically, Medicaid is a safety net for poor families with dependent children, disabled and blind adults, and the elderly. In 2005, the poverty guide was $9570 for a single person and $12 830 for a couple (Federal Register 2005). The respective numbers in 1996 were $7740 and $10 300.

For people aged 65 years and over, Medicaid financed 15% of healthcare in 1999 (Keehan et al 2004). In 2002, 17.9% of the US population was enrolled in the Medicaid program. The total cost including contributions from federal and state Medicaid programs was $297.5 billion in 2004 (CMS 2005).

An important feature of the Medicaid program is the coverage of long-term care, which amounted to $39.3 billion for 1.8 million beneficiaries in 2002 (Hoffman et al 2005).

THE OLDER AMERICANS ACT

Like the Medicare and Medicaid legislation, the Older Americans Act (OAA) was passed in 1965. It established the Administration on Aging, which organizes and directs the delivery of community-based services at the state level and represents a federal grant program. The OAA supports education, research and training. It has been the impetus for states to establish local agencies concerned with aging. These programs are often involved in establishing social services, nutritional services and senior center programs.

CONCLUSION

From its inception, Medicare has been surrounded with controversy over costs, paperwork, fraud and types of services rendered. The great achievement of this mammoth system is that many, many patients have received quality healthcare services that may not have been available to them in the past. The changing demographics of the aging population, including the increasing wealth of a large percentage of Medicare recipients, are likely to be considerations in determining the services to be rendered to the postwar baby boomers when they reach retirement and Medicare age.

References

Binstock R, Post S 1991 Too Old For Health Care? Controversies in Medicine, Law Economics and Ethics. The Johns Hopkins University Press, Baltimore, MD

Centers for Medicare & Medicaid Services (CMS) 2005 Statistics. US Department of Health and Human Services. Available: http://www.cms.hhs.gov/MedicareMedicaidStatSupp/downloads/2005_CMS_Statistics.pdf. Accessed 4 March, 2006

Centers for Medicare & Medicaid Services (CMS) News 2006 Healthcare Spending Growth Rate Continues to Decline in 2004. Available: http://www.cms.hhs.gov/apps/media/press/release.asp?Counter=1750. Accessed 19 January, 2006

Federal Register 2005 Vol. 70, No. 33, p 8373–8375. Available: http://aspe.hhs.gov/poverty/05poverty.shtml. Accessed March 4 2006

Hoffman E, Klees B, Curtis C 2005 Brief Summaries of Medicare & Medicaid, Title XVIII and Title XIX of the Social Security Act. Office of the Actuary, Centers for Medicare & Medicaid Services, Department of Health and Human Services, Baltimore, MD

Hubert H, Bloch D, Oehlert et al 2002 Lifestyle habits and compression of morbidity. J Gerontol 57A:347–351

Keehan S, Lazenby H, Zezza M et al 2004 Health Care Financing Review/Web Exclusive; Age Estimates in the National Health Accounts, Vol. 1, No. 1 Centers for Medicare & Medicaid Services, Department of Health and Human Services, Baltimore, MD

Moon M 1995 Medicare Now and in the Future. Urban Institute Press, Washington, DC

Poen MM 1996 Harry S Truman versus the Medical Lobby: The Genesis of Medicare. University of Missouri Press, Columbia, MO

Chapter 78

The end of life

Timothy L. Kauffman

INTRODUCTION

Death and Dying

Death is a finite moment
known only to God
Dying is a process that
Everyone does differently and uniquely.
Death is a victory
A gift from Jesus on the cross
Dying is a plethora of emotions
frustration
inconsistent days
some joyful
some angry
some, maybe many, in pain
or some days when you just sense
an overall loss of wellness
Death is the final goodbye to life on earth
as we know it
Dying is the goodbyes to people, events, yes, even things close to you.
The hardest and most overwhelming goodbye to me is leaving my children
Their careers I'll not see develop and flourish
Their weddings I'll never participate in
The grandchildren I'll never hold or spoil and of course other immediate family, friends, colleagues, places
I've traveled, forests, waterfalls, lakes, flowers, mountains, rustic roads, parks, oceans, my cats, Tabitha and Magnum, my stuffed animals, and more and more.

Death is our greatest victory
propelling us to a peace beyond our own understanding.
Dying is the vehicle that transports us, not always a smooth and tranquil ride but at journey's end remains the promise of a safe arrival.
Lynn Phillippi, written at Linen & Lace B&B, June 26, 1997

These words were composed by Lynn Phillippi who wrote Chapter 65 in the first edition of this book. Struggling with her own medical problems and shortly before her own death, Lynn Phillippi composed these words as well as her other contribution to the first edition, which was revised for Chapter 63 of this edition. As Lynn noted, death is but a finite moment, and each person's death is different and unique. As healthcare providers to geriatric patients, we are faced with the reality of patients dying, but the process and timing of that moment are not always simple or clearly delineated. Therein lies a difficult and ethical problem, especially with the acute care model dictated by the US Medicare system. That is, when should rehabilitation services be stopped? This question does not concern medical or nursing services because Medicare requirements are not the same as rehabilitation, which is '. . .performed with the expectation of restoring the patient's level of function which has been lost or reduced by injury or illness'. But the dying process is often protracted, filled with repetitive losses and rebounds as the progressive decline and downward spiral transpire, so rehabilitation should be refined to meet the changing needs of increasingly frail and debilitated patients. In these commonly occurring cases, the purposes of rehabilitation are to assist the patient and other caregivers with quality of life issues such as pain control, positioning, mobility, handling, and toileting, and to provide dignity to a human being and his or her family.

THE END OF LIFE

When does the end of life start – after the second stroke or when a terminal illness is diagnosed, or when a person is admitted to an extended care facility or when a doctor says so. . .? In an abstract way, the end of life may start at the time of birth, and luck, choice, and genetics determine how long the involution will be. Most healthcare providers in the field of geriatrics recognize when a patient is approaching the end of life; but most also realize that some patients will 'hang on' for days, months or even years. Therefore, to withdraw rehabilitation services too early or to deny those services may approach neglect or abuse, especially if rehabilitation specialists are not consulted.

Admittedly, constraints such as patient potential exist, but the decision should be arrived at by the family, care providers, physicians and rehabilitation specialists with due consideration given to pathology, family and patient desires, availability of services and financial realities. Included among the family's and patient's desires are sociological differences, for the end of life is surrounded by a variety of habits, beliefs, customs and values. Culture and religion are crucial considerations that influence the provision of healthcare to people as they approach death.

PALLIATIVE CARE

When a patient has little or no potential or refuses rehabilitative care, then respect, dignity and physical as well as emotional comfort must be given freely by all ethical people who come into contact with this human being. At such a time, rehabilitation for the purpose of restoring or recovering function is obviously not appropriate; however, palliative care is. Palliation simply means moderating the intensity of pain or offering care or services that will allow for a better quality of life at the time when life is ending. Often, care is directed toward the dying patient's family as much as it is given to the patient. For example, the family might need help in accepting the harsh and sad reality of the impending expiration.

In palliative care, an interdisciplinary team including nurses, social workers, physical therapists, pastoral counselors, family therapists and physicians usually provides the better services. Family members are crucial members of this team. The desired outcome is a 'good death', which is defined as '. . .one that is free from avoidable distress and suffering for the patients, families and caregivers: in general accord with the patients' and families' wishes; and reasonably consistent with clinical, cultural and ethical standards' (Field & Cassel 1997).

Emanuel and associates (2001) developed the needs at the end-of-life screening tool (NEST), which is concerned with four areas: (i) needs that are social, financial, caregiving and access to care; (ii) existential needs that are spiritual, purpose, distress and settledness; (iii) symptoms that are physical and mental; and (iv) therapeutic needs that are relationship, information and goals of care (Emanuel et al 2001). These categories of care may be helpful for all members of the team and may enable a 'good death' (Della-Santina & Bernstein 2004). Emanuel et al (2004) reported that talking in a structured interview with terminally ill patients and their caregivers caused little or no stress in nearly 90% of their subjects and that nearly 50% found it to be helpful. These researchers found the interview to be helpful, especially for ethnic minorities and persons who were anxious. Over 50% of dying patients who were having difficulty in coming to closure with family and friends reported that the discussion was helpful.

Appropriate services from a physical or occupational therapist may help with proper positioning or mobility in bed, with sitting, and with assisting to toilet. Speech therapy may be helpful for teaching swallowing, mouth care and communication modifications. Perhaps at this stage of life, the end, the ability to communicate at any level is a most crucial need, especially for the sake of family and intimate friends.

Palliative care is not something that is done only at the end of life. Efforts to moderate the intensity of pain and minimize functional limitations and impairment would have been made prior to clinical recognition that the patient has poor rehabilitative potential and is approaching the end of life. So rehabilitative and palliative care are not mutually exclusive but are on a continuum, with the emphasis on curative recovery of function lost lying at one end of the spectrum and on comfort and moderating the intensity of pain lying at the other, when restoration is unlikely or impossible.

This concept of the continuum of rehabilitation/palliation fits well within the parameters of the *Guide to Physical Therapist Practice* (1997), especially with the roles of the physical therapist in consultation and communication. The interventions of coordination and communication are particularly pertinent, as they can be used to coordinate care of the patient with family, significant others, caregivers and other professionals. This involves instruction in proper procedures and techniques but holds quality of life issues and palliation as the focus. The American Physical Therapy Association (APTA 2005) recently released an Emerging PT Practice: No. 13, which validates the purpose of physical therapy care at the end of life in the hospice setting.

THE ROLE OF REHABILITATION

Because each individual patient and family approaches the dying process with a different set of medical, spiritual and physical needs, the role of rehabilitation must be varied. In the early stages, mobility is an important treatment consideration, and thus typical gait, balance and therapeutic strengthening exercises may be appropriate. The use of assistive devices for balance, safety, pain reduction and joint protection may enable the patient to maintain a sense of independence and involvement in life's activities. Joint protection with the use of an orthotic or splint may enhance functional capacity and, as a patient becomes more confined to bed, it may be used to prevent painful and disfiguring contractures, swelling or pressure areas.

Therapeutic exercise to maintain breathing capacity and exercise tolerance is useful. The inability to breathe is frightening and can usually be controlled until the very last days or hours of life. Exercise tolerance should be aimed at sitting up on the bedside or in an easy chair or wheelchair. The world looks better from an upright posture, and the patient may be able to eat or at least sit at a meal with family and friends. Breathing and eating may be easier in the upright position.

Adaptive equipment for eating, dressing and bathing may help to maintain independence and a sense of self-worth. A wheelchair is most useful for transport and to conserve energy; however, it can cause injury or at least pain and fatigue if it is ill-fitted. Pressure areas can occur, and edema may result in dependent extremities. A poorly fitted wheelchair or prolonged sitting encourages kyphosis of the spine, which can cause back pain, reduce chest expansion for breathing and compress the abdomen, making eating more difficult.

Pain management for the terminally ill patient usually involves medication, especially narcotics. Some patients and their families choose not to use these types of medications because of their beliefs or because of the lightheadedness or drowsiness that results. The physical modalities of the various heat or cold applications and electrical stimulation are beneficial, although realistic expectations are requisite. The effects of the portable and easily used transcutaneous electrical nerve stimulator (TENS) are less potent and not identical to the effects of a dose of morphine, but they are of value. The physical modalities are described in more detail in Chapter 68, Conservative Interventions for Pain Control.

Range of motion exercises help to control pain and to prevent contractures, stiffness and pressure areas. These can often be taught to family members; that way, they have an opportunity to participate in the care of their loved one rather than being just bystanders. Further, these exercises require physical contact, which is an important human need that may be lost to the dying patient because of medical interventions or simply because family members do not know whether or not handling will cause harm. Gentle massage is therapeutic too, both physically and emotionally.

EMOTIONS

When providing medical care, be it curative or palliative, it is vital to remember that patients and their families have real emotions that must be considered. Bereavement is a process that starts before death and continues after it. The family and intimate friends are facing a loss, sometimes one that they are not ready to accept, and denial is a common coping mechanism. Denial may be used by the patient, too, and that can impede the more important acts of completing one's life work, settling one's affairs and saying goodbyes. When working with a patient and family members at a time when all of them may be in various stages of denial, it is necessary to be honest, but not brutally so. Empathy and honesty help, especially when they come from all members of the healthcare team and from clergy (Faulkner 1995).

Anger and frustration are also commonly encountered in a dying patient and may be directed at family members, at God, or at some or all of the medical care providers. Fear and guilt may also be present, for death is an unknown. Several of the world's major religions have taught the concept of sin, and the dying person may have a sense of guilt about the commissions or omissions of life, and may regret the inability to do something about them in the last remaining days. Again, empathy, honesty and dignity are important. At the end of life, a person should feel that he or she is okay and is valued by the medical providers as a human being until death and then as a memory.

Many patients and families are most appreciative of anything that can be done to provide additional comfort, dignity and worth. Therein lies the inner strength to continue to work with patients and their families as life completes its journey.

HOSPICE

The hospice concept developed in the 1960s in the UK; in the US, it is now a Medicare Part A program, which usually starts when a patient is determined by a physician to have less than 6 months left to live. A wide variety of physical capabilities and needs are found among hospice patients. In the early stages of hospice care, rehabilitation services may indeed be curative and, in the end, only palliative. The blending of one phase into the other is usually gradual, but the consultation and care provided by rehabilitation specialists as members of the hospice team will maintain the quality of life at its optimal level (Della-Santina & Bernstein 2004, APTA 2005).

IMPENDING DEATH

Certain signs indicate that death will occur soon. In the final days, the patient may become increasingly somnolent and diaphoretic, and intake of fluids and food may nearly cease. Parenteral nutrition is not advocated at this time; however, oral care and the use of lip salve and ice chips is palliative (Merck 2000). The toes and fingers as well as the nose and ears may become cyanotic as the circulation and oxygen perfusion decline. The death rattle, a frequent cause of distress for family members, results from bronchial congestion or palatal relaxation. If desired, clergy should be consulted, and the family can be present and hold hands or touch or rub the loved one to say final goodbyes. Peace, dignity and respect must prevail.

CONCLUSION

As Lynn Phillippi wrote, 'Death is the final goodbye to life on earth'. It is an individual experience inherent in life. Knowing what stops life allows a better understanding of what life is. Healthcare providers to aging and dying patients participate in this universal college frequently. Rehabilitative services, curative and palliative, enhance the quality of life for the dying patient and for the patient's family.

The following words were written as I sat at the funeral of a patient I had treated, off and on, for 8 years, both curatively and palliatively.

The Meaning of Life

What is the meaning of life?
The answer is unclear;
And it is not the same for all.
Part of the answer is in death
When it is not.
Death begets life
For it is the aging, the passage
    of time that nourishes the young;
Without someone before us,
    there can be none behind us.

Life is not easy.
It is filled with problems,
    heartaches, sadness, Yet
    there is joy abundant.
Sometimes it is hard to find. Accept
the bad, for it is life, too. But search
and focus on the good,
    the beauty.
It passes every day.

Those who precede us and those
    who pass through life with us
    are ALWAYS present.
They live with us forever
    in our thoughts,
    our actions,
    our lives.

In life, there is no absolute beginning
    and no absolute ending;
    there is only conception and there is death
    which mark these times.
But what preceded and followed these events,
    both conception and death?

Are the lives of loved ones
    both giving and receiving love;
    sharing learning and living.
We are our parents, our spouses,
    our children, our grandparents, and
    grandchildren,
    and others who enter our lives
    sharing, learning, living, loving.

The meaning of life is the here and now,
    which are built upon what preceded and
    provide for what follows;
The meaning of life is to experience it,
    the good and the bad,
But most important is to focus
    on the beauty of its experiences.

Tim Kauffman, March, 1993

References

American Physical Therapy Association (APTA) 2005 Hospice Care: Emerging PT Practice, No. 13, Rehabilitation. Oncology 23(2):24–26

Della-Santina C, Bernstein R 2004 Whole patient assessment, goal planning, and inflection points: their role in achieving quality end-of-life care. Clin Geriatr Med 20:595–2004

Emanuel L, Alpert H, Emanuel E 2001 Concise screening questions for clinical assessments of terminal care: the needs near the end-of-life screening tool. J Palliat Med 4:465–474

Emanuel E, Fairclough D, Wolfe P et al 2004 Talking with terminally ill patients and their caregivers about death, dying, and bereavement. Arch Intern Med 164:1999–2004

Faulkner A 1995 Working with Bereaved People. Churchill Livingstone, London

Field M, Cassel C 1997 Approaching Death: Improving Care at the End of Life. National Academy Press, Washington, DC

Guide to Physical Therapist Practice. Phys Ther 1997:77(11).

Merck 2000 Manual of Geriatrics, 3rd edn. Merck Research Laboratories, Whitehouse Station, NJ, p 115–127

UNIT 11

The rehabilitation team

Chapter 79

Caregivers: the sustaining force

Cheryl Anderson

The focus of most medical care and concern in dealing with frail elderly patients is on the elder and their medical treatments. However, this is a small fraction of the overall care provision for most chronically ill elders. Well over 90% of all care to the elderly and disabled is provided by an informal network of family, friends, and faith (Family Caregiver Alliance 2004). This invisible network of support and help sustains most elders through their aging years.

INFORMAL NETWORKS

Dissecting the major realms of this invisible caregiver network, family is usually primary. Family includes the spouse, children and siblings. Generally, the family is faced with determining the type of living arrangements and has the responsibility of most formal decisions. Friends may be lifelong acquaintances or neighbors who may find their simple acts of kindness turn into an ongoing, often reluctant role. Shoveling a heavy snowfall may gradually turn into routine home maintenance, to transportation, to medical advocate and some form of communication conduit with the family. It is difficult for these good Samaritans to say they wish to decrease or terminate their services. The third variable, faith, is generally a more distant role than family and friends. However, the rise of parish nursing programs is a method for faith communities to acknowledge their own important role in caregiving.

The informal caregiver network is faced with multiple, conflicting issues. In the case of spouses, friends and some faith providers, the caregiver is often at least as old as the person requiring help. These people are often ill equipped to deal with comorbid conditions of aging elders. This informal network begins to fail when chronic illnesses progress and difficult behaviors arise, causing a frail elder to wear out their caregivers and begin to outlive their own assets. Such is the testament for many admissions to skilled nursing facilities.

As part of the clinical team treating frail elders, therapists must develop a broader perspective of whom and what supports each patient. Given the multiple demands and stresses that equate with caregiving, therapists should monitor and assess the well-being of the caregivers for older patients. Often, the overwhelming burden of caregiving places a risk on the caregiver becoming a patient too.

It is well documented that caregivers are at a high risk of developing disorders such as depression and anxiety, which may contribute to hostility toward, and even abuse of, the difficult or demented elder. Furthermore, the risk of caregivers developing depression and their own physically debilitating symptoms increases with increased caregiver burden (Schultz et al 1995).

SOCIETAL VIEWPOINTS

Societal pressures and the stigma of skilled nursing facilities place pressure on informal caregivers to provide care to the elder in home and community settings. There is a general belief that all senior citizens desire to grow old and eventually die in their lifelong home. This, like most stereotypes, is false for many. However, this belief is pervasive, influencing public policy in multiple modes.

Families are increasingly faced with caregiver concerns for their elderly relatives. Although about 3.4% of the American public reside in a skilled nursing facility at any one time, another 3% reside in assisted living facilities, while another 5–8% receive care through home- and community-based services (HCBS) (University of Maryland 2005). Many HCBS are actually provided by the same informal network that already existed.

The landmark 1999 passage of the National Family Caregiver Support Program acknowledged the prominent public policy issue associated with aging and long-term care and the factors associated with informal caregivers (US Department of Health and Human Services 2003). This legislation laid the groundwork for HCBS programs that focused funding needs on frail elders while continuing to ignore the actual needs of the caregivers who provide that care.

HCBS-type systems put a face on the invisible caregiver network. The mission of HCBS is to keep the elderly in their own homes and community for as long as possible. HCBS are driven to decrease institutionalization. This legislative policy is the main force credited with the closure of nursing home beds in lieu of community alternatives. On the face of public policy, this is what the public wanted. However, the silent burdens actually increased for the caregivers. Given that society was pressuring toward no institutionalization, the family was left to grapple with the questions of 'then what?' and 'how?'.

A positive outcome of HCBS-type care is monetary. Funding is now available to pay people who provide care, including the family. There are restrictions on who may be paid for what services, e.g. a spouse cannot be paid for providing activities of daily living (ADL) support but a daughter may be reimbursed. Many caregivers question these policy changes, as they would provide care whether paid or not. HCBS funding is provided through a combination of federal and state dollars by formulas generally managed through state Medicaid programs.

Families face difficult pressures. With child-bearing occurring later in life, many dual-income, middle-aged couples have school-aged children at home. Further, these couples often have their own 70+ aged parents and their 90+ aged grandparents to worry about. The stress of caregiving for the aged is falling squarely on the busiest people in American society.

CLINICIAN VIEWPOINT

Surprisingly to many clinicians, families provide the vast majority of long-term care needed by frail elderly. Clinicians generally recognize families as decision-makers and short-term caregivers following acute incidents. However, the rise in elders living longer with multiple comorbidities increases familial responsibilities beyond most expectations. The rehabilitation team should acknowledge this factor. Treatment that focuses on a frail elder being discharged to their home or a community source will be dependent on others, most probably a family member, for care.

Minnesota (MN) has long studied this phenomenon. The 2005 report to the legislature completed by the MN Department of Human Services found that one in four adults in MN was involved in some level of caregiving for older relatives. The dollar value of informal care far outweighed the other sources of funds spent caring for MN elders. This longitudinal study found that $6.84 billion was spent in 2004 for all care provided for MN seniors. The cost breakdown found that Medicare accounted for 7%, Medicaid and other state programs for 13%, out-of-pocket 11%, private insurance 1%, with 67% provided through informal care (MN Department of Human Services 2005).

COGNITION AS THE DECISION DRIVER

The most debilitating factor for caregivers is cognitive decline. Notably, the majority of patients with Alzheimer's disease live outside institutions, creating considerable serious psychological morbidity among their caregivers. Research continues to focus on methods of dealing with cognitive decline. However, the day-to-day challenges are far outside the researchers' microscope. Families find themselves forced to understand a dizzying array of services and placements provided by mismatched incentives and awkward systems.

THE MANY ROLES OF THE CAREGIVER

Caregivers have many roles to perform in the care of an aging person. Some people are natural-born caregivers requiring little instruction, while others have no idea how to help or where to begin. Furthermore, the more helpful of these caregivers may also be the most disabling. In the effort to ensure that the elder does not have to exert too much physically or have increased pain, a softhearted caregiver may not allow the elder to reach maximal rehabilitation potential. The caregiver may view the exercises as too hard, too time consuming

or not necessary. They may rush to do things that the frail elder may actually be able to do independently. For the healthcare provider, this situation may create an ethical dilemma because the caregiver rejected the care. In this case, the healthcare provider must offer the appropriate services and also respect the caregiver with one exception, which is that no abuse is taking place.

The roles that the caregiver may assume run a gamut. The following sections describe several of these roles.

Medical advocate

The route to being a caregiver is insidious, creeping into one's life in a slow or innocuous fashion. Advocating for appropriate medical care is one of the first formal steps an informal caregiver may begin assuming. As the physical presence, caregivers play an integral role in treatment decisions and their implementation. Caregivers begin the processes through their role as transporter and information source. This includes bringing frail elderly to appointments, assisting with diagnosis, providing the oral history and accurately conveying the current abilities of their loved one. Caregivers bear the burden for final decisions including what treatments may be implemented, when to begin or end treatments and end of life issues. Caregivers become increasingly responsible for making medical decisions as the elder's physical and cognitive status deteriorates. For these reasons, it is very important for caregivers to fully understand the nature of each chronic or debilitating condition and the possible treatment approaches, benefits, limitations and potential side effects. As caregiving may last anything from 2 to 20 years, this is a long-term partnership that requires respect of the caregivers' abilities.

Difficulties and disagreements often arise as different people may assume this role at varying times. Distant living children may hold legal title to Power of Attorney or Health Care Guardian; however, others may make the daily small decisions.

Clinical partner

For a frail elder to reach maximal rehabilitation potential, the caregiver needs to be seen as a clinical partner. Caregivers need to have realistic expectations about what benefits can be realized and how they may be a part of the success or failure. If the caregiver does not fully understand and support the treatment plan, the elder's care may suffer. The therapist needs to be able to effectively communicate with each caregiver and insure that the regime may fit into the schedule of daily life for both the elder and their caregiver. Overzealous treatment programs, multiple exercises and lengthy care plans will certainly meet with failure for all involved. The focus on function, mobility, movement and recognition of what life is like in the home setting will help each therapist to be realistic in assisting the caregiver to be a clinical partner.

Personal care attendant

One of the most difficult tasks for caregivers is providing ADL support. Bathing and grooming may fall to those ill equipped to deal with another's personal needs. Incontinence problems are disdainful to deal with and are often a leading driver toward institutionalization. Feeding assistance and specific meal preparations become burdensome and time-consuming tasks for many caregivers.

Guardian

Caregivers are burdened with the responsibility of preventing harm from befalling a frail elder. Parenting the parent is a term that is often heard. One expects to parent their child for about 20 years. One rarely expects to do the same for their own mother or father (or grandparent). Guardian duty is certainly a graded responsibility depending on the cognitive and physical abilities of the elder.

Guardians insure that the physical environment inside and outside the home remains safe. It may begin as yard work and snow shoveling, and progress to the laundry and housework. Soon meal preparation, inside safety and sleep routines require attention.

While therapists may make treatment recommendations, the day-to-day quality of life is the responsibility of the caregiver. The caregivers' efforts may be focused on continuity, dignity, pleasure, social interaction and a stable environment, while the therapist's are toward increased functional ability.

Activities and social director

The family is often faced with being the main social interaction for the frail elder. The weekly visit, grocery shopping and medical appointments often progress to becoming their confidante and friend. It is a difficult role that seems to creep in slowly until a family realizes that the burdens of providing social outlets have fallen solely on their shoulders.

The wise therapist will assist families in determining other sources of care and respite. Community resources may be accessed to relieve some of this burden, and elder visiting networks may also provide the needed companionship for housebound elders.

Chief cook and bottle washer

A sudden, acute illness causes most to rush to the aid of the ill or injured. The first steps home often find many willing secondary-type caregivers including friends or faith-based/ parish nursing people who are not usually involved in day-to-day caregiving. These caregivers bring in food and offer household help. Unfortunately, the rush quickly turns to a trickle with a few or one left to fill in the gaps of services required to run a home. For a married couple, it is the spouse who takes on most of the duties the two previously shared. In the case of a widow or widower, children step in as long as possible supported by lifelong family friends including the faith community. Recognizing the long-term nature of this role early may help caregivers to talk and plan how this role will be filled. Most communities do have formal services that may be accessed for meals, house maintenance and yard work. Relinquishing these tasks to formal, paid providers may assist in decreasing the caregiver burden.

THE STAGES OF CAREGIVING

Caregiving may be viewed as a linear process beginning from the insidious start to heavy involvement to death of the elder. Seminal work by Pfeiffer (2005) has been done in the stages of caregiving. His research describes seven distinct states of caregiving. Table 79.1 outlines each stage.

The seven stages described by Pfeiffer are important for therapists and for caregivers to understand. Although he applied much of his research to Alzheimer's patients, it is an applicable model for most caregivers. Each stage describes a new responsibility for caregivers and legitimizes the multiple, conflicting emotions felt at each stage.

Stage 1: Coping – the stage of disbelief. The diagnosis is given; the incident happened; a hospitalization occurred. All create an acute awareness that life for this elder and their networks will never be the same. Internalizing Stage 1 leads to Stage 2.

Table 79.1	The stages of caregiving
Stage 1	Coping with the initial impact
Stage 2	Deciding whether a family member can take on the caregiver role
Stage 3	The long stretch of at-home caregiving provision
Stage 4	Considering residential placement
Stage 5	Caregiving during residential placement
Stage 6	Death of the patient – grief and relief
Stage 7	Resuming life – healing and renewal

Stage 2: Deciding who will be the caregiver. This may be a lengthy stage with multiple versions of caregivers. This stage seems to meld into Stage 3.

Stage 3: The long stretch of at-home caregiving. This is the strength of the invisible caregiver network formed by family, friends and faith. Multiple incidents may occur during this phase. The ebbs and flows of chronic illnesses will be found. It is the stage when caregivers grow weary and are at risk of becoming patients themselves.

Stage 4: Considering residential placement. Stage 4, a watershed decision, may be viewed tragically by society and welcomed by caregivers. Nursing home placement is a relief to many. The caregiver is allowed to rest, to resume activities and to be assured that others can provide 24/7 care. Handing the baton of care from overwrought caregivers to a formal system is difficult even when welcomed. Although it may appear that this is the end of the informal network, it is not. The network changes and adapts to the newer, often lesser demands and provides more nurturing and care vs. meeting physical needs.

Stage 5: Caregiving during residential placement. This stage recognizes the caregiving changes following placement. Daily or weekly routines will develop for caregivers and the elder.

Stage 6: The eventual death of the elder that brings grief and relief. Most deaths are grieved even when expected. A sense of guilt may pervade those who have borne the brunt of care provision and now find the relief they desired. This is the stage where the faith community may provide the most support to the informal caregivers.

Stage 7: Resuming life. Stage 7 is intertwined with Stage 6. Finding a sense of renewal in one's own life and healing from the long bout of burdens from caregiving.

Staging systems are helpful methods of describing processes and emotions that may be in place for caregivers of elders. However, not all people will progress neatly through stages and staging systems will not always accurately describe the process for all.

CAREGIVER RECOGNITION

Caregivers need to be recognized as an integral component in successful rehabilitation. Therapists need to fully understand the breadth and depth of the care delivery system, noting particularly that most care is not found in the medical arena. Therapists need to analyze each patient and their networks before determining how to integrate rehabilitation programs.

Each patient is an individual, as are his or her caregivers. No system, no matter how well developed or planned, can adequately address all individual needs. In the drive to do the right thing, empathy toward the caregivers needs to become a prerequisite characteristic.

References

Family Caregiver Alliance 2004 The State of the States in Family Caregiver Support: A 50-State Survey. Family Caregiver Alliance, Washington, DC

MN Department of Human Services 2005 Financing long-term care for Minnesota's baby boomers. A report to the Minnesota Legislature. Available: http://www.dhs.state.mn.us/main/groups/aging/documents/pub/dhs_id_025734.hcsp. Accessed December 15 2005

Pfeiffer EA 2005 Caring for the caregiver. Available: http://www.medscape.com/viewarticle/465785_22. Accessed December 15 2005

Schultz R, O'Brien AT, Bookwala J, Fleissner K 1995 Psychiatric and physical morbidity effects of dementia caregiving: prevalence, correlates, and causes. Gerontologist 35(6):771–791

University of Maryland 2005 Partnership for long-term care. Available: http://www.hhp.umd.edu/AGING/index.html. Accessed December 15 2005

US Department of Health and Human Services 2003 The Older Americans Act, National Family Caregiver Support Program: Compassion in Action. US Administration on Aging, Washington, DC

Chapter **80**

Interdisciplinary geriatric assessment

Michael Moran, David C. Martin, Margaret Basiliadis and Timothy L. Kauffman

INTRODUCTION

Many approaches to the care of the geriatric patient have been lumped under the rubric of 'geriatric assessment'. Indeed, in terms of process and outcome, geriatric assessment is one of the most widely studied aspects of geriatric healthcare. By 2006, there were thousands of published reports on geriatric assessment, and numerous meta-analyses had been performed or were under way.

The American Geriatrics Society (AGS) Core Writing Group of the Task Force on the Future of Geriatric Medicine has outlined a series of core attributes and competencies for geriatric medicine. These include 'coordinated care that includes communication among providers' and 'interdisciplinary team care with shared responsibility for patient care processes and outcomes' (Besdine et al 2005). The goal of this chapter is to examine the philosophical underpinnings of the interdisciplinary approach to geriatric medicine, to examine some of the models of how geriatric assessment has been operationalized and to point out some of the weaknesses and future directions of research for this model of healthcare.

PHILOSOPHICAL UNDERPINNINGS OF GERIATRIC ASSESSMENT

Secondary aging must be distinguished from primary aging

Physiologists often divide the problems of aging into two categories – primary aging and secondary aging. Primary aging includes those physiological changes that can be ascribed solely to the passage of time. Several theories have been set forth to explain the changes caused only by aging. These include denaturation of proteins through cross-linking, cumulative damage from free radicals and an internal biological clock that is genetically determined. This last theory gained

credibility from cross-species studies that related longevity to the number of cell doublings that could occur in cell culture. The number of cell doublings proved to be species-specific and varied directly with the longevity of the species. (See Chapter 1 for additional information about theories of aging.)

An exciting finding could further elucidate the exact nature of this biological clock. This finding is the discovery that repeating basepairs at the ends of strands of DNA, called telomeres, prevent unraveling of the DNA strands and preserve the genetic integrity through their repeated replication. The telomeres 'harden' the DNA strand in a fashion similar to the way in which the plastic caps on the ends of shoelaces prevent the shoestring from unraveling. The length and stability of telomeres could be the physiological basis of the biological clock.

Secondary aging involves those decrements in function that can be ascribed to disease processes. Primary and secondary aging are sometimes difficult to distinguish from each other. For example, it was once thought that there was a substantive decline in cardiac output that was age related and due to primary aging. However, Pugh & Wei (2001) reported that cardiac output is actually well preserved into advanced age.

Likewise, in the era before autopsy studies had been done upon people with dementia, it was believed that dementia was simply a primary process of the senium rather than secondary aging. Autopsy series later disclosed that cognitive losses could be explained by specific pathologies such as multiple strokes or the senile plaques and neurofibrillary tangles of Alzheimer's disease. It is now known that, even though speed of effortful mental processing slows with aging, in the absence of disease, cognition remains well preserved (Weaver et al 2006).

How do these principles relate to geriatric assessment? It is the role of geriatric assessment to tease out the effects of secondary aging and to reverse them through specific treatments, to ameliorate them through interventions that may improve, although not cure, the underlying condition or to assist the patient to function better by marshaling support services or altering the patient's environment to make that environment more conducive to the patient's needs.

Coexistence of multiple diseases and the cascade of illness

When clinicians are first trained in medicine, they are commonly taught to think in terms of the 'chief complaint'. This approach proves to be much too restrictive in the practice of geriatric medicine. Here, the most common scenario is one of multiple, coexisting pathologies that are all conspiring to harm the patient's functional ability. Many patients presenting for geriatric assessment may have more than four significant medical problems that need to be addressed.

An example of the cascade effect of multiple problems might be the patient who presents with delirium. Such a change in mental status is a final common pathway for many medical and psychiatric conditions. In this example, the pathology might be traced back as follows: the patient has some moderate renal insufficiency and prostatic hypertrophy. The prostatic hypertrophy leads to urinary retention, which further worsens renal function, which leads to azotemia and anorexia, which leads to reduced fluid and nutritional intake, which leads to even further worsening of renal function and a relentless downward spiral. This interrelationship of organ system function causes a cascade of illness that affects many organs.

A challenge of geriatric assessment is to trace the cascade of events back to find key points in each patient's unique pathophysiology where treatment may halt or reverse the downward spiral. Because of the complexity of this process, an interdisciplinary approach is often most successful. Also, there is no substitute for seasoned and experienced clinicians making expert diagnoses. The challenges of treating the frail elderly led Franklin Williams, a past director of the National Institutes on Aging, to coin the phrase 'the fruition of the clinician' in respect of the practice of geriatric medicine.

As any cohort ages, variability increases

As noted earlier, it is often impossible to predict the specific decline of any particular organ system on the basis of aging alone. Likewise, it is impossible to predict the physiological function of any individual based on age alone. One may speak of chronological age vs. physiological age. To speak of a young 80-year-old or an old 65-year-old does not sound like an oxymoron to the geriatric practitioner.

What can be predicted is that, as people age, they become less and less like each other. (Anyone who has attended a 25-year class reunion has probably experienced this first hand.) No two persons age identically. Some encounter diseases, others suffer traumatic injuries and others cope with both. Lifetime habits, choices and fortune add to the genetic variability of aging individuals.

The increasing diversity that comes with age has a direct effect on geriatric assessment. For geriatric assessment to work well, it is crucial that both diagnostic and therapeutic approaches be individualized for each patient. Attempting a 'cookbook' approach to the solution of clinical problems in such a diverse group could easily lead to iatrogenic harm. The recent trend toward the creation and application of clinical pathways or clinical guidelines in the treatment of specific conditions must proceed carefully and contain greater flexibility when dealing with issues in geriatric medicine.

Again, the interdisciplinary approach, because of its greater clinical diversity, can better account for the pluralism of this unique population.

Diminished homeostatic reserve blocks recovery

Perhaps the best definition of aging is 'increasing susceptibility to the forces of mortality due to decreased homeostatic reserve'. Homeostasis concerns the body's ability to maintain itself in a steady state and to get itself back on track whenever there is perturbation from that steady state. Ability to maintain a constant temperature, constant blood pressure, and constant blood glucose level are all examples of homeostasis.

When homeostatic reserves are constrained, there is diminished likelihood of survival with any extreme stress. A key principle in geriatric assessment is to recognize that homeostatic reserves are diminished and that patients are more sensitive to both the disease processes and the iatrogenic effects of intervention. This should lead to a more conservative and individualized approach in the application of therapeutic maneuvers and drug therapies.

These issues are especially important in geriatric rehabilitation. A common scenario is the elderly patient who has suffered a hip fracture and requires surgical repair. With postoperative pain and analgesia, the patient often suffers such setbacks as postoperative delirium, fever, anemia from blood loss, atelectasis and hypoxemia. Thus, the rehabilitation measures may be delayed for several days by intercurrent illness. While at bedrest, the patient may be losing in the order of 2–5% of muscle strength (Gillis 2005) and 1–2% of aerobic capacity daily. Whereas younger people may surmount these losses, in the geriatric patient who is already marginally compensated, these losses become highly significant and make rehabilitation and recovery all the more difficult.

In this setting, the patient might not cope well physically or psychologically with the arduous exercise demands of rehabilitation. The twice-daily treatments of up to 4 hours imposed by government regulations may be too rigorous for some of these more frail individuals. Sometimes, rehabilitation must occur at a more gradual pace and in the long-term care setting.

Diseases present in an atypical fashion

Among geriatric patients, the common presentations of illness are often replaced by the less specific and more global findings of increased confusion, weakness, anorexia and tendency to fall. One sees such phenomena as 'silent myocardial infarction', 'afebrile pneumonia' and 'depression without sadness'. The first manifestation of urosepsis might be falling, or the presenting symptom of a myocardial infarction might be increased agitation. In geriatric assessment, the clinician must cast a wider net in attempting to make diagnoses.

Other diseases typically present only in the elderly or much more frequently in the elderly, and the index of suspicion for these problems must remain higher. These disorders include such entities as polymyalgia rheumatica, Parkinson's disease and hypothyroidism.

Diseases are underreported

Geriatric patients commonly underreport their problems (Doughty 2003, Tariq et al 2003). Sometimes, cognitive impairment gets in the way of an accurate relating of historical information. At other times, the patient is embarrassed to bring up certain problems. This may account for the fact that incontinence is so underreported. At other times, depression may lead to a sense of hopelessness about the possibility of getting help; or patients may have acquired some of the ageist bias from the society in which they live and may feel that their problems are to be expected at their time of life and they should not complain.

The process of geriatric assessment strives for accurate and reliable historical information by collecting data through collateral interviews with caregivers and loved ones as well as with the patient himself or herself. The patient is also typically interviewed by several professionals. A patient might relate something to a nurse or social worker that would not have been mentioned to a doctor.

Self-report questionnaires and structured assessment tools to measure cognition, affect and morale can yield quite useful information if they are administered carefully and in a nonthreatening manner. These tools add additional important information to the historical database.

THE PROCESS OF GERIATRIC ASSESSMENT

The process of geriatric assessment typically involves an interdisciplinary approach. The most consistent team members to have formed the traditional core of this assessment process have included the geriatrician or geriatric nurse practitioner, nurse and social worker. Ancillary team members have included the occupational therapist, physical therapist, psychiatrist, nutritionist, speech therapist, exercise physiologist, recreational therapist and respiratory therapist. One of the very first outpatient assessment programs even employed an architect because of the frequency with which changes in the patient's home environment were being recommended.

In the following case study, an example of the geriatric team in action may help to illustrate many of the principles of geriatric assessment:

Case study

Mrs A was an 85-year-old widowed woman who was living with and being cared for by her 54-year-old daughter. She was referred by her daughter for outpatient geriatric assessment. The patient had been suffering from gradual and progressive memory loss for the preceding 3 years. Three weeks previously, she had become more apathetic and withdrawn, and had ceased to be able to climb the stairs because of arthritic complaints. On intake, she was being treated with amitriptyline 25 mg at night for depression.

On further questioning, it was learned that the patient was becoming delusional, believing that people on the television screen were real. Her functional status a month earlier had been much better and her incontinence was new. She complained of a feeling of profound weakness. The social worker learned that the daughter was extremely resentful that the caregiving burden had fallen to her and was not being shared by her two siblings. She felt guilty about her resentment, and this made her caregiving even more difficult.

Medical workup disclosed moderate degenerative joint changes, moderate hearing loss and dysphoric mood. The patient made seven depressive responses on the Geriatric Depression Scale and scored 20/30 on the Folstein Mini-Mental Examination. She remembered zero out of three objects on early recall. Mobility testing showed profound weakness, with difficulty arising from the examination chair and broadening of the support base. Screening laboratory tests showed a mild anemia with a hemoglobin of 11.3 g/dL and a mean corpuscular volume (MCV) of 81. The serum cobalamin level was low normal at 200 pg/mL. The sedimentation rate was markedly elevated at 110 mm/h. Other blood parameters were normal. A magnetic resonance imaging (MRI) scan showed periventricular hyperintensity and multiple lacunae. Soon after the initial assessment, the patient was begun on 15 mg of prednisone daily for a presumptive diagnosis of polymyalgia rheumatica. In addition, she was begun on cobalamin injections. The amitriptyline was discontinued. When the patient was returned to the clinic for a family conference, her mobility had improved dramatically, as had her pain symptoms. The incontinence had resolved because the patient was now mobile enough to get to the bathroom. The delusions had also disappeared, but the patient remained dysphoric. The family was educated and counseled about the spectrum of the patient's problems. It was pointed out that her cognitive loss might not be due to Alzheimer's disease, as she had been told previously, and that the prognosis was uncertain. It was decided to continue to monitor the patient's mood for another month and to consider treating her with one of the newer selective serotonin uptake inhibitors if her mood remained depressed. The patient was referred to an adult daycare program. She began to attend 3 days per week.

Six months later, the patient was being maintained on 5 mg of prednisone daily. Her mobility remained good and the sedimentation rate was 26 mm/h. The patient had been started on sertraline 50 mg daily, and her mood had improved. The hemoglobin had risen to 13.0 g/dL. She was still occasionally delusional and the score on the Mini-Mental examination had not improved. The patient's daughter, however, was feeling greatly relieved, and she perceived her mother to be functioning at a much higher level of cognition, even though this could not be objectively demonstrated. The daughter was planning to have her mother enter a 1-week respite program while the family went on a week-long vacation.

This case illustrates several key principles of geriatric assessment. This patient was suffering primarily from an illness (polymyalgia rheumatica) that is found exclusively in the elderly population. In the absence of any symptoms suggesting cranial arteritis, many clinicians would institute an empiric trial of corticosteroid therapy without doing a temporal artery biopsy and gauge the response to therapy. A dramatic response, as was seen in this case, helps to confirm the diagnosis.

The next most important problems, those of the cognitive impairment and dysphoria, reveal how multiple coexisting pathologies can conspire to create dysfunction. The suddenness of the onset of the patient's delusions and cognitive decline suggested either a vascular process or a reaction to the anticholinergic effects of the amitriptyline. The low cobalamin level is also a not uncommon finding and could also be contributing to the cognitive loss. The use of oral rather than parenteral replacement therapy for a low cobalamin level is debatable, but the decision was made to institute parenteral replacement just in case the patient could not adequately absorb the vitamin.

In many instances of geriatric assessment, the caregiver becomes as much a client as the patient. Predictable respite is one effective means of reducing caregiver stress, and referral to an adult daycare program is an ideal way to provide predictable respite. When alleviated of some of the caregiving burden, the daughter could once again enjoy her relationship with her mother.

The perception on the part of family members that the patient was functioning much better cognitively even though objective improvement could not be measured represents another phenomenon deserving of mention. Significant disparity between 'perceived' and 'measured' improvement often exists.

In order to coordinate and implement the various recommendations of the separate professionals involved in the interdisciplinary approach, a team conference is typically held after the assessment. The care plan is crafted with input from the various team members. Often, a family conference is held with the patient and all involved family members and caregivers. The purpose of this conference is to educate the patient and caregivers, to make official recommendations, and to answer questions. It also provides yet another opportunity to assess for caregiver burden and to move to alleviate it if it is clinically significant.

The interdisciplinary model of geriatric assessment has been applied to a variety of settings (Phillips 2005). The most common have been adult medical–surgical hospital wards, outpatient clinics, inpatient geropsychiatry units, nursing homes, rehabilitation hospitals, patient homes and hospital-based consulting services. There are also more complex models that involve many team members and are found in the inpatient and consultation models.

From many outcome studies (Barnes 2006, Covinsky 2006, Jacobs 2006) that have been performed on the various manifestations of geriatric assessment, one can make several generalizations. First, and perhaps most important, is that assessment without implementation is of almost no value. The programs with the most robust outcomes have been those with direct links to rehabilitation services and those in which the geriatric team had direct responsibility for the implementation of care plans. Second, not all geriatric patients can be expected to benefit from geriatric assessment. Patients who have relatively high function and those who are hopelessly ill are less likely to derive benefit, so many programs attempt to target those who would be most likely to benefit. On the other hand, one would also not wish to be too quick to judge a patient as hopelessly ill, because geriatric assessment has scored some of its greatest successes in patients who had previously been written off by the traditional healthcare system.

In terms of traditionally measured outcomes (such as mortality, functional status, frequencies of hospitalization and nursing home placement), research study results are mixed. Because of the mixed models of geriatric assessment and differing sites of practice, meta-analyses and generalizations about the value of geriatric assessment are difficult. Nevertheless, some reviewers (Jouanny 2005) have felt that the data are convincing in terms of reduction in mortality, lowered rates of nursing home placement and lowered levels of caregiver burden.

DIRECTIONS FOR FUTURE RESEARCH

The technology of geriatric assessment has been under attack because it is viewed as labor intensive and inadequately reimbursed. Were the data of research studies more conclusive with regard to outcomes, it would be easier to advocate the widespread application of interdisciplinary geriatric assessment. The main challenge in the light of what has been learned seems to be selective application of this interdisciplinary approach, targeting those subjects and contexts in which geriatric assessment is determined to be cost effective.

Other areas of active research in this field include investigation into the optimal place to perform geriatric assessment. Some intriguing studies suggest that the optimal site may be in the patient's own home (Nikolaus & Bach 2003). Other important questions also have to be answered. Do data that have been collected largely through interview reflect what the patient is actually able to perform? Do data on functional status, which are often garnered by physical therapy and occupational therapy in a laboratory setting, correlate well with what the patient can do in his or her own home?

The development of critical pathways, or clinical algorithms, is a process that is being repeated at virtually every acute care hospital in an effort to standardize care and reduce costs. As healthcare systems become globalized to include the entire continuum, these pathways must become more extended. They will cease to be disease- or organ-specific and, rather, will evolve into a 'syndromic' approach. To work effectively, these pathways must take into account the various principles of geriatric assessment that have been under discussion. The effects of the application of such pathways on outcomes have been positive (Smyth 2001, Endo et al 2004).

Many other important questions about the approach to treating the geriatric patient must be addressed. Some of these are the following: What is the value of treating dysphoric mood that falls short of full-blown depression? Some data suggest that patients with dysphoria may be inappropriately high utilizers of healthcare resources. How stable are people's advance directives? Do they change when patients are more immediately confronted with life-threatening situations and the issues are more immediate and less abstract than when the directive was originally formulated? How valuable are exercise prescriptions in later life? What are some of the long-term effects of nutrition on health? Higher folate intakes may have an antiatherogenic effect mediated through homocysteine levels. Are there ways to ameliorate the effects of bedrest deconditioning and the development of delirium that so often add to the morbidity of hospitalization of geriatric patients? Is there a role for anticipatory conditioning prior to elective hospitalizations or procedures (so-called prehabilitation)?

CONCLUSION

It remains for the upcoming generation of researchers and practitioners to improve the knowledge base and give good health and meaning to the later stages of peoples' lives. Not enough students are entering this important field, yet it can be among the most rewarding and challenging of endeavors.

To recapitulate the previous clinical scenario of the 85-year-old woman with both physical and cognitive impairments, recall that the patient's subjective improvement vastly surpassed what could be measured objectively. When a patient is marginally compensated and just barely able to get by, then slight improvements in condition are often perceived as dramatic, even when the degree of improvement can scarcely be measured by our crude assessment tools. This magnified effect of intervention on the patient's and family's perceptions of health and well-being can be one of the most gratifying aspects of serving a frail geriatric population.

It is hoped that the information in this book will help to enable accomplishment of the AGS Task Force goals for geriatric medicine. They include: (i) 'continuity and seamlessness across all sites and providers' and (ii) 'appropriateness of care within the context of the goals of the individual patient and the values of society'. But to achieve this, new models must be developed for healthcare delivery especially in the United States, which is largely determined by the Medicare system. In this system, benefits are not uniform and obstacles exist within the fee-for-service model that encourages payment for units of care but not for case/disease management (Besdine et al 2005).

References

Barnes DE 2006 Depressive symptoms, vascular disease, and mild cognitive impairment: findings from the cardiovascular health study. Arch Gen Psychiat 63(3):273–279

Besdine R, Boult C, Brangman et al 2005 Caring for older Americans: the future of geriatric medicine. J Am Geriatr Soc 53 (suppl6):S245–S256

Covinsky KE 2006 Development and validation of an index to predict activity of daily living dependence in community dwelling elders. Med Care 44(2):149–157

Doughty DB 2003 Promoting continence: simple strategies with major impact. Ostomy/Wound Manage 49(12):46–52

Endo H, Nippon R, Igakkai Z 2004 Comprehensive geriatric medicine. Jap J Geriatr 41(4):375–377

Gillis A 2005 Deconditioning in the hospitalized elderly. Can Nursing 101(6):16–20

Jacobs LG 2006 Warfarin pharmacology, clinical management, and evaluation of hemorrhagic risk for the elderly. Clin Geriatr Med 22(1):17–32

Jouanny P 2005 Pharmacological treatment in severe dementia. Psychol Neuropsychiat Vieill 3(suppl1):S51–S55

Nikolaus T, Bach M 2003 Preventing falls in community dwelling frail older people using a home intervention team (HIT): results from the randomized falls-HIT trial. J Am Geriatr Soc 51(3):300–305

Phillips SL 2005 Pain management in a long term care setting: an interdisciplinary approach. Ann Long Term Care 13(6):34–36

Pugh KG, Wei JY 2001 Clinical implications of physiological changes in the aging heart. Drugs Aging 18(4):263–276

Smyth C 2001 Creating order out of chaos: models of GNP practice with hospitalized older adults. Clin Excellence Nurse Pract: Int J NPACE 5(2):88–95

Tariq SH, Morley JE, Prather CM 2003 Fecal incontinence in the elderly patient. Am J Med 115(3):217

Weaver CJ, Maruff P, Collie A, Masters C 2006 Mild memory impairment in healthy older adults is distinct from normal aging. Brain Cognition 60(2):146–155

Chapter 81

Gerontological and geriatric nursing

Brenda Hage

INTRODUCTION

The nursing profession has a long history of providing healthcare to sick older people. Initially, geriatric nursing focused on physical care, comfort measures and palliation. The care was often given almost entirely by nurses and their assistants in nursing homes or in people's own homes. As knowledge, technology, public policy, and societal expectations changed, the scope, types of geriatric services and quality of nursing care also changed. The establishment of the first formal standards for nursing care for older adults, adopted in 1970 by the American Nurses Association (ANA), was a landmark initiative for nurses in geriatrics. It provided a link to nursing science, which is defined by the ANA as the deliberate problem-solving process, grounded in the biopsychosocial sciences, of diagnosing and treating actual or potential health problems.

As these practice standards were reviewed and modified over time, patient-centered care, family participation and nursing services related to the prevention of disease and disability and the promotion of good health for older adults were articulated more explicitly as major components of geriatric nursing practice. This paved the way for the use of the term 'gerontological nursing' to refer to a domain in the continuum of the science and practice of nursing that is devoted to the complex care of older adults and their families and to balancing the effects of normal aging and pathology. Today, the term 'geriatric nursing' indicates specialized clinical care for the medical problems of the sick and chronically ill elderly in various interdisciplinary patient care settings. Nurses with advanced training who practice in this area are known as geriatric nurse practitioners or geriatric clinical specialists.

An overall goal for gerontological and geriatric nursing is to provide humanistic healthcare to older adults and their families by paying careful attention to individual circumstances, needs and goals. Preventing impairment, restoring function and maintaining an enduring state of health and well-being and quality of life are embedded in these goals. A key strategy that is used to meet these goals is the application of the nursing process that consists of assessment, planning, intervention and evaluation within the context of healthcare issues presented by the elder and their family.

As a discipline, nursing has agreed to a social contract to make its services available 24 hours a day. Thus, gerontological and geriatric nurses have critical roles in the collaboration of the healthcare team, as they must be involved in planning, implementing and evaluating patient care. The nurses' roles and functions include nursing management and other therapeutic activities for direct patient care, case management, patient and family health education and counseling, administration, advocacy, public policy development, and education and research.

DIRECT PATIENT CARE

To ensure seamless care, continuous leadership and accountability are requisite. Professional nurses act on these responsibilities in acute care units, ambulatory care clinics, long-term care facilities, homecare agencies and other sites where the need for geriatric care can be fulfilled.

At least three different types of nursing expertise, using different levels of critical thinking and clinical decision-making skills, are available to older patients to assist them in meeting their healthcare needs:

1. Staff nurses have clinical, technical and humanistic skill in one-to-one interaction so they can strengthen and support the biopsychosocial processes of recovery, rehabilitation, healing, preventing disease and disability, and dying with dignity. Nurses functioning in this role practice in acute care settings, skilled nursing facilities, home health settings and hospices, and a smaller number practice in ambulatory care clinics or doctors' offices.

2. Advanced practice nursing roles in gerontological nursing primarily include clinical specialists and nurse practitioners. These master's degree or doctorally prepared nurses function in a variety of roles to support this challenging patient population.

(i) Geriatric clinical nurse specialists have expertise in working with complex nursing care problems and draw from their advanced skills in hands-on clinical care, critical analysis and decision-making, teaching, counseling, and coordination and follow-up of interdisciplinary care plans. They practice in acute and long-term care settings and may be consultants to community clinics and home-based geriatric care programs. They may also conduct research, evaluate program outcomes, and coordinate quality improvement activities.

(ii) Geriatric nurse practitioners have expertise in performing comprehensive physical assessments, interpreting symptoms and physiological abnormalities, and developing treatment, management and follow-up plans for medical problems, in partnership with the primary care physician and other team members. Their practice is closely linked with primary care services in ambulatory clinics, although a growing number of these nurses are providing services to elderly patients in long-term care facilities, adult day health programs, and physicians' offices as well as inpatient settings.

THE FOUR STEPS OF NURSING

The four-step nursing process guides the nurse to individualize, contextualize and prioritize problem areas. The steps consist of assessment, planning, intervention and evaluation.

Step 1: Assessment

Biopsychosocial data about geriatric patients are collected by means of interviews, record reviews, direct observations and other approaches, as time allows, to build a composite picture of the multiple and often competing needs of the geriatric patient and the informal caregiver. For example, the federally mandated multidisciplinary assessment called the Minimum Data Set (Burke & Walsh 1997) is used in nursing homes by long-term care nurses to record assessment data as part of the team approach to care planning and treatment.

Data from nursing assessments are necessary to identify problems in the order of clinical significance at a specific time and according to the urgent need for nursing interventions. The information may include general and specific data on the presenting problems as defined by the patient and the caregiver, medical diagnoses, prescribed medical treatments, status of physical and mental functions, alternate healthcare resources, patient goals and expectations, safety risks, self-care abilities for recovery, including the ability to perform activities of daily living, and other information that a nurse considers clinically relevant to the case or situation. Identifying nursing diagnoses and prioritizing these problem areas are the major intended process outcomes.

Since 1973, the North American Nursing Diagnosis Association (NANDA) has continued to develop a taxonomy of nursing diagnoses, and currently there are approximately 130 approved classifications of patient care problems in nine categories. In 1987, the Center for Nursing Classification and Clinical Effectiveness at the College of Nursing, University of Iowa, developed taxonomies for classifying and organizing nursing interventions and nursing outcomes through the use of the Nursing Intervention Classification (NIC). This was followed by the development of Nursing Outcomes Classification (NOC) coding systems in 1992. The NIC/NOC codes are linked to the NANDA diagnoses and serve to document the effectiveness of nursing interventions and outcomes (McCloskey et al 2004, Moorhead et al 2004). Refinement of the NIC/NOC classification systems has been ongoing. The use of nursing taxonomies facilitates the capture of nursing data useful for evaluation, quality improvement, and research activities.

It is important for members of healthcare teams to be aware that some problem areas that demand priority nursing interventions may not always be parallel to or target directly the 'curing' goals of a medical plan.

Step 2: Planning

The nursing care plan incorporates specific nursing interventions and activities to treat specific nursing diagnoses or deal with problem areas such as changes in food intake, impaired capacity for personal care, risk of accidental injuries due to general weakness and mild dementia, grief unrelated to the health problem, and other needs of the geriatric patient and the caregiver. Included in the plan are nursing actions to insure the continuity of all prescribed medical treatments and other intervention modalities for the geriatric patient. Clinical judgment is an important nursing skill in this process because it enables an accurate identification of the nursing diagnosis.

Step 3: Implementation

The process of implementation utilizes the collective efforts of members of the nursing staff, including auxiliary nursing personnel, and directs them so that the nursing care plan can be carried out. Safe and compassionate approaches that are clinically and technically appropriate are used to achieve the desired clinical outcomes. Nursing actions may include activities such as checking vital signs, changing the position of an immobilized elderly patient, orienting an elder with a memory deficit to time, place, and activity, interviewing a family caregiver prior to homecare, consulting other healthcare professionals, advocating for an elder to obtain a local community resource, and other actions aimed at resolving a nursing problem or reducing the impact of a nursing diagnosis.

Step 4: Evaluation

A patient's physical, verbal and behavioral responses, informal caregivers' reports and observations by healthcare providers from other disciplines are important aspects of the feedback mechanism that helps the nursing staff to maintain a dynamic, flexible care plan. Critical analysis of information obtained while nursing interventions are in progress may be used to modify nursing interventions, redirect patient and family participation in the overall treatment and management plan, re-examine the healthcare team's understanding of the clinical problem, determine cost benefits, realign leadership and support the standards of quality patient care.

CASE MANAGEMENT

The nurse case manager looks after a group of elderly patients and informal caregivers. As a rule, frailty, multiple chronic illnesses, unstable functional status, complex psychosocial and financial situations, and other multilayered clinical issues trigger the need for this type of professional nurse. Advanced skills in clinical decision-making, communication, resource identification, referral, management, systems analysis and cost analysis are essential for effective case management. The role of a nurse case manager involves consulting with healthcare providers; meeting with patients, family members and other support systems; advocating for need-specific health and social services; planning for discharge; insuring safe termination of services; facilitating shared decision-making; and recording appropriate documentation. Case managers may also negotiate a change in health benefit with third-party payers to insure that the older patient's needs are being optimally addressed. As healthcare delivery systems change, the number of nurse case managers for older people is expected to increase, particularly in community-based programs such as home-based services, adult day health programs, and respite and hospice services. For example, in the home health arena, the nurse is the ideal team leader; in that role, the nurse can coordinate the case and facilitate the completion of required documentation by interdisciplinary care providers, institutions, physicians in group or private practice and payers. With the growing trend toward managed care, the nurse in such a role might be called a case manager. Other administrative functions may also be part of the geriatric nurse case manager's responsibility in the practice sites mentioned earlier.

HEALTH EDUCATION AND COUNSELING FOR PATIENTS AND FAMILIES

A major focus of the teaching and counseling done by gerontological and geriatric nurses relates to the implementation of treatment and management prescribed by healthcare providers in acute care, homecare, or community care. Teaching patients before they are discharged home or to another site of care helps to prepare the patient and the family. Education in ways of preventing disease, disability, and complications of existing chronic health conditions becomes increasingly necessary as the shift to community care expands. Teaching and counseling by these nurses take place across the continuum of care of the elderly. This function may be combined with direct patient care and case management functions.

ADMINISTRATION

Professional roles for administrative nurses include director of nursing services in a skilled nursing facility and administrator in a variety of settings, such as homecare, adult day health, respite care, hospice, and other community care programs for older adults. Some nurse entrepreneurs take on the challenge of administering small board-and-care (i.e. personal care) homes. The legislative mandates of Medicare and Medicaid, regulations, and the standards of care, to name a few, are complex bodies of information that the geriatric nurse administrator is able to translate into practice in order to support quality standards of care and insure fiscal responsibility.

ADVOCACY AND PUBLIC POLICY DEVELOPMENT

Although nurse activism is found among all types of practitioners of nursing, some nurses in gerontology and geriatrics build careers in advocacy dedicated to shaping and changing public policy. Their expertise in the legislative process and their analyses of public policies may be applied to issues related to healthcare access for the aging population and other relevant concerns. They find employment in governmental agencies, in the offices of public officials, with advocacy organizations, or with other entities oriented toward public policy issues and aging.

EDUCATION AND RESEARCH

With the increasing number of education programs in gerontological and geriatric nursing being taught in colleges and universities, the need for faculty members with doctoral and master's degrees in gerontology and geriatrics will continue to grow. Clinical specialists, nurse practitioners and nursing administrators predominate in the faculties of many nursing schools across the country. Gerontological and geriatric nurses with doctoral degrees have teaching and research responsibilities. They are prepared to function as principal investigators in research projects and clinical trials and to establish research programs in gerontological and geriatric nursing science. Generating evidence-based nursing practice is an important commitment of these nurse researchers. Some of the domains of nursing research are sleep disturbances, agitation, pet therapy, family caregiving, falling behavior, sensory disabilities, use of technology to support aging in place and self-care deficits. The body of knowledge produced by their studies contributes to improving healthcare for older people and to advancing the science of aging. In addition, these researchers create opportunities for other nurses to experience the research process as assistants, graduate students or participants in the study.

CONCLUSION

Gerontological and geriatric nurses have a variety of roles and functions. With the trend toward downsizing and the shift to managed care programs, these roles and functions are being fused and structured in different ways. New personnel who deliver direct bedside care but have limited formal education and training are being introduced into the clinical arena. The challenge to nursing, in particular to nurses in gerontology and geriatrics, is to maintain the standards of healthcare for older adults, especially those who are disempowered by chronic disability, socioeconomic status, racial or cultural factors, environmental situations, low health literacy or technological illiteracy, and lack of technology access. Also, the aging of the baby boomers, a social and historical phenomenon, is already shifting the focus of healthcare from the cure model to the prevention model. The high incidence of chronic disease in this population requires new approaches to assisting older adults in the development of self-management skills needed to deal effectively with these problems. It is clear that new expertise and more advanced practice nurses will be needed in this specialty.

References

Burke M, Walsh M (eds) 1997 Gerontologic Nursing: Holistic Care of the Older Adult. Mosby Year Book, St Louis, MO

McCloskey Dochterman J, Bulacheck GM (eds) 2004 Nursing Intervention Classification (NIC), 4th edn. Mosby, Philadelphia, PA

Moorhead S, Johnson M, Maas M (eds) 2004 Nursing Outcomes Classification (NOC), 3rd edn. Mosby, Philadelphia, PA

Chapter **82**

Geriatric occupational therapy

Molly Mika

INTRODUCTION

Occupation may be defined as any meaningful and purposeful activity or series of activities in which an individual engages. According to the occupational therapy practice framework of the American Occupational Therapy Association (AOTA), areas of occupation include activities of daily living (eating, dressing, toileting, etc.), instrumental activities of daily living (homemaking, meal preparation, money management, etc.), education, work, play, leisure, and social participation (AOTA 2002). Disease, dysfunction and loss associated with advanced age threaten the older adult's satisfactory engagement in occupations. Occupational therapy (OT) practitioners, consisting of both occupational therapists and occupational therapy assistants, therapeutically use meaningful and purposeful activities to insure and enhance an individual's participation in chosen occupations.

OT practitioners serve older adults in various settings including a variety of inpatient settings such as acute care hospitals, rehabilitation centers, skilled nursing facilities and psychiatric centers. Community-based occupational therapy may be provided in outpatient settings, clients' homes or in adult daycare and senior centers (Boyt Schell et al 2003a). Occupational therapy professionals may fulfill the roles of direct service provider, administrator, consultant, educator and researcher.

OCCUPATIONAL THERAPY ASSESSMENT

In order to provide effective, efficient therapeutic intervention, occupational therapists conduct a thorough twofold assessment of their clients. The therapist conducts an occupational profile (a client-centered interview) designed to gather pertinent information regarding the individual's occupational history and preferences, the various contexts in which the client engages in occupation, and the client's values, beliefs and goals regarding his or her current functional performance (AOTA 2002, Boyt Schell et al 2003b).

Additionally, the occupational therapy clinician conducts an analysis of the client's occupational performance (AOTA 2002, Boyt Schell et al 2003b). He or she observes the older adult engaging in a valued occupation, such as eating, dressing, moving in bed or preparing a meal, to identify the client's functional strengths and limitations. The clinician then performs standardized and/or non-standardized tests to specifically pinpoint the client factors, such as decreased strength or decreased ability to initiate a task, contributing to any functional limitations.

Occupational therapists and the interdisciplinary team members share their assessment findings with one another in order to develop a comprehensive treatment plan. In some settings, such as hospitals and home healthcare, interdisciplinary team members contribute their findings to a joint team evaluation. Using the Functional Independence Measure (FIM), in hospitals across the United States for example, enables healthcare providers to establish a baseline level of performance for each client and provides all team members with a method of tracking a client's progress in primary areas of daily functioning (Uniform Data System for Medical Rehabilitation 1993). While the FIM tool may be entirely conducted by any treatment team member, occupational therapists are often responsible for completing the self-care and transfers portion of the assessment.

Through joint and discipline-specific evaluation, the occupational therapist and the treatment team members, in collaboration with the older adult, prepare for the client's discharge either home or to the next level of service.

OCCUPATIONAL THERAPY INTERVENTION

Upon completion of the OT assessment, the OT practitioner begins intervention planning and implementation. Practitioners may employ a combination of interventions including the therapeutic use of self, the therapeutic use of occupations and activities, education and consultation with either individuals or groups (AOTA 2002).

Additionally, based on the etiology of the client's deficits, practitioners use a combination of the following treatment approaches: create/promote, establish/restore, maintain, modify and prevent. (This approach is used when a client's pathological condition, Alzheimer's or Parkinson's disease for example, is progressive in nature. In these situations, the absence of OT intervention would result in significant decline in a client's functional performance, thereby increasing his or her burden of care.)

The following case illustrates how occupational therapy might be applied in geriatrics.

Case study

Arlene's physician referred her to home healthcare services including nursing, physical therapy, and occupational therapy. The physician's orders for occupational therapy included training in activities of daily living, transfers, instrumental activities of daily living (homemaking), increasing left upper extremity active range of motion (ROM) and left upper extremity strengthening.

Arlene, an 83-year-old female, recently fractured her left distal humerus, her dominant extremity, when she fell trying to get to the bathroom one night. While the doctor performed no surgery or casting to Arlene's left arm, he had immobilized it with a simple sling for 6 weeks. He has removed the sling and has ordered therapeutic services through a home health agency. Arlene has diabetes and experiences atrial fibrillation. Her right middle finger was surgically amputated 1 year ago. Arlene has type II diabetes and undergoes kidney dialysis three times per week.

Occupational profile

Arlene resides in a two-story home with her husband and adult son. Her husband uses compressed oxygen 24 hours per day and her son works full time in a warehouse. Prior to her fall and subsequent left humeral fracture Arlene slept in her bedroom and used the bathroom on the second floor of her home. Arlene currently does not access her second story because she cannot use the single handrail when descending the stairs because of left upper extremity pain and ROM limitations. She sleeps in a rented hospital bed on the first floor. As there is no bathroom on the first floor, Arlene toilets using a portable commode and sponge bathes in the kitchen. She relies on her son to empty the commode and for assistance with bathing and dressing. Arlene reports significant limitations when attempting her favorite occupations, cooking and baking.

Arlene reports that she longs to sleep in her bed upstairs as well as use the second-story bathroom. She also wishes to prepare a simple lunch for herself and her husband without the assistance of her son.

Arlene uses a straight cane when ambulating throughout her home and requires supervision to do so as her compromised endurance and dynamic standing balance put her at risk of future falls.

Analysis of occupational performance

The occupational therapist observed Arlene's performance in functional mobility (transferring to and from the bed, the commode, a kitchen chair and a reclining chair) and in self-care (item retrieval required for grooming in the kitchen and hand washing). Arlene required minimal assistance (a helper contributed approximately 25% of the effort necessary for Arlene to engage in the tasks) with transfers and moderate assistance (a helper contributed approximately 50% of the effort necessary for Arlene to engage in the tasks) with most self-care tasks. The therapist also assessed Arlene's left upper extremity status and function, including pain and edema (excess swelling that had accumulated in Arlene's hand as a result of sustained immobilization and now interfered with her mobility) evaluation, active/passive ROM and muscle strength measurement. Moderate edema of Arlene's left hand and wrist was noted. She experienced moderate pain during gentle passive ROM of her shoulder and elbow and had significant active and passive ROM and strength limitations throughout her left upper extremity. Additionally, the therapist assessed Arlene's home in order to make recommendations to insure the client's safety and to optimize her future occupational performance. The occupational therapist noted obstacles such as clear oxygen tubing strewn on the floor in multiple rooms.

The occupational therapist, in collaboration with Arlene, set the following long-term goals:

1. Arlene will perform all self-care with supervision only within 5 weeks.
2. Arlene will prepare a simple lunch for her husband independently within 5 weeks.

The occupational therapist set corresponding short-term goals for each long-term goal. For example, in order to meet long-term goal number one, Arlene would first meet the following short-term goal:

Arlene will comb her hair using her left hand with minimal assistance within 2 weeks.

Occupational therapy intervention

Arlene's occupational therapist used a variety of intervention approaches to insure Arlene's goal accomplishment.

Prevention: As Arlene's humeral fracture resulted from a fall, the occupational therapist educated her and her family in fall prevention. To increase visibility, yellow duct tape was applied to the clear oxygen tubing at 6-inch intervals. Additional lighting in hallways, especially for night use, was also recommended.

Restoration: The occupational therapist instructed Arlene in left upper extremity active assistive ROM exercises. Additionally, she engaged Arlene in therapeutic activities and occupations designed to increase shoulder, elbow, wrist and finger strength and ROM. For example, Arlene used her right hand to assist the left hand in pressing out a graham cracker pie crust and later cleaned the table using her left upper extremity, stretching to reach a bit further with each swipe of the dishcloth.

Modify: The occupational therapist introduced Arlene to adaptive dressing equipment, a sock aid and shoe horn to assist her with lower extremity dressing. Arlene is not expected to fully regain the function of her left upper extremity, but would still like to don her socks and shoes independently.

An OT consultant, hired by the manager of a high-rise apartment building for independent seniors, uses the create/promote approach when instituting a work simplification and energy conservation program in the setting so that seniors might not become overly fatigued when shopping or preparing meals. The create/promote approach targets the well population with the aim of enhancing quality of life through participation in occupation.

An OT practitioner uses the establish/restore approach to intervention when he/she facilitates a patient's functional skills that were lost as a result of a particular condition. An OT practitioner teaching a stroke survivor how to use a spoon again uses the establish/restore approach to intervention.

Occupational therapists often work with families whose loved ones have dementia. As a client with dementia is forgetful and will progressively decline in functional performance, the occupational therapist uses the maintain approach to intervention when he/she suggests ways in which the family could structure the home environment to support or preserve the client's current abilities. For example, to maintain an older adult's independence with dressing himself, an occupational therapist might post signs with pictures of simple sequences to remind the client to put on his socks before putting on his shoes.

When using the modify approach to treatment, OT practitioners alter tasks or environments to insure the client's success in functional performance. For example, an OT practitioner would recommend showering while seated on a tub bench for an older adult who has sustained bilateral lower extremity amputations.

Finally, OT practitioners concern themselves with preventing further disability among their clients. Older adults recovering from lower extremity joint replacement, for instance, would benefit from a fall prevention program.

CONCLUSION

Occupational therapy practitioners work closely with a number of different healthcare professionals in caring for geriatric clients. They use therapeutic occupation and activities as their primary modality in meeting their patients' needs. Finally, regardless of the setting, occupational therapists and assistants, upon completion of a thorough assessment, insure clients participate as fully as possible by employing a variety of treatment approaches including creation/promotion, restoration/establishment, maintenance, modification and prevention.

References

American Occupational Therapy Association (AOTA) 2002 Occupational therapy practice framework: domain and process. Am J Occup Ther 56:609–639

Boyt Schell BA, Cohn ES, Crepeau EB 2003a Occupational therapy practice today. In: Neistadt ME, Crepeau EB (eds) Willard and Spackman's Occupational Therapy, 10th edn. J.B. Lippincott, Philadelphia, PA

Boyt Schell BA, Cohn ES, Neistadt ME 2003b Introduction to evaluation and interviewing: section one: overview of evaluation. In: Neistadt ME, Crepeau EB (eds) Willard and Spackman's Occupational Therapy, 10th edn. J.B. Lippincott, Philadelphia, PA

Uniform Data System for Medical Rehabilitation 1993 Guide for the Uniform Data Set for Medical Rehabilitation (Adult FIM). UB Foundation Activities, Buffalo, NY

Chapter 83

Geriatric physical therapy

William H. Staples

CHAPTER CONTENTS

INTRODUCTION

This chapter is designed to introduce the reader to current physical therapy practice and its importance in the rehabilitation process. Physical therapy is an integral part of the rehabilitation process of the older adult. As the population ages, physical therapists will play a pivotal role in the recovery of geriatric clients who have experienced disease or illness.

The American Physical Therapy Association (APTA)'s *Guide to Physical Therapist Practice* provides the following definition: 'Physical therapy is a dynamic profession with an established theoretical base and widespread clinical applications in the restoration, maintenance, and promotion of optimal physical function' (APTA 2003). The World Confederation for Physical Therapy (WCPT), a nonprofit organization comprising 92 member organizations representing over 250 000 physical therapists worldwide, states that 'the aim of physical therapists is to identify and maximize human movement potential within the spheres of promotion, prevention, treatment, and rehabilitation, in partnership with their clients' (World Confederation for Physical Therapy 2005).

The primary goal of geriatric physical therapy is to prevent, maintain or rehabilitate an impairment or functional limitation, which is accomplished with the application of evidence-based scientific principles. The rehabilitative process should be geared to assist the older person to achieve the highest level of function possible within their environment. Physical therapy tries to focus on functional mobility while maintaining safety, enabling the older adult to enjoy a longer life by living it more independently and with less pain. The WCPT has a subgroup called the International Association of Physical Therapists working with Older People, whose goal is to serve as the international resource for physical therapists working with the elderly.

Physical therapists are healthcare professionals involved in the examination and evaluation of individuals with neuromuscular, musculoskeletal, cardiopulmonary and integumentary disorders. The physical therapist can then determine a physical therapy diagnosis and develop an individualized intervention plan to achieve short- and long-term goals for improved function. Physical therapists do not limit their skills to treating people who are ill. A significant portion of time is spent working on health promotion and prevention of primary and secondary problems to avert an initial injury or secondary impairment that would lead to subsequent loss of movement and function.

The physical therapist is a graduate of a college or university physical therapist education program, which in the US is accredited by the Commission on Accreditation in Physical Therapy Education (CAPTE), and has passed a licensing examination that is regulated by each state. The physical therapist assistant holds an Associate's Degree from a college program also accredited by CAPTE. The WCPT currently recommends a minimum of 4 years of university-level studies to achieve professional recognition. Physical therapist assistants are licensed in most states through examination. They are not permitted to perform evaluations, but can perform many of the treatment activities under the supervision of a physical therapist. Supervision requirements vary from state to state.

The APTA has set forth a goal that, by the year 2020, physical therapy will be provided by physical therapists who are doctors of physical therapy (APTA 2005). As of 2006, 78% of 209 CAPTE accredited physical therapist education programs offered the Doctor of Physical Therapy (DPT) degree. It is anticipated that, by the year 2008, 95% of US physical therapy programs will be offering the DPT degree.

Geriatric physical therapy can be practiced in a variety of settings including acute care hospitals, rehabilitation centers, skilled nursing facilities, continuing care communities, home healthcare agencies and outpatient clinics. Geriatric physical therapy is committed to combating and minimizing the accumulative disabling effects of physical illness in association with the aging process. This is performed by hastening convalescence and reducing institutionalization, education of the patient and caregivers, contributing to the comfort and well-being of the patient, and assisting the individual to return to optimal living within their capabilities. Geriatric physical therapy has been recognized as an area of specialization that requires a specific set of advanced skills and knowledge that addresses the aging process. Specialists in geriatric physical therapy understand the differences between 'normal' aging and pathological changes that commonly occur in the older adult. Assisting the geriatric client can be an arduous task because of multisystem involvement and multiple comorbidities. Special considerations such as psychosocial issues, reimbursement, environmental, frailty, nutritional, pharmacological and cultural factors must be accounted for in a successful rehabilitation process. The American Board of Physical Therapy Specialties first recognized individuals as board-certified geriatric clinical specialists (GCSs) in 1992. To become a GCS, one must be a licensed physical therapist, spend a prescribed number of hours in direct patient care with the elderly, and pass a rigorous written examination. The WCPT (2005) supports the specialization process.

REFERRALS TO PHYSICAL THERAPY

There are many reasons to seek out the knowledge and skills of a physical therapist. Box 83.1 is a useful, but not entirely inclusive, list

---

Box 83.1   Possible indications for geriatric physical therapy referral

- Recent fall or history of falls
- Deficits in strength or range of motion
- Loss of mobility or ambulation requiring an assistive device
- Musculoskeletal pain
- Difficulty with transfers
- Orthotic or prosthetic needs
- Open wound
- Neurological disorder
- Balance deficits
- Decreased endurance for ADLs
- Bed bound status
- Need for adaptive equipment to enhance safety and function

---

of possible indications for a physical therapy referral. Physical therapists understand a vast array of problems that affect physical function and general health. They utilize screening to enable them to refer to other appropriate healthcare practitioners if the therapist is serving as a portal to the healthcare system. Physical therapy is a rapidly evolving profession. In most states, an individual can have direct access to a physical therapist for evaluation and treatment without first seeing a physician for a referral. The APTA's Vision Sentence states that physical therapists will be 'recognized by consumers and other health care professionals as the practitioners of choice to whom consumers have direct access for the diagnosis of, interventions for, and prevention of impairments, functional limitations, and disabilities related to movement, function, and health' (APTA 2005).

Many older people do seek out a physician as the traditional first stop in the healthcare process, with subsequent referral for physical therapy, although this may be underutilized. Johnson et al (1994) determined that almost half the patients who were hospitalized and found to be deficient in ambulatory or transfer skills compared with status at admission did not receive physical therapy services. Interestingly, those patients who received physical therapy in the hospital were significantly more likely to receive it in the postacute period. It is possible to infer that elderly medical patients develop functional disabilities during hospitalization that are not appropriately recognized. Routine physical screening of all elderly patients should be performed by nursing staff to determine if there has been any loss of physical performance. Freburger et al (2003) found that, even after controlling for diagnosis, illness severity, and physical therapy supply, referrals to physical therapy were much less likely from primary care physicians in comparison with orthopedic surgeons. This lack of referrals affects the quality of care received and may eventually result in an increased cost if a treatable condition worsens. Delays in care can also lead to decreased functional outcomes and frustration for clients and patients.

In a hospital, the physician is traditionally in charge of the patient as he or she has admitting privileges. The therapist may very well be an employee who is assigned the case through a scheduling rotation or

based on their specific skills (e.g. GCS), and does not usually have the authority to seek older persons in need of services without a referral from the physician. The physician has traditionally served as the 'gatekeeper' to the healthcare system.

Outside the hospital, a great number of states do allow direct access, although the majority of therapists still receive referrals from a physician, physician's assistant or nurse practitioner. Direct access varies considerably in terms of legal, practice and reimbursement models. Some limitations or barriers to receiving physical therapy services result from legal issues, but other reasons include lack of public and healthcare provider education. Additionally, most secondary payers such as the federal government and private insurance carriers limit reimbursement without a physician referral.

Interestingly, Miller et al (2005) found that over 66% of physician orders or referrals to physical therapy for geriatric clientele specified only 'evaluate and treat' or 'PT consult'. This finding does indicate some degree of physician confidence in the expertise and decision-making skills of physical therapists.

ASSESSMENT OF THE GERIATRIC PATIENT

Evaluation of clients, whether referred or by direct access, should include a history as well as a physical examination using various tests and measures (see Box 83.2). The examination should also include a

---

Box 83.2   Tests and measures provided by physical therapists (APTA 2003)

- Aerobic capacity/endurance
- Anthropometric characteristics
- Arousal, attention, and cognition
- Assistive and adaptive devices
- Circulation (arterial, venous, lymphatic)
- Cranial and peripheral nerve integrity
- Environmental, home, and work (job/school/play) barriers
- Ergonomics and body mechanics
- Gait, locomotion, and balance
- Integumentary integrity
- Joint integrity and mobility
- Motor function (motor control and motor learning)
- Muscle performance (including strength, power, and endurance)
- Neuromotor development and sensory integration
- Orthotic, protective, and supportive devices
- Pain
- Posture
- Prosthetic requirements
- Range of motion (including muscle length)
- Reflex integrity
- Self-care and home management (including activities of daily living and instrumental activities of daily living)
- Sensory integrity
- Ventilation and respiration/gas exchange
- Work (job/school/play), community, and leisure integration or reintegration (including instrumental activities of daily living)

systems review for screening purposes to rule out any pathological conditions that need to be referred to other health professionals. The therapist then evaluates the data collected and makes clinical judgments based on this information to establish a physical therapy diagnosis. The geriatric physical therapist is able to interpret the data gathered into categories, syndromes or clusters to determine the appropriate intervention strategies. This can be quite a challenge in older adults because they present with more complex problems. The aging process has taken some toll on the body, and multiple pathologies may exist that may exaggerate, or hide, underlying conditions. The experienced therapist will attempt to determine, where possible, which problems are age related and which are due to pathology.

The examination of Mrs S (see Case study) reveals that she has had several recent falls, history of osteoarthritis, hypertension and atherosclerotic heart disease. She was taking Lasix, acetaminophen (paracetamol) and Evista prior to the hospitalization and she has begun to take them again. She is unsure of what medications she was given in the hospital. Tests and measures reveal overall left hip strength of 3+/5; a mild kyphosis; independent gait with a standard walker, weight-bearing as tolerated at approximately 75%, limited due to pain rated at 3/10; difficulty with activities of daily living (ADLs); decreased balance (Tinetti score of 20/28); limited endurance as she is only able to ambulate 80 feet in 2 minutes before requiring a rest period; and she is hard of hearing. Vital signs at rest: blood pressure (BP) 140/82, heart rate (HR) 74, respiration rate (RR) 20. Vital signs after gait: BP 150/86, HR 110, RR 28. She has not been on a regular exercise program.

The physical therapist must now analyze these data. There is a myriad of factors that will need to be considered before progressing to the next steps of goal setting and selection of interventions. The geriatric therapist has to screen for a possible lower extremity blood clot because of recent surgery and recognize that Evista has a tendency to promote clots. The physician will need to be contacted regarding medications. Knowing that the best predictor of a fall is a previous fall, the therapist must try to determine the underlying cause of her falls. The Performance-Oriented Assessment of Mobility, commonly called the Tinetti assessment, was chosen by the therapist because of the patient's ability to use an assistive device. Additionally, the therapist felt that the Berg Balance Scale would be too difficult for the patient to perform safely. The Tinetti score (see Table 83.1) indicates that she remains at a moderate risk of falling. Is the cause external (environmental, such as loose carpeting) or internal (possibly orthostatic hypotension caused by taking Lasix as an antihypertensive medication)? Is she able to get in and out of her apartment independently in case of emergency or able to shop for food? Will she require a call alert, home health aide, Meals on Wheels or other services? These factors must be accounted for in order to insure a successful rehabilitation process.

Case study

Mrs S is an 82-year-old retired school teacher who lives alone in a two-storey walk-up apartment. She had fallen at home, fracturing the left femoral head. After a 5-day hospitalization for a left hemiarthroplasty, followed by a 2-week stay at a skilled nursing facility, she was referred to a home health agency. The physical therapist is scheduled to open this case the day after her return home.

GOAL SETTING AND INTERVENTIONS

Improved function must be the priority focus of interventions provided by the geriatric physical therapist. Functional goals are established with the patient, and sometimes with family or caregiver, in order to determine the appropriate treatment interventions. The skills of the therapist are utilized to provide appropriate treatment strategies and techniques. For this case study, the long-term goal of return to being an independent functioning, community-dwelling individual was determined. To meet this long-term goal, several short-term goals were set. These included:

- Safe and independent gait, with full weight bearing left lower extremity with a walker, progressing to a cane and stair climbing as appropriate.
- Increase lower extremity strength to 4/5 to enable progression to cane.
- Increase Tinetti score to 24/28 to decrease risk of falls.
- Independent with ADLs to decrease outside care and expense.
- Increase endurance and ambulatory velocity to 100 feet (30.48 m) in 1 minute with a perceived exertion level not to exceed '5' on a 0/10 scale or '13' on the 0/20 Borg Rating of Perceived Exertion Scale.

Table 83.1   The Tinetti assessment tool

Gait tests	Maximum score is 12
Balance tests	Maximum score is 16
Totals	Maximum score is 28
Score	19 or below = high risk of falls
Score	20–24 = moderate risk of falls
Score	25 and above = low risk of falls

Table 83.2   Case study evaluation and interventions

Evaluation findings	Interventions
Decreased hip strength	Progressive resistance exercise
	80% 1 rep max, 8–12 repeats without pain
Decreased balance	Balance exercise at kitchen counter or heavy chair, progress with less upper extremity support
History of falls	External: loose rugs, cords, pets
	Internal: check BP sit to stand and provide education
Diminished gait status	Gait training with appropriate assistive device including stair climbing. May need to order cane or quad cane
Decreased endurance	Increased ambulatory distance, while monitoring vital signs, home exercise program. Monitor through use of target heart rate or perceived exertion
Other needs	Raised toilet seat, grab bars for bathroom, are banisters adequate in stairwell?

The therapist must monitor and continually assess the client's progress in the short-term goals in order to update them and progress toward the long-term goal. Modification of the interventions must be made if outcomes are not being successfully achieved. Additionally, the therapist must provide preventative and wellness education to this client regarding the importance of regular exercise, osteoporosis and posture.

In order to achieve the long-term functional goal, interventions are planned to improve Mrs S's impairments. These interventions will be tailored to meet this individual's needs and tolerance (see Table 83.2).

In addition to the above noted interventions, the physical therapist may identify the need for additional services. Referrals were made to occupational therapy for ADL training and to social services in order to arrange Meals on Wheels. Geriatric patients, i n particular, benefit from a team approach. The elderly are commonly affected by a variety of interacting problems that can be better solved with input from several points of view. It is essential that members of the team communicate with each other in order to achieve a positive outcome.

CONCLUSION

The geriatric population is a unique group to work with because of the aging and disease processes that interact to produce a wide variation in each individual. Physical therapists, as healthcare providers, are also health educators and health promoters, and will continue to play an ever more important role in the provision of healthcare services. Time should be spent to teach, counsel and modify the behaviors of individuals that, if left unattended, would lead to dysfunction. Some of the concerns that can affect the older adult, such as nutritional concerns, psychosocial problems, and limited finances, may fall outside the immediate practice of physical therapists, but must be addressed in order to maximize therapeutic outcomes. The geriatric practitioner must also understand reimbursement issues to better serve their clientele. Rather than working in a vacuum, communication and teamwork must be utilized for the best overall care of the patient or client. Geriatric rehabilitation offers a huge challenge to the talent and creativity of each therapist. As the geriatric population continues to grow, so will the challenges.

References

American Physical Therapy Association (APTA) 2003 Guide to physical therapist practice, 2nd edn. APTA, Alexandria, VA

American Physical Therapy Association (APTA) 2005 Vision Sentence for Physical Therapy 2020 and APTA Vision Statement for Physical Therapy 2020. Available: http://www.apta.org. Accessed 15 September 2005

Freburger JK, Holmes GM, Carey TS 2003 Physician referrals to physical therapy for the treatment of musculoskeletal conditions. Arch Phys Med Rehabil 84:1839–1849

Johnson JH, Sager MA, Horn G et al 1994 Referral patterns to physical therapy in elderly hospitalized for acute medical illness. Phys Occup Ther Geriatr 12:1–12

Miller EW, Ross K, Grant S et al 2005 Geriatric referral patterns for physical therapy: a descriptive analysis. J Geriatr Phys Ther 28:20–27

World Confederation for Physical Therapy. Available: http://www.wcpt.org/. Accessed 16 September 2005

Chapter 84

Providing social services to the older client

James Siberski

INTRODUCTION

Internationally, older adults are confronted with numerous challenges as they age (Lemme 2006). In addition to normal age-related changes, there are frequently disease states that must also be addressed in order to age successfully. The social service provider plays an important role in assisting older adults to adjust to age-related changes through adaptive changes and devices, and to adjust to the disease state when required, through the rehabilitative process. It is recognized that not all elderly people will require rehabilitation. Some will need treatment, time and perhaps education to return to their previously healthy state. The social service provider can contribute to positive outcomes.

As a member of the rehabilitative team, the social service provider performs a key role. In order to succeed, the team needs specific information from the social worker or geriatric care manager. Initially, this individual completes a comprehensive social work assessment and social history providing important data that will be incorporated into the rehabilitative care plan and enable theolder client to achieve his or her goals. While various forms are available (see Form 84.1) for completing this task, in many settings, the format is dictated by the agency or department. As a result of education and training, professional social service providers are efficient at completing an assessment, taking a social history, determining needs and strengths, and developing discipline-specific goals. In assessing the elderly, additional considerations must be entertained in order to facilitate optimal care/services placement.

ADDITIONAL CONSIDERATIONS

Additional considerations, which include goal incongruence, cure vs. care, client and family perceptions, personality, activities and diversity issues, can either assist or detract from the success of the rehabilitative process.

Goal incongruence

In the rehabilitative process, the team often determines that the appropriate placement is a structured living arrangement, whereas the older client believes that the appropriate living arrangement is their home. This goal incongruence between team and client is not restricted to just placement but can include driving, employment, financial management and other issues of autonomy. Unresolved goal incongruence hinders the rehabilitative process. In addressing this issue, the social worker should capitalize on the client's motivation to go home by communicating that several steps are necessary to attain this goal. By graphically demonstrating the intervening steps toward the goal (see Fig. 84.1), the social worker utilizes the client's motivation to achieve the rehabilitative team's goal as well as his or her own personal goal. In Figure 84.1, several possible steps are identified in a rehabilitation process to capitalize on a patient's motivation to return to their own home. Step one is attending therapy until X% of function is gained. Step two is learning to use adaptive devices. Step three is discussing the required supports and home adaptations with the social worker and family. Step four is placement in a personal care home for a period of 6 months in order to demonstrate the ability to do X. Step five is to return home. While returning home may not even be an attainable goal, the social worker should avoid making it an issue in order not to detract from the rehabilitative process.

Cure vs. care

The social service assessment should address the older client's desire for care or for cure. Many clients will want a cure. Other clients will want a purpose in their lives and that purpose may be the caregiver–client interaction. The rehabilitative team needs to be aware that older clients need care to achieve cure. Care is also the opportunity for such things as intimate touch by the physical therapist, occupational therapist, nurse or physician. Care also gives purpose to the day. The older client needs to go to the outpatient clinic on Monday; to cardiac rehabilitation on Tuesday; to the pharmacy on Wednesday, etc. The older client's regular interaction with the social worker or home health aide is an opportunity to socialize and to feel valued by the provider. In contrast, cure, by eliminating therapy or treatment, creates a loss of the caregiver–client interactions. Recognizing this situation, the rehabilitative team can then plan around the loss if, indeed, care is the focal issue, so that the client will not be excessively concerned.

Form 84.1   Social work assessment form

Room #: _____ Admission date: _____   _____

Name: _____   Age: _____   DOB _____

Address: _____   Hospital admitted from: _____

_____   Insurance info.: _____

Phone: _____   Physician: _____

Rehab. DX: _____   Other DX: _____

Employment status: _____   Employer: _____

Income source(s): _____   Work phone: _____

FAMILY/CAREGIVER

Marital status: M S D W Sep.   Spouse name: _____

Others in household: Name: _____ Age: _____   Empl. _____

Other contact: Name: _____   Phone: _____

Address: _____   _____

Name: _____   Phone: _____

HOME/ENVIRONMENT

Type of home: Own: _____ Rent: _____ No. of floors: _____ No. of steps: _____

Primary entry: _____ No. of steps: _____ Handrails: _____

Bedroom location: _____ Bath location: _____ Handrails: _____

Mental status and emotional reaction: _____

Alert? _____ Oriented? _____ Depressed? _____

Equipment at home: _____ Anticipated equipment needs: _____

Home health agency? _____ Other community services? _____

Patient family goals: _____

Plan: _____ Comments: _____

Social worker: _____ Date: _____

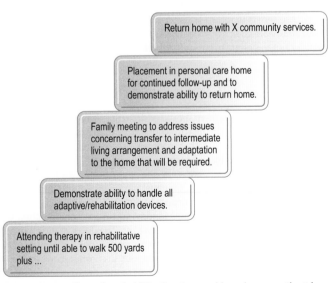

Figure 84.1   Steps in rehabilitation to consider when a patient is motivated to return home.

Client, family and others' views of rehabilitation

The social service provider needs to assess both the client's and the family's view of the expected outcomes of rehabilitation. If the prevailing view is that the rehabilitative plan will not help or that the client is doomed to fail, the client's potential for success is seriously impaired. The social worker must provide education, appropriate for reading and comprehension level, and perhaps even involve other team members in the education process.

Personality

Knowledge of the client's personality in their youth is beneficial in determining possible issues and appropriate team approaches prior to therapy (Hoyer & Roodin 2003). Someone who was guarded at age 40 tends to be more guarded, if not suspicious, as they age, especially when under stress. As an overly friendly approach would increase suspicion and hinder therapy, the social worker should employ a passive friendly approach. This would entail briefly discussing the rehabilitation process and then pulling back and letting the client ponder the information. Next, could be one or two more short visits by the social worker, asking if there are any questions or concerns, followed by gently asking the client what are their thoughts and when might they be ready to start the rehabilitation process? This process can take a bit more time but yields more positive results. If someone had always demanded perfection, and with therapy, could not expect 100% return to function, the social worker would also need to address this in therapy.

Activities

An assessment of the older individual's activities and activity style enables one to get a good understanding of the severity of the client's condition and its impact on the client's life. The passionate reader, who after completing therapy has 50% mobility, may be satisfied, whereas the passionate walker would be upset. The social worker needs to address this situation by first discovering the needs met by walking, e.g. stress reduction, and then by providing either alternative methods to meet the needs or by modifying the walking pattern, e.g. a slower pace, a shorter distance or a different frequency. This might require the involvement of other members of the rehabilitation team. A bright light at the end of the rehabilitation tunnel will motivate the older person to work harder and ultimately experience better results from rehabilitation.

Diversity

Social service providers need to be cognizant of ethnic diversity and cultures. African–Americans, Pacific Asian Americans, American Indians and Hispanic Americans all have different belief systems. The older American Indian will approach rehabilitation differently from the African–American. The manner in which the team approaches, addresses, and instructs the client is important to the outcome of therapy (Quadagno 2005). The social worker should educate the team as to how to address diverse populations as well as their cultural beliefs in terms of medical care and, in fact, if they are even accepting of traditional medical care.

THE GERIATRIC CARE MANAGER

A geriatric care manager (GCM), as defined by the National Association of Professional Geriatric Care Managers, is a health and human services professional, such as a gerontologist, social worker, counselor or nurse, with a specialized body of knowledge and experience related to aging and elder care issues. The GCM assists older adults and persons with disabilities in attaining their maximum functional potential. They strive to respect the autonomy of the individual and to deliver care coordination and support services with sensitivity, in order to preserve the dignity and the respect of the individual. In addition, the GCM is an experienced guide and resource for families of older adults and others with chronic needs. As time progresses and as baby boomers age, the rehabilitative team will work hand in hand with this newly emerging professional. Clinical journals, business publications and weekly news magazines frequently discuss the current concept of care management for older individuals. The GCM can be quite helpful to the social worker in terms of assessment and understanding of the older person in need of rehabilitation. The role of the GCM will develop internationally as the older population grows. The title of GCM could vary from country to country as the profession matures. At present, no international organization exists.

When discharge approaches, the social worker and the rehabilitation team need to consider the post rehabilitation requirements and needs of the client and family. Those requirements and needs include the home, durable medical equipment, home health and community services.

The home

A home visit by members of the rehabilitation team allows family members to be interviewed in a familiar, nonthreatening setting. It allows therapists to evaluate the home for barriers and adaptations that may be needed. Occasionally, a home may be dangerous or inappropriate for a patient's return. Extreme clutter, filth, lack of utilities or disrepair may require community intervention. The social worker will have to refer these rare situations to the Protective Service Unit of the Area Agency on Aging or some other appropriate agency. A first-hand view of the home environment helps the social worker to prepare the family for the patient's return and also helps to coordinate community services for the patient's return home.

DURABLE MEDICAL EQUIPMENT

Most rehabilitation patients require the use of assistive devices, if only for a short time. Ordering durable medical equipment (DME) in a managed care climate requires knowledge of preferred provider relations and limits of coverage. Patients and families rely on social workers for this knowledge.

Basic items such as canes, walkers and wheelchairs are covered by most insurance carriers for appropriate patients. Larger items such as lifts, continuous passive motion units and even hospital beds are less readily available and may not be covered at all. Items such as lift chairs or stair glides are rarely, if ever, covered by insurance. Some DME suppliers have previously used lift chairs and stair glides, as well as other items available at reduced cost.

Those patients injured under workers' compensation or automobile plans may be covered for special items. Each individual has to be reviewed separately.

Some rehabilitation facilities or agencies for the disabled may employ an equipment adaptor. This professional person modifies and customizes medical equipment to individual needs. This can be a very helpful service for the geriatric patient.

Home health

Medicare and most major insurance plans cover rehabilitative and nursing services in the home after the patient has been discharged from a facility if a skilled service (a physical therapist or a registered nurse) is ordered by a physician. In some cases, a nurse's aide may be covered for personal care, such as bathing. As with DME, many carriers are now requiring the use of preferred providers for home health services.

It should be noted that rural areas are often underserved by home health rehabilitative services. This can delay the initiation of care in the home.

Many people are under the impression that Medicare or other insurance companies provide for private nurses or aides in a patient's home. Medicare has never covered this service, and most other plans have long since discontinued such benefits. There are many agencies that offer this help for a fee.

Community services

The following are useful community services that have traditionally helped older people to remain at home; however, as public funds for these programs have dwindled, agencies have initiated fee-for-service arrangements. This has resulted in shorter waiting lists and faster start-up for services. Of course, it has also resulted in increased costs to the older consumer.

Area Agency on Aging (AAA)

This is a local, public agency funded by federal and state monies; the agencies were created to provide support for older people in their homes. Some of the services offered include homemakers, personal care aides, friendly visitors, Meals on Wheels (MOW), and so forth. A means test determines eligibility, and the services are generally limited to 1 or 2 hours a week. Some AAA offer personal attendant care or Title XX (Lamp II or Options) programs designed to help the most physically challenged individuals stay at home. Agencies on Aging are generally run by county governments. Phone numbers and addresses can be found in the blue pages of the telephone book.

Chore

Chore services may be available through AAA or another public agency. This useful program can help to build ramps, attach handrails, or provide other minor adaptations. All materials are purchased by the individual receiving the service.

Meals on Wheels

This is perhaps the best known service. MOW provides a full meal for the homebound individual 5 days a week or more. A fee is generally charged for this service. This agency is also listed in the blue pages of the telephone book.

Transportation

Adequate transportation services are the most common need of the elderly, especially for the geriatric rehabilitation patient. Most communities offer some type of subsidized transportation for eligible individuals. These programs function as a cross between a bus and a taxi. The vehicles, usually modified vans, travel specified routes but require advance notification of appointments. Vans equipped with wheelchair lifts are available, but extra notice may have to be given. Ambulance transport for routine medical appointments is rarely covered by insurance and is very expensive. Many ambulance providers offer wheelchair van service at more reasonable rates.

PLACEMENT

Despite the best efforts and the fervent hopes of all, the goal of returning home may not be possible for all patients. Inadequate progress in therapy or insufficient support at home may make nursing home, assistive living or other appropriate placement the only appropriate course of action. The social worker has to be sensitive to feelings of guilt, abandonment and hopelessness as he or she guides the patient and family through the application process. Furthermore, if the realities of modern healthcare make the first choice of a facility unachievable, the social worker must be frank and straightforward in dealing with placement issues. At all times, lines of communication must be kept open to make the patient's transition as smooth as possible.

CONCLUSION

While the social assessment and history provide a good basis for the rehabilitative process, it is important to be cognizant of the older person's special needs. Assessing and evaluating these additional considerations enhances the social worker's or social service provider's opportunity for positive outcomes from the rehabilitative effort. The social worker's counseling skills, knowledge of community resources and ability to provide education throughout the rehabilitation process help the client and family cope with the process and reach their rehabilitation goals.

RESOURCES

National (USA): http://nihseniorhealth.gov/ (National senior health net)

National Alliance for Caregiving
Suite 642
4720 Montgomery Lane
Bethesda, MD 20814
(301) 718–8444
http://www.caregiving.org

National Family Caregivers Association
Suite 500
10400 Connecticut Avenue
Kensington, MD 20895
(800) 896–3650
http://www.nfacares.org

National Association for Home Care
228 7th Street, NE
Washington, DC 20003
(202) 547–7424
http://www.nahc.org
http://www.caremanager.org/(geriatric care managers)

National Council on the Aging
Suite 200
409 3rd Street, SW
Washington, DC 20024
(202) 479–1200
http://www.ncoa.org

International:

International Society for Aging and Physical Activity:
www.isapa.org
International Council on Active Aging® (ICAA): www.icaa.cc
International Conference on Aging, Disability and Independence (ICADI): www.ittatc.org

References

Hoyer JW, Roodin P 2003 Adult Development and Aging, 5th edn. McGraw Hill, Boston

Lemme BH 2005 Development in Adulthood, 4th edn. Allyn & Bacon, Boston

Quadagno J 2005 Aging and the Life Course: An Introduction to Social Gerontology, 3rd edn. McGraw Hill,

Index

Note: Page numbers in *italics* refer to figures, tables and boxes.